Haematology and Blood Transfusion
29
Hämatologie und Bluttransfusion

Edited by
H. Heimpel, Ulm · D. Huhn, Berlin
C. Mueller-Eckhardt, Gießen
G. Ruhenstroth-Bauer, München

Modern Trends in Human Leukemia VI

New Results in Clinical and Biological Research Including Pediatric Oncology

Organized on behalf of the Deutsche Gesellschaft für Hämatologie und Onkologie. Wilsede, June 17–20, 1984

Wilsede Joint Meeting on Pediatric Oncology III
Hamburg, June 21/22, 1984

Edited by
Rolf Neth, Robert C. Gallo, Melvyn F. Greaves, and Gritta Janka

With 178 Figures and 127 Tables

Springer-Verlag
Berlin Heidelberg New York Tokyo

Dr. Rolf Neth, Universitäts-Krankenhaus Eppendorf
Medizinische Klinik, Abteilung für klinische Chemie,
Martinistraße 52, 2000 Hamburg 20, FRG

Dr. Robert C. Gallo, National Cancer Institute, Laboratory
of Tumor Cell Biology, Bethesda, MD 20205, USA

Dr. Melvyn F. Greaves, Leukaemia Research Fund Centre, Institute of
Cancer Research, Chester Beatty Laboratories, Fulham Road,
London SW3 6JB, UK

Dr. Gritta Janka, Universitäts-Kinderklinik,
Abteilung für Hämatologie und Onkologie,
Martinistraße 52, 2000 Hamburg 20, FRG

Supplement to

BLUT – Journal Experimental and Clinical Hematology

Organ of the *Deutsche Gesellschaft für Hämatologie und Onkologie* der *Deutschen Gesellschaft für Bluttransfusion und Immunhämatologie* and of the *Österreichische Gesellschaft für Hämatologie und Onkologie*

ISBN 3-540-15329-2 Springer-Verlag Berlin Heidelberg New York Tokyo
ISBN 0-387-15329-2 Springer-Verlag New York Heidelberg Berlin Tokyo

Library of Congress Cataloging in Publication Data. Main entry under title: Modern trends in human leukemia VI.
(Haematology and blood transfusion = Hämatologie und Bluttransfusion ; 29)
"Supplement to Blut" – T.p. verso.
Includes index.
1. Leukemia–Congresses. 2. Leukemia in children–Congresses. I. Neth, Rolf. II. Deutsche Gesellschaft für Hämatologie und Onkologie. III. Wilsede Joint Meeting on Pediatric Oncology (3rd : 1984 : Hamburg, Germany) IV. Blut. Supplement. V. Title: Modern trends in human leukemia 6. VI. Series: Haematology and blood transfusion ; 29. [DNLM: 1. Leukemia–Congresses. W1 HA1655 v.29 / WH 250 M6891 1984]
RC643.M623 1985 616.99′419 85-2848
ISBN 0-387-15329-2 (U.S.)

Typesetting, printing and binding: Triltsch, Würzburg
2127/3130/543210

Scientific Organisation of the Sessions

New Strategies in Leukemia Diagnostic and Therapy

Bertino, Joseph R., Yale University School of Medicine, Section of Medical Oncology, Department of Internal Medicine, New Haven, Connecticut 06510-8032, USA
Kersey, John H., University Hospitals and Clinics, 420 Delaware Street S.E., Minneapolis, Minnesota 55455, USA

Round Table Discussion on Clinical Aspects

Clarkson, Bayard, Memorial Sloan-Kettering Cancer Center, 1275 York Avenue, New York, New York 10021, USA
Lister, T. Andrew, Imperial Cancer Research Fund, Dept. Medical Oncology, St. Bartholomew's Hospital, West Smithfield, London, EC1A 7BE, England
Henderson, Edward S., Roswell Park Memorial Institute, Dept. of Health, 666 Elm Street, Buffalo, New York 14263, USA
Murphy, Sharon, St. Jude Children's Research Hospital, 332 North Lauderdale, Memphis, Tennessee 38101, USA

Mechanism of Malignant Transformation

Cellular Human Oncogenes, Chromosomes and Viruses, Implication for Leukemia and Lymphoma

Burny, Arsène, Université Libre de Bruxelles, Dept. de Biologie Moleculaire, Laboratoire de Chimie Biologique, Rue des Chevaux, 67, 1640 Rhode-Saint-Genèse, Belgium
Cooper, Geoffrey M., Sidney Farber Cancer Institute, 44 Binney Street, Boston, Massachusetts 02115, USA

Special Session

Gallo, Robert C., National Cancer Institute, Bethesda, Maryland 20205, USA
Greaves, Melvyn F., Leukaemia Research Fund Centre, Institute of Cancer Research, Chester Beatty Laboratories, Fulham Road, London SW3 6JB, Great Britain

Blood Cell Growth and Differentiation

Dexter, T. Michael, Paterson Laboratories, Christie Hospital & Holt Radium Institute, Wilmslow Road, Manchester M20 9BX, England
Moore, Malcolm A. S., Sloan-Kettering Institute for Cancer Research, Donald S. Walker Laboratory, 145 Boston Post Rd., Rye, N.Y. 10580, USA

Immunological Aspects in Malignancy

Klein, Jan, Max-Planck-Institut für Biologie, Abteilung Immungenetik, Correnssstrasse 42, 7400 Tübingen, FRG
Mitchison, N. Avrion, Department of Zoology, University College London, Gower Street, London WC1E 6BT, England

Wilsede Joint Meeting in Pediatric Hematology and Oncology III

Janka, Gritta, Abteilung für pädiatrische Hämatologie und Onkologie, Universitätskinderklinik, Martinistrasse 52, 2000 Hamburg 20, FRG
Kabisch, Hartmut, Abteilung für pädiatrische Hämatologie und Onkologie, Universitätskinderklinik, Martinistrasse 52, 2000 Hamburg 20, FRG

Local Organisation

Mannweiler, Klaus, Heinrich-Pette-Institut für experimentelle Virologie und Immunologie an der Universität Hamburg, Martinistrasse 52, 2000 Hamburg 20, FRG
Neth, Rolf, Universitätskrankenhaus Eppendorf, Medizinische Klinik, Abteilung für klinische Chemie, Martinistrasse 52, 2000 Hamburg 20, FRG

Contents

---

[1] presented in the Wilsede Joint Meeting on Pediatric Oncology III

[2] Wilsede Meeting and Special Lecture for the Wilsede Joint Meeting on Pediatric Oncology III

Mechanism of Malignant Transformation

Cellular Human Oncogens, Chromosomes and Viruses, Implication for Leukemia and Lymphoma

[1] Henry Kaplan Award for the best poster Clinical Session

---

[1] Henry Kaplan Award for the best poster Virological Session

Cellbiology

[1] Henry Kaplan Award for the best poster Cellbiological Session

Immunological Aspects in Malignancy

[1] Henry Kaplan Award for the best poster Immunological Session

Participants of the Meeting

Anders, Fritz, Genetisches Institut, Heinrich-Buff-Ring 58–62, 6300 Giessen, FRG
Aoki, Tadao, Shinrakuen Hospital, Nishiariakecho 1–27, Niigatashi, Japan
Bauer, Heinz, Institut für Virologie, Frankfurter Strasse 107, 6300 Giessen, FRG
Beato, Miguel, Institut für Physiologische Chemie I, Emil-Mannkopff-Strasse 1–2, D-3550 Marburg, FRG
Bertino, Joseph R., Yale University School of Medicine, 333 Cedar Street, New Haven, Connecticut 06510, USA
Beug, Hartmut, European Molecular Biology Laboratory, Meyerhofstrasse 1, 6900 Heidelberg, FRG
Bloomfield, Clara Derber, Coleman Leukemia Research and Treatment Center, Sect. Medical Oncology, 420 Delaware Street S.E., Minneapolis, Minnesota 55455, USA
Blume, Karl G., Dept. Hematology and Bone Marrow Transplantation, City of Hope National Med. Center, 1500 East Duarte Road, Duarte, California 91010, USA
Boguslawska-Jaworska, Janina, Institute of Pediatrics, Dept. Hematology, ul. Smoluchowskiego 32/4, 50-373 Wroclaw, Poland
Bosco, John, Dept. Medicine, University of Malaya, Kuala Lumpur, Malaysia
Brandeis, Werner, Kinderklinik, Sektion Onkologie/Immunologie, Im Neuenheimer Feld 150, 6900 Heidelberg, FRG
Browne, Marcia T.*, Pediatric Branch, Clinical Oncology Program, Div. of Cancer Treatment, National Cancer Institute, National Institutes of Health, Bethesda, Maryland, USA
Burny, Arsène, Laboratoire de Chimie Biologique, 67 Rue des Chevaux, 1640 Rhode-St.-Genèse, Belgium
Castaigne, S., Service d'Hématologie du Pr Boiron, Hopital St. Louis, Paris, France
Chieco-Bianchi, Luigi, Instituto di Anatomia Patologica, Cattedra di Oncologia, Via Gattamelata 64, 35128 Padova, Italy
Clark, Edward A., Genetic Systems Corporation, 3005 First Avenue, Seattle, Washington 98121, USA
Clarkson, Bayard, Memorial Sloan-Kettering Cancer Center, 1275 York Avenue, New York, N.Y. 10021, USA
Conez, Dominique, Département de Biologie Moléculaire, Laboratoire de Chimie Biologique, 67 Rue des Chevaux, 1640 Rhode-St.-Genèse, Belgium
Cooper, Geoffrey M., Sidney Farber Cancer Institute, Lab. Molecular Carcinogenesis, 44 Binney Street, Boston, Massachusetts 02115, USA
Coutinho, Antonio, Institut Pasteur, 28, Rue du Dr. Roux, 75724 Paris Cedex 15, France
Cowling, Graham J., Searle Research & Development, Lane End Road, High Wycombe, Bucks HP12 4HL, England
Croce, Carlo M., The Wistar Institute, 36th Street at Spruce, Philadelphia, Pennsylvania, USA

Dalgleish, Angus, Institute of Cancer Research, Chester Beatty Laboratories, Fulham Road, London SW3 6JB, England

Deinhard, Friedrich, Max v. Pettenkofer-Institut für Hygiene und Mikrobiologie, Pettenkoferstrasse 9 a, 8000 München 2, FRG

Dexter, T. Michael, Christie Hospital & Holt Radium Institute, Dept. Experimental Haematology, Wilmslow Road, Manchester M20 9BX, England

Dube, Shyam, Dept. Pharmacology, Sterling Hall of Medicine, 333 Cedar Street, New Haven, Connecticut 06510, USA

Duesberg, Peter H., Dept. Molecular Biology, Wendell M. Stanley Hall, Bergeley, California 94720, USA

Eaves, Connie, Terry Fox Laboratories, B.C. Cancer Research Center, 601 West 10th Avenue, Vancouver, B.C. V52 IL3, Canada

Elstner, Elena, Universitätsklinik f. Innere Med., Schumannstrasse 20/22, 1040 Berlin, GDR

Feldman, Michael, The Weizman Institute of Science, Dept. Cell Biology, 76100 Rehovot, Israel

Francis, Gillian E., The Royal Free Hospital, Pond Street, Hamstead, London NW3 2QG, England

Gaedicke, Gerhard, Universitätskinderklinik, Prittwitzstrasse 43, 7900 Ulm, FRG

Gaffin, Stephen L.*, Dept. of Physiology, University of Natal Med. School, P.O. Box 17039, 4013 Congella, South Africa

Gallo, Robert C., National Cancer Institute, Bethesda, Maryland 20205, USA

Ganser, Arnold, Zentrum für Innere Medizin, Abteilung für Innere Medizin III, Hämatologie und Onkologie, Steinhövelstr. 9, 7900 Ulm, FRG

Gissmann, Lutz, Deutsches Krebsforschungszentrum, Im Neuenheimer Feld 280, 6900 Heidelberg, FRG

Goldmann, Shraga Felix*, Abt. Transplantationsimmunologie der DRK-Blutspendezentrale, Oberer Eselsberg 10, 7900 Ulm, FRG

Gough, Nicholas M., Ludwig Institute for Cancer Research, Melbourne, Victoria 3050, Australia

Gramatzki, Martin, Institut und Poliklinik für Klinische Immunologie und Rheumatologie, Krankenhausstrasse 12, 8520 Erlangen, FRG

Greaves, Melvyn F., Imperial Cancer Research Fund Laboratories, Membrane Immunology Laboratory, London WC2A 3PX, England

Greene, Warner C., National Institutes of Health, Building 10, Room 4N117, Bethesda, Maryland 20205, USA

Haas, R. J., Dr. v. Haunersches Kinderspital, Abt. Hämatologie & Onkologie, Lindwurmstrasse 4, 8000 München 2, FRG

Hahn, Beatrice, National Cancer Institute, Bethesda, Maryland 20205, USA

Harel, Jacques, Institut Gustave-Roussy, 39–53, Rue Camille Desmoulins, 94805 Villejuif, France

Harłozińska-Smyrka, Antonia, Akademia Medyczna, Katedra I Zaklad Anatomii Pathologicznej, 50-368 Wrocław, Poland

zur Hausen, Harald, Deutsches Krebsforschungszentrum, Im Neuenheimer Feld 280, 6900 Heidelberg, FRG

Hayman, Michael, Imperial Cancer Research Fund Laboratories, Dominion House, London EC1A 7BE, England

Hehlmann, Rüdiger, Medizinische Klinik, Pettenkoferstrasse 8 a, 8000 München 2, FRG

von der Helm, Klaus, Max v. Pettenkofer-Institut für Hygiene und Mikrobiologie, Pettenkoferstrasse 9 a, 8000 München 2, FRG

Henderson, Edward S., Roswell Park Memorial Institute, Medicine A, 666 Elm Street, Buffalo, N.Y. 14263, USA

Higi, M.*, Klinik Dr. Schedel, 8391 Kellberg-Passau, FRG

Hoelzer, Dieter, Zentrum der Inneren Medizin, Abteilung für Hämatologie, Universität Frankfurt, Theodor-Stern-Kai 7, 6000 Frankfurt/Main 70, FRG

Hofschneider, Peter-Hans, Max-Planck-Institut für Biochemie, 8033 Martinsried, FRG

Hossfeld, Dieter, II. Medizinische Univ. Klinik, Abt. Onkologie und Hämatologie, Martinistrasse 52, 2000 Hamburg 20, FRG

Hrodek, Otto, 2nd Dept. of Pediatrics, V úvalu 84, Prague 5 – Motol, Czechoslovakia

Hyjek, Elzbieta, Katedra Onkologii AM, ul. Gagarina 4, 93-509 Lodz, Poland

Jacobs, Allan, Dept. Haematology, Heath Park, Cardiff CF4 4XN, England

Jacobs, Peter, Dept. Haematology – Research Centre, Anzio Road, Observatory 7925, Cape Town, South Africa

Jacquemin, Paul, Institut Pasteur du Brabant, 642 Rue Engeland, 1180 Brussels, Belgium

Janka, Gritta, Universitäts-Kinderklinik, Abt. für Hämatologie und Onkologie, Martinistrasse 52, 2000 Hamburg 20, FRG

Janossy, George, The Royal Free Hospital, Academic Dept. Immunology, Pond Street, London NW3 2QG, England

Johnson, Gregory R., Cancer Research Unit, Walter & Eliza Hall Institute, P.O. Royal Melbourne Hospital, 3050 Melbourne, Australia

Kabisch, Hartmut, Universitäts-Kinderklinik, Martinistrasse 52, 2000 Hamburg 20, FRG

Kalden, Joachim, Institut und Poliklinik für Klinische Immunologie und Rheumatologie, Krankenhausstrasse 12, 8520 Erlangen, FRG

Kaneko, Yutaro, Shinrakuen Hospital, Nishiariakecho 1–27, Niigatashi, Japan

Kanki, Phyllis J., Dept. Cancer Biology, 665 Huntington Avenue, Boston, Massachusetts 02115, USA

Karpowicz, Marek, Instytut Hematologii, Klinika Chorob Wewnetrznych, ul. Chocimska 5, 00-957 Warsaw, Poland

Kersey, John H., University Hospitals and Clinics, 420 Delaware Street S.E., Minneapolis, Minnesota 55455, USA

Killmann, Sven-Age, Rigshospitalet, 9 Blegdamsvej, 2100 Copenhagen, Denmark

Kirsten, Werner, Dept. Pathology, 950 East 59th Street, Chicago, Illinois 60637, USA

Kisseljov, Fjodor L., Institute of Cancerogenesis, Dept. Viral Molecular Biology, Kashirskoe sh. 24, Moscow, USSR

Klein, Jan, Max-Planck-Institut für Biologie, Abt. Immungenetik, Corrensstrasse 42, 7400 Tübingen, FRG

Koeffler, Phillip H., UCLA School of Medicine, Division Hematology/Oncology, 11-240 Louis Factor Bldg., Los Angeles, California 90024, USA

Koutecky, Josef, Dept. Pediatric Oncology, V úvalu 84, Prague 5, Czechoslovakia

Kramer, Gisela, Clayton Foundation Biochemical Institute, Dept. Chemistry, Austin, Texas 78712, USA

Kyewski, Bruno A., Deutsches Krebsforschungszentrum, Im Neuenheimer Feld 280, 6900 Heidelberg, FRG

Lane, Mary Ann, Sidney Farber Cancer Institute, Lab. Molecular Carcinogenesis, 44 Binney Street, Boston, Massachusetts 02115, USA

Lange-Wantzin, Gunhild, Finseninstitutet, Dermatologisk afdeling, Strandboulevarden 49, 2100 Copenhagen, Denmark

Lapin, Boris A., Institute of Experimental Pathology and Therapy, Gora Trapetziya, Sukhumi, USSR

Letowska, Magdalena, Instytut Hematologii, Ul. Chocimska 5, 00-957 Warsaw, Poland

Lindner, Stephan Georg, Universitäts-Kinderklinik, Martinistrasse 52, 2000 Hamburg 20, FRG

Lister, T. Andrew, Imperial Cancer Research Fund, Dept. Medical Oncology, St. Bartholomew's Hospital, London EC1A 7BE, England

Mannweiler, Klaus, Heinrich-Pette-Institut für Experimentelle Virologie und Immunologie, Martinistrasse 52, 2000 Hamburg 20, FRG

Manzari, Vittorio, Instituto di Patologia Generale, Viale Regina Elena 324, 00161 Rome, Italy

Martin, Paul J., Fred Hutchinson Cancer Research Center, 1124 Columbia Street, Seattle, Washington 98104, USA

McCredie, Kenneth B., M. D. Anderson Hospital and Tumor Institute, Dept. Developmental Therapeutics, 6723 Bertner Avenue, Houston, Texas 77030, USA

Micheel, Burkhard, Forschungszentrum für Molekularbiologie und Medizin, Bereich Experimentelle und Klinische Immunologie, Lindenberger Weg 80, 1115 Berlin-Buch, GDR

Minowada, Jun, Edward J. Hines, Jr. Veterans Administration Hospital, Hines, Illinois 60141, USA

Mitchison, N. Avrion, Dept. Zoology, Tumour Immunology Unit, Gower Street, London WC1E 6BT, England

Mölling, Karin, Max-Planck-Institut für Molekulare Genetik, Ihnestrasse 63–73, 1000 Berlin 33, FRG

Moore, Malcolm A. S., Sloan-Kettering Institute for Cancer Research, Donald S. Walker Laboratory, 145 Boston Post Rd., Rye, N.Y. 10580, USA

Moroni, Christoph, Friedrich Miescher Institut, 4002 Basel, Switzerland

Muller-Berat, C. Nicole, Statens Seruminstitut, 80, Amager Boulevard, 2300 Copenhagen, Denmark

Munk, Klaus, Deutsches Krebsforschungszentrum, Im Neuenheimer Feld 280, 6900 Heidelberg, FRG

Murphy, Sharon, St. Jude Children's Research Hospital, Memphis, Tennessee 38101, USA

Neth, Rolf, II. Medizinische Universitätsklinik, Abt. Klinische Chemie, Martinistrasse 52, 2000 Hamburg 20, FRG

Obłakowski, Piotr, Instytut Hematologii, ul. Chocimska 5, 00-957 Warsaw, Poland

Ohno, Susumu, City of Hope Research Center, 1450 East Duarte Road, Duarte, California 91010, USA

Olsson, Inge, Lund Hospital, Research Dept. 2, 22185 Lund, Sweden

Papas, Takis S., National Cancer Institute, Lab. Molecular Oncology, Frederick, Maryland 21701, USA

Parks, Wade P., Dept. Microbiology & Immunology, 1550 N.W. 10th Avenue, Miami, Florida 33101, USA

Pawlita, Michael, Deutsches Krebsforschungszentrum, Im Neuenheimer Feld 280, 6900 Heidelberg

Petrakova, Alena, Research Institute of Child Development, Dept. Genetics, V úvalu 84, 15006 Prague, Czechoslovakia

Poglod, Ryszard, Instytut Hematologii, ul. Chocimska 5, 00-957 Warsaw, Poland

Popovic, Mikulas, National Cancer Institute, Bethesda, Maryland 20205, USA

Rabe, Klaus, Katholisches Marienkrankenhaus, Alfredstrasse 9, 2000 Hamburg 76, FRG

Rickard, Karyl A.*, Depts of Pediatric Nutrition and Dietetics, Pediatric Hematology, Oncology and Pediatric Surgery, James Whitcomb Riley Hospital for children, Indiana University Sch. of Medicine, 702 Barnhill Drive, Indianapolis, Indiana 46223, USA

Ritter, Jörg, Kinderklinik, Abt. Hämatologie und Onkologie, Robert-Koch-Strasse, 4400 Münster, FRG

Rosenthal, David S., Brigham & Women's Hospital, Hematology Division, 75 Francis Street, Boston, Massachusetts 02115, USA

Rübsamen-Waigmann, Helga, Paul-Ehrlich-Institut, Paul-Ehrlich-Strasse 42–44, 6000 Frankfurt 70, FRG

Sachs, Leo, The Weizman Institute of Science, Dept. Genetics, Rehovot 76100, Israel

Santos, George W., The Johns Hopkins Oncology Center, Bone Marrow Transplantation Program, 600 North Wolfe Street, Baltimore, Maryland 21205, USA

Sarngadharan, Magallasserie, National Cancer Institute, Bethesda, Maryland 20205, USA

Schiffer, Charles A., University of Maryland Cancer Center, Div. Hematologic Malignancies, 22nd South Greene Street, Baltimore, Maryland 21201, USA

Schubert, Johannes, St.-Joseph-Hospital, Wiener Strasse 1, 2050 Bremerhaven, FRG

Seeburg, Peter H., Genentech., Inc., Dept. Molecular Biology, 460 Point San Bruno Boulevard, South San Francisco, CA 94080, USA

Sherman, Linda, Scripps Clinic & Research Foundation, 10666 N. Torrey Pines Road, La Jolla, California 92037, USA

Siebenlist, Ulrich, National Institutes of Health, Lab. Clinical Investigation, Bethesda, Maryland 20205, USA
Singer, Jack W., Veterans Administration, Medical Oncology, 4435 Beacon Avenue South, Seattle, Washington 98108, USA
Skrobowska-Wozniak, Anna, Instytut Pediatrii AM, ul. Marszalkowska 24, 00-579 Warsaw, Poland
Stehelin, Dominique, Institut Pasteur, Laboratoire d'Oncologie Moléculair, 15 rue Camille Guérin, 59019 Lille, France
Stein, Harald, Universitätsklinikum Steglitz, Institut für Pathologie, Hindenburgdamm 30, 1000 Berlin 45, FRG
Strauss, Ronald, DeGowin Memorial Blood Center, University of Iowa, Iowa City, 52242, USA
Thomsen, Kristian, Finseninstitutet, Dermatologisk afedeling, Strandboulevarden 49, 2100 Copenhagen, Denmark
Tiefenbach, Aleksander, Pediatric Dept., Salata 4, 41000 Zagreb, Yugoslavia
Trainin, Ze'ev, Kimron Veterinary Institute, Beit Dagan, Israel
Vogel, Carl-Wilhelm, Dept. Biochemistry, 3900 Reservoir Road, N.W., Washington, D.C. 20007, USA
Weh, Hans-Josef, II. Medizinische Klinik, Abt. Hämatologie/Onkologie, Martinistrasse 52, 2000 Hamburg 20, FRG
Weissman, Irving L., Dept. Pathology, Stanford, California 94305, USA
Wilson, E. Lynette, Dept. Clinical Science and Immunology, Observatory, Cape Town, South Africa
Witz, Isaac, Tel Aviv University, Dept. Microbiology, Tel-Aviv, Israel
Wozniak, Leszek, Katedra Onkologii Akademii Medycznej, ul. Gagarin 4, 93-509 Lodz, Poland
Yohn, David S., Comprehensive Cancer Center, 410 West 12th Avenue, Columbus, Ohio 43210, USA
Yoshida, Mitsuaki, Cancer Institute, Kami-Ikebukuro, Toshima-ku, Tokyo 170, Japan
Young, Bryan D., The Beatson Institute for Cancer Research, Wolfson Laboratory for Molecular Pathology, Garscube Estate, Switchback Road, Glasgow G61 1BD, England
Young, Lowell S.*, Department of Medicine, Division of Infectious Diseases, UCLA Medical Center, Los Angeles, CA 90024, USA
Ziegler-Heitbrock, H. W. Löns, Institut für Immunologie, Schillerstrasse 42, 8000 München 2, FRG
Zintl, Felix, Universitäts-Kinderklinik, Abt. Hämatologie/Onkologie/Immunologie, Kochstrasse 2, 6900 Jena, GDR

* Participants of the Wilsede Joint Meeting on Pediatric Oncology III

Wilsede Scholarship Holders

Bartram, Claus Rainer, Universitätskinderklinik, Prittwitzstrasse 43, 7900 Ulm, FRG

Benter, Thomas, Max-Planck-Institut für Molekulare Genetik, Ihnestrasse 63–73, 1000 Berlin 33, FRG

Bevan, Philip, Dept. Haematological Medicine, Hills Road, Cambridge CB2 1TS, England

Chan, Li Chong, Membrane Immunology Laboratories, Imperial Cancer Research Fund, Lincoln's Inn Fields, London WC2A 3PX, England

Darbyshire, Philip, Dept. Haematology, Royal Hospital for Sick Children, St. Michael's Hill, Bristol BS2 8BJ, England

Davies, Sally, Courtauld Institute of Biochemistry, Mortimer Street, London W1P 7PN, England

Dhaliwal, H. S., Medical Oncology Unit, St. Bartholomew's Hospital, West Smithfield, London EC1A 7BE, England

Doldi, Kristin, Institut und Poliklinik für klinische Immunologie und Rheumatologie, Krankenhausstrasse 12, 8520 Erlangen, FRG

Drexler, Hans G., Hines Veterans Administration Medical Center, Hines, Illinois 60141, USA

Euler, Hans-Hartwig, II. Medizinische- und Poliklinik, Metzstrasse 53/57, 2300 Kiel, FRG

Erber, Wendy, Dept. Haematology, John Radcliffe Hospital, Oxford, OX3 9DU, England

Fauser, Axel A., Medizinische Universitätsklinik, Hugstetter Strasse 55, 7800 Freiburg i. Br., FRG

Furley, Andrew, Membrane Immunology Laboratories, Imperial Cancer Research Fund, Lincoln's Inn Fields, London WC2A 3PX, England

Gerhartz, Heinrich, Medizinische Klinik III, Marchioninistrasse 15, 8000 München 70, FRG

Heil, Gerhard, Abt. Innere Medizin III, Schwerpunkte Hämatologie/Onkologie, Steinhövelstrasse 9, 7900 Ulm, FRG

Jansen, Hans, W., Max-Planck-Institut für Molekulare Genetik, Ihnestrasse 63–73, 1000 Berlin 33, FRG

Matutes, Estella, MRC Leukaemia Unit, Ducane Road, London W12 OHS, England

Meyer-Hofmann, Helmut, Medizinische Universitätsklinik I, Joseph-Stelzmann-Strasse 9, 5000 Köln 41, FRG

Müller, Dorith, Tenovus Research Laboratory, Southampton General Hospital, Tremona Road, Southampton SO9 4XY, England

Nerl, Christoph, I. Medizinische Klinik, Hämatologie/Immunologie/Onkologie, Kölner Platz 1, 8000 München 40, FRG

Platzer, Erich, Dept. Developmental Hematopoiesis, Memorial Sloan-Kettering Cancer Center, 1275 York Avenue, New York, N.Y. 10021, USA

Prümmer, Otto, Abt. Klinische Physiologie und Arbeitsmedizin, Oberer Eselsberg, 7900 Ulm, FRG

Rooney, Cliona, Dept. Cancer Studies, Vincent Drive, Birmingham B15 2TJ, England
Rückle, Heide, Medizinische Poliklinik, Klinikstrasse 8, 8700 Würzburg, FRG
Sieverts, Hauke, Kinderklinik der RWTH Aachen, Goethestrasse 27–29, 5100 Aachen, FRG
Standen, Graham R., Dept. Haematology, Heath Park, Cardiff CF4 4XN, England
Walden, Peter, Max-Planck-Institut für Biologie, Abt. Immungenetik, Correnssstrasse 42, 7400 Tübingen, FRG
Wernicke, Dorothee, Max v. Pettenkofer-Institut für Hygiene und Mikrobiologie, Pettenkoferstrasse 9a, D-8000 München 2, FRG
Whetton, Anthony, Paterson Laboratories, Christie Hospital and Holt Radium Institute, Manchester M20 9BX, England
Wittmann, Peter, Max-Planck-Institut für Immunbiologie, Stübeweg 51, 7800 Freiburg, FRG

Nicht müde werden
sondern dem Wunder
leise
wie einem Vogel
die Hand hinhalten.

Hilde Domin in "Hier"
Fischer Verlag 1964
Fotos Regina Völz

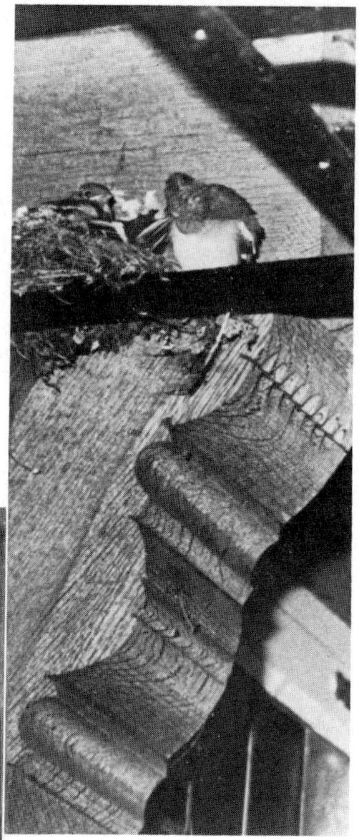

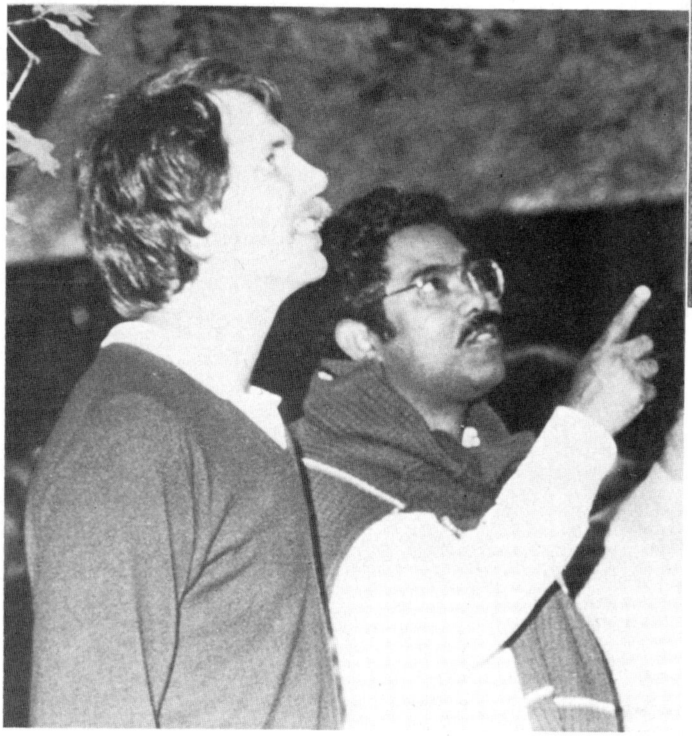

Participants of the Wilsede Meeting enjoy the sight of the birds over the entrance of "De Emmenhof"

Wilsede, June 1984

Preface

In June 1984 a total of 169 physicians, scientists and students assembled in the now familiar and much-loved lair in the Wilsede Luneberg Heath near Hamburg, Germany, for the sixth biennial conference on Modern Trends in Human Leukaemia. This meeting, conducted by Prof. Rolf Neth in his own inimitable style, has established itself as one of the major events in the all too crowded programme of international conferences on leukaemia, cancer and related topics.

Some may ponder why, with its "rustic" setting – flies, equine deposits, and lack of easy exit –, Wilsede has such an irresistible and persistent lure for so many of the world's top practitioners of leukaemia research? The answer is, I suspect, a cocktail of Rolf's extraordinary charm, the pleasure of meeting friends and colleagues in a uniquely informal and relaxed atmosphere and the special style of the proceedings themselves, which focus on the evaluation of ideas and hypotheses rather than the cataloguing of data. Indeed the sixth Wilsede meeting maintained the usual high standard of highly original presentations, with Anders (the "fish" man), Duesberg, Ohno, Mitchison and Coutinho, and others providing incisive challenges to "conventional wisdom" and great entertainment. Carlo Croce sang a marvellous aria on the *myc* gene and Bob Gallo managed to get in a few words about quite an interesting-looking human retrovirus. It all looked pretty good to me, although Peter Duesberg expressed some powerful reservations about the significance of these latter findings. The two Fred Stohlman memorial lectures (this year by Duesberg and Mitchison) again provided highspots of the meeting.

On a sober and sad note, this meeting was marred by the loss during the preceding year of three outstanding scientists who have helped make Wilsede the success that it is: Henry Kaplan, Dick Gershon and Sol Spiegelmann. All three epitomised what is best about the Wilsede meeting and science itself, with their striking originality, debating skill and warm friendship. They will be sadly missed. As a token of respect to Henry Kaplan, the Henry Kaplan Awards for the best posters by young investigators were introduced at the sixth meeting.

Ken McCredie was presented with a special award to mark both the sheer audacity of his presentation and his special affection for the wild life of the Luneberg Heath.

The Wilsede meetings have proved the ideal forum for practising physicians and basic scientists to meet together and discuss new innovations from molecular biology to treatment strategies. The "educational" component of Wilsede, enjoyed by both students and golden oldies alike, is not

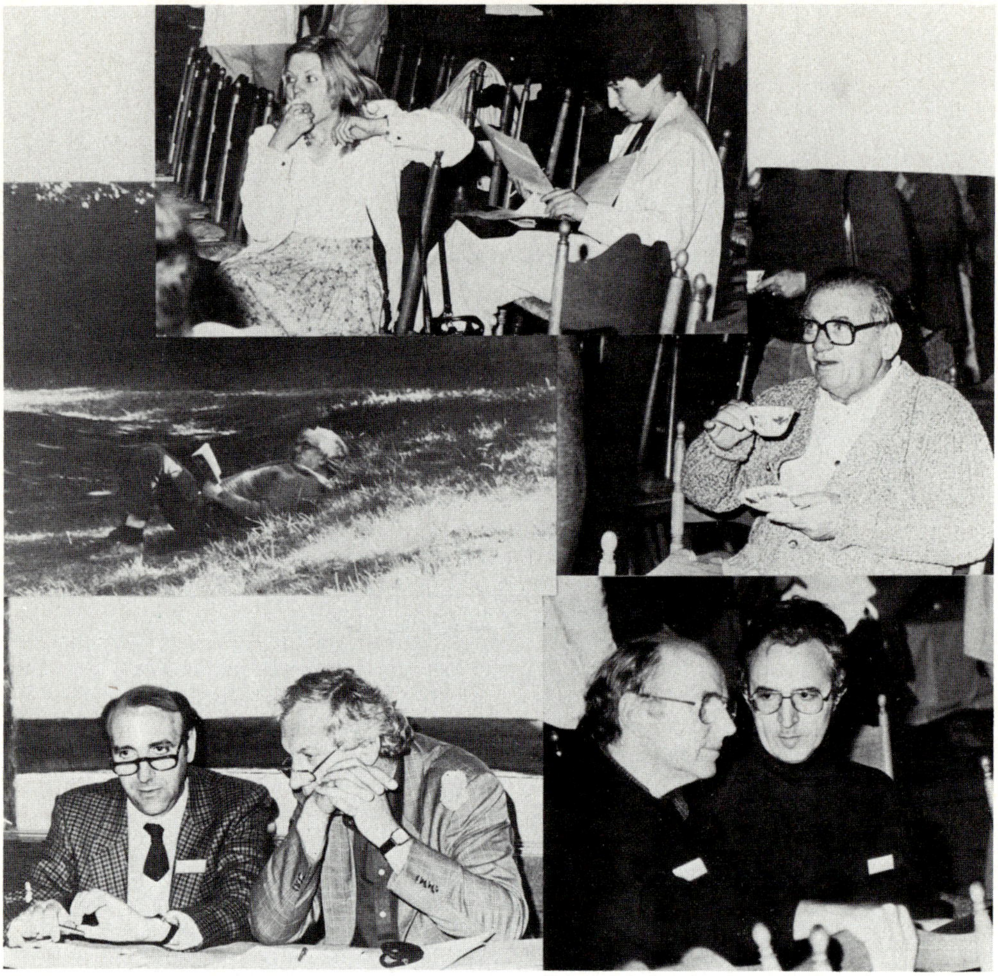

to be underestimated; in an increasingly specialised, technical and rapidly developing research arena it serves a vital function. If, as we all hope, the exciting discoveries in (proto-)oncogenes in leukaemia and monoclonal antibody manipulation of leukaemic cells are to lead to new forms of diagnosis, monitoring and treatment of leukaemia and lymphoma, then Wilsede is the place which will foster the creative skills required.

As in previous Wilsede meetings, the organisers wish to express their thanks to the session chairmen for their help with the programme and emphasise their continued gratitude to Dr. Alfred Toepfer and his associates for keeping the *Naturschutzpark Lüneburger Heide* the delightful and unspoilt place that it is. We are particularly fortunate that the future of these meetings has now been assured by a generous biennial grant of DM 100 000 from the Erich und Gertrud Roggenbuck-Stiftung zur Krebshilfe, Hamburg, to be administered by the Dean of the Faculty of Medicine at the University of Hamburg, Prof. Karl H. Hölzer.

M. F. Greaves

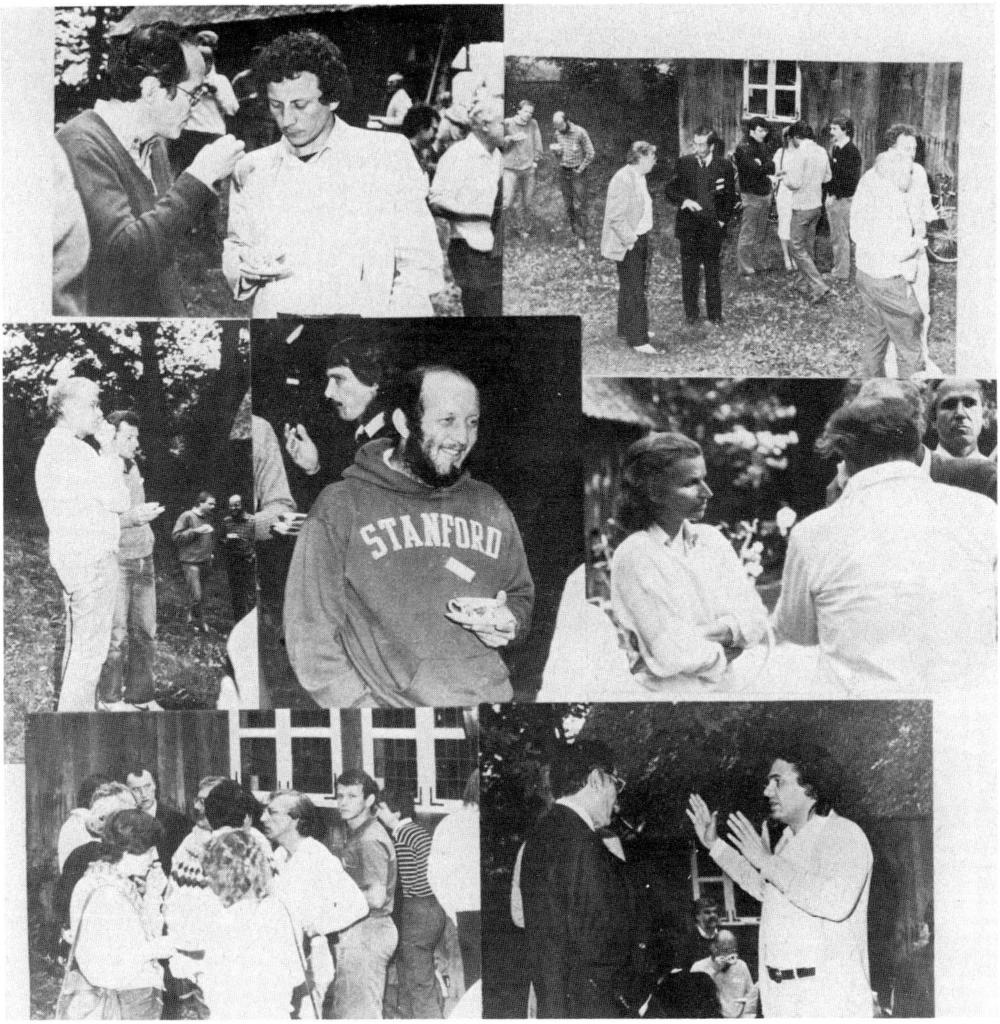

Personal and scientific night discussion
Wilsede, June 1984

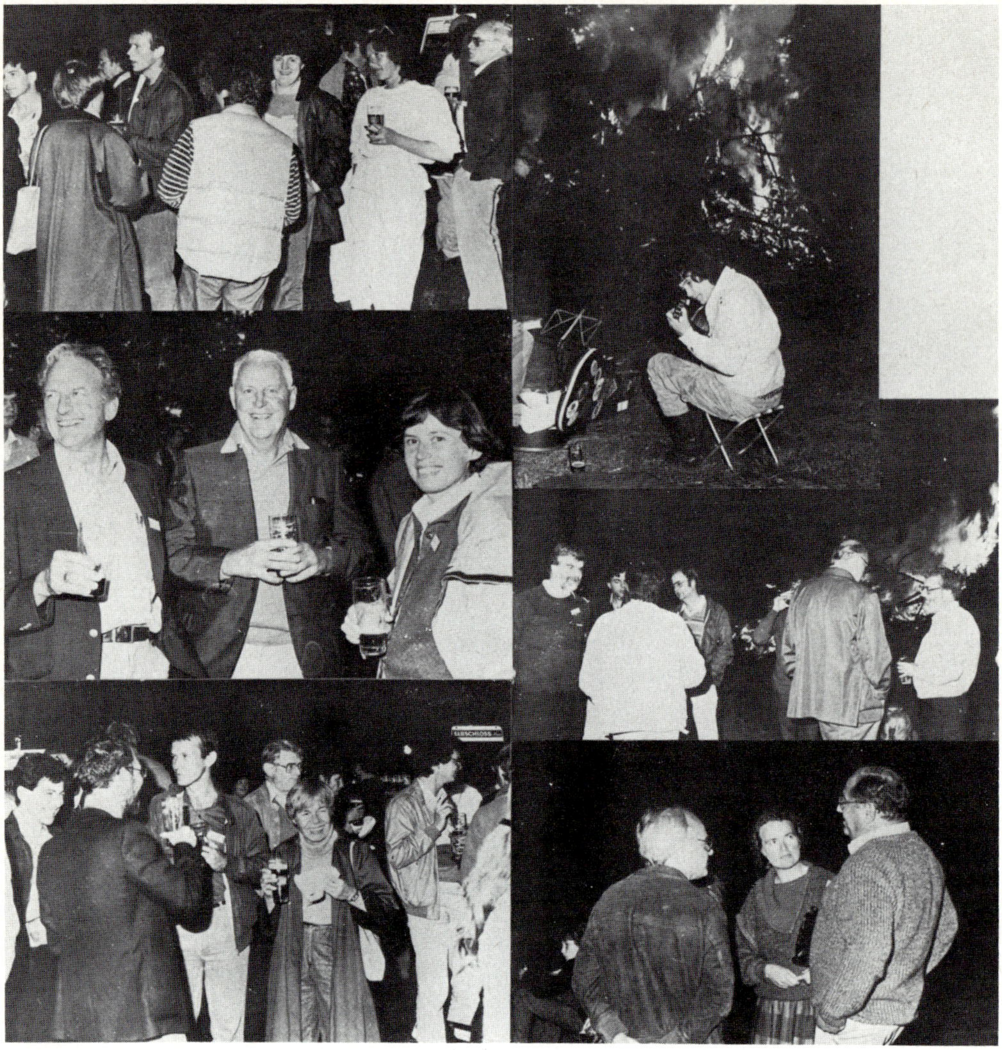

Personal and scientific discussion around and in "De Emmenhof"
Wilsede, June 1984

Acknowledgments

We should like to thank all who made this workshop possible:

Deutsche Forschungsgemeinschaft
Deutsche Krebshilfe
Erich und Gertrud Roggenbuck-Stiftung zur Krebshilfe, Hamburg
Freie und Hansestadt Hamburg
Hamburger Landesverband für Krebsbekämpfung und Krebsforschung e.V. Hamburg
Hamburgische Wissenschaftliche Stiftung
Leukemia Research Fund, Great Britain
Leukemia Society of America
Paul Martini Stiftung
Werner Otto Stiftung Hamburg

For generous hospitality we thank the Stiftung F.V.S. zu Hamburg, Verein Naturschutzpark e.V. Hamburg, the Amerikahaus in Hamburg and the Freie und Hansestadt Hamburg.

Frederick Stohlman Jr.
Memorial Lecture

Wilsede, June 21, 1978

Memorial Tribute to Dr. Frederick Stohlman Presented by William C. Moloney

Gallo, Robert C.: Cellular and Virological Studies Directed to the Pathogenesis of the Human Myelogenous Leukemias

Pinkel, Donald: Treatment of Childhood Acute Lymphocytic Leukemia

Wilsede, June 18, 1980

Klein, George: The Relative Role of Viral Transformation and Specific Cytogenetic Changes in the Development of Murine and Human Lymphomas

Kaplan, Henry S.: On the Biology and Immunology of Hodgkin's Disease

Wilsede, June 21, 1982

Greaves, Melvyn F.: Immunobiology of Lymphoid Malignancy

Thomas, E. Donnall: Bone Marrow Transplantation in Leukemia

Wilsede, June 17, 1984

Klein, Jan: Introduction for N. Avrion Mitchison

Mitchison, N. Avrion: Repertoire purging by medium-concentration self-macromolecules is the major factor determining helper and suppressor repertoire differences

June 18, 1984

Gallo, Robert C.: Introduction for Peter H. Duesberg

Duesberg, Peter H.: Are Activated Proto-*Onc* Genes Cancer Genes?

Haematology and Blood Transfusion Vol. 29
Modern Trends in Human Leukemia VI
Edited by Neth, Gallo, Greaves, Janka

Introduction for N. A. Mitchison

J. Klein[1]

Ladies and Gentlemen,

When I started in immunology, Professor Mitchison was already a legend. Not because he was that much older than I, but because he had made important discoveries early in his scientific career and because even at that time, more than 25 years ago, there were many interesting stories circulating about him. I shall skip the stories and concentrate on Professor Mitchison's scientific contributions.

When you are asked to introduce a famous person and you have to ask yourself what he has actually done, sometimes you may have difficult a time answering this question. Not so when you are asked to introduce Av Mitchison! If anything, you find you have just the opposite problem of choosing a few representative contributions from amongst the many he has made. I have chosen four, which I would now like to mention.

The first contribution he made in 1954, while working solo (at that time you could still work alone and publish papers without 15 other people coauthoring them). He asked a simple question: What is responsible for the rejection of a transplanted tumor? And to answer it he did a simple experiment. He took lymphocytes and serum separately from a mouse that had just rejected a tumor graft, and transferred each into another mouse, which he then grafted with the same tumor. He observed that the mouse that received the cells rejected the tumor, whereas the mouse that received the serum did not. He concluded that tissue grafts are rejected by lymphocytes and not by antibodies, and this conclusion you now find in every immunology textbook, not as an isolated fact, but as a discovery that brought about the era of cellular immunology.

The second discovery I would like to mention you might not even have heard of. It, too, was made in 1954, and it, too, was very simple. Av noticed that when you want to induce an immune response against bacteria, you have to put the bacteria on a cell. As far as I know this was the first experimental demonstration of the requirement for antigen presentation by cells, and it marked the beginning of a path that led – by way of Lawrence and Kindred to Zinkernagel and Doherty – to the discovery of Mhc restriction. Again, it was not an isolated fact that Av discovered, but the beginning of an era.

The third discovery was made by Av, I believe, in 1964. It was the finding that if you injected small amounts of bovine serum albumin into mice and you did it often over a long time, the mice, instead of being immunized, built up a tolerance to this antigen. This experiment represented the discovery of low-zone tolerance, another milestone in cellular immunology.

Finally, the fourth discovery has to do with haptens and carriers. As you know, haptens are small molecules, and when you place them on the large carrier molecules you can make antibodies against them.

1 Max-Planck-Institut für Biologie, Abt. Immungenetik, Corrensstraße 42, 7400 Tübingen, FRG

What Av did was to immunize one set of mice with a hapten and another set with a carrier, and then mix lymphocytes from the two sets of animals and inoculate immunized recipients with the mixture. He observed that these recipients then produced hapten- specific antibodies as if they were immunized by the hapten-carrier complex itself. This finding showed that there were two kinds of cells, one recognizing the hapten and the other the carrier. From here it was only a small step to the discovery of T and B lymphocytes and of T–B collaboration.

I have selected these four examples because each of them marks the beginning of something momentous; each opens a new pathway in immunology. These were not discoveries that were in the air – that anybody could have made but which Av made because he was quicker or luckier. They were unexpected, highly original discoveries that inspired a whole generation of immunologists. They did not follow the beaten track; they opened up new tracks.

However, making original discoveries is not the only way in which Av has made his presence felt in immunology. The other way is through his intellectual influence on his fellow immunologists. This effect is difficult to express in any objective terms and for this reason I can only tell you how Av has influenced me.

I rarely, if ever, read any of the many proceedings of meetings that are published, simply because I do not find them inspiring. I do, however, make one exception – I read the contributions by Av Mitchison. I read these because I know that they are not mere conglomerations of data either already published or in print in one immunology journal or another. I know that they will contain an intelligent assessment of the topic they deal with, and that they will make me think about it in a different way from the way I might have thought earlier.

Also, when I discuss ideas with people and they tell me "I think you are wrong," without being able to tell me why, I do not lose much sleep over it. However, if Av tells me "I think you are wrong," I get nervous. I know of no better compliment I can pay to a person's intellect.

And with these words, ladies and gentlemen, I present to you one of the most original and most inspiring of contemporary immunologists, Professor Avrion Mitchison.

Haematology and Blood Transfusion Vol. 29
Modern Trends in Human Leukemia VI
Edited by Neth, Gallo, Greaves, Janka

Repertoire Purging by Medium Concentration Self-Macromolecules is the Major Factor Determining Helper and Suppressor Repertoire Differences

N. A. Mitchison [1]

Interest in helper and suppressor epitopes has been growing rapidly. It is now generally accepted that most antigens present structures (epitopes) to the immune system which are recognized preferentially by different sets of lymphocytes, as shown in Fig. 1. These sets belong to the effector compartment containing B cells, Tc cells (cytotoxic cells), and delayed-type hypersensitivity-mediating T cells (not shown), or to the regulatory compartment containing Th and Ts cells (helper and suppressors). Structures preferentially recognized by Th cells are termed helper epitopes, and so on, and the balance of the two types of regulatory epitope is known to be an important factor in determining the outcome of at least some immune responses. The presence of even a single suppressor epitope may be enough to prevent a response from occurring. The fullest analysis of an antigen along these lines has been carried out on lysozyme [1] and β-galactosidase [18, 9], and other antigens which have been examined in this way include ferredoxin [19] and tumour antigens [5, 7]. Note however that cleavage of serum albumin does not yield fragments with distinct helper and suppressor epitopes [2, 4].

Understanding the nature of helper and suppressor epitopes is a matter of importance to leukaemia research because it could link tumour idiotype to membership of a lymphocyte set, and also because of its relevance to any future tumour immunotherapy. It is important to immunological diseases at large, because it is likely to help explain why particular types of antigen tend to generate a harmful response. And at the present time it is most obviously important to development of the new generation of vaccines. This is an area of great excitement because these vaccines, based on bioengineering, promise to control and eventually eradicate the major tropical diseases. Of course one needs to exercise caution in evaluating this promise and as yet engineered vaccines are only just entering veterinary trials, but there is no doubt that this hope has given new heart to vaccine research. What is now being done, world-wide, is to take a parasite such as the plasmodium of malaria, clone cDNA into an expression vector, and screen for antibody-defined antigens [6, 7]. A complementary approach is to screen for antibody-reactive synthetic peptides [11]. Both

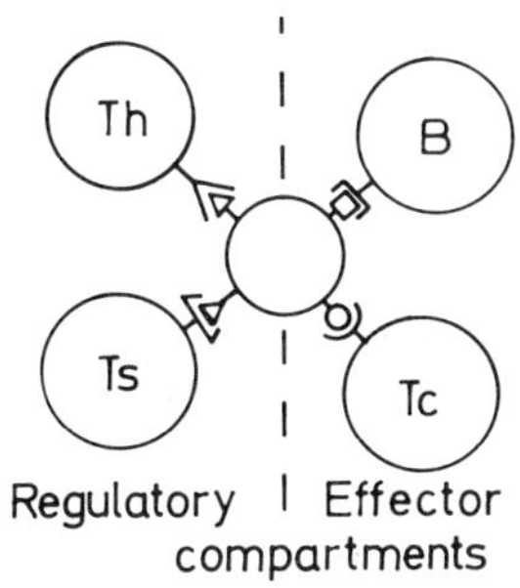

Fig. 1. How a vaccine looks to T cells. Th–Ts repertoire differences are potentially valuable

1 Imperial Cancer Research Fund Tumour Immunology Unit, Department of Zoology, University College London, Gower Street, London, WC1E 6BT, England

of these strategies concentrate initially on the ability of vaccine molecules to interact with the effector compartment, simply because antibodies and to a lesser extent cytotoxic T cell clones are the only practical screening agents. But in the long run this is too limited an approach, particularly for the major tropical diseases all of which are long-term and characteristically display an ineffective host response. Surely the main hope is for a vaccine which can perturb this balance between parasite and host, through manipulation of the regulatory compartment.

The nature of suppressor and helper epitopes is still poorly understood. I wish here to offer a contribution towards a general theory of what makes them different from one another. Any discussion of the problem should start with a distinction between differences based on antigen processing and differences based on the receptor repertoire of lymphocytes. As regards the former, interpretations have tended to diverge, with some authors emphasizing the importance of relatively crude factors such as the gross anatomical localization of antigen, while others emphasize the importance of the interaction of fragments of antigen with particular cell receptors. Thus chemical modification can greatly effect anatomical localization [3], and the route of immunization or form in which a determinent is administered can greatly influence which sets of lymphocyte respond [14]. On the other hand it has been suggested that peptide fragments of antigens associate selectively with particular major histocompatibility complex components, and thus determine which regulatory cells respond to "aggretope selection" [10]. Or suppressor cells may resemble B cells rather than helper cells in their interaction with antigen, and consequently tend to respond to conformational rather than sequence determinants [12]. These are fascinating questions, but we have little hard information with which to answer them.

In contrast there is something more definite to say about repertoire differences between helper and suppressor cells, even if at present this is of a rather general character. Thanks to recent advances in our understanding of the interactions of four

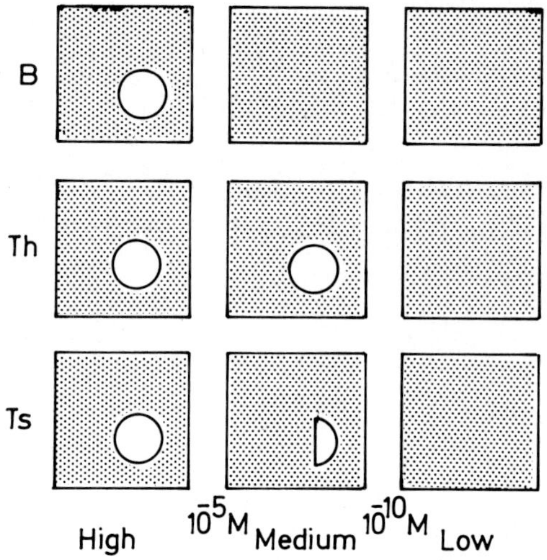

Fig. 2. Only medium concentration self-macromolecules generate Th–Ts repertoire differences (see text for details)

proteins with the immune system as they occur naturally, we can begin to define what is probably the main factor responsible for moulding this repertoire difference. The proteins in question are C5, a complement component, F, a liver and serum protein of unknown function, AFP, α-fetoprotein, and Tg, thyroglobulin. The argument is summarized in Fig. 2, which requires some explanation. Each stippled area represents the repertoire of antigen receptors for a set of lymphocytes (each dot representing, as it were, a single clone of cells). The circles represent holes punched out of the repertoire by tolerance of a single self-protein; it is assumed that self-tolerance results from purging the repertoire of clones reactive with self-proteins. The top row describes what happens to B cells: their repertoire is purged only by proteins which occur in the body at high concentrations, over 10^{-5} *M*, such as serum albumin or the constant part of immunoglobulin. The next row deals with helper T cells: their repertoire is purged by proteins occurring down to lower levels of concentration, 10^{-10} *M*, but no doubt there are still other molecules which occur at concentrations too low to be noticed at all by the immune system, and for which no purging occurs. Thyroglobulin is an example at the bor-

Table 1. Documentation of reactivity of the main lymphocyte sets to four medium concentration self-proteins

	C5	F	AFP	Tg
B cells	+ ±	+ +	+ +	+ +
Th cells	–	–	–	–
Ts cells	+	+		+
Concentration in body fluid (M)	10^{-7} M	10^{-6} M	10^{-9} M	10^{-15} M
References	[5]; Y. Borel, personal communication	[12, 20]	[15, 16]	[17, 18]

derline between the medium and low ranges of concentration: it purges the helper cell repertoire to a significant extent, but incompletely. At the bottom come suppressor T cells: their repertoire is no more than partially purged by proteins occuring at medium concentrations, as exemplified by the proteins F and C5. The important point is that purging of helper and suppressor cells occurs down to different levels, and that this difference defines a medium concentration range at which their repertoires must differ. No other factor can be identified which is known to generate a difference between their repertoires. This does not mean that other factors do not operate, but simply that at present we do not know what they are. For instance at the time of writing there is a suspicion, but at present no more than that, that helper and suppressor T cells draw from different sets of V genes. The evidence for the medium concentration range that is crucial to this argument is cited in Table 1 for the four proteins C5, F, AFP and Tg, and is discussed in greater detail elsewhere [13].

What are the practical consequences? It is ironic that this, the only definite piece of information which we have about the helper-suppressor epitope difference should produce so little in the way of practical advice about how to design a particular epitope. Even if we knew the full three-dimensional structure of the proteins listed in Table 1 we would only be a little nearer this goal. From this point of view research on differential antigen processing perhaps has more to offer, even if so far its achievements have been small. For the time being immunologists will be kept busy cloning genes and synthesizing peptides of potential value in vaccines. More and more of these new products will enter immunization trials without much rhyme or reason, and as they do so we shall no doubt acquire empirical information about which kinds of structure are good immunogens as distinct from ones which merely react well with antibodies. It will be important to have some kind of theoretical framework into which this information will fit. I believe that medium concentration self-proteins as defined here will be an important part of that framework.

References

1. Adorini L, Harvey MA, Miller A, Sercarz EE (1979) Fine specificty of regulatory T cells. II. Suppressor and helper T cells are induced by different regions of hen egg-white lysozyme in a genetically non-responder mouse strain. J Exp Med 150:293–306
2. Benjamin DC, Daigle CA, Riley RL (1983) The antigenic structure of bovine serum albumin: T-cell, B-cell, and Ia determinants. In: Celada F, Schumacher VE, Sercarz EE (eds) Protein confrontation as an immunological signal. Plenum, New York, pp 261–280
3. Dailey MO, Hunter RL (1974) The role of lipid in the induction of hapten-specific delayed hypersensitivity and contact sensitivity. J Immunol 112:1526–1534
4. Ferguson TA, Peters T Jr, Reed R, Pesce AJ, Michael JG (1983) Immunoregulatory properties of antigenic fragments from bovine serum albumin. Cell Immunol 78:1–12
5. Harris DE, Cairns L, Rosen FS, Borel Y (1982) A natural model of immunologic tolerance. Tolerance to murine C5 is me-

diated by T cells, and antigen is required to maintain unresponsiveness. J Exp Med 156:567–584
6. Kemp DJ, Koppel RL, Cowman AF, Saint RB, Brown GV, Anders RF (1983) Expression of Plasmodium falciparum blood stage antigens in Escherichia coli: detection with antibodies from immune humans. Proc Natl Acad Sci USA 80:3787–3791
7. Klein BY, Sharon R, Tarcic N, Naor D (1982) Induction of antitumour reactive cells or suppressor cells by different molecular species isolated from the same nonimmunogenic tumour. Immunobiology 163:7–21
8. Kong YM, Okayasu I, Giraldo AA, Beisel KW, Sundiale RS, Rose NR, David D, Audibert F, Chedid L (1982) Tolerance to thyroglobulin by activating suppressor mechanisms. Ann NY Acad Sci 392:191–209
9. Krzych U, Fowler AV, Miller A, Sercarz EE (1982) Repertoires of T cells directed against a large protein antigen, β-galactosidase. I Helper cells have a more restricted repertoire than proliferative cells. J Immunol 128:1529–1534
10. Krzych U, Fowler A, Sercarz EE (1983) Antigen structures used by regulatory T cells in the interaction among T suppressor, T helper, and B cells. In: Celada F, Schumacher VE, Sercarz EE (eds) Protein confrontation an immunological signal. Plenum, New York, p 395–408
11. Lerner RA (1983) Synthetic vaccines. Sci Am 248:66–74
12. Lukic ML, Mitchison NA, Self- and allospecific suppressor T cells evoked by intravenous injection of F protein. Eur J Immunol 14:8:766–768
13. Mitchison NA, Lukic ML, Nardi N, Proteins at the margin between being tolerated and being noticed. In: Proc Ninth Int Covocation on Immunology. Karger, Basel
14. Plak W, Rozycka D, Askenase PW, Gershon RK (1980) Role of antigen presenting cells in the development and persistence of contact hypersensitivity. J Exp Med 151:362–375
15. Ruoslahti E, Wigzell H (1975) Breakage of tolerance to alpha-foetoprotein in monkeys. Nature 255:716–717
16. Ruoslahti E, Pihko H, Becker M, Mäkelä M (1975) Rabbit alpha-foetoprotein: normal levels and breakage of tolerance with haptenated homologous alpha-fetoprotein. Eur J Immunol 5:7–10
17. Romball CG, Weigle WO (1984) T cell competence in heterologous and homologous thyroglobulins during the induction of experimental autoimmune thyroiditis. Eur J Immunol 14:10:887–893
18. Turkin D. Sercarz EE (1977) Key antigenic determinants in regulation of the immune response. Proc Nat Acad Sci USA 74:3934–3987
19. Weaver M, Singhai R, Sikora L, Levy JC (1983) Identification of an idiotypic marker of a major regulatory T cell of the immune response in B10.BR mice to ferredoxin. The relationship of idiotypic regulation to conventional hapten-carrier effects. J Exp Med 157:285–300
20. Wedderburn L, Lukic ML, Edwards S, Kahan MC, Nardi N, Mitchison NA (1984) Single-step immunosorbent preparation of F protein from mouse liver with conservation of the alloantigenic site, and determination of concentration in liver and serum. Mol Immunol 21:10:979–984

Haematology and Blood Transfusion Vol. 29
Modern Trends in Human Leukemia VI
Edited by Neth, Gallo, Greaves, Janka

Introduction for P. H. Duesberg

R. C. Gallo[1]

It is time now to introduce my friend Peter Duesberg. Where do I begin? At NIH, Peter is sometimes known as the battling bulldog. He gets his teeth into something and 1 year, 5 years, 10 years, 20 years later those teeth are still sunk in. I should be serious a bit, shouldn't I? Peter, of course, was born here in Germany. He was educated at Tübingen and he came to the United States 20 years ago at the age of 27. I've known Peter now for about 15 years. When I first met him, he was already doing molecular virology, and I was already involved in retroviruses. Peter first began work on the molecular virology of parainfluenza and influenza viruses. He was the first to show that parainfluenza had a singular RNA genome and that influenza virus had multiple RNAs. This was the first time a virus was shown to have a segmented genome, thus explaining the rather distinctive ability of that virus to undergo frequent recombination by reassortment.

He began working with retroviruses around 1966, and he was among the first, or perhaps even the very first, to characterize their structural proteins. He was involved in the first work that provided a genetic map of retroviruses. Surely, this is one of the most important of his many biochemical contributions, that is, the order of the genes, *gag, pol, env,* and some aspect of the nature of their nucleotide sequences. We now know that this fundamental result is applicable to all retroviruses, including HTLV-I, II, and III. So, the application of biochemical methods to the mapping of retroviral genes was first and primarily carried out by Peter. Some of this work also ultimately became critical to the taxonomy of retroviruses.

He carried out the first restriction endonuclease mapping of a provirus. This was in the late 1970s. He was the first, or one of the first, to demonstrate repetitive sequences at the ends of the proviruses, which were the beginning of our understanding of the LTRs that we talk about routinely today. He was involved in the first publications which demonstrated that these viruses replicate via a circular proviral DNA form. After reverse transcriptase was discovered (it was about that time I began to know Peter fairly well), Peter did some of the early characterization of this DNA polymerase. His publications with his colleagues were the first reports showing that reverse transcriptase utilized a primer mechanism, not just a template, but a primer to initiate DNA synthesis, and he was the first to show that the primer was a 4S molecule. But actually, although listing this as one of his major accomplishments, I remember Peter telling me when he did those experiments he didn't know what a primer actually was!

The next major phase of his work involved his classic studies with Peter Vogt; Vogt the biologist, Peter the biochemist. This really led to the first molecular and genetically defined transforming gene, the *sarc* gene. A great deal of this brilliant and original work, the real critical aspects, was

1 National Cancer Institute, Bethesda, Maryland 20205, USA

carried out by this extraordinarily effective collaboration through the 1970s. Of course, Peter also worked on a number of other *onc* genes, describing several for the first time, mostly in avian systems but also in murine systems. Most recently this has been in collaboration with Takas Papas at NCI.

These are some of Peter's contributions. There are many more. However, there are things about him that stand out as much as his science. Peter Duesberg is a man of extraordinary energy, unusual honesty, enormous sense of humor, and a rare critical sense. This critical sense often makes us look twice, then a third time, at a conclusion many of us believed to be foregone. However, his critiques are sometimes a major problem for the casual observer. When is he truly debating? When is he only being the devil's advocate? When is he being the devil himself? The casual observer is also often at a loss to determine which of the many weapons he possesses he is using. Peter, it is hard for us to tell when you are using your machine gun or your slingshot, or simply exercising your vocal cords. In any event you are an extraordinary scientist, a man who makes life more interesting and pleasurable to many of us; and it is my good fortune to know you as a friend.

Haematology and Blood Transfusion Vol. 29
Modern Trends in Human Leukemia VI
Edited by Neth, Gallo, Greaves, Janka

Are Activated Proto-*onc* Genes Cancer Genes? *

P. H. Duesberg [1], M. Nunn [2], Nancy Kan [3], D. Watson [3], P. H. Seeburg [4], and T. Papas [3]

A. Introduction

The main objective of cancer molecular biology is to identify cancer genes. Despite fierce efforts, this objective has still not been met [1–3]. As yet the only known cancer genes are the transforming *onc* genes of retroviruses. Typically these viruses initiate and maintain cancers with autonomous transforming genes that are dominant in susceptible cells [5]. The discovery of single gene determinants of cancer in retroviruses has become a precedent that has infected cancer gene research. It has made retroviral *onc* genes the favorite models of cellular oncogenes, although the relevance of single-gene models to virus-negative tumors is as yet unknown. Fortunately, *onc* genes are either detrimental or at least useless to the viability of the virus and thus are not maintained by retroviruses. They are the products of rare, genetic accidents, generated by illegitimate recombinations between retroviruses and cellular genes, termed proto-*onc* genes. About 20 different proto-*onc* genes corresponding to 20 different retroviral *onc* genes are known [5]. At this time the normal function of proto-*onc* genes has not yet been determined. One of them is structurally related to a growth factor, another is related to a growth factor receptor [6], and two appear to be yeast cell cycle genes [6, 7].

It is now widely believed that, upon transcriptional or mutational "activation," proto-*onc* genes function like viral *onc* genes. Activation is assumed to be the conversion of a nononcogenic proto-*onc* gene into a carcinogenic variant. Indeed, mutationally altered or transcriptionally activated proto-*onc* genes have been found in certain tumors. However, the known mutationally or transcriptionally altered proto-*onc* genes are structurally different from viral *onc* genes and have not been shown to be the causes of tumors.

Consistent with the single gene models set by retroviral *onc* genes, it has been proposed, recently, that molecularly defined or cloned DNA species from some tumors are autonomous cancer genes, because these DNAs are capable of transforming the morphology of certain preneoplastic cell lines [4]. Despite the popularity of this view, there is no convincing evidence to date that these DNA species can also transform normal cells in culture or that they are the causes of tumors in animals (see below).

Circumstantial evidence suggests that most cancers are not caused by single genes but are the products of multiple genes that have been formally divided into initiation

---

* This lecture was also presented at the "International Conference on RNA Tumor Viruses in Human Cancer," Denver, Colorado, United States, 10–14 June, 1984. A portion of this lecture will also be printed as part of a review in *Science,* May 10, 1985

1 Department of Molecular Biology, University of California, Berkeley, CA 94720, USA
2 The Salk Institute, P. O. Box 85800, San Diego, CA 92138-9216, USA
3 Laboratory of Molecular Oncology, National Cancer Institute, Frederick Cancer Research Facility, Frederick, MD 21701, USA
4 Genentech, Inc., 460 Point San Bruno Boulevard, South San Francisco, CA 90007, USA

and maintenance genes [1–3]. Retroviruses without *onc* genes (leukemia viruses) and DNA viruses are thought to function either as initiation or as maintenance genes in multigene carcinogenesis because these viruses enhance the cancer risk of infected animals.

Recently it has been proposed that activated proto-*onc* genes play a role in multigene carcinogenesis, rather than being autonomous cancer genes. Here the evidence for the views that activated proto-*onc* genes are sufficient (one gene-one cancer hypothesis) or at least necessary (multigene-one cancer hypothesis) is reviewed. It is concluded, that there is as yet no adequate functional evidence for oncogenicity and no consistent correlation between any proto-*onc* alteration and a certain tumor. To date viral *onc* genes are the only proven examples of "activated" proto-*onc* genes.

B. Retroviral *onc* Genes and Normal Proto-*onc* Genes

Retroviruses with *onc* genes are the fastest-acting, obligatory carcinogens known to date. Such viruses have only been isolated from animals with neoplasms, while all other retroviruses and all DNA viruses with oncogenic potential are regularly isolated from animals without neoplasms. This is consistent with single-gene carcinogenesis by retroviruses with *onc* genes and possible multigene carcinogenesis with all other viruses. Indeed, retroviral *onc* genes are the only genes known that initiate and maintain cancers per se. That they are necessary for transformation has been proven genetically with temperature-sensitive (*ts*) mutants of Rous (RSV) [8], Kirsten (KiSV) [9], and Fujinami sarcoma viruses [10, 11]; with avian erythroblastosis virus [12]; and with deletion mutants of these and other retroviruses [13–19]. The most convincing argument, that they are also sufficient to initiate and maintain neoplastic transformation, is that all susceptible cells infected by retroviruses with *onc* genes become transformed as soon as they are infected. This high transformation efficiency virtually excludes selection of preneoplastic cells initiated by another gene.

The structural characteristic of retroviral *onc* genes is a specific sequence that is unrelated to the three essential virion genes *gag, pol,* and *env*. This *onc*-specific sequence of retroviruses is related to one or several proto-*onc* genes. Typically the *onc*-specific sequence replaces essential virion genes and thus renders the virus replication-defective, or it is added to the essential genes as in the case of RSV and is readily deleted [5, 13, 14, 20]. Since *onc* sequences are parasitic and have no survival value for the virus, *onc* genes are readily lost by spontaneous deletion [5, 20]. Therefore, viruses with *onc* genes are subject to extinction unless maintained in laboratories.

About 17 of the 20 known viral *onc* genes are hybrids of coding regions from proto-*onc* genes linked to coding regions from essential retroviral genes [20]. The remaining viral *onc* genes consist of coding regions from proto-*onc* genes linked to retroviral control elements. The identification of hybrid *onc* genes provided the first unambiguous clues that viral *onc* genes and corresponding cellular proto-*onc* genes are different, since proto-*onc* genes are neither related to nor linked in the cell to elements of essential retrovirus genes [21, 22]. Sequence comparisons of cloned genes have since confirmed and extended that all proto-*onc* genes and corresponding viral *onc* genes are not isogenic [5, 20]. The known viral *onc* genes are subsets of proto-*onc* genes linked to regulatory and coding elements of virion genes.

In our laboratories we are studying the structural and functional relationships between viral *onc* genes and corresponding proto-*onc* genes, with particular emphasis on the *onc* genes of the following avian carcinoma, sarcoma, and leukemia viruses. The *onc* gene of avian carcinoma virus MC29 was the first among viral *onc* genes to be diagnosed as a hybrid gene [21, 23] (Fig. 1). About one-half of its information (1.5 kb) is derived from the *gag* gene of retroviruses; the other half (1.6 kb), termed *myc,* is derived from the proto-*myc* gene [22]. The gene is defined by a 110-kilodalton *Δgag-myc* protein, termed p110 [21, 24]. The proto-*myc* gene of the chicken has at least three exons. The boundaries of the

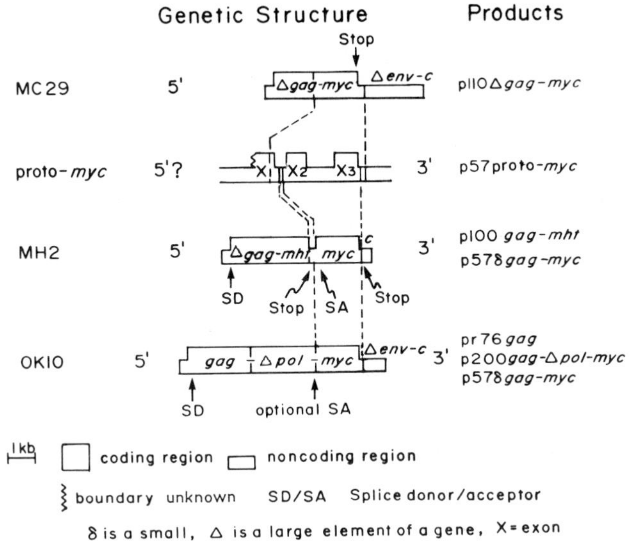

Fig. 1. Comparison of the genetic structures and gene products of the *myc*-related genes of MC29, MH2, OK10, and chicken proto-*myc*

first exon are as yet undefined [25–27]. The *myc* region of MC29 derives four codons possibly from the 3′ end of the first exon and includes the second and third proto-*myc* exons (Fig. 1). Three other avian carcinoma viruses, MH2, OK10, and CMII, also have *onc* genes with *myc* sequences [24]. The *myc*-related gene of MH2 is derived from the second and third proto-*myc* exon and includes the splice acceptor of the first proto-*myc* intron [25, 28, 29] (Fig. 1). It also appears to be a hybrid consisting of six *gag* codons up to the splice donor of the *gag* gene [30]. It is expressed via a subgenomic mRNA as a p57 *myc*-related protein product [31–33]. In addition, MH2 contains a second potential transforming gene, *Δgag-mht*. The *mht* sequence is very closely related to the *onc* gene of murine sarcoma virus MSV 3611 [28, 29]. It is as yet unclear whether both genes are necessary for transforming function. The *myc* sequence of OK10, like that of MH2, is derived from the second and third proto-*myc* exons and includes the splice acceptor of the first proto-*myc* intron (Fig. 1) (J. Hayflick, P. Seeburg, R. Ohlsson, S. Pfeifer, D. Watson, T. Papas and P. Duesberg, unpublished). It is expressed via a subgenomic mRNA as a p57 protein [32–34]. At the same time, the *myc* sequence of OK10 is also part of a large hybrid *onc* gene, *gag-Δpol-myc,* similar to the hybrid *myc* gene of MC29 [24]. This gene is defined by a 200-kilodalton protein termed p200 [24]. Again, it remains to be determined whether both of these two *onc* gene products are necessary for transforming function. The *myc* sequence of CMII is part of a *Δgag-myc* hybrid gene similar to that of MC29 [24]. Thus, all *myc*-related viral *onc* genes are subsets of proto-*myc* linked to large or small retroviral coding regions and regulatory elements. As yet, no virus with a *myc*-related *onc* gene has been isolated from a mammalian species. However, a *myc* containing feline provirus with unknown biological activity was recently detected by hybridization of lymphoma DNA from a feline-leukemia-virus-infected cat [35].

The results of similar comparisons between the *Δgag-fps* genes of Fujinami, PRCII, and PRCIIp sarcoma viruses and cellular proto-*fps* are summarized in Fig. 2 [19, 36, 37]. In these cases, the sarcoma viruses share with proto-*fps* a 2- to 3-kb *fps* domain, including probably the 3′ translation stop codon. However, the viral genes each initiate with retroviral *gag* regions, whereas proto-*fps* initiates with a proto-*fps*-specific exon(s) [36] (Fig. 2).

Analysis of the *onc* genes of the leukemia viruses avian myeloblastosis (AMV) and erythroblastosis virus (E26), and of proto-*myb,* the common cellular prototype of the *myb* sequence shared by these viruses, is al-

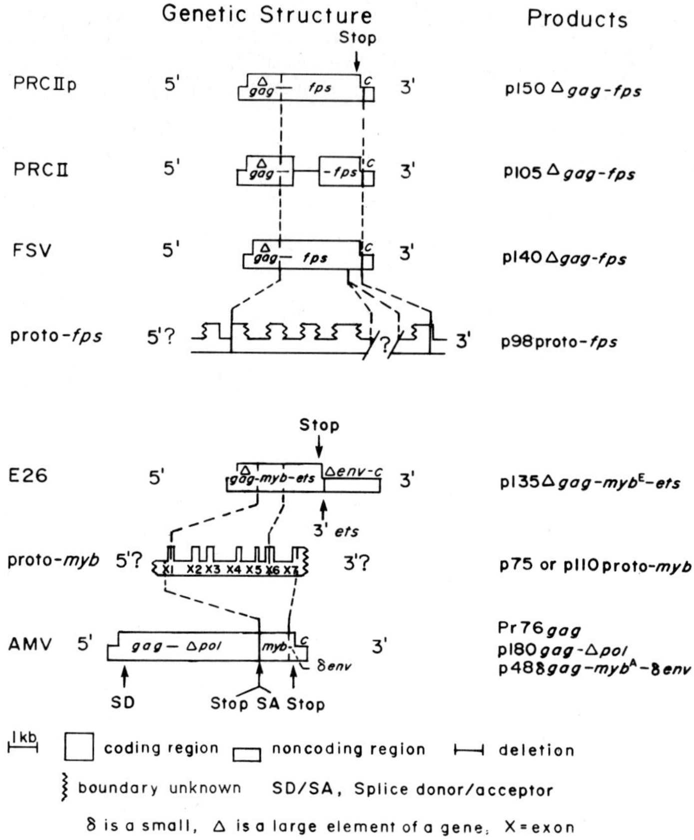

Fig. 2. Comparison of the genetic structures and gene products of the *fps*-related genes of avian Fujinami, PRCIIp and PRCII sarcoma viruses, and the chicken proto-*fps* gene (*top*) and of the *myb*-related genes of avian leukemia viruses E26 and AMV and the chicken proto-*myb* gene (*bottom*)

so schematically summarized in Fig. 2. Unlike the *myc*- and *fps*-containing *onc* genes, the *onc* genes of each of these viruses share an internal domain with the cellular prototype [38, 39]. In E26, the *myb* region is flanked by a *gag*-related region at its 5′ end and by a newly discovered *onc*-specific domain, termed *ets*, at its 3′ end to form a tripartite *onc* gene [40, 41]. In AMV, the *myb* region includes a proto-*myb* splice acceptor that is presumably served in the virus by the splice donor of *Δgag* [30]. The *myb* region of AMV is flanked at its 3′ end by an element derived from the *env* gene of retroviruses. It is concluded that the *onc*-specific sequences of each of these carcinoma, sarcoma, and leukemia viruses are subsets of proto-*onc* genes linked to elements of essential retrovirus genes.

Other examples of hybrid *onc* genes have been described [5, 16, 20, 24]. Since in all the cases studied proto-*onc* genes are not related and not linked to essential genes of retroviruses, all viral hybrid *onc* genes are by definition structurally different from proto-*onc* genes. The coding regions of a few viral *onc* genes, possibly the *src* gene of RSV and probably the *onc* genes of Harvey, Kirsten sarcoma viruses (termed Ha- and Ki-*ras*), are derived entirely from proto-*onc* sequences (see below and Fig. 4). Nevertheless, even these *onc* genes differ from proto- *onc* genes in extensive deletions and point mutations. The *src* gene of RSV is a hybrid of genetic elements derived from two proto-*src* genes [5, 42] and possibly five codons from a retrovirus [139].

Two arguments indicate that these qualitative differences between *onc* and proto-*onc* genes are essential for transforming function of the viral genes: There is the overwhelming evidence that many proto-*onc* genes are regularly expressed in normal cells without altering the normal phenotype [5, 43]. There is more indirect evidence that proto-*onc* sequences cloned in retroviral or plasmid vectors do not transform normal, diploid cells. For example, phage or plasmid vectors carrying the viral *src*-related region, but not a complete complement of the major proto-*src* gene [44–47] or proto-*fos*, the precursor of the transforming gene of FBJ (Finkel-Biskis-Jinkins) murine osteosarcoma virus [48], or proto-*fps/fes*, the precursors of avian Fujinami and feline sarcoma viruses [49] (W.-H. Lee and P. H. Duesberg, unpublished), or proto-*myc*, the precursor of avian MC29 virus (T. Robins, P. Duesberg, and G. Vande Woude, unpublished), do not transform cells in culture. The *src*-related region of the major proto-*src* gene also fails to transform in a RSV vector [50]. Further, proto-*src* and proto-Ha-*ras* (the precursor of Ha-MuSV) fail to transform in a reticuloendotheliosis virus vector while the corresponding viral *onc* genes have transforming function [51].

Apparent exceptions are proto-*mos* and proto-*ras* which, after ligation to retroviral promoters, transform the preneoplastic NIH 3T3 cell line [52, 53]. The proto-*mos* and *ras* regions used in these constructions are essentially the same as those found in Moloney and Harvey sarcoma viruses but are not complete proto-*onc* genes (see below and Fig. 2). Conceivably, the proto-*onc* regions that were not included into these constructions and are not in the viruses might in the cell suppress transforming potential of the complete proto-*onc* genes. Moreover, it will be detailed below that transforming function in 3T3 cells is not a reliable measure of transforming function in diploid embryo cells or in the animal. Neither the proto-*ras* nor the proto-*mos* construction were found to transform diploid embryo cells [54, 55] (G. Vande Woude, personal communication). Thus, normal proto-*onc* genes and viral *onc* genes are related, but are structurally and functionally different. The question is now whether there are conditions under which proto-*onc* genes can cause cancer.

C. The Search for Activation of Proto-*onc* Genes to Cancer Genes

The only clear, although indirect, proof for activation of proto-*onc* genes to cancer genes is based on the rare cases in which proto-*onc* genes functioned as accidental parents of retroviral *onc* genes. It has been deduced from structural analyses of retroviral genes and proto-*onc* genes that viral *onc* genes were generated by transduction of specific domains from proto-*onc* genes [5, 20]. Because no significant sequence homology exists between retroviruses and proto-*onc* genes, such transductions must procede via two rare, nonhomologous recombinations [5, 25][5]. It is probably for this reason that viral transductions or "activations" are extremely rare, even though all cells contain proto- *onc* genes and many animal species contain retroviruses without *onc* genes. Only 50–100 sporadic cancers from which retroviruses with *onc* genes were isolated have been reported and no experimentally reproducible system of transduction has ever been described [56–58]. Thus, retroviruses with *onc* genes are the causes of rare, natural tumors rather than laboratory artifacts.

Their role as accidental progenitors of viral *onc* genes has made proto-*onc* genes the focus of the search for cellular cancer genes. Their possible function in cancer was initially tested in many laboratories in view of a "one gene–one cancer" and more recently in view of a "multigene–one cancer" hypothesis. The one gene–one cancer hypothesis is similar to postulates that activation of inactive cellular oncogenes is sufficient to cause cancer the oncogene hypothesis of Huebner and Todaro [59]. Some investigators have postulated that activation is the result of increased dosage of a given proto-*onc* gene product. This view, termed the quantitative model, received support from early experiments which suggested that the *src* gene of RSV or the *myc* gene of MC29 and the corresponding proto-*onc* genes were equivalents [60–64]. In the meantime, significant structural and functional differences between these genes have been found [5, 43, 44–47, 50] (see above).

5 In addition, it appears that only a few cellular genes are proto-*onc* genes or can function as progenitors of viral *onc* genes since the same proto-*onc* sequences have been found in different isolates [29]

Others have suggested that proto-*onc* genes are activated by mutations or rearrangements in the primary DNA sequence [65, 66]. This view is termed the qualitative model [5].

The multigene–one cancer hypothesis postulates that an activated proto-*onc* gene is necessary, but unlike the corresponding viral gene, not sufficient to cause cancer. A quantitatively or qualitatively activated proto-*onc* gene is postulated to function either as initiation or as maintenance gene together with another proto-*onc* gene, in a multistep process [54, 55, 67–73]. This hypothesis fits the view of how virus-negative tumors are thought to arise in general and provides identifiable candidates to test the hypothesis. However, since retroviral *onc* genes have yet to be dissociated into initiation and maintenance functions, this hypothesis is without viral precedent.

Two kinds of assays have been performed to test these hypotheses. One assay correlates transcriptional activation and mutation of proto-*onc* genes with cancer; the other directly measures transforming function of proto-*onc* genes upon transfection into certain recipient cells, typically the preneoplastic mouse NIH 3T3 cell line [4, 54, 55]. Such experiments have most frequently linked cancers with alterations of proto-*myc* and proto-*ras*.

I. Is Proto-*myc* Activation the Cause of B-Cell Lymphomas?

Based on the observation that transcription of the cellular proto-*myc* is enhanced in retroviral lymphomas of chicken, it has been postulated that transcriptional activation of proto-*myc* is the cause of B-cell lymphoma [64, 74]. Chicken B-cell lymphoma is a clonal cancer that appears in a small fraction of animals infected by one of the avian leukosis viruses (which have no *onc* genes) after latent periods of over 6 months [58]. The hypothesis, termed downstream promotion, postulates that the gene is activated by the promoter of a retrovirus integrated upstream (Fig. 3) and that activated proto-*myc* functions like the transforming gene of MC29 [64]. Subsequently, samples were found in which the retrovirus is integrated 3′ of proto-*myc* or 5′ in the opposite transcriptional direction. In these cases, the virus is thought to function like an enhancer of proto-*myc* [74] (Fig. 3).

However, proto-*myc* differs structurally from the 3-kb *Δgag-myc* gene of MC29 as diagrammed in Figs. 1 and 3 [25, 26]. Further, it has been argued previously [5] that the hypothesis fails to explain the origin of about 20% of viral lymphomas in which proto-*myc* is not activated [64]; the discrepancies between the phenotype of the disease and the cancers caused by MC29; the clonality of the tumors, defined by a single integration site of the retrovirus with regard to proto-*myc;* and the long latent period of the disease. Given about 10^6 kb of chicken DNA and activation of proto-*myc* by retrovirus integration within about 5 kb of proto-*myc* [27, 74], one in 2×10^5 infections should generate the first tumor cell. Since the chicken probably has over 10^7 uncommitted B cells and many more virus particles, the critical carcinogenic integration event should occur after a short latent period. The tumor should also not be clonal, since integration by retroviruses is not site specific and there could be numerous infections during the latent period of about 6 months. Further, the model has not been confirmed in murine [75, 76], feline [35], and bovine [77] leukemia. Instead, the high percentage of virus-negative feline [35] and bovine [78] lymphomas indicates that a retrovirus is not even necessary for the disease.

Recently, it was suggested that a mutation, rather than a virus, may have activated avian proto-*myc* because mutations have been observed in viral lymphoma [79]. However, the proto-*myc* mutations have not been shown to be the cause of the viral lymphoma.

Activation of proto-*myc* has also been postulated to cause the retrovirus-negative, human Burkitt's lymphomas, and mouse plasmacytomas. In these cases, chromosome translocation has been proposed as a mechanism of activating proto-*myc* function [70, 71, 80, 81]. The human proto-*myc* is related to that of the chicken from which carcinoma viruses have been derived (Fig. 3). The two genes have unique first exons, similar second exons with unique re-

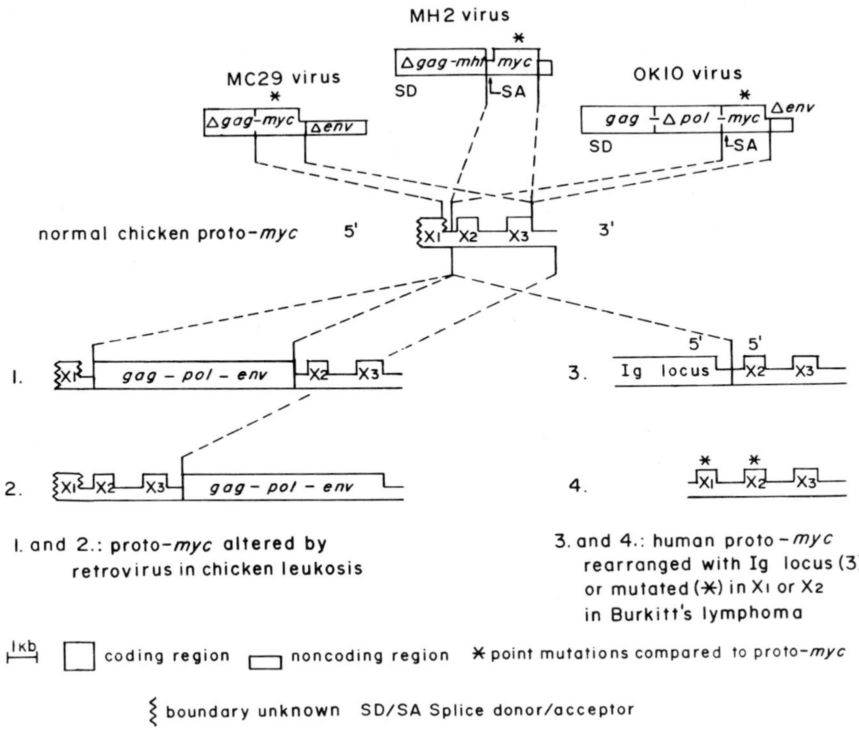

Fig. 3. *Myc*-related genes in avian carcinoma viruses and in normal and lymphoma cells. The common and specific *myc* domains of avian carcinoma viruses MC29 [25, 26], MH2 [28, 29], and OK10 [24, and unpublished], of normal chicken proto-*myc* [25, 71], and of the proto-*myc* genes of avian leukosis [57, 67] and human Burkitt's lymphoma [70, 71, 80] are graphically compared. Proto-*myc* has three exons (X1, X2, X3) the first of which is thought to be noncoding [25, 81]. The proto-*myc* genes of chicken and man are related but not identical: Their first exons are essentially unrelated; there are major unique sequence elements in each of their second exons and minor differences between the third exons [25]. *Gag, pol,* and *env* are the three essential virion genes of retroviruses and *Δ* marks incomplete complements of these genes

gions, and colinear third exons [25]. In man, proto-*myc* is located on chromosome 8 and an element of this chromosome is reciprocally translocated in many Burkitt's lymphoma lines to immunoglobulin (Ig) loci of chromosome 14 and less frequently of chromosome 2 or 22. Since the crossover points of chromosome 8 are near proto-*myc,* translocation was initially suspected to activate proto-*myc* transcriptionally by rearranging proto-*myc* (Fig. 1) or by altering its immediate environment and thus bringing it under the influence of new promoters or enhancers [80]. However, in many lymphomas rearranged proto-*myc* is not linked to a new promoter; instead the first presumably noncoding exon is replaced by the Ig locus, linked to it 5′–5′ in the opposite transcriptional orientation [80] (Fig. 3). Further this model cannot explain how proto-*myc* would be activated when the complete proto-*myc* gene, including its known promoters and flanking regions, is translocated [70, 72, 82], or recent observations that in a significant minority of Burkitt's lymphomas proto-*myc* remains in its original chromosomal location while a region 3′ of proto-*myc* is translocated [83–87]. Despite these inconsistencies, proto-*myc* is thought to function as a cellular oncogene in these tumors.

Moreover, there is no consensus at this time whether proto-*myc* expression is enhanced in Burkitt's lymphoma cells, as compared with normal control cells. Some investigators report elevated expression compared with normal B-lymphoblasts or lines [88], while others report essentially normal levels of proto-*myc* mRNA [70, 82, 86, 87, 89–92]. Further, enhanced proto-*myc* transcription is not specific for B-cell lymphomas, since high levels of proto-*myc* expression are seen in non-Burkitt's lymphomas [91], in other tumors [73], and in chemically transformed fibroblast cell lines in which proto-*myc* is not translocated or rearranged [43]. The view that enhanced expression of proto-*myc* may be sufficient to cause Burkitt's lymphoma is also challenged by the observations that proto-*myc* transcription either reaches cell cycle-dependent peak levels in certain cell lines [43, 93] or maintains constitutively high levels in embryo cells similar to those in tumor cells [F. Cuzin (Nice), M. Bywater (Uppsala), and A. Braithwaite (Canberra), personal communications].

The possibility that mutations of proto-*myc* may correlate with Burkitt's lymphoma has also been investigated. In some Burkitt's cell lines mutations have been observed in translocated, but unrearranged, proto-*myc* [93, 94] (Fig. 3). Initially it was proposed that these mutations may activate proto-*myc* by altering the gene product [94], but in at least one Burkitt's lymphoma line the coding sequence corresponding to proto-*myc* exons 2 and 3 was identical to that of the normal gene [82] (Fig. 3). Recently it has been proposed that mutations in the first noncoding exon may activate the gene [92, 95]. However, there is no functional evidence for this view and an activating mutation that is characteristic of Burkitt's lymphomas has not been identified. It is also an open question at this time whether the first human proto-*myc* exon is indeed noncoding [82] or has possibly a large, open reading frame capable of encoding a major protein [25, 95a]. A sequence comparison between translocated proto-*myc* of a mouse plasmacytoma with the germline proto-*myc* found the two genes to be identical except for one nucleotide difference in the first exon. It was concluded that proto-*myc* mutations are not required for oncogenesis [96].

Therefore, no translocation, rearrangement, elevated expression, or characteristic mutation of proto-*myc* is common to all Burkitt's lymphomas investigated. This casts doubt on the concept that any of the known proto-*myc* alterations are a sufficient cause (or even necessary) for Burkitt's lymphoma.

The question of whether proto-*myc* has transforming function has been tested directly using the 3T3 cell transformation assay with DNA from chicken or human B-cell lymphomas. However, no *myc*-related DNA was detected even though its presumed functional equivalent, the *Δgag-myc* gene of MC29, is capable of transforming 3T3 cells [97, 98] and other rodent cell lines [99]. Instead, another DNA sequence, termed *Blym*, was identified by the assay [67, 100]. Based on these results, the role of proto-*myc* in lymphomas has been interpreted in terms of a two-gene hypothesis. It has been suggested that activated proto-*myc* is necessary but not sufficient to cause the lymphoma [68, 70]. It is postulated to have a transient early function that generates a lymphoma maintenance gene, *Blym*. This gene appears to be the DNA that transforms 3T3 cells and is thought to maintain the B-cell tumor. There is no proof for this postulated role of proto-*myc* as a lymphoma initiation gene, because the 3T3 cell-transformation assay does not measure proto-*myc* initiation function, and because there is no evidence that the two genes jointly (or alone) transform B cells. Furthermore, the hypothesis does not address the question why proto-*myc* should have any transforming function at all, if it is not like MC29. (MC29 does not require a second gene to transform a susceptible cell.) It is also not known whether *Blym* is altered in primary Burkitt's lymphomas, since all of the transfection experiments were done with DNA from cell lines.

It is conceivable that chromosome translocation involving the proto-*myc* chromosome 8 may be a specific but not a necessary consequence, rather than the cause of the lymphoma [101]. Human B-cell lymphomas with translocations that do not involve chromosome 8 have indeed been described [102, 103]. In the case of clonal myeloid leukemias with consistent translocations, like the Philadelphia chromosome, it has been convincingly argued that translocation is preceded by clonal proliferation of certain stem cells with the same isoenzyme markers as leukemic cells but without chromosomal or clinical abnormalities [104].

Perhaps primary Burkitt's lymphomas should be analysed now and more emphasis should be given to the question of whether proto-*myc* alteration contributes to Burkitt's lymphoma, rather than to speculation about possible mechanisms.

II. Proto-*ras* Mutations, the Cause of Human and Rodent Carcinomas?

Use of the 3T3 cell assay to measure transforming function of DNA from a human bladder carcinoma cell line has identified DNA homologous to the *ras* gene of Harvey sarcoma virus [66, 105] (Fig. 4). Based on the viral model, the proto-Ha-*ras* gene is thought to be a potential cancer gene because it encodes a 21-kilodalton protein, p21, which is colinear with an *onc* gene product p21 of Ha-MuSV [106] (Fig. 4). The proto-Ha-*ras* gene from the bladder carcinoma cell line differs from normal proto-Ha-*ras* in a point mutation which alters the 12th p21 codon in exon 1 from normal *gly* to *val* [66, 107]. This mutation does not cause overproduction of the *ras* gene product (p21) in the 3T3 cell line [66] and does not change known biochemical properties of p21 [108]. The single-base change is thought to activate the gene to a functional equivalent of Ha-MuSV and to be the cause of the carcinoma because it is the apparent cause for 3T3 cell-transforming function [66, 109]. However, this mutation has not been found in over 60 primary human carcinomas, including 10 bladder, 9 colon, and 10 lung carcinomas [110], in 8 other lung carcinomas [111], and in 14 additional bladder and 9 kidney carcinomas (R. Muschel and G. Khoury, personal communication). Further, the mutated human proto-Ha-*ras*, which transforms 3T3 cells, does not transform primary rat embryo cells [54, 69] and, more significantly, does not transform human embryo cell [112]. Transformation of primary cells would be expected from a gene that causes tumors in animals. Thus the mutated proto-*ras* gene does not correspond to the viral model which transforms primary mouse, rat [113,

Fig. 4. Comparison of the genetic structures and p21 gene products of the human proto-Ha-*ras* gene [106, 107] and the 5.5-kb RNA genome of Harvey sarcorma virus (Ha-MuSV) [132]. Ha-MuSV is a genetic hybrid of the rat proto-*ras* gene, a 30S defective retrovirus RNA from rat cells and of Moloney leukemia virus [107, 135]

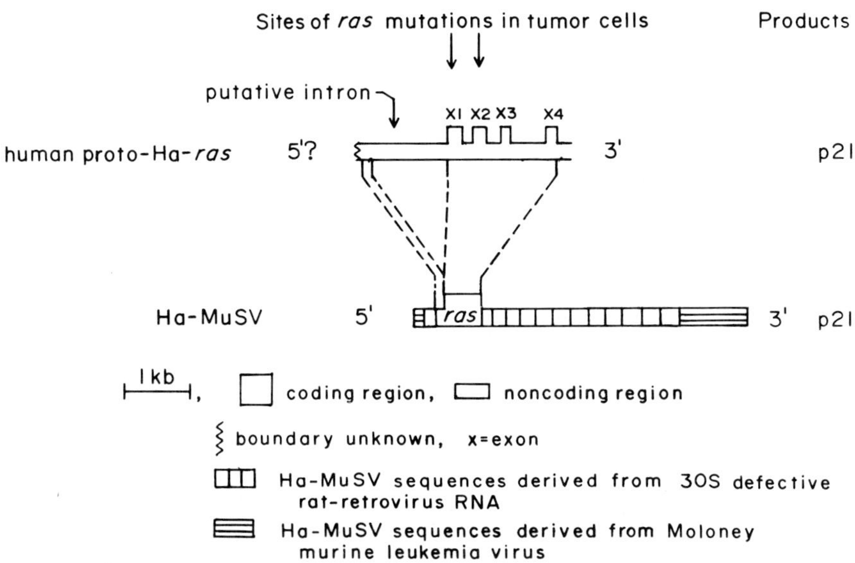

114], and human cells [115–119]. In addition, the *val* in the 12th codon of 3T3 cell transforming proto-*ras* is different for the *arg* of the viral counterpart [107].

Other mutations have since been found to confer 3T3 cell-transforming function to proto-Ha-*ras* DNA. Porto-Ha-*ras* with a mutation in codon 61 was isolated from a human tumor cell line [120]. 3T3 cell-transforming proto-Ha-*ras* DNAs were also isolated from 2 out of 23 primary urinary tract tumors analyzed. One of these contained a mutation in codon 61; the other was not identified [121]. The mutations were not found in the normal tissue of the respective patients. Nevertheless, this does not prove that 3T3 cell-transforming function of proto-*ras* was necessary for tumor formation since each was associated with only 1 out of 23 histologically indistinguishable tumors.

A 3T3 cell-transforming mouse proto-Ha-*ras* DNA was also found in some (not all) chemically induced benign papillomas and malignant carcinomas of mice [122]. Since only a small (5%–7%) portion of the benign tumors progressed to carcinomas, it would appear that 3T3 cell-transforming proto-*ras* was not sufficient to cause the carcinomas, and since not all carcinomas contained the mutation, it would appear that it was not necessary either. A high proportion, i.e., 14 out of 17 methylnitrosourea-induced mammary carcinomas of rats, were found to contain 3T3 cell-transforming proto-Ha-*ras* DNA (M. Barbacid, personal communication). This suggests that the mutation is not necessary for the tumor, although it may be important for tumor progression. The original study reported nine out of nine positives [123]. Moreover, the hormone dependence and high tissue specificity of the carcinogen in this study suggest that other genes must be involved, because mutated proto-*ras* has been found in association with other tumors and transforms 3T3 cells without hormones. It is plausible that other genes, which may be involved in tumorigenesis but which do not register in the 3T3 assay, were also altered by the carcinogen.

In an effort to explain why mutated proto-Ha-*ras* transforms preneoplastic 3T3 cells, but not rat or human embryo cells, it has recently been proposed that mutated proto-Ha-*ras* is only one of at least two activated genes that are necessary to induce cancer [54, 55, 69]. This two-gene hypothesis has been tested by transfecting primary rat cells with a mixture of the mutated human proto-Ha-*ras* and either MC29 provirus or activated proto-*myc* from mouse plasmacytoma [54], or the EIA gene of adenovirus [69] as helper genes. None of these genes were able to transform rat embryo cells by themselves, but some cells were transformed by the artificial mixed doubles. The study that used the adenovirus virus helper gene showed that proto-*ras* expression varied from high to normal levels in transformed cells and that normal proto-*ras* was inactive in the assay [69]. The study that used *myc*-related helper genes did not show that the transformants contained and expressed the added DNAs. It also did not test whether unaltered forms of proto-*myc* or proto-*ras* were sufficient for a mixture of these genes to register in this assay. This appears to be a particularly relevant question since a proto-*myc* clone from a mouse plasmacytoma with an SV40 enhancer at its 3′ end but without its natural promoter [71] was reported to be active [54] although such a construction is not expected to activate proto-*myc*.

The *myc*-related genes were proposed to convert rat embryo cells to cells that are capable of dividing indefinitely, like 3T3 cells, a function termed immortalization [54, 55]. The supposed immortalization function of MC29 or of activated proto-*myc* was not demonstrated independently. The proposal did not explain why an immortalization gene was necessary. Obviously immortalization is necessary to maintain cells in culture. However, immortalization is not necessary for focus formation and probably not for tumor formation since embryo cells are capable of sufficient rounds of mitoses (up to 50) in cell culture and in the animal [124]. In the avian system, MC29 transforms primary cells and causes tumors in chicken independently without the benefit of secondary oncogenes, and most MC29 tumor cells are not immortal if tested in cell culture. The failure of maintaining cells from many human tumors in cell culture, under conditions where cells from similar tumors survive, also suggests that immortality may not be an essential criterion of a tumor cell [125, 125 a]. There is also no precedent for a function of proto-*ras* in a multistep transformation mechanism, because the transforming genes of Harvey of Kirsten sarcoma viruses transform rat and mouse embryo cells [113, 114] or human embryo cells [115–119] with single-hit kinetics and without helper genes. Moreover, there is no precedent for the artifical mixtures of the two activated proto-*onc* genes in any natural tumors.

Other 3T3 cell-transforming proto-*ras* genes, namely proto-Ki-*ras*, which is more closely related to the *ras* gene of Kirsten sarcoma virus than to Harvey virus, and N-*ras*, which is related to both viruses, have also been found in tumors or cell lines [126]. Proto-Ki-*ras* encodes a p21 protein that is related to the p21 protein encoded by proto-Ha-*ras* [107, 126, 127]. One group has found 3T3 cell-transforming proto-Ki-*ras* DNA in three primary human tumors and five tumor cell lines out of 96 samples tested [111, 128]. The same group also found 3T3 cell-transforming proto-Ki-*ras* DNA in one out of eight lung carcinomas tested [111]. The DNA from this tumor, but not that from normal tissue of the same patient, had a mutation in the 12th codon. Obviously the low percentage of 3T3 cell-positives among these tumors raises the question of whether the mutations were necessary for tumorigenesis.

In a study of human melanomas, only one of five different metastases from the same human melanoma patient was found to contain 3T3 cell-transforming proto-Ki-*ras* DNA [129]. A 3T3 cell-transforming Ki-*ras* DNA was also detected in a metastatic variant but not in a primary methylcholanthrene-induced T-cell lymphoma of mice [130]. An example of a spontaneous proto-*ras* mutation appearing in tumor cells cultured in vitro has just been described [131]. This suggests that these proto-*ras* mutations were consequences rather than the causes of these tumors. The view that *ras* mutation is a consequence of tumorigenesis is also consistent with the results that only one *ras* allele is mutated in some primary tumors [111, 121, 127] whereas both alleles are mutated in typical tumor-cell lines [110, 111].

Since 3T3 cell-transforming or mutated proto-*ras* genes are only rarely associated with human and murine tumors and since mutated proto-Ha-*ras* does not transform human or rat embryo cells [54, 69, 112] (proto-Ki-*ras* was not tested), there is as yet no proof that mutated proto-*ras* is sufficient or even necessary for any of the above tumors.

The failure of the mutated proto-Ha- or Ki-*ras* to behave like the viral model suggests that structural differences between the cellular and viral genes are responsible (Fig. 4). The 5′ end of proto-Ha-*ras* is not as yet defined [107]. Proto-Ha-*ras* differs from the 5.5-kb RNA genome of Harvey sarcoma virus [132] in a cell-specific 1-kb DNA region 5′ of exon 1 that is preceded by a virus-related region [107] and in the sizes (1.2 and 5 kb) of the proto-*ras* transcripts compared with the genomic viral 5.5-kb mRNA [58, 133, 134]. The cell-specific proto-Ha-*ras* region is thought to be an intron but it may have another function. The base changes that confer 3T3 cell-transforming function to proto-Ha-*ras* are different from those that set apart viral *ras* genes from proto-*ras* [66, 107, 126] (Fig. 4). Proto-Ha-*ras* with 3T3 cell-transforming function further differs from the viral *ras* and from normal proto-Ha-*ras* in point mutations in exons 1 or 2 [66, 107] (Fig. 4). Moreover, only about 10% of the genomes of Harvey and Kirsten sarcoma viruses are *ras* related. Each viral RNA contains about 3 kb of genetic information, derived from a rat 30S defective retrovirus RNA [135] which may contribute to the oncogenicity of these viruses (Fig. 4). Further, it has been argued that mutated proto-*ras* is a recessive transforming gene, because both *ras* alleles are mutated in typical tumor-cell lines, although only one allele is mutated in some primary tumors [111, 127]. By contrast, the viral *onc* gene is dominant. A definitive answer to the question whether *ras* mutations are dominant or recessive 3T3 cell-transforming genes could be obtained by simultaneous transformation with mutated and normal *ras* genes. Finally, Ha- and Ki- MuSV are not obvious models for proto-*ras* genes with hypothetical carcinoma function, since these viruses cause predominantly sarcomas.

D. Conclusions

I. Does the 3T3 Assay Detect Cancer Genes?

The preponderance of 3T3 cell-transformation negatives among the above-described tumors suggests that either no genes have caused the negative tumors or that the assay failed to detect them. That only *ras*-related proto-*onc* genes have been detected in human tumors signals another limitation of the 3T3 assay. Since the proto-*ras* mutations found by the 3T3 assay do not transform primary cells, it is possible that they are not relevant for tumor formation. Available data suggest that these are coincidential or consequential rather than cancer causative mutations occurring in tumor cells, because the mutations are not consistently correlated with specific tumors and because in some cases they precede tumor formation and in other they evolve during tumor progression. Despite its effectiveness to transform 3T3 cells, it would follow that mutated proto-*ras* is not a dominant singular cancer gene, similar to a viral *onc* gene, and that the test is insufficient to determine whether proto-*onc* genes cause tumors in animals. The efficiency of the assay to identify cancer genes unrelated to proto-*onc* genes [4] remains to be determined.

II. Are Altered Proto-*onc* Genes Sufficient Causes of Cancer?

Clearly, proto-*onc* genes are sometimes mutationally or transcriptionally altered in tumor cells. However, no altered proto-*onc* gene has been found that looks like a viral *onc* gene. More importantly, no altered proto-*onc* gene from tumors investigated functions like a viral *onc* gene. Altered proto-*myc* has no transforming function in known assay systems, and altered proto-*ras* transform 3T3 cells but does not transform rodent or human embryo cells. Thus, altered proto-*onc* genes are structurally and functionally different from viral *onc* genes. Moreover, alterd proto-*onc* genes are not consistently associated with specific tumors. Since there is no functional evidence that altered proto-*onc* genes transform embryo cells or cause tumors and no consistent correlation between altered proto-*onc* genes and a specific tumor, the one-gene hypothesis (that altered proto-*onc* genes are sufficient to cause tumors) is without support. As yet, viral *onc* genes are the only "activated" proto-*onc* genes that are sufficient to cause tumors.

III. Are Altered Proto-*onc* Genes Necessary to Cause Cancer?

The observations that altered proto-*onc* genes do not behave like viral *onc* genes and that in some tumors multiple proto-*onc* genes are altered [73] have been interpreted in terms of a multigene hypothesis. Altered proto-*myc* has been proposed to cooperate with the *Blym* gene to cause chicken and human B-cell lymphoma [68]. Altered proto-*ras* has been proposed to cause carcinomas with other genes, and reported to cooperate in an artificial system with altered proto-*myc* to transform rat embryo cells in culture [54, 55]. However, there are several reservations about a role of altered proto-*myc* or proto-*ras* in multigene carcinogenesis: (a) There is no functional evidence that a combination of altered *myc* and *Blym* from lymphomas or that altered *ras,* together with another gene from carcinomas, transforms appropriate normal test cells. An artificial combination of altered *ras* in combination with an *myc*-related or an adenovirus gene was reported to transform primary rat cells. However, it was not reported whether both genes are present and functional in all transformants, and there is no evidence that these artificial *ras*-helper genes are models for the hypothetical helper genes in tumors with altered *ras.* (b) The observations that proto-*myc* alterations are not consistently associated with B-cell lymphomas and that proto-*ras* mutations are only rarely associated with specific carcinomas argue that at least one of two hypothetically synergistic cancer genes is not necessary for these tumors. As yet, no multigene complements that include one or two proto-*onc* genes have been shown to be consistently associated with specific tumors. (c) The proposals that altered proto-*onc* genes play role in a multigene carcinogenesis are a significant departure from the original view that they were equivalents of viral *onc* genes. The proposals speculate that altered proto-*onc* genes are necessary but not sufficient for tumor formation and behave like functional subsets of viral *onc* genes. They do not address the question why these genes are assumed to have unique oncogenic functions that are different from those of the viral models. The ad hoc assumption is without precedent since it is not known whether viral *onc* genes can be dissociated into complementary or helper-gene-dependent genetic subsets. Since there is no functional proof for multiple, synergistic transforming genes and no consistent correlation between at least one altered proto-*onc* gene and a specific tumor, the view that proto-*onc* genes are necessary for multigene carcinogenesis is still unproven.

IV. Prospects

It may be argued that the proto-*onc* gene alterations that are associated with some cancers play a nonspecific but causative role in carcinogenesis that could be substituted for by another gene. To support this view, it would be necessary to know which other genes could substitute for the role that altered proto-*onc* genes are thought to play in the origin of cancer. Further, one would have to know whether proto-*onc* gene alterations are more typical of cancer cells than alterations of other genes and which other genes characteristically undergo alterations in tumor cells. It is likely that unknown events, additional to the known alterations of resident proto-*onc* genes, are required for the development of cancer [5, 136].

The fact that proto-*onc* genes share common domains with viral *onc* genes remains a persuasive argument that proto-*onc* genes may, under certain conditions, be changed into cancer genes. The evidence that most normal proto-*onc* genes are expressed in normal cells suggests that cell- specific domains of proto-*onc* genes may suppress potential oncogenic function. Thus, mutation or removal of suppressors could activate a proto-*onc* gene, as has been predicted for Burkitt's lymphoma. Clearly, the identification of such suppressors would depend on a complete genetic definition of proto-*onc* genes. To date, we do not know both termini of any proto- *onc* gene (except for human proto-*myc* [79], which is not a protoype of a know oncogenic virus). In addition, virus-specific *onc* gene elements may also be essential to activate a proto-*onc* gene. In this case, a retrovirus without an *onc* gene (chronic leukemia virus) could activate a proto-*onc* gene by a single illegitimate recombination which would form a hybrid *onc* gene. Such an event would be more probable than the generation of a retrovirus with an *onc* gene, for which at least two illegitimate recombinations are necessary.

DNA technology has made it possible to convert nontransforming DNA from viral or cellular sources to DNA species that transform cell lines or embryo cells. Examples are the proto-*mos* and proto-*ras* retroviral LTR recombinants that transform 3T3 cells [49, 50]; the proto-*ras*, *myc*, and adenovirus DNA combinations that transform rat embryo cells [51, 66]; or an LTR-mutant proto-*ras*-SV40 construction that transforms rat embryo cells [137]. Another example is a synthetic gene that consists of a mouse proto-*myc* gene in which all or part of the first exon is replaced by the LTR of mouse mammary tumor virus. Upon introduction into the germ line, this gene was expressed in 11 transgenic mice. Only two of these developed mammary tumors after two pregnancies, and not in all mammary glands. It was suggested that the gene may be necessary but not sufficient for the development of these tumors [138]. Both the level of expression and the integrity of proto-*onc* genes were altered in these constructions, since only subsets of proto-*onc* genes were included. In order to assess the relevance of such iatrogenic transformations to cancer, it would be helpful to determine whether the number of DNA species that can be converted to transforming variants is large or small, and it would be necessary to determine whether any such DNAs ever occur in natural tumors. The most important challenge now is to develop functional assays for cellular cancer genes.

Acknowledgements. I specifically thank my colleagues M. Botchan, G. S. Martin, H. Rubin, M. Carey, W. Phares, S. Pfaff, and C. Romerdahl for encouragement and many critical comments and L. Brownstein for typing numerous drafts of this manuscript. The work from my laboratory is supported by NIH grant CA 11426 from the National Cancer Institute and by grant CTR 1547 from The Council for Tobacco Research – USA, Inc.

References

1. Rous P (1967) The callenge to man of the neoplastic cell. Science 157:25
1a. Berenblum I (1981) Sequential aspects of chemical carcinogenesis: skin. In: Becker F (ed) Cancer, vol 1. Plenum, New York
2. Knudson AG (1981) Genetic influences in human tumors. In: Becker F (ed) Cancer, vol 1. Plenum New York
3. Foulds L (1969) Neoplastic development, vols 1 and 2. Academic, New York
4. Cooper GM (1982) Cellular transforming genes. Science 218:801
5. Duesberg PH (1983) Retroviral transforming genes in normal cells? Nature 304:219
6. Heldin C-H, Westermark B (1984) Growth factors: mechanism of action and relation to oncogenes. Cell 37:9
7. Peterson TA, Yochem J, Byers B, Nunn MF, Duesberg PH, Doolittle RF, Reed SI (1984) A relationship between the yeast cell cycle genes *CDC4* and *CDC36* and the *ets* sequence of oncogenic virus E26. Nature 309:556
8. Martin GS (1970) Rous sarcoma virus: a function required for the maintenance of the transformed state. Nature 221:1021
9. Shih TY, Weeks MO, Young MA, Scolnick EM (1979) p21 of Kirsten murine sarcoma virus is thermolabile in a viral mutant temperature sensitive for the maintenance of transformation. J Virol 31:546
10. Pawson A, Guyden J, Kung T-H, Radke K, Gilmore T, Martin GS (1980) A strain of Fujinami sarcoma virus which is temperature-sensitive in protein phosphorylation and cellular transformation. Cell 22:767
11. Lee W-H, Bister K, Moscovici C, Duesberg PH (1981) Temperature-sensitive mutants of Fujinami sarcoma virus: tumorigenicity and reversible phosphorylation of the transforming p140 protein. J Virol 38:1064
12. Palmieri S, Beug H, Graf T (1982) Isolation and characterization of four new temperature-sensitive mutants of avian erythroblastosis virus (AEV). Virology 123:296
13. Duesberg PH, Vogt PK (1970) Differences between the ribonucleic acids of transforming and nontransforming avian tumor viruses, Proc Natl Acad Sci USA 67:1673
14. Martin GS, Duesberg PH (1972) The *a*-subunit in the RNA of transforming avian tumor viruses: I. Occurrence in different virus strains. II. Spontaneous loss resulting in nontransforming variants. Virology 47:494
15. Wei C-M, Lowy DR, Scolnick EM (1980) Mapping of transforming region of the Harvey murine sarcoma virus genome by using insertion-deletion mutants constructed in vitro. Proc Natl Acad Sci USA 77:4674
16. Goff SP, Baltimore D (1982) The cellular oncogene of the Abelson murine leukemia virus genome. In: Klein G (ed) Advances in viral oncology, vol 1. Raven, New York
17. Srinivasan A, Dunn CY, Yuasa Y, Devare SG, Reddy EP, Aaronson SA (1982) Abelson murine leukemia virus: structural requirements for transforming gene function. Proc Natl Acad Sci USA 79:5508
18. Evans LH, Duesberg PH (1982) Isolation of a transformation-defective deletion mutant of Moloney murine sarcoma virus. J Virol 41:735
19. Duesberg PH, Phares W, Lee WH (1983) The low tumorigenic potential of PRCII, among viruses of the Fujinami sarcoma virus subgroup, corresponds to an internal *fps* deletion of the transforming gene. Virology 131:144
20. Duesberg PH (1980) Transforming genes of retroviruses. Cold Spring Harbor Symp Quant Biol 44:13
21. Mellon P, Pawson A, Bister K, Martin GS, Duesberg PH (1978) Specific RNA sequences and gene products of MC29 avian acute leukemia virus. Proc Natl Acad Sci USA 75:5874
22. Robins T, Bister K, Garon C, Papas T, Duesberg PH (1982) Structural relationship between a normal chicken DNA locus and the transforming gene of the avian acute leukemia virus MC29. J Virol 41:635
23. Duesberg PH, Bister K, Vogt PK (1977) The RNA of avian acute leukemia virus MC29. Proc Natl Acad Sci USA 74:4320
24. Bister K, Duesberg PH (1982) Genetic structure and transforming genes of avian retroviruses. In: Klein G (ed) Advances in viral oncology, vol 1. Raven, New York
25. Papas TS, Kan NK, Watson DK, Flordellis CS, Psallidopoulos MC, Lautenberger J, Samuel KP, Duesberg PH (1984) *myc*-Related genes in viruses and cells. In: Vande Woude GF, Levine AJ, Topp WC, Watson JD (eds) Cancer cells 2/oncogenes and viral genes. Cold Spring Harbor Laboratory, Cold Spring Harbor

26. Watson DK, Reddy EP, Duesberg PH, Papas TS (1983) Nucleotide sequence analysis of the chicken c-*myc* gene reveals homologous and unique coding regions by comparison with the transforming gene of avian myelocytomatosis virus MC29, *Δgag-myc*. Proc Natl Acad Sci USA 80:2146
27. Shih C-K, Linial M, Goodenow MM, Hayward WS (1984) Nucleotide sequence 5′ of the chicken c-*myc* coding region: localization of a noncoding exon that is absent from *myc* transcripts in most avian leukosis virus-induced lymphomas. Proc Natl Acad Sci USA 81:4697
28. Kan NC, Flordellis CS, Mark GE, Duesberg PH, Papas TS (1984) Nucleotide sequence of avian carcinoma virus MH2: two potential *onc* genes, one related to avian virus MC29, the other to murine sarcoma virus 3611. Proc Natl Acad Sci USA 81:3000
29. Kan NC, Flordellis CS, Mark GE, Duesberg PH, Papas TS (1984) A common *onc* gene sequence transduced by avian carcinoma virus MH2 and by murine sarcoma virus 3611. Science 223:813
30. Schwartz DE, Tizard R, Gilberg W (1983) Nucleotide sequence of Rous sarcoma virus. Cell 32:853
31. Pachl C, Biegalke B, Linial M (1983) RNA and protein encoded by MH2 virus: evidence for subgenomic expression of v-*myc*. J Virol 45:133
32. Hann SR, Abrams HD, Rohrschneider LR, Eisenman RN (1983) Proteins encoded by v-*myc* and c-*myc* oncogenes: identification and localization in acute leukemia virus transformants and bursal lymphoma cell lines. Cell 34:781
33. Alitalo K, Ramsay G, Bishop JM, Pfeiffer SO, Colby WW, Levinson AD (1983) Identification of nuclear proteins encoded by viral and cellular *myc* oncogenes. Nature 306:274
34. Chiswell DJ, Ramsey G, Hayman MJ (1981) Two virus-specific RNA species are present in cells transformed by defective leukemia virus OK10. J Virol 40:301
35. Levy LS, Gardner MB, Casey JW (1984) Isolation of a feline leukaemia provirus containing the oncogene *myc* from a feline lymphosarcoma. Nature 308:853
36. Seeburg PH, Lee W-H, Nunn MF, Duesberg PH (1984) The 5′ ends of the transforming gene of Fujinami sarcoma virus and of the cellular proto-*fps* gene are not colinear. Virology 133:460
37. Lee W-H, Phares W, Duesberg PH (1983) Structural relationship between chicken DNA locus, proto-*fps*, and the transforming gene of Fujinami sarcoma virus (*Δgag-fps*). Virology 129:79
38. Rushlow KE, Lautenberger JA, Papas TS, Baluda MA, Perbal B, Chirikjian JG, Reddy EP (1982) Nucleotide sequence of the transforming gene of avian myeloblastosis virus. Science 216:1421
39. Klempnauer K-H, Gonda TS, Bishop JM (1982) Nucleotide sequence of the retroviral leukemia gene v-*myb* and its progenitor c-*myb:* the architecture of a transduced oncogene. Cell 31:453
40. Nunn MF, Seeburg PH, Moscovici C, Duesberg PH (1983) Tripartite structure of the avian erythroblastosis virus E26 transforming gene. Nature 306:391
41. Nunn M, Weiher H, Bullock P, Duesberg PH (1984) Avian erythroblastosis virus E26: nucleotide sequence of the tripartite *onc* gene and of the LTR, and analysis of the cellular prototype of the viral *ets* sequence. Virology 139, 330:339
42. Takeya T, Hanafusa H (1983) Structure and sequence of the cellular gene homologous to the *src* gene of RSV and the mechanism of the generation of the viral transforming gene. Cell 32:881
43. Campisi J, Gray HE, Bardee AB, Dean M, Sonenshein GE (1984) Cell-cycle control of c-*myc* but not c-*ras* expression is lost following chemical transformation. Cell 36:241
44. Takeya T, Hanafusa H (1982) DNA sequence of the viral and cellular *src* gene of chickens. II. Comparison of the *src* genes of two strains of avian sarcoma virus and of the cellular homolog. J Virol 44:12
45. Parker RC, Varmus HE, Bishop JM (1984) Expression of v-*src* and chicken c-*src* in rat cells demonstrates qualitative differences between $pp60^{v\text{-}src}$ and $pp60^{c\text{-}src}$. Cell 37:131
46. Parsons JT, Bryant D, Wilkerson V, Gilmartin G, Parsons SJ (1984) Site-directed mutagenesis of Rous sarcoma virus $pp60^{src}$: identification of functional domains required for transformation, In: Vande Woude GF, Levine AJ, Topp WC, Watson JD (eds) Cancer cells 2/oncogenes and viral genes. Cold Spring Harbor Laboratory, Cold Spring Harbor
47. Shalloway D, Coussens PM, Yaciuk P (1984) *c-src* and *src* homolog overexpression in mouse cells. In: Vande Woude GF, Levine AJ, Topp WC, Watson JD (eds) Cancer cells 2/oncogenes and viral genes. Cold Spring Harbor Laboratory, Cold Spring Harbor
48. Miller AD, Curran T, Verma IM (1984) c-*fos* Protein can induce cellular transfor-

mation: a novel mechanism of activation of a cellular oncogene. Cell 36:51
49. Sodroski JG, Goh WC, Haseltine WA (1984) Transforming potential of a human protooncogene (c-*fps/fes*) locus. Proc Natl Acad Sci USA 81:3039
50. Iba H, Takeya T, Cross FR, Hanafusa T, Hanafusa H (1984) Rous sarcoma virus variants that carry the cellular *src* gene instead of the viral *src* gene cannot transform chicken embryo fibroblasts. Proc Natl Acad Sci USA 81:4424
51. Wilhelmsen KC, Tarpley WG, Temin HM (1984) Identification of some of the parameters governing transformation by oncogenes in retroviruses. In: Vande Woude GF, Levine AJ, Topp WC, Watson JD (eds) Cancer cells 2/oncogenes and viral genes. Cold Spring Harbor Laboratory, Cold Spring Harbor
52. Blair DG, Oskarsson M, Wood TG, McClements WC, Fischinger PJ, Vande Woude GF (1981) Activation of the transforming potential of a normal cell sequence: a molecular model for oncogenesis. Science 212:941
53. Chang EH, Furth ME, Scolnick EM, Lowy DR (1982) Tumorigenic transformation of mammalian cells induced by a normal human gene homologous to the oncogene of Harvey murine sarcoma virus. Nature 297:479
54. Land H, Parada LF, Weinberg RA (1983) Tumorigenic conversion of primary embryo fibroblasts requires at least two cooperating oncogenes. Nature 304:596
55. Land H, Parada LF, Weinberg RA (1983) Cellular oncogenes and multistep carcinogenesis. Science 222:771
56. Gross L (1970) Oncogenic viruses. Pergamon, New York
57. Tooze J (ed) (1973) The molecular biology of tumour viruses. Cold Spring Harbor Laboratory, Cold Spring Harbor
58. Weiss RA, Teich NM, Varmus H, Coffin JM (eds) (1982) Molecular biology of tumor viruses: RNA tumor viruses. Cold Spring Harbor Laboratory, Cold Spring Harbor
59. Huebner RJ, Todaro GJ (1969) Oncogenes of RNA tumor viruses as determinants of cancer. Proc Natl Acad Sci USA 64:1087
60. Bishop JM, Courtneidge SA, Levinson AD, Oppermann H, Quintrell N, Sheiness DK, Weiss SR, Varmus HE (1980) Origin and function of avian retrovirus transforming genes. Cold Spring Harbor Symp Quant Biol 44:919
61. Bishop JM (1981) Enemies within: the genesis of retrovirus oncogenes. Cell 23:5
62. Wang L-H, Snyder P, Hanafusa T, Moscovici C, Hanafusa H (1980) Comparative analysis of cellular and viral sequences related to sarcomagenic cell transformation. Cold Spring Harbor Symp Quant Biol 44:766
63. Karess RE, Hayward WS, Hanafusa H (1980) Transforming proteins encoded by the cellular information of recovered avian sarcoma viruses. Cold Spring Harbor Symp Quant Biol 44:765
64. Hayward WS, Neel BG, Astrin SM (1981) Activation of a cellular *onc* gene by promoter insertion in ALV-induced lymphoid leukosis. Nature 290:475
65. Klein G (1981) The role of gene dosage and genetic transposition in carcinogenesis. Nature 294:313
66. Tabin CJ, Bradley SM, Bargmann CI, Weinberg RA, Papageorge AG, Scolnick EM, Dhar R, Lowy DR, Chang EH (1982) Mechanism of activation of a human oncogene. Nature 300:143
67. Cooper GM, Neiman PE (1981) Two distinct candidate transforming genes of lymphoid leukosis virus-induced neoplasms. Nature 292:857
68. Diamond A, Cooper GM, Ritz J, Lane M-A (1983) Identification and molecular cloning of the human *Blym* transforming gene activated in Burkitt's lymphomas. Nature 305:112
69. Ruley HE (1983) Adenovirus early region 1A enables viral and cellular transforming genes to transform primary cells in culture. Nature 304:602
70. Leder P, Battey J, Lenoir G, Moudling C, Murphy W, Potter H, Stewart T, Taub R (1983) Translocations among antibody genes in human cancer. Science 222:765
71. Adams JM, Gerondakis S, Webb E, Carcoran LM, Cory S (1983) Cellular *myc* oncogene is altered by chromosome translocation to an immunoglobulin locus in murine plasmacytoma and is rearranged similarly in human Burkitt lymphomas. Proc Natl Acad Sci USA 80:1982
72. Klein G, Klein E (1984) Oncogene activation and tumor progression. Carcinogenesis 5:429
73. Slamon DJ, deKernion JB, Verma IM, Cline MJ (1984) Expression of cellular oncogenes in human malignancies. Science 224:256
74. Payne GS, Bishop JM, Varmus HE (1982) Multiple arrangements of viral DNA and an activated host oncogene in bursal lymphomas. Nature 295:209
75. Tsichlis PN, Strauss PG, Hu LF (1983) A common region for proviral DNA integra-

tion in MoMuLV-induced rat thymic lymphomas. Nature 302:445
76. Yoshimura FK, Levine KL (1983) AKR thymic lymphomas involving mink cell focus-inducing leukemia viruses have a common region of provirus integration. J Virol 45:576
77. Kettmann R, Deschamps J, Cleuter Y, Couez D, Burny A, Marbaix G (1982) Leukemogenesis by bovine leukemia virus: proviral DNA integration and lack of RNA expression of viral long terminal repeat and 3′ proximate cellular sequences. Proc Natl Acad Sci USA 79:2465
78. Miller JM, Miller LD, Olson C, Gillette KS (1969) Virus-like particles in phytohemagglutinin-stimulated lymphocyte cultures with reference to bovine lymphosarcoma. J Natl Cancer Inst 43:1297
79. Westaway D, Payne G, Varmus HE (1984) Proviral deletions and oncogene base-substitutions in insertionally mutagenized c-*myc* alleles may contribute to the progression of avian bursal tumors. Proc Natl Acad Sci USA 81:843
80. Klein G (1983) Specific chromosomal translocations and the genesis of B-cell-derived tumors in mice and men. Cell 32:311
81. Rowley JD (1983) Human oncogene locations and chromosome aberrations. Nature 301:290
82. Battey J, Moulding C, Taub R, Murphy W, Stewart T, Potter H, Lenoir G, Leder P (1983) The human c-*myc* oncogene: structural consequences of translocation into the IgH locus in Burkitt lymphoma. Cell 34:779
83. Gelmann E, Psallidopoulos MC, Papas TS, Dalla-Favera R (1983) Identification of reciprocal translocation sites within the c-*myc* oncogene and immunoglobulin μ locus in a Burkitt lymphoma. Nature 306:799
84. Croce CM, Thierfelder W, Erikson J, Nishikura K, Finan J, Lenoir GM, Nowell PC (1983) Transcriptional activation of an unrearranged and untranslocated c-*myc* oncogene by translocation of a $C\lambda$ locus in Burkitt lymphoma cells. Proc Natl Acad Sci USA 80:6922
85. Erikson J, Ar-Rushidi A, Drwinga HL, Nowell PC, Croce CM (1983) Transcriptional activation of the translocated c-*myc* oncogene in Burkitt lymphoma. Proc Natl Acad Sci USA 80:820
86. Hollis GF, Mitchell KF, Battey J, Potter H, Taub R, Lenoir GM, Leder P (1984) A variant translocation places the λ immunoglobulin genes 3′ to the c-*myc* oncogene in Burkitt's lymphoma. Nature 307:752
87. Davis M, Malcolm S, Rabbitts TH (1984) Chromosome translocation can occur on either side of the c-*myc* oncogene in Burkitt lymphoma cells. Nature 308:286
88. Erikson J, Nishikura K, Ar-Rushdi A, Finan J, Emanuel B, Lenoir G, Nowell PC, Croce CM (1983) Translocation of an immunoglobulin $\varkappa$ locus to a region 3′ of an unrearranged c-*myc* oncogene enhances c-*myc* transcription. Proc Natl Acad Sci USA 80:7581
89. Westin EH, Wong-Staal F, Gelmann EP, Dalla Favera R, Papas TS, Lautenberger JA, Eva A, Reddy EP, Tronick SR, Aaronson SA, Gallo RC (1982) Expression of cellular homologues of retroviral *onc* genes in human hematopoietic cells. Proc Natl Acad Sci USA 79:2490
90. Maguire RT, Robins TS, Thorgersson SS, Heilman CA (1983) Expression of cellular *myc* and *mos* genes in undifferentiated B-cell lymphomas of Burkitt and non-Burkitt types. Proc Natl Acad Sci USA 80:1947
91. Hamlyn PH, Rabbitts TH (1983) Translocation joins c-*myc* and immunoglobulin $\gamma 1$ genes in a Burkitt lymphoma revealing a third exon in the c-*myc* oncogene. Nature 304:135
92. Taub R, Moulding C, Battey J, Murphy W, Vasicek T, Lenoir GM, Leder P (1984) Activation and somatic mutation of the translocated c-*myc* gene in Burkitt lymhoma cells. Cell 36:339
93. Kelly K, Cochran BH, Stiles CD, Leder P (1983) Cell-specific regulation of the c-*myc* gene by lymphocyte mitogens and platelet derived growth factor. Cell 35:603
94. Rabbitts TH, Hamlyn PH, Baer R (1983) Altered nucleotide sequences of a translocated c-*myc* gene in Burkitt lymphoma. Nature 306:760
95. Rabbitts TH, Forster A, Hamlyn P, Baer R (1984) Effect of somatic mutation within translocated c-*myc* genes in Burkitt's lymphoma. Nature 309:593
95a. Gazin C, Dupont de Dinechin S, Hampe A, Masson J-M, Martin P, Stehelin D, Galibert F (1984) Nucleotide sequence of the human c-*myc* locus: provocative open reading frame within the first exon. EMBO, J 3:383
96. Stanton LW, Fahrlander PD, Tesser PM, Marcu KB (1984) Nucleotide sequence comparison of normal and translocated murine m-*myc* genes. Nature 310:423
97. Copeland NG, Cooper GM (1980) Transfection by DNAs of avian erythroblastosis virus and avian myelocytomatosis virus strain MC29. J Virol 33:1199

98. Lautenberger JA, Schulz RA, Garon CF, Tsichlis PH, Papas TS (1981) Molecular cloning of avian myeloblastosis virus (MC29) transforming sequences. Proc Natl Acad Sci USA 78:1518
99. Quade K (1979) Transformation of mammalian cells by avian myelocytomatosis virus and avian erythroblastosis virus. Virology 98:461
100. Goubin G, Goldman DS, Luce J, Neiman PE, Cooper GM (1983) Molecular cloning and nucleotide sequence of a transforming gene detected by transfection of chicken B-cell lymphoma DNA. Nature 302:114
101. Rubin H (1984) Chromosome aberrations and oncogenes: cause or consequence in cancer. Nature 309:518
102. Erikson J, Finan J, Tsujimoto Y, Nowell PC, Croce C (1984) The chromosome 14 breakpoint in neoplastic B cells with the t (11; 14) translocation involves the immunoglobulin heavy chain locus. Proc Natl Acad Sci USA 81:4144
103. Yunis JJ, Oken MD, Kaplan ME, Ensurd KM, Howe RR, Theologides A (1982) Distinctive chromosomal abnormalities in histologic subtypes of non-Hodgkin's lymphoma. N Engl J Med 307:1231
104. Fialkow RJ, Singer JW (1984) Tracing development and cell lineages in human hemopoietic neoplasia. In: Proceedings of the Dahlem Workshop on Leukemia. Springer, Berlin Heidelberg New York Tokyo (in press)
105. Der JC, Krontiris TG, Cooper GM (1982) Transforming genes of human bladder and lung carcinoma cell lines are homologous to the *ras* genes of Harvey and Kirsten sarcoma viruses. Proc Natl Acad Sci USA 79:3637
106. Ellis RW, Lowy DR, Scolnick EM (1982) The viral and cellular p21 (*ras*) gene family. In: Klein G (ed) Advances in viral oncology, vol 1. Raven, New York
107. Capon DJ, Chen EY, Levinson AD, Seeburg PH, Goeddel DV (1983) Complete nucleotide sequences of the T24 human bladder carcinoma oncogene and its normal homologue. Nature 302:33
108. Finkel T, Channing JD, Cooper GM (1984) Activation of *ras* genes in human tumors does not affect localization, modification, or nucleotide binding properties of p21. Cell 37:151
109. Reddy EP, Reynolds RK, Santos E, Barbacid M (1982) A point mutation is responsible for the acquisition of transforming properties by the T24 human bladder carcinoma oncogene. Nature 300:149
110. Feinberg AP, Vogelstein B, Droller MJ, Baylin SB, Nelkin BD (1983) Mutation affecting the 12th amino acid of the c-Ha-*ras* oncogene product occurs infrequently in human cancer. Science 220:1175
111. Santos E, Martin-Zanca D, Reddy EP, Pierotti MA, Della Porta G, Barbacid M (1984) Malignant activation of a K-*ras* oncogene in lung carcinoma but not in normal tissue of the same patient. Science 223:661
112. Sager R, Tanaka K, Lau CC, Ebina Y, Anisowicz A (1983) Resistance of human cells to tumorigenesis induced by cloned transforming genes. Proc Natl Acad Sci USA 80:7601
113. Harvey JJ, East J (1971) The murine sarcoma virus (MSV). Int Rev Exp Pathol 10:265
114. Levy JA (1973) Demonstration of differences in murine sarcoma virus foci formed in mouse and rat cells under a soft agar overlay. J Natl Cancer Inst 46:1001
115. Aaronson SA, Todaro GI (1970) Transformation and virus growth by murine sarcoma virus in human cells. Nature 225:458
116. Aaronson SA, Weaver CA (1971) Characterization of murine sarcoma virus (Kirsten) transformation of mouse and human cells. J Gen Virol 13:245
117. Klement V, Friedman M, McAllister R, Nelson-Rees W, Huebner RJ (1971) Differences in susceptibility of human cells to mouse sarcoma virus. J Natl Cancer Inst 47:65
118. Pfeffer LM, Kopeolvich L (1977) Differential genetic susceptibility of cultured human skin fibroblasts to transformation by Kirsten murine sarcoma virus. Cell 10:313
119. Levy JA (1975) Host range of murine xenotropic virus: replication in avian cells. Nature 253:140
120. Yuasa Y, Srivastava SK, Dunn CY, Rhim JS, Reddy EP, Aaronson SA (1983) Acquisition of transforming properties by alternative point mutations within c-*bas*/*has* human proto-oncogene. Nature 303:775
121. Fujita J, Yoshida O, Yuasa Y, Rhim JS, Hatanaka M, Aaronson SA (1984) Ha-*ras* oncogenes are activated by somatic alterations in human urinary tract tumors. Nature 309:464
122. Balmain A, Ramsden M, Bowden GT, Smith J (1984) Activation of the mouse cellular Harvey-*ras* gene in chemically induced benign skin papillomas. Nature 307:658
123. Sukumar S, Notario V, Martin-Zanca D, Barbacid M (1983) Induction of mammary

carcinomas in rats by nitroso-methylurea involves malignant activation of H-*ras*-l locus by single point mutations. Nature 306:658
124. Holliday R (1983) Cancer and cell senescence. Nature 306:742
125. Fogh J (ed) (1975) Human tumor cells in vitro. Plenum, New York
125a. Salmon SE (1980) Cloning of human tumor stem cells. Alan R Liss, NY
126. Wigler M, Fasano O, Taparowsky E, Powers S, Kataoka T, Brinbaum D, Shimizu KF, Goldfarb M (1984) Structure and activation of ras genes. In: Vande Woude GF, Levine AJ, Topp WC, Watson JD (eds) Cancer cells 2/oncogenes and viral genes. Cold Spring Harbor Laboratory, Cold Spring Harbor
127. Capon DJ, Seeburg PH, McGrath JP, Hayflick JS, Edman U, Levinson AD, Goeddel DV (1983) Activation of Ki-*ras* 2 gene in human colon and lung carcinomas by two different point mutations. Nature 304:507
128. Pulciani S, Santos E, Lauver AV, Long LK, Aaronson SA, Barbacid M (1982) Oncogenes in solid human tumors. Nature 300:539
129. Albino AP, Le Strange R, Oliff AI, Furth ME, Old LJ (1984) Transforming *ras* genes from human melanoma: a manifestation of tumor heterogeneity? Nature 308:69
130. Vousden KM, Marshall CJ (1984) Three different activated *ras* genes in mouse tumours; evidence for oncogene activation during progression of a mouse lymphoma. EMBO J 3:913
131. Tainsky MA, Cooper CS, Giovanella BC, Vande Woude GF (1984) An activated ras^{N} gene: detected in late but not early passage human Pa1 teratocarcinoma cells. Science 225:643
132. Maisel J, Klement V, Lai MMC, Ostertag W, Duesberg PH (1973) Ribonucleic acid components of murine sarcoma and leukemia viruses. Proc Natl Acad Sci USA 70:3536
133. Ellis RW, Defeo D, Furth ME, Scolnick EM (1982) Mouse cells contain two distinct *ras* gene mRNA species that can be translated into a p21 *onc* protein. Mol Cell Biol 2:1339
134. Parada LF, Tabin C, Shih C, Weinberg RA (1982) Human EJ bladder carcinoma oncogene is homologue of Harvey sarcoma *ras* gene. Nature 297:474
135. Scolnick EM, Vass WC, Howk, Duesberg PH (1979) Defective retrovirus-like 30S RNA species of rat and mouse cells are infectious if packaged by Type C helper virus. J Virol 9:964
136. Temin HM (1983) We still don't understand cancer. Nature 302:656
137. Spandidos DA, Wilkie NM (1984) Malignant transformation of early passage rodent cells by a single mutated human oncogene. Nature 310:469
138. Stewart TA, Pattengale PK, Leder P (1984) Spontaneous mammary adenocarcinoma in transgenic mice that carry and express MTV/*myc* fusion genes. Cell 38:627–637
139. Bizub D, Katz RA, Skalka AM (1984) Nucleotide sequence of noncoding regions in Rous-associated Virus-2: comparisons delineate conserved regions important in republication and oncogenesis. J Virol 49:557–565

New Strategies in Leukemia Diagnostic and Therapy

Haematology and Blood Transfusion Vol. 29
Modern Trends in Human Leukemia VI
Edited by Neth, Gallo, Greaves, Janka

Allogeneic Marrow Transplantation from HLA-Identical Siblings in the Acute Leukemias: Baltimore Experience

G. W. Santos[1]

A. Introduction

Allogeneic bone marrow transplantation in the treatment of acute leukemia has shown remarkable therapeutic progress in recent years. Long-term remissions and possible cure rates of 50% or higher have been obtained by a number of centers in acute nonlymphocytic leukemia (ANL), particularily when patients were transplanted in their first remission [1–9]. Most reported series of allogeneic marrow transplantation in acute lymphocytic leukemia (ALL) performed in the second remission have shown long-term disease-free survival of 20%–30%. Data for patients in their third and subsequent remissions are less good [10–14]. The recent report from the Memorial Sloan Kettering group [15] and the Baltimore group [16] has shown a therapeutic improvement over the previously reported series of ALL transplanted in their second remission. In the present communication, we wish to update our results of allogeneic marrow transplantation in patients with ANL and ALL who received marrow grafts from genotypically HLA-identical siblings.

B. Material and Methods

I. Informed Consent

All protocols were reviewed and approved by The Johns Hopkins University Institutional Review Board.

1 Johns Hopkins Oncology Center, 600 North Wolfe Street, Baltimore, MD 21205, USA

II. Patient Selection

To be eligible for these studies, patients had to have a diagnosis of ANL or ALL confirmed by examination of a marrow aspirate. In addition, for ANL, they had to have a negative history for central nervous system leukemia and, for both ANL and ALL, a spinal fluid free of leukemic cells on cytocentrifuge examination at admission. All data were analyzed as of 15 April 1984.

A total of 27 patients with ANL were transplanted in their first remission and 28 patients in their subsequent remissions and early relapse; 18 patients with ALL were transplanted to the second remission and 16 in their third remission. The characteristics of each patient group are noted in Table 1.

III. Marrow Grafts

Marrow aspiration was performed under general anesthesia. The technical aspects of

Table 1. Characteristics of patients with ANL and ALL

Diagnosis	Remission	Number	Median age (range) (years)
ANL	1st	27	24 (9–41)
ANL	2nd, 3rd, and early relapse	28	25 (5–39)
ALL	2nd	18	13 (3–31)
ALL	3rd	16	12 (6–22)

the marrow collection and administration were as described previously [17].

IV. Preparation for Engraftment

Patients with ANL were prepared with oral busulfan (BU) given in divided doses over a 4-day period for a total dose of 16 mg/kg. This was followed by cyclophosphamide (CY) given intravenously (i.v.) at a dose of 50 mg/kg for four consecutive daily doses. Patients with ALL were prepared with CY given i.v. at a dose of 50 mg/kg for four consecutive daily doses followed by low dose rate total body irradiation (TBI) of 300 rad/day for four consecutive daily doses (lungs shielded for the third dose). All patients received one intrathecal injection of methotrexate (10 mg/m^2, but not more than a total of 12 mg) before cytoreductive therapy.

V. Treatment After Marrow Grafting

Patients were given CY or cyclosporine prophylactically to prevent graft-versus-host disease. Prophylaxis for central nervous system leukemia was given 50–80 days after marrow transplantation as five intrathecal doses of methotrexate (10 mg/m^2) over 10–14 days.

C. Results

Analysis by Kaplan-Meier plots for patients with ANL revealed an actuarial 3-year disease-free survival and median duration of living survivors (range) for patients transplanted in the first remission of 44% and 33.4 months (2.4–61.3 months) respectively. Similar analysis of patients transplanted in second and subsequent remission and early relapse revealed an actuarial 3-year disease-free survival of 43%. The median survival for the survivors was 15.7 months with a range of 4.9–46.5 months. The 3-year probability of disease-free survival (for both groups of ANL patients combined) for those aged 20 years or younger and older patients was 61% and 35%, respectively. There was only one leukemic relapse in this entire series. This occurred 1 year after transplantation in a 36-year-old male transplanted in his third remission. Of 18 patients with ALL transplanted in their second remission, 9 survive in continuous remission from 1.2 to 49 months (median 19.2 months). The probability of a 2-year disease-free survival is 48%. There have been no relapses in this group. Of 16 patients (6 in continuous remission) with ALL transplanted in their third remission, 8 survive for 2.3–46.8 months (median 22.3 months) with a projected 2-year survival of 46%. Six relapses were seen. The projected 2-year probability of remission was 44%. The causes of deaths in both the ANL and ALL series of patients were similar. Some 80% of the deaths were related to graft-versus-host disease and viral infections.

D. Discussion

Our initial series of patients transplanted for ANL following preparative treatment with BU and CY have been previously reported [8]. The present extension of that study with additional time and more patient entry continues to show promise. In particular, the very uncommon relapses (1 of 55 patients) suggests that this regimen may well have a more profound antileukemic effect than other reported treatments. Other possible practical or future advantages for this preparative treatment have been noted previously.

The studies in ALL are not quite so advanced, but already it appears that the transplantation of patients with ALL following the CY–TBI protocol outlined here results in a therapeutic response better than most reported series and at the moment is at least similar to the Memorial–Sloan Kettering experience using hyperfractionated TBI followed by CY [15]. Because of the high relapse rate of ALL patients in the third remission, we are currently preparing patients for transplantation with BU and CY as outlined for ANL.

Graft-versus-host disease and viral infections continue to be a major cause of death. A number of laboratories in transplant centers are intensively investigating approaches to the prevention and treatment of these complications. Some of these studies already show considerable promise. It is reasonable to assume therefore, that within the next few years disease-free survivals following allogeneic marrow transplantation may increase by 20%–30%.

Acknowledgements. This work was supported by PHS Grants CA-15396 and CAO-6973 awarded by The National Cancer Institute, DHHS.

References

1. Thomas ED, Buckner CD, Clift RA et al. (1979) Marrow transplantation for acute nonlymphoblastic leukemia in first remission. N Engl J Med 301:597–599
2. Forman SJ, Spruce WE, Farbstein MJ et al. (1983) Bone marrow ablation followed by allogeneic marrow grafting during first complete remission of acute nonlymphocytic leukemia. Blood 61:439–442
3. Powles RL, Morgenstern G, Clink HM et al. (1980) The place of bone-marrow transplantation in acute myelogenous leukaemia. Lancet 1:1047–1050
4. Kersey JH, Ramsey NKC, Kim T et al. (1982) Allogeneic bone-marrow transplantation in acute non-lymphocytic leukemia: A pilot study. Blood 60:400–403
5. Zwaan FE, Hermans J, for the E.B.M.T. Leukaemia Working Party (1982) Bone-marrow transplantation for leukaemia. European results in 264 cases. Exp Hematol 10 (suppl 10):64–69
6. Mannon P, Vernant JP, Roden M et al. (1980) Marrow transplantation for acute nonlymphoblastic leukemia in first remission. Blut 41:220–225
7. Gale RP, Kay HEM, Rimm AA et al. (1982) Bone-marrow transplantation for acute leukaemia in first remission. Lancet 2:1006–1009
8. Santos GW, Tutschka PJ, Brookmeyer R et al. (1983) Marrow transplantation for acute non-lymphocytic leukemia following treatment with busulfan and cyclophosphamide. N Engl J Med 309:1347–1353
9. Dinsmore R, Kirkpatrick D, Flumenberg N, Gulati S, Kapoor N, Brochstein J, Shank B, Reid A, Groshen S, O'Reilly R (1984) Allogeneic bone-marrow transplantation for patients with acute non-lymphocytic leukemia. Blood 63:649–656
10. Thomas ED, Sanders JE, Flournoy N et al. (1979) Marrow transplantation for patients with acute lymphoblastic leukemia in remission. Blood 54:468–476
11. Johnson FL, Thomas ED, Clark BS, Chard RL, Hartmann JR, Storb R (1981) A comparison of marrow transplantation to chemotherapy for children with acute lymphoblastic leukemia in second or subsequent remission. N Engl J Med 305:846–851
12. Scott EP, Forman SJ, Spruce WE et al. (1983) Bone-marrow ablation followed by allogeneic bone-marrow transplantation for patients with high-risk acute lymphoblastic leukemia during complete remission. Transplant Proc 15:1395–1396
13. Kendra JR, Joshi R, Desai M et al. (1983) Bone-marrow transplantation for acute lymphoblastic leukemia with matched allogeneic donors. Exp Hematol 11 (suppl 13):9 (abstract)
14. Woods WG, Nesbitt NE, Ramsey NKC et al. (1983) Intensive therapy followed by bone-marrow transplantation for patients with acute lymphocytic leukemia in second or subsequent remission: Determination of prognostic factors (A report from the University of Minnesota Bone Marrow Transplantation Team). Blood 61:1182–1189
15. Dinsmore R, Kirkpatrick D, Flomenberg N et al. (1983) Allogeneic bone-marrow transplantation for patients with acute lymphoblastic leukemia. Blood 62:381–388
16. Santos GW (1983) Allogeneic and syngeneic marrow transplantation for acute lymphocytic leukemia (ALL) in remission. Blood 62:229
17. Thomas E, Storb R (1970) Technique for human marrow grafting. Blood 36:507–515

Haematology and Blood Transfusion Vol. 29
Modern Trends in Human Leukemia VI
Edited by Neth, Gallo, Greaves, Janka

Monoclonal Antibodies and Immunotoxins in Bone Marrow Transplantation: Purging Marrow of ALL or GVHD Cells with Preservation of Stem Cells *

J. H. Kersey, D. Vallera, N. Ramsay, A. Filipovich, R. Youle, D. Neville, R. Stong and T. LeBien

A. Introduction

Bone marrow transplantation is now in frequent use for the treatment of a number of hematologic diseases, including severe immune deficiencies, aplastic anemias, and acute and chronic leukemias. In allogeneic transplantation, a problem remains with graft versus host disease-producing immunocompetent cells which contaminate the marrow. In autologous transplantation for treatment of the leukemias, residual leukemic cells may result in the return of unwanted cells to the recipient. Thus, an objective for both autologous and allogeneic marrow transplantation has become the removal of these unwanted cells prior to infusion into the recipient.

In our institutions, the approach to the problem of purging marrow of unwanted leukemic or GVHD-producing cells has been the development of monoclonal antibodies that bind to surfaces of leukemic or GVHD-producing cells. Such monoclonal antibodies have several advantages over alternative means of purging marrow. First, an advantage over pharmacologic means is that the antibodies are highly specific for molecular determinants that are characteristic of particular cells. Second, these monoclonal antibodies have the advantage over previously produced heteroantisera in that large quantities of highly specific antibody may be produced in a very standardized manner.

The current approach taken by ourselves and others is to utilize antibodies which are well characterized with respect to binding of unwanted cells, but do not bind to stem cells. Highly specific reagents can be used in this way to treat marrow in vitro without the need to administer potentially toxic substances to patients in vivo. An additional reason for the in vitro use of such reagents is to avoid the uncertain and often toxic effects of agents administered in vivo. With the use of antibodies in vitro, an adequate killing mechanism must be provided. In vivo killing mechanisms, such as through complement activation, are not sufficiently dependable to be reliable, as we observed in our earlier studies of marrow purging [1]. Thus, our recent studies have focused on in vitro killing. We have used antibody plus rabbit serum as a complement source [2], or alternatively, antibody conjugated to the potent toxin, ricin, derived from the castor bean [3]. These antibody–ricin conjugates which represent a new class of pharmacologic reagents have been developed at the National Institute of Mental Health [4, 5]. We have found both complement and ricin-mediated killing to be effective in vitro [2, 3] and studies are currently underway comparing the two forms of cell killing. Antibody–ricin immunotoxin conjugates have an advantage over antibody alone in that they can be produced in standardized form without reliance on the complex complement cascade. Not all antibodies produce effective ricin conjugates, however, in that high affinity antibodies are generally required for efficient specific killing [6].

---

* University of Minnesota Hospitals and Clinics, 420 Delaware Street S.E., Minneapolis, Minnesota 55455, USA

Table 1. Monoclonal antibodies and immunotoxins for marrow transplantation; purging bone marrow of ALL or GVHD-producing cells

Antibody	References	Cluster designation	Structure detected	Used with rabbit complement	Used as ricin conjugate	Autologous: removal of leukemic cells	Allogeneic: removal of mature t lymphoid cells
BA-1	[19]	CD 24	gp 45/55[a]	Yes	No	80% of B lineage	No
BA-2	[20]	CD 9	p24	Yes	No	70% of B lineage	No
BA-3	[21]	CD 10	gp100(CALLA)	Yes	No	70% of B lineage	No
TA-1	[12, 13]	–	gp170/95	No	Yes	95% of T lineage	Yes
UCHT1	[14]	CD 3	P19/29	No	Yes	25% of T lineage	Yes
T101	[15]	CD 5	p65	No	Yes	95% of T lineage	Yes

[a] S. J. Pirruccello and T. W. LeBien, 1985. J. Immunol., in press

B. T Lineage Antibodies for Removal of GVHD-Producing T Lymphocytes from Allogeneic Marrow or Leukemic T Lymphocytes from Autologous Marrow

A major use for monoclonal antibodies is to purge marrow of GVHD-producing T lymphocytes. A great deal of evidence has accumulated to indicate the T lymphocyte-depleted marrow can result in effective engraftment without GVHD, despite transplantation across major transplantation barriers in the rodent [7, 8]. In our studies, marrow has been effectively depleted of T lymphocytes in mice by antibody plus complement [8] or in more recent experiments by antibody conjugated to ricin [9]. The ricin molecule is composed of two chains, A and B. The A chain is responsible for killing via inhibition of protein synthesis at the level of the 60 *S* ribosome. Conjugates containing B chain generally kill more effectively and exhibit more efficient cell killing per occupied receptor than conjugates made with A chain alone [10]. Ricin B chain binds to branched galactosyl residues on the cell surface; conjugates containing B chain are made specific for the target cell by blocking ricin binding to non-target cells with lactose [11]. In our clinical studies, intact ricin is currently in use. Ricin used in these experiments is conjugated using a heterobifunctional cross-linker resulting in a thioether linkage [5].

We have extensively studied three anti-T lymphocyte antibodies, each of which binds to a unique determinant on T cell surfaces (Table 1). The antibody TA-1 binds to a gp170/95 kilodaltons structure as previously described [12, 13]. The antibody UCHT1 is a CD3 antibody which binds to a p19/29 kilodalton structure as previously described [14]. The third antibody, T101, is a CD5 antibody, which binds to a p65 kilodalton structure as previously described [15]. These three antibodies have been conjugated to ricin as already discussed. The antibody–ricin immunotoxin conjugates have been studied extensively relative to inhibition of T cell function in the PHA assay, the generation of cytotoxic T lymphocytes, and the inhibition of stem cell growth [3]. These studies indicate that while each of these conjugates individually are effective in cellular killing, T lymphocyte activity can be further reduced by about 1 log when the conjugates are used as an equal part mixture, designated TUT.

Based on preclinical studies suggesting the high efficiency of the TUT–ricin immunotoxin cocktail for T cell removal, we have proceeded to phase I–II clinical studies in which HLA-matched sibling donor marrow has been treated in vitro with the TUT–ricin cocktail prior to administration to sibling recipients [16]. Preliminary results indicate that marrow engraftment is extremely prompt, indicating no undue toxicity to marrow stem cells. No toxicity has been observed in the patients following administration of the immunotoxin-treated marrow [16]. To date, a total of eight patients have been followed for a sufficient period for evaluation (Filipovich et al., in preparation). Severe GVHD was observed in none of the patients and two developed steroid-responsive Grade 1–2 GVHD. Of concern was the fact that one patient, who showed prompt engraftment, subsequently had graft failure, presumably due to rejection. Based on these preliminary observations a phase III trial of TUT immunotoxin-treated marrow in HLA-matched combinations appears warranted.

Preclinical studies have been performed using T antibodies conjugated to ricin for autologous marrow transplantation in T cell acute leukemia. These studies indicate that the antibodies T101 and TA-1 bind to most T cell leukemias and that killing in a clonogenic assay is extremely effective, particularly with T101, where greater than 5 log of killing was observed [17]. Three patients with acute T cell leukemia have had autologous marrow treated with the T cell antibody–ricin conjugates and in each case prompt engraftment was observed (Kersey et al., in preparation). The first patient treated in this manner had skin nodules prior to intensive treatment with total body irradiation and cyclophosphamide. She subsequently relapsed in the skin, suggesting, that the relapse occurred from inadequate treatment of leukemia in vivo, rather than from inadequate removal of leukemia cells from the marrow. This case illustrates that when adequate control is obtained of leukemia in vivo, efficacy of marrow cleanup will be easier to ascertain. Phase I–II studies of T cell antibody–ricin conjugates for transplantation in T leukemia continue in our institution.

C. B Lineage-Associated Antibodies for Autologous Transplantation in ALL

The vast majority of cases of acute lymphoblastic leukemia appear to be derived from B lineage progenitor cells based on studies of immunoglobulin gene rearrangement and immunoglobulin gene expression; consistent with these observations are the data indicating that B lineage-associated antibodies bind to these leukemias [18]. Three B lineage-associated ALL antibodies have been produced and extensively studied at Minnesota. These are BA-1, BA-2, and BA-3 (Table 1). BA-1 binds to about 85% of cases of ALL, but does not bind to multipotent stem cells [19]. BA-2 is an anti-p24 antibody that binds to most B lineage ALL, but not stem cells [20]. BA-3 is an anti-gp100/CALLA antibody [21]. The three antibodies have been recently shown to be very effective as a cocktail with complement for the killing of ALL cells in a clonogenic assay [22].

Based on the preclinical studies describing the efficacy of that cocktail of BA-1, 2, 3 for removal of clonogenic cells in the presence of complement, we have begun phase I–II clinical trials in ALL. High risk patients whose leukemic cells are BA-1, 2, or 3 positive are eligible. Patients are generally those who have previously relapsed and are back in remission. Remission marrow is treated and stored while the patient recieves intensive therapy and total body irradiation and cyclophosphamide. To date, 21 patients have been treated and followed at least 2 months. Preliminary analysis indicates that patients have generally had prompt engraftment, consistent with the in vitro studies demonstrating lack of stem cell reactivity of the cocktail of BA-1, 2, 3 plus complement (Ramsay et al., 1985, Blood, in press). The only toxicity of the treatment was observed in several patients early in the study who recieved marrow that was contaminated with gram-positive organisms, presumably a consequence of marrow collection and manipulation. This is currently an ongoing study in our institution and similar to studies under way elsewhere.

D. Conclusions

Extensive preclinical studies have been performed with the use of monoclonal antibodies and antibody–ricin immunotoxin conjugates for purging marrow of unwanted cells. Purging of marrow has now been used in phase I–II clinical trials for both autologous and allogeneic marrow transplantation. The lack of in vivo toxicity of antibody or ricin and the lack of apparent stem cell toxicity is encouraging. Efficacy of marrow purging for removal of GVHD-producing cells in allogeneic transplantation or leukemic cells in autologous transplantation will be determined following additional clinical studies.

Acknowledgments. The authors thank Hybritech, Inc., San Diego, for sufficient quantities of BA-1, 2, 3, TA-1, and T101 and Peter Beverly for UCHT1 used in the studies described herein. These studies were supported in part by Hybritech, Incorporated and the following grants from the National Cancer Institute: PO1-CA-21737, RO1-CA-25097, and RO1-CA-31685. T. LeBien is a scholar of the Leukemia Society of America, A. Filipovich is a Clinical Investigator of the NIH.

References

1. Filipovich AH, Ramsay NKC, Warkentin P, McGlave PB, Goldstein G, Kersey JH (1982) Pretreatment of donor bone marrow with monoclonal antibody OKT3 for prevention of acute graft-versus-host disease in allogeneic histocompatible bone marrow transplantation. Lancet I/8284:1266–1269
2. LeBien TW, Ash RC, Zanjani ED, Kersey JH (1983) In vitro destruction of leukemic cells using a cocktail of monoclonal antibodies. In: Neth R (ed) Modern trends in human leukemia V. Springer, Berlin Heidelberg New York, pp 112–115
3. Vallera DA, Ash RC, Zanjani ED, Kersey JH, LeBien TW, Beverly PCL, Neville DM Jr, Youle RJ (1983) Anti-T-cell reagents for human bone marrow transplantation: ricin linked to three monoclonal antibodies. Science 222:512–515
4. Youle RJ, Neville DM Jr (1980) Anti-thy 1.2 monoclonal antibody linked to ricin is a potent cell-type-specific toxin. Proc Natl Acad Sci USA 77:5483–5486
5. U.S. Patent No 4,539, 457, Anti-thy 1.2 monoclonal antibody–ricin hybrid utilized as a tumor suppressant. Neville DM Jr, Youle RJ
   U.S. Patent No 4,440,747, Monoclonal antibody–ricin as a treatment of animal graft versus host disease. Neville DM Jr, Youle RJ
6. Neville DM Jr, Youle RJ (1982) Monoclonal antibody–ricin or ricin A chain hybrids: kinetic analysis of cell killing for tumor therapy. Immunol Rev 62:135
7. Rodt HV, Thierfelder S, Eulitz M (1972) Suppression of acute secondary disease by heterologous anti-brain serum. Blut 25:385 –389
8. Vallera DA, Soderling CCB, Carlson GJ, Kersey JH (1981) Bone marrow transplantation across major histocompatibility barriers in mice: the effect of elimination of T cells from donor grafts by treatment with monoclonal thy 1.2 plus complement or antibody alone. Transplantation 31:218–222
9. Vallera DA, Youle RJ, Neville DM Jr, Kersey JH (1982) Bone marrow transplantation across major histocompatibility barriers V. Protection of mice from lethal GVHD by pretreatment of donor cells with monoclonal anti-thy 1.2 coupled to the toxin lectin ricin. J Exp Med 155:949–954
10. Youle RJ, Neville DM Jr (1979) Receptor-mediated transport of the hybrid protein ricin-diphtheria toxin fragment A with subsequent ADP-ribosylation of intracellular elongation factor II. J Biol Chem 24:11089
11. Youle RJ, Murray JJ, Neville DM Jr (1979) Ricin linked to monophosphopentamannose bind to fibroblasts lysozomes hydrolase receptors resulting in a cell-type specific toxin. Proc Natl Acad Sci USA 76:5559
12. LeBien TW, Kersey JH (1980) A monoclonal antibody (TA-1) reactive with human T lymphocytes and monocytes. J Immunol 125: 2208–2214
13. LeBien TW, Bradley JG, Koller B (1983) Preliminary structural characterization of the leukocyte cell surface molecule recognized by monoclonal antibody TA-1. J Immunol 130:1833–1836
14. Beverley PCL, Callard RE (1981) Distinctive functional characteristics of human T lymphocytes defined by E rosetting or a monoclonal anti-T cell antibody. Eur J Immunol 11:329
15. Royston I, Majda A, Baird SM, Meserve BL, Griffiths JC (1979) Monoclonal antibody specific for human T lymphocyte-identification of normal and malignant T-cells. Blood 54:1069
16. Filipovich AH, Vallera DA, Youle RJ, Quinones RA, Neville DM Jr, Kersey JH (1984) Ex vivo treatment of donor bone marrow with anti-T-cell immunotoxins for the prevention of graft versus host disease. Lancet 1:469–471
17. Stong RC, Youle RJ, Vallera DA (1984) Elimination of clonogenic T-leukemic cells from human bone marrow using anti-M_r 65 000 protein immunotoxins. Cancer Res 4: 3000 –3006
18. Korsmeyer SJ, Arnold A, Bakhshi A, Ravetch JV, Siebenlist U, Hieter PA, Sharrow SO, LeBien TW, Kersey JH, Poplack DG, Leder P, Waldmann TA (1983) Immunoglobulin gene rearrangement and cell surface antigen expression in acute lympho-

cytic leukemias of T cell and B cell precursor origins. J Clin Invest 71:301–313
19. Abramson CS, Kersey JH, LeBien TW (1981) A monoclonal antibody (BA-1) reactive with cells of human B lymphocyte lineage. J Immunol 126:83–88
20. Kersey JH, LeBien TW, Abramson CS, Newman R, Sutherland R, Greaves M (1981) p24: a human leukemia-associated and lymphohemopoietic progenitor cell surface structure identified with monoclonal antibody. J Exp Med 153:726–731
21. LeBien TW, Boue DR, Bradley JG, Kersey JH (1982) Antibody affinity may influence antigenic modulation of the common acute lymphoblastic antigen in vitro. J Immunol 129:2287–2292
22. LeBien TW, Stepan DE, Bartholomew RM, Stong RC, Anderson JM (1985) Utilization of a colony assay to assess the variables influencing elimination of leukemic cells from human bone marrow with monoclonal antibodies and complement. Blood (in press)

Haematology and Blood Transfusion Vol. 29
Modern Trends in Human Leukemia VI
Edited by Neth, Gallo, Greaves, Janka

Bone Marrow Transplantation for Acute Leukemia *

K. G. Blume, S. J. Forman, R. A. Krance, M. Henke, D. O. Findley, and L. R. Hill

Between May 1976 and December 1983, 200 patients underwent bone marrow transplantation (BMT) for hematologic malignancies at our center; 164 had acute leukemia. After administration of high dose radiochemotherapy for marrow ablation and immunosuppression, these 164 patients received marrow grafts from histocompatible sibling donors. Graft-versus-host disease prophylaxis (and therapy) consisted of either methotrexate and prednisone or cyclosporin A and prednisone. All patients have been followed for a minimum of 3 months after BMT. Results are summarized in Table 1 and Fig. 1.

* City of Hope National Medical Center Duarte, California 91010, USA

A total of 92 patients had acute myeloblastic leukemia (AML); 53 of them were in first complete remission (CR), 12 were in second or third CR, and 27 were in relapse at the time of BMT. The 53 patients with AML who were in first CR had the following subtypes according to FAB criteria: M1 4 patients; M2 19 patients; M3 6 patients; M4 17 patients, M5 6 patients; M6 1 patient. Actuarial survival in continued CR without further chemotherapy for the three groups of patients is 51%, 17%, and 19%, respectively, with a follow-up ranging from 6 to 89 months (median 34, 13, and 25 months).

A total of 72 patients had acute lymphoblastic leukemia (ALL); 21 of them were in first CR, 30 were in second CR, and 21 in relapse at the time of BMT. The 21

Table 1. Allogeneic BMT for 164 patients with ANLL or ALL at the City of Hope National Medical Center since May 1976

	Remission status at BMT	1st CR	2nd and 3rd CR	Relapse
ANLL	Number of patients transplanted	53	12	27
(N=92)	Age at BMT median/range (years)	27/1–41	29/15–38	27/2–54
	Relapse after BMT (%)	7 (13)	3 (25)	9 (33)
	Time to relapse: median/range (months)	8/5–19	6/4–9	4/1–14
	Patients alive in continued CR (%)	29 (55)	2 (17)	7 (26)
	Age of survivors; median/range (years)	25/1–39	33/28–38	23/2–39
ALL	Number of patients transplanted	21	30	21
(N=72)	Age at BMT: median/range (years)	26/2–41	20/8–48	17/5–36
	Relapse after BMT (%)	1 (5)	9 (30)	9 (43)
	Time to relapse: median/range (months)	3	5/3–17	10/2–38
	Patients alive in continued CR (%)	13 (62)	14 (47)	6 (29)
	Age of survivors: median/range (years)	25/2–31	24/8–33	19/5–32

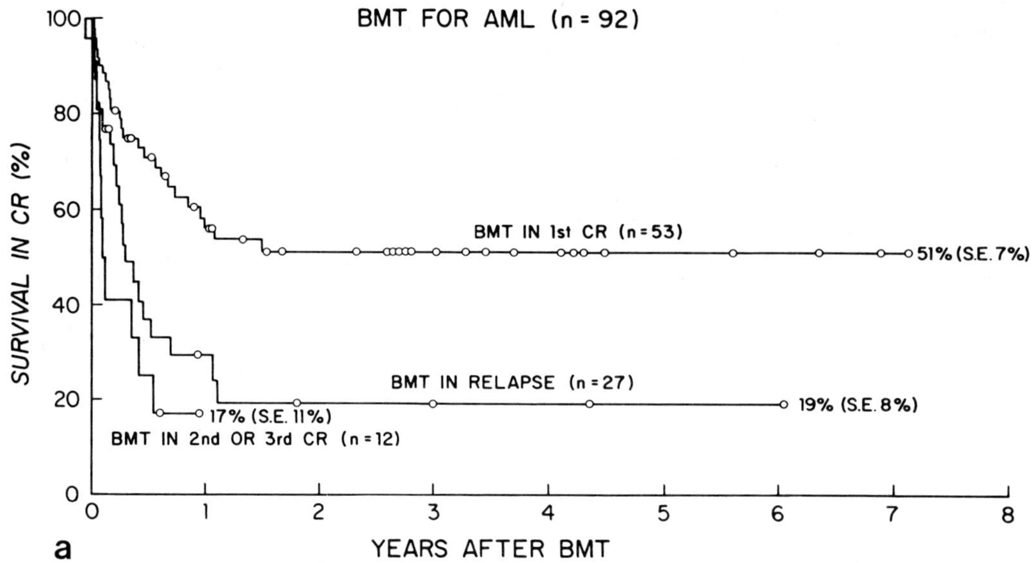

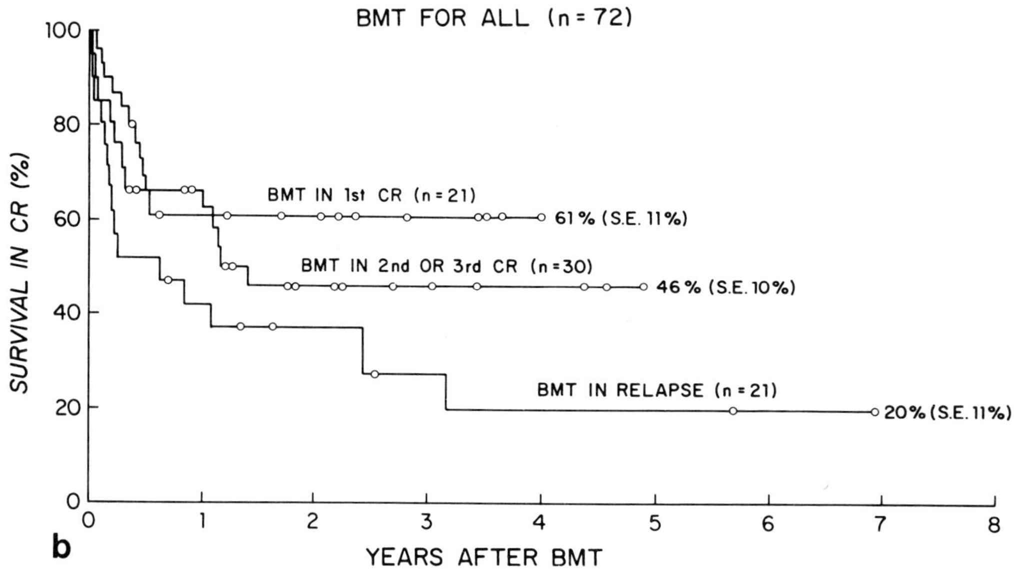

Fig. 1 a, b. Allogenic BMT for 164 patients with **a** AML and **b** ALL at the City of Hope National Medical Center. Date of analysis 9 February 1984

patients with ALL who were in first CR had the following subtypes of their disease: T cell 9 patients; CALLA-positive 5 patients; null 3 patients; not classified 4 patients. Actuarial survival in continued CR for the three groups of patients is 61%, 46%, and 20%, respectively, with a follow-up ranging from 7 to 62 months (median 30, 29, and 27 months).

Age, pre-BMT remission status, and extramedullary leukemic involvement at any time prior to BMT are the major factors which determine outcome of BMT for patients with acute leukemia [1–8].

References

1. Blume KG, Beutler E, Bross KJ, Chillar RK, Ellington OB, Fahey JL, Farbstein MJ, Forman SJ, Schmidt GM, Scott EP, Spruce WE, Turner MA, Wolf JL (1980) Bone marrow ablation and allogeneic marrow transplantation in acute leukemia. N Engl J Med 302:1041
2. Blume KG, Spruce WE, Forman SJ, Bross KJ, Beutler E, Farbstein MJ, Fahey JL, Schmidt GM, Scott EP, Wolf JL (1981) Bone marrow ablation and marrow transplantation in acute leukemia: Influence of clinical pretransplant condition. Transplant Proc 13:252
3. Woods WG, Nesbit ME, Ramsay NKC, Krivit W, Kim TH, Goldman A, McGlave PB, Kersey JH (1983) Intensive therapy followed by bone marrow transplantation for patients with acute lymphocytic leukemia in second or subsequent remission: Determination of prognostic factors (A report from the University of Minnesota Bone Marrow Transplantation Team). Blood 61:1182
4. Santos GW, Tutschka PJ, Brookmeyer R, Saral R, Beschorner WE, Bias WB, Braine HG, Burns WH, Elfenbein GJ, Kaizer H, Mellits D, Sensenbrenner LL, Stuart RK, Yeager AM (1983) Marrow transplantation for acute nonlymphocytic leukemia after treatment with busulfan and cyclophosphamide. N Engl J Med 309:1347
5. Dinsmore R, Kirkpatrick D, Flomenberg N, Gulati S, Shank B, O'Reilly RJ (1983) Allogeneic marrow transplantation for acute lymphoblastic leukemia in remission: The importance of early transplantation. Transplant Proc 15:1397
6. Thomas ED (1983) Marrow transplantation for malignant diseases. J Clin Oncol 1:517
7. Buckner CD, Clift RA (1984) Marrow transplantation for acute lymphoblastic leukemia. Semin Hematol 21:43
8. Spruce WE, Forman SJ, Krance RA, Farbstein MJ, Wolf JL, Scott EP, Nademanee AP, Fahey JL, Henke M, Blume KG (1983) Outcome of bone marrow transplantation in patients with extramedullary involvement of acute leukemia. Blut 48:75

Haematology and Blood Transfusion Vol. 29
Modern Trends in Human Leukemia VI
Edited by Neth, Gallo, Greaves, Janka

T Cell Depletion of Donor Marrow for Prevention of Acute Graft-Versus-Host Disease*

P. J. Martin, J. A. Hansen, R. Storb, and E. D. Thomas

Allogeneic bone marrow transplantation can provide curative therapy for patients with acute leukemia or aplastic anemia. However, acute graft-versus-host disease (GVHD) occurs in a high proportion of patients, even when the donor is an HLA genotypically identical sibling. Observations that GVHD can be prevented in rodent models by removing mature T cells from the donor marrow have prompted similar investigations in human bone marrow transplantation. These investigations have been facilitated recently by the availability of monoclonal antibodies that recognize surface molecules expressed by T lymphocytes and not by hematopoietic precursors. In Seattle, 20 patients 31–50 years of age with hematologic malignancies received HLA identical allogeneic bone marrow grafts depleted of T lymphocytes with the use of monoclonal antibodies and rabbit serum complement. The patients were prepared for transplantation with cyclophosphamide (60 mg/kg, two doses) and fractionated total body irradiation. Cyclosporine was administered after transplantation for prophylaxis of GVHD.

Treatment of marrow resulted in 2–3 log depletion of T cells. Engraftment of granulocytes to > $1000/mm^3$ was achieved at a median of 21 days, a time period comparable to that required for engraftment in historical controls who received unmodified marrow. Engraftment of lymphocytes, however, was delayed 3–4 days compared with historical controls. None of the patients who received T-depleted bone marrow developed grade III or IV acute GVHD and only three patients had grade II disease. These results represented a statistically significant decrease in acute GVHD compared with results in similar historical control patients who received unmodified donor marrow.

Despite the decreased incidence of GVHD, survival was not improved in our patients because of an increased incidence of graft failure which to date has been fatal in three patients. Graft failure represents a highly unusual outcome after HLA identical marrow transplantation in patients with hematologic malignancies. Also, the reduced incidence of GVHD in our study was not associated with a decrease in the mortality from CMV interstitial pneumonia. In previous studies, acute GVHD has been identified as a prognostic factor predictive of death from CMV interstitial pneumonia [1].

In the current study, five of the patients have had graft failure which was transient in one patient, but apparently irreversible in the others. It was noteworthy that all 5 patients who had difficulty with engraftment were in a group of 11 patients who were conditioned for transplantation with 12.0 Gy fractionated total body irradiation. In contrast, none of the nine patients who were conditioned with 15.75 Gy fractionated total body irradiation had difficulty with engraftment. The increased

* Fred Hutchinson Cancer Research Center, Puget Sound Blood Center, Seattle, WA 98104 and the Department of Medicine, Division of Oncology, University of Washington, Seattle, WA 98195, USA

radiation administered to these patients may have been sufficient to overcome graft resistance caused either by disparity in minor histocompatibility antigens of the donor and recipient or by allosensitization associated with previous transfusions.

Our data suggest that lymphocytes may play a role in facilitating sustained engraftment after marrow transplantation. In recipients of conventional unmodified marrow, a graft-versus-host reaction may suppress or eliminate residual host hematopoietic and lymphoid cells, thereby preventing host cell-mediated effects such as graft rejection from occurring. In favor of this hypothesis are observations by Deeg et al. that thoracic duct lymphocytes can facilitate engraftment in dogs given marrow grafts from unrelated DLA nonidentical donors [2] and that cyclosporine can abrogate the graft enhancing effects of buffy coat cells in dogs given marrow grafts from unrelated DLA nonidentical donors [3]. It remains to be determined whether changes in the pre- or posttransplant regimens can decrease the graft failure associated with T cell depletion of donor marrow. Alternatively, it may be possible to distinguish between T cells that cause GVHD and those required to facilitate sustained engraftment.

Acknowledgments. The authors thank Pauline Marsden for assistance in preparation of the manuscript. This investigation was supported by contract N00014-82-K-0660 from the Office of Naval Research, Department of Defense, and grants CA 18029, CA 30924, and CA 29548 awarded by the National Cancer Institute, Department of Health and Human Services. Dr. Thomas is the recipient of Research Career Award AI-02425 from the National Institutes of Allergy and Infectious Disease.

References

1. Neiman PE, Reeves W, Ray G et al. (1977) A prospective analysis of interstitial pneumonia and opportunistic viral infection among recipients of allogeneic bone marrow grafts. J Infect Dis 136:754
2. Deeg HJ, Storb R, Weiden PL et al. (1979) Abrogation of resistance to and enhancement of DLA-nonidentical unrelated marrow grafts in lethally irradiated dogs by thoracic duct lymphocytes. Blood 53:552
3. Deeg HJ, Storb R, Weiden PL et al. (1982) Cyclosporin A and methotrexate in canine marrow transplantation: engraftment, graft-versus-host disease, and induction of tolerance. Transplantation 34:30

Haematology and Blood Transfusion Vol. 29
Modern Trends in Human Leukemia VI
Edited by Neth, Gallo, Greaves, Janka

Long-Term Survivors of Adult Acute Nonlymphocytic Leukemia: Fact or Fiction? *

D. S. Rosenthal, S. E. Emerson, J. M. Rappeport, W. C. Moloney, and R. I. Handin

A. Introduction

From 1970 to 1982, 157 consecutive patients with de novo acute nonlymphocytic leukemia (ANLL) were treated and followed by the Hematology Unit at the Brigham and Women's Hospital, Boston, Massachusetts. It was in 1970, with the addition of cytosine arabinoside and daunorubicin, that remission induction (RI) rates significantly increased from 30% to greater than 50% [1]. During the past decade, major emphasis has been placed on an attempt to prolong disease-free survival with intensive chemotherapy programs and more recently with allogeneic and syngeneic bone marrow transplantation [2, 3]. Since 1970, we have attempted to treat our patients with more aggressive remission and maintenance consolidation (RC) programs.

B. Patients and Chemotherapy Protocols

During the 12-year period ending 1982, 157 consecutive patients were followed and treated for de novo ANLL. All patients with a previously known hematologic dis-

* Division of Hematology, Department of Medicine, Brigham and Women's Hospital and Harvard Medical School, Boston, Mass. USA

Fig. 1 A–D. Chemotherapy of adult ANLL 1970–1982. Four major programs were in effect: COD (**A**), DAC 1 (**B**), VAPA (**C**), and DAC II (**D**)

INDUCTION RI

	CYTOSAR	ANTHRACYCLINE	OTHER	
A	2 mgm/kg IV x3-6d, bolus	1 mgm/kg IV (DNR) x3-6d, bolus	Onc	→ CR → Continued Rx
B	2 mgm/kg 24 hr. continuous IV 5-7d	1 mgm/kg IV (DNR) x3d, bolus	–	→ CR → Continued Rx
C	100 mgm/M² 24 hr. continuous IV 7d	30 mgm/M² (ADR) x3d	Onc pred	→ CR → ARAC + ADR → Continued Rx
D	200 mgm/M² 24 hr. continuous IV 7d	45 mgm/M² (DNR) x3d	–	→ CR → ARAC + DNR → Continued Rx

order or who had previous chemotherapy were excluded from this study. In order to have at least a 2-year follow-up on all patients from date of RI therapy, only patients treated prior to June 1982 were analyzed. Four major protocols were in effect during this 12-year period (Table 1, Fig. 1). From 1970 to 1974 (program A), RI was the COD program, using intravenous bolus infusions of cytosar, oncovin, and daunorubicin [4]. RC utilized an ambulatory program of 5 days of cyclophosphamide, oncovin, cytosar, and prednisone (COAP) every 28 days, continuing indefinitely. Program B (DAC I), in effect from 1974 to 1977, had RI consisting of 24 h of continuous intravenous infusion of cytosar for 5–7 days with three bolus infusions of daunorubicin. The RC alternated COAP with cytosar and daunorubicin (to a maximum dose of 700 mg/m²). RI of program C (1977–1980) was similar to program B, but RC (VAPA) was an attempt to give 14 months of very intensive chemotherapy utilizing higher doses of cytosar plus non-cross-resistant agents [2]. Program D (DAC II), evaluated from 1980 to 1982, involved more intensive RI with twice the dose of continuous intravenous cytosar used in previous RI. The RC period was shortened to 8–12 months, but the drug doses remained high.

C. Results

A total of 50 patients were treated with the COD program (A); 32 patients with DAC I

Table 1. ANLL treatment protocols

Year	Program	Median age	CR/total number	(%)	Alive	CCR[c]
1970–74	A	43	31/50	(62)	0	0
1974–77	B	54	15/32	(46)	1	1
1977–80[a]	C	46	22/41	(54)	4	4
1980–82[b]	D	49	25/34	(74)	13	0
			93/157	(59)	18	15

[a] In 1977–80, 3/22 BMT in first remission 1/3 in CCR (65 + months)
[b] In 1980–82, 1/25 BMT in first remission 1/1 in CCR (30 + months)
[c] CCR continuous CR

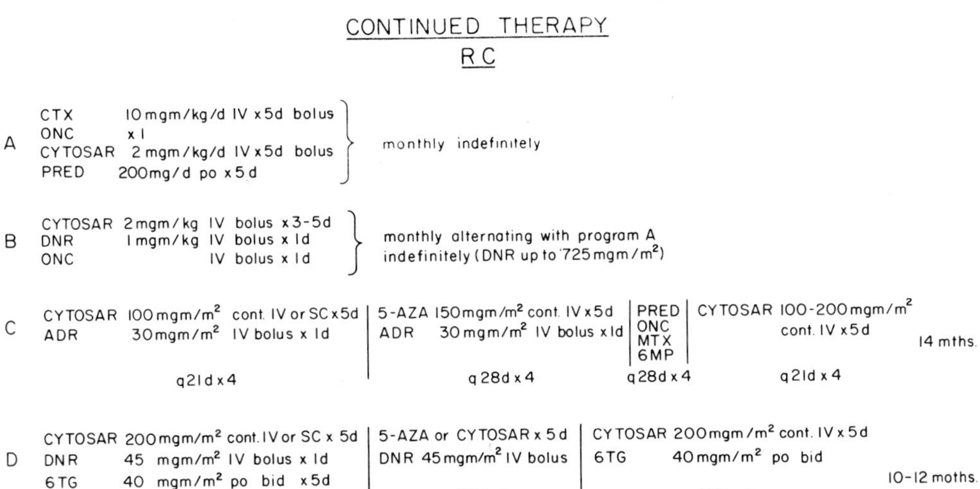

Table 2. Therapy of long-term survivors

CCR/total CR	RI	RC	CCR (months)
1/15	DAC I	2 years COAP, CAT	1 (96)
4/22	VAPA	16 months – full VAPA	2 (56, 54)
		BMT	1 (65)
		16 months – ½ dose VAPA	1 (61)
10/25	DAC II	12 months DNR, Arac-C 6-TG, 5-Aza	2 (37, 39)
		9 months DNR, Ara-C, 6-TG, 5-Aza	1 (47)
		12 months DNR, Ara-C 6-TG	4 (22, 30, 34, 34)
		8 months DNR, Ara-C, 6-TG	1 (26)
		BMT	1 (30)
		2 months DNR, Ara-C, 6-TG	1 (35)

(B); 41 patients with VAPA (age < 50 years) or with modified VAPA (age > 50 years) (C); and 34 patients with DAC II (D) (see Table 1). Of the 157 patients, 93 (59%) achieved complete remission (CR). CR rates have been 62% in program A, 46% in B, 54% in C, and 74% in D. Currently, 18 of the 93 CR patients are still alive (19%) and 15 of the 93 (16%) still in continuous complete remission. The longest survivor is 96 months and is the only survivor of program A and B. Four patients from program C are still in CR (54–65 months), one of whom received a marrow transplant (BMT) while in first remission. Ten patients are still in CR from program D, one for 22 months, six for 26–35 months, and three for 37–47 months. One of the ten patients received a BMT. Table 2 illustrates the actual therapy of the 15 long-term survivors. Although the RI programs were usually carried out per protocol, there were many CR patients who did not receive the full RC programs. In fact, two were removed from protocol for allogeneic BMT during the first 3 months after RI and four had significantly reduced length of treatment owing to toxicity.

Survival curves from programs A, B, and C demonstrated a long-term disease-free status of less than 20% (Fig. 2). Program D with the shortest follow-up demonstrates by life table analysis a disease-free survival of 38%. However, since relapses in the previous programs have occurred as late as 2–3 years after CR, the length of follow-up for program D is too short to predict an increased percentage of long-term survivors.

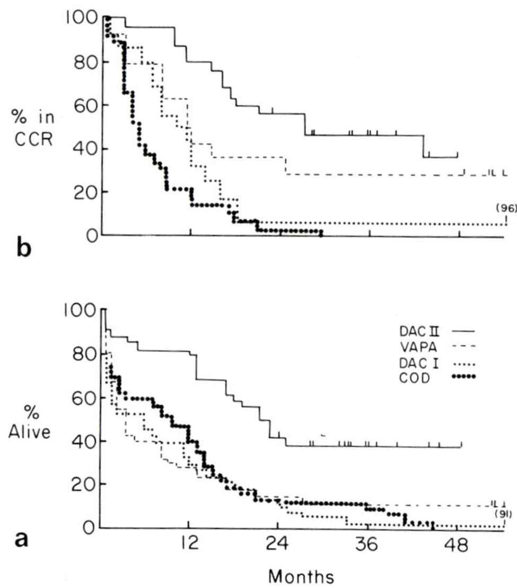

Fig. 2a, b. Actual survival curves for **a** total group and **b** disease-free survival for all complete remissions broken down according to treatment program

D. Summary and Conclusions

From 1970 to 1982, remission rates from large series of patients with a median age of approximately 50 years continue to exceed 50% and in series of younger patients may be as high as 75% [1]. These improved results have been due to the combination of cytosar and an anthracycline in RI programs. The current major question is whether or not "consolidation" therapy has improved long-term disease-free survival

[5–7]. Our current results, covering the decade 1970–1980 and using more and more intensive RC programs, do not demonstrate an increase in the percentage of long-term survivors. The results from 1980 to 1982 are encouraging, but must be tempered by the fact that late relapses of adult ANLL are becoming more frequent and 2-year follow-up is much too short an evaluation period. In addition, the prolonged survival in program D may be due to the more intensive RI program and not at all related to the RC. At the present time, our experience lends no support to the theory that more intensive RC programs meaningfully prolong long-term survival.

References

1. Gale RPL (1979) Advances in the treatment of acute myelogenous leukemia. N Engl J Med 300:1189–1199
2. Weinstein HJ, Mayer RT, Rosenthal DS, Camitta BM, Coral FS, Nathan DG, Frei E III (1980) Treatment of acute myelogenous leukemia in children and adults. N Engl J Med 303:473–478
3. Thomas ED, Buckner CD, Clift RA et al. (1979) Marrow transplantation for acute nonlymphoblastic leukemia in first remission. N Engl J Med 301:597–599
4. Rosenthal DS, Moloney WC (1972) The treatment of acute granulocytic leukemia in adults. N Engl J Med 286:1176–1178
5. Sauter C, Fopp M, Imbach P, Tschopp L, Berchtold LW, Gratwohl A, Maurice P, Von-Fliedner V, Cavalli F (1984) Acute myelogenous leukemia: Maintenance chemotherapy after early consolidation treatment does not prolong survival. Lancet 1:379–382
6. Marcus RE, Catovsky D, Goldman JM, Worsley AM, Galton DAG (1984) Maintenance and consolidation therapy in AML. Lancet 1:686–687
7. Emerson S, Rosenthal DS, Moloney WC, Handin RI (1983) Limited impact of intensive combination chemotherapy in adult acute myelogenous leukemia. Blood 62:201 a

Haematology and Blood Transfusion Vol. 29
Modern Trends in Human Leukemia VI
Edited by Neth, Gallo, Greaves, Janka

Risk Groups in a Multicenter Pilot Study for Treatment of Acute Lymphoblastic and Acute Undifferentiated Leukemia in Adults*

D. Hoelzer, E. Thiel, H. Löffler, H. Bodenstein, T. Büchner, R. Engelhardt, A. Ganser, D. Messerer, H. Rühl, and T. Zwingers

A. Introduction

The German Multicenter Trial for Adult Acute Lymphoblastic (ALL) and Acute Undifferentiated (AUL) Leukemia was undertaken to improve remission duration by using a modified form of an intensified induction regimen successful in childhood ALL (Riehm et al. 1980). The results from the pilot study, with a total of 162 patients and a median observation time of 4½ years, now allow some conclusions regarding prognostic factors which influence the achievement of complete remission or the length of remission.

B. Treatment

The concept of this therapeutic trial was to eradicate as much as possible of the initial tumor cell load by an eight-drug induction therapy and a similarly intensive early consolidation therapy after 3 months, whereas the maintenance therapy is conventional with 6-mercaptopurine and methotrexate. The 8-week induction regimen consists of two phases: In the first 4 weeks prednisone 60 mg/m² PO daily, vincristine 1.5 mg/m² IV once weekly, daunorubicin 25 mg/m² IV once weekly, and l-asparaginase 5000 units/m² IV on days 1–14; and in the second 4 weeks cyclophosphamide 650 mg/m² IV 3 doses at 2-week intervals, cytosine arabinoside 75 mg/m² IV on 4 days per week for 4 weeks, and 6-mercaptopurine 60 mg/m² PO daily for 4 weeks. CNS prophylaxis consists in methotrexate 10 mg/m² intrathecally each week and CNS irradiation with 24 Gy. A 6-week reinduction course is given after 3 months and is similar to the induction regimen, adriamycin being substituted for daunorubicin, dexamethasone for prednisone, and thioguanine for 6-mercaptopurine; L-asparaginase is omitted. Maintenance therapy with 6-mercaptopurine 60 mg/m² PO daily and methotrexate 20 mg/m² PO or IV once weekly is continued for 2 years. Further details of the therapy and of the diagnostic procedure have been described previously (Hoelzer et al. 1984).

C. Results

From October 1978 to June 1981 a total of 162 adult patients from 25 hospitals entered the study, and 126 (77.8%) achieved complete remission. At the evaluation date, 30 November 1983, the median survival time for all patients was 23.4 months and that for complete remitters was 34 months. Median remission duration was 20.5 months. The probability of being in complete remission at 4½ years is 0.397. Cell marker analysis identified c-ALL in 56.4%, null-AL (defined as being non-B-ALL, non-T-ALL, cALLA⁻) in 25.6%, T-ALL in 15.4%, B-ALL in 0%, and mixed leukemia in 2.6%. The best results were achieved in patients with T-ALL, for whom the prob-

* German Multicenter Trial for Adult ALL/AUL, FRG. Supported by the Bundesministerium für Forschung und Technologie, Contract No. 01 ZW 450

Table 1. Prognostic factors for remission duration: Pilot study

Factor		*n* (126)	MRD (months)	In continuous CR	P-value
Age	≦35 years	98	24.9	42.9%	0.0150
	>35 years	28	12.7	28.6%	
Leukocyte count	≦30 000/µl	85	28.0	44.7%	0.0314
	>30 000/µl	41	14.8	29.3%	
Time to achieve CR	Within 4 weeks	94	28.2	42.6%	0.0285
	After 4 weeks	32	11.8	31.3%	
Immunological subtype	c-ALL	32	23.4	48.8%	0.0143
	T-ALL	11	m.n.r.[a]	63.6%	
	null-AL	16	12.7	12.5%	
Low-risk group		19	m.n.r.[a]	79.0%	0.0000
High-risk group		40	11.8	20.0%	

[a] Median not reached

ability of being in continuous complete remission at 4½ years is 0.636.

D. Prognostic Factors and Risk Groups

Regarding the complete remission rate, none of the initial laboratory or clinical features, such as age, leukocyte count, hepatosplenomegaly, mediastinal tumor, CNS involvement, or other organ infiltration, had an unfavorable influence on the achievement of complete remission. The adverse effect of older age, high initial leukocyte count, and hepatosplenomegaly, which have been shown in other studies to have an unfavorable influence on the achievement of complete remission, could not be confirmed in the large number of patients in this study (Hoelzer et al. 1984).

I. Prognostic Factors

Prognostic factors for remission duration (Table 1) were time required to achieve remission, initial leukocyte count, immunological subtype, and age.

Age. The difference in remission duration for patients above and below 35 years of age was evident. In earlier studies (Hoelzer 1984) higher age was also found to exert an unfavorable influence on the survival time and remission duration. This multicenter ALL/AUL study has proved that results for older patients who did not require any essential omissions or reductions in the therapy program were similar to those for younger patients. The main problem is that for many of the older patients it is not possible to carry out the complete therapy schedule.

Leukocyte Count. In this therapy study, as in other ALL studies in adults (Schauer et al. 1983) or children, a high initial leukocyte count was found to be unfavorable for a long remission.

Immunological Subtype. The best prognosis in this study was for the subtype T-ALL, for which the median remission duration has not yet been reached. This finding is remarkable, since up to now patients with T-ALL, who frequently have a high initial leukocyte count, a mediastinal tumor, or CNS involvement, have had a poor prognosis. The worst prognosis, in keeping with findings from another study (Lister et al. 1979), was for patients with null-AL, who had a median remission duration of 13 months. Of the patients with c-ALL, 44% were disease-free at the evaluation date.

Time Required to Achieve Complete Remission. The length of treatment required to achieve complete remission had the strongest influence on remission duration. Late response to therapy probably reflects a primarily more resistant population of leukemic cells. Other adult ALL therapy studies have also shown that of a total of 70% remission patients, only 50% achieved remission within 4 weeks (Hoelzer 1984). In childhood ALL the proportion of patients who reach complete remission after prolonged treatment is very low (< 5%). For them, it is also true that late response to therapy is correlated with a very poor prognosis (Frei and Sallan 1978).

II. Definition of Risk Groups

On the basis of these factors found to have prognostic significance for remission duration in the pilot study, it was possible to define groups of patients exposed to different degrees of risk. Those defined as low-risk patients are the ones who have none of the four risk factors, in comparison to high-risk patients who have one or more of the four risk factors. At the last evaluation date of 30 November 1983, 79% of the low-risk patients were still in first remission, whereas only 20% of the high-risk patients were still free of disease.

E. Risk-Adapted Therapy Protocol

The study group has developed a new risk-adapted therapy protocol based on the results of the pilot study, which was activated on 1 July 1983. According to this, in addition to the intensive induction therapy and consolidation therapy, high-risk patients will receive further cycles of consolidation therapy with VM-26 and cytosine arabinoside, to improve results in this group. In addition, the high-risk patients are to be considered for allogeneic bone marrow transplantation in first remission if a suitable donor is available. After establishment of the method, autologous bone marrow transplantation also appears to be useful for these patients. The low-risk patients will be treated according to the present protocol with no essential changes. It is to be expected that in this group, even with chemotherapy alone, more than 50% will reach the 5-year limit without disease and might thereby be considered as cured.

References

Frei E, Sallan SE (1978) Acute lymphoblastic leukemia: treatment. Cancer 42:828–838

Hoelzer D (1984) Current status of ALL/AUL therapy in adults. In: Thiel E, Thierfelder S (eds) Leukemia. Springer, Berlin Heidelberg New York Tokyo, pp 182–203 (Recent results in cancer research, vol 93)

Hoelzer D, Thiel E, Löffler H, Bodenstein H, Plaumann L, Büchner T, Urbanitz D, Koch P, Heimpel H, Engelhardt R, Müller U, Wendt FC, Sodomann H, Rühl H, Herrmann F, Kaboth W, Dietzfelbinger H, Pralle H, Lunscken C, Hellriegel K-P, Spors S, Nowrousian RM, Fischer J, Fülle H, Mitrou PS, Pfreundschuh M, Görg C, Emmerich B, Queisser W, Meyer P, Labedzki L, Essers U, König H, Mainzer K, Herrmann R, Messerer D, Zwingers T (1984) Intensified therapy in acute lymphoblastic and acute undifferentiated leukemia in adults. Blood 64:38–46

Lister TA, Roberts MM, Brearly RL, Woodruff RK, Greaves MF (1979) Prognostic significance of cell surface phenotype in adult acute lymphoblastic leukaemia. Cancer Immunol Immunother 6:227–230

Riehm H, Gadner H, Henze G, Langermann H-J, Odenwald E (1980) The Berlin childhood acute lymphoblastic leukemia therapy study, 1970–1976. Am J Pediatr Hematol Oncol 2:299–306

Schauer P, Arlin ZA, Mertelsmann R, Cirrincione C, Friedman A, Gee TS, Dowling M, Kempin S, Straus DJ, Koziner B, McKenzie S, Thaler HT, Dufour P, Little C, Dellaquila C, Ellis S, Clarkson B (1983) Treatment of acute lymphoblastic leukemia in adults: Results of the L-10 and L-10M protocols. J Clin Oncol 1:462–470

Haematology and Blood Transfusion Vol. 29
Modern Trends in Human Leukemia VI
Edited by Neth, Gallo, Greaves, Janka

New Approaches to the Treatment of Chronic Myelogenous Leukemia *

K. B. McCredie, H. Kantarjian, M. J. Keating, J. P. Hester, and E. J. Freireich

A number of therapeutic strategies have been introduced for the management and treatment of the benign phase of CML. Eighty years ago, radiation therapy was the only available treatment and splenic irradiation was continued for a period in excess of 20 years when in 1924, Minot and colleagues published the now classic paper demonstrating that, although therapy could reduce morbidity of the disease, the median duration of survival with or without therapy was the same. Because of symptomatic relief, radiation therapy or ^{32}P were the methods of choice until the introduction of busulfan in the early 1950s. The initial study with busulfan showed median survival of 42 months and did not appear to be a significant improvement over radiation therapy, although symptomatic improvement was again seen and this is still true today. A number of other agents have been used in an attempt to delay the onset of blast crisis and prolong survival, the most commonly used being hydroxyurea, dibromomannitol, melphalan, and 6-mercaptopurine. In addition, nitrogen mustard, cyclophosphamide, and vinca alkaloids have been used in an attempt to manage the disease.

Because of the relatively prolonged nature of the disease and the ease of administering an oral single agent medication, very little progress has been made in its management. More recently, however, with the introduction of newer chemotherapeutic agents and combination chemotherapy, attempts have been made to treat the benign phase of the disease aggressively, particularly in an attempt to eradicate the Philadelphia chromosome and the abnormal neoplastic clone. Although more than 50% of patients can get a significant reduction in the number of abnormal chromosomes identified after aggressive combination chemotherapy, the majority of the patients have recurrent Philadelphia chromosome within 3–12 months from the discontinuation of this form of aggressive therapy. Preliminary reports suggest, however, that with this aggressive therapy there has been an associated prolongation of median duration of survival.

Other modalities of therapy include bone marrow transplantation: isogeneic, allogeneic and autologous. However, transplantation performed in the later stages of the disease, particularly in the blast phase, has been almost uniformly unsuccessful because of the resistant nature of the underlying disease and recurrence is almost inevitable in spite of the regimen used. Investigators are now looking at the possibility of transplantation in the benign phase of the disease and preliminary data, particularly from identical twins, is encouraging with disease-free survivors in excess of 24 months without evidence of a recurring Philadelphia-positive clone.

In addition to allogeneic transplantation, autologous transplantation in the benign phase of the disease has been attempted and although engraftment does occur, the abnormal clone is not eradicated and the

* The University of Texas System Cancer Center, M. D. Anderson Hospital and Tumor Institute, Houston, TX USA

disease makes recurrence almost inevitable. More recently, a number of institutions have adopted the approach of aggressive chemotherapy in an attempt to eradicate the Philadelphia chromosome and store the bone marrow of these patients for use in transplantation in the early phase with normal hemopoietic stem cells without the Philadelphia chromosome.

We previously demonstrated that leukocyte interferon (HuIFN-α) had a significant antiproliferative effect on in vitro colony proliferation. In addition to its antiproliferative effect, it appeared to block differentiation. In search of new modalities of treatment of chronic granulocytic leukemia, a pilot study was embarked on to investigate the potential of using HuIFN-α prepared in the State Serum Institute of the Finnish Red Cross Center, Helsinki, Finland. This material was partially purified to a specific activity of $1-3 \times 10^6$ U per milligram protein. The initial pilot study was performed on seven patients with Philadelphia-positive chronic myelogenous leukemia utilizing a schedule of 3×10^6 U/day up to a maximum 9×10^6 U/day. Following hematologic remission, the patients were maintained on doses of 3×10^6 U/day or every other day. Five of the initial patients responded to interferon, judged by a reduction in the white cell count, platelet count, normalization of serum B12 and LDH, and a reduction in the bone marrow cellularity for pretreatment values of 100% –70%, or less. ME ratios returned to normal and there was a modest reduction of 10%–35% in Philadelphia chromosome-positive cells in the bone marrow aspirate.

With these encouraging results, the phase II program was developed utilizing the same doses of HuIFN-α and a further 25 evaluable patients have been entered. A majority of these were previously untreated and the remainder had minimal treatment with a single agent. Of the 25 patients, 22 responded with normalization of the peripheral blood, and a decrease in the mean white cell count from 112 000 to 5000 µl. There was a decrease in marrow cellularity and serum B12 levels returned to normal, as did serum LDH. One patient developed blast transformation after 2 months on HuIFN-α. Of 11 patients who have been treated for months or more, 7 show a modest decline in the Philadelphia-positive cells in the bone marrow from 100% to a median of 65% (range 10–92% diploid cells). Human interferon is effective in causing a block in myeloid proliferation in the chronic phase of chronic granulocytic leukemia, with normalization of the peripheral blood and reduction in marrow cellularity and return of other parameters to normal. These changes can be maintained with reduced doses of HuIFN-α.

It is clear in this pilot study that the possibility of combining HuIFN-α with intensive chemotherapy is worthwhile, using the intensive chemotherapy to reduce the complement of Philadelphia-positive cells toward zero and maintaining this status with HuIFN-α maintenance therapy. Further activity and significantly more biologic effect may be obtainable with the more purified forms of interferon now becoming available, utilizing cell lines and recombinant techniques.

References

1. Talpaz M, McCredie KB, Mavligit GM, Gutterman JU Leukocyte interferon-induced myeloid cytoreduction in chronic myelogenous leukemia. Blood 62 (3):689–692
2. Kantarjian H, Vellekoop L, McCredie K, Hester J, Keating M, Trujillo J, Freireich E (1984) Intensive chemotherapy (ROAP 10) and splenectomy in the management of chronic myelogenous leukemia. Proc Am Soc Clin Onco 3:200

Haematology and Blood Transfusion Vol. 29
Modern Trends in Human Leukemia VI
Edited by Neth, Gallo, Greaves, Janka

The Feasibility of Opal/High Dose Ara-C Treatment of Adult Acute Lymphoblastic Leukaemia *

M. J. Barnett, A. Z. S. Rohatiner, M. A. Richards, J. H. Waxman, T. S. Ganesan, A. Miller, R. Biruls, and T. A. Lister

A. Introduction

Studies conducted at St. Bartholomew's Hospital between 1972 and 1982 into the treatment of acute lymphoblastic leukaemia (ALL) in adults showed a complete remission (CR) rate of 65% (73/112) using a combination of vincristine, prednisolone, adriamycin, and L-asparaginase, with CR frequency being highest in young patients and lowest in those with L3 morphology. The duration of remission correlated closely with blast cell count at presentation and the surface phenotype of the blast cells, being significantly longest in patients with low blast counts of common ALL antigen (CALLA) positivity. Central nervous system (CNS) relapse alone was relatively frequent in those patients in whom the cerebrospinal fluid (CSF) was positive at the first lumbar puncture (3/13) despite craniospinal or cranial irradiation and intrathecal therapy. However, by far the greatest problem was bone marrow relapse alone, or in association with relapse at other sites, e.g. CSF, testis, skin (43/53) and was not reduced by introducing escalating doses of adriamycin and cyclophosphamide into the early therapy [1].

Recent experience with the use of high dose cytosine arabinoside (Ara-C) in the treatment of both ALL in relapse and the lymphoid blast crisis of chronic myeloid leukaemia has been encouraging with a response being achieved in 9/14 patients after one cycle (Barnett MJ, unpublished observations), and supporting our initial results [2]. In addition, pharmacokinetic studies of the concentration of Ara-C in the plasma and CSF have shown that, when given intravenously in high doses, prolonged levels of the drug can be achieved in the CSF, which should be effective in the treatment of CNS leukaemia [3].

In December, 1982 an open study commenced with the intention of exploiting the systemic and CSF activity of high dose Ara-C in the initial therapy of adults with ALL at St. Bartholomew's Hospital. Preliminary results to demonstrate the feasibility of the programme are presented below.

B. Patients and Methods

A total of 13 previously untreated patients have so far been entered into the study (Table 1), using the treatment regimen shown in Fig. 1. Ara-C was infused over 3 h every 12 h at a dose of 2 g/m^2, a total of 12 doses being given over 6 days. All patients received prophylactic nonabsorbable antibiotics and prednisolone eyedrops were prescribed every 2 h for 10 days from the commencement of the Ara-C. Maintenance therapy comprises oral 6-mercaptopurine (daily), cyclophosphamide and methotrexate (weekly) for 3 years. During this time intrathecal injections of methotrexate or Ara-C are given every 2 months.

C. Results

All 13 patients received the treatment programme as planned at least to the com-

* ICRF Department of Medical Oncology, St. Bartholomew's Hospital, London. EC1A 7BE, England

pletion of the Ara-C. The Ara-C was stopped after 11 doses in one patient, and after 10 doses in two patients owing to the development of severe skin reactions in two and nystagmus in the third. There was no evidence of leukaemia in 8/13 patients prior to administration of Ara-C. Seven patients entered CR, the eighth dying of pseudomembranous colitis without peripheral blood recovery on day 19 following Ara-C administration. Five patients had residual leukaemia prior to Ara-C administration, of the three evaluable for response, two had obvious residual leukaemia following Ara-C treatment, and in the third, in whom the bone marrow was heavily infiltrated before Ara-C treatment, there was no detectable leukaemia afterwards, but persistent cyto-

Table 1. Patients ($N = 13$)

Sex	M:F	8:5
Age (years)	Range	18–55
	Mean	36
	Median	34
Blast count ($\times 10^9$/l)	Range	0–279
	Mean	34
	Median	2.1
Morphology	L1	3
	L2	10
	L3	0
Phenotype	C-ALL	2
	N-ALL	5
	T-ALL	2
	B-ALL	1
	Uncertain	2
	Untested	1
CSF	Positive	0
	Negative	12
	Untested	1

Table 2. Toxicity and myelosuppression

Ara-C Toxicity		No. of patients
Nausea and vomiting		11
Skin	Blistering reaction (palms and soles)	7
	Macular rash	4
Diarrhoea		8
Ocular discomfort		4
Neuro-logical	Tremor	2
	Nystagmus	1
	Grand mal fits (see text)	1

Duration of myelosuppression neutrophils ($\times 10^9$/l)

		0–0.1	0.1–0.5	0.5–1.0
Time (days)	Mean	12	2	2
	Range	(7–19)	(0–5)	(1–3)

NB: These data relate to 9 patients and exclude one (see text) in whom the duration of myelosuppression was

	0–0.1	0.1–0.5	0.5–1.0
Time (days)	13	22	34

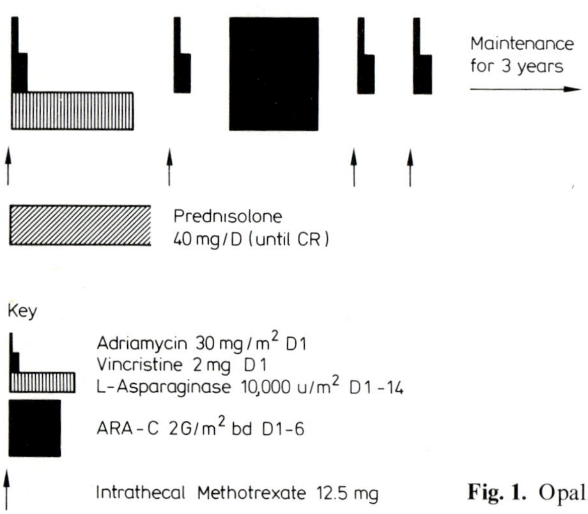

Fig. 1. Opal/high dose Ara-C regimen

penia, and recovery of the peripheral blood coincided with recurrent leukaemia. Two patients died before peripheral blood recovery, one on day 14 with *Pseudomonas* septicaemia and the other, who died on day 13, had bronchopneumonia and bone marrow infiltration at post-mortem examination. Of the seven patients entering CR, six remain in remission, one having had bone marrow relapse.

Toxicity related to the Ara-C is shown in Table 2. One patient, a 22-year-old female, developed grand mal epileptic fits on day 19 following Ara-C treatment and a CT head scan showed patchy areas of low attenuation in the occipital and parietal lobes. A repeat scan 5 weeks later was normal and she recovered completely with no sequelae.

D. Discussion

The major problem in the treatment of ALL with conventional therapy is bone marrow relapse. High dose Ara-C has been used to intensify the initial systemic therapy, as well as providing CNS prophylaxis and thus obviating the need for cranial irradiation. In the limited number of patients entered into the study so far, the CR rate was 55% (7/13) compared with 65% (73/112) in the previous study. The low CR rate is disappointing, particularly as at least three of the five patients who had leukaemia prior to the Ara-C treatment had persistent leukaemia afterwards, and none entered CR. However, the patient population in this study has a median age 8 years older than the previous one, and also an unusual membrane phenotype distribution.

Although the toxicity from high dose Ara-C was considerable, except for the high incidence of severe skin reactions which was unexpected, it was predictable from our previous experience. It is certainly feasible to administer high dose Ara-C in close proximity to the conventional combination chemotherapy. Whether or not the toxicity is acceptable will be determined by the effect of the regimen on long-term survival.

Acknowledgments. We are pleased to acknowledge the contribution of the medical and nursing staff of Dalziel and Annie Zunz Wards, St. Bartholomew's Hospital. The immunological phenotype was determined in the ICRF Membrane Immunology laboratory (Dr. M. F. Greaves). The manuscript was typed by Jane Ashby.

References

1. Lister TA, Amess JAL, Rohatiner AZS, Henry G, Greaves MF (1983) The treatment of adult acute lymphoblastic leukaemia (ALL). ASCO C-661
2. Rohatiner AZS, Slevin ML, Dhaliwal HS, Malpas JS, Lister TA (1984) High-dose cytosine arabinoside: response to therapy in acute leukaemia and non-Hodgkin's lymphoma. Cancer Chemother Pharmacol 12:90–93
3. Slevin ML, Piall EM, Aherne GW, Johnston A, Lister TA (1982) The pharmacokinetics of cytosine arabinoside in the plasma and cerebrospinal fluid during conventional and high-dose therapy. Med Pediatr Oncol 1:157–168

Haematology and Blood Transfusion Vol. 29
Modern Trends in Human Leukemia VI
Edited by Neth, Gallo, Greaves, Janka

Treatment of Leukemia with Low Dose Ara-C: A Study of 159 Cases *

S. Castaigne, H. Tilly, F. Sigaux, M. T. Daniel, and L. Degos

A. Introduction

The management of acute leukemia has been transformed by the advent of major antimitotic agents. Intensive combination drug therapy has given excellent results for many patients, but in certain cases it remains dangerous (acute leukemia in elderly patients) or ineffective (refractory anemia with excess blasts (RAEB), secondary leukemia, leukemic relapse). Allogeneic bone marrow grafts are also limited by the particular conditions required (compatibility of MHC, age).

In vitro studies by Lotem and Sachs [1] demonstrated the differentiation of leukemic cells from normal cells, raising new hopes of therapeutic possibilities. In recognition of this, clinical trials with low dose cytosine arabinoside (LD Ara-C) were undertaken. Success was obtained for one case of RAEB and two cases of acute nonlymphoblastic leukemia (ANLL) unresponsive to combination chemotherapy [2]. The first substantial series (23 patients) showed that it was possible to obtain complete remission in all categories of leukemia [3].

Several clinical trials with LD Ara-C have recently been reported, but the small number of patients in each series (less than 20) and the contradictory results render a conclusive judgement impossible. Thus, a number of questions have yet to be answered. What is the efficacy of LD Ara-C and which category of patients can benefit from it? What is the hematologic and extrahematologic tolerance to the treatment? By what mechanism does LD Ara-C produce its effects? That is why this report presents the results obtained by 12 centers in 159 cases, including some cases which have been published previously [2, 3].

B. Patients and Methods

The series was made up of 159 patients suffering from acute leukemia (AL) or myelodysplastic syndrome (MDS). A total of 12 centers took part in the study: Brest, Dijon, Hamburg, Montpellier, Nantes, Paris Beaujon, Paris Pitié-Salpétrière, Paris St. Louis, Praz Coutant, Rennes, Rouen, and Tours. Patients whose treatment commenced before June 1983 were included in the series.

The aim of the study was first of all to determine the response to the treatment (complete or partial remission, or no response) and to note the main incidents observed. Second, a more detailed questionnaire enabled us to study the results obtained for ANLL in patients over 65 years of age. All patients were treated with Ara-C as the sole agent, administered in two daily subcutaneous injections. The dose was generally 10 mg/m^2 every 12 h. The duration of treatment varied for the different groups, with a median of 19 days. The treatment was used for cases in which combination drug therapy was contraindicated for various reasons (age, failure of previous treatment, relapse, MDS). One

* Service d'Hématologie du Pr BOIRON – Hôpital St Louis Paris, France

Table 1. Results of therapy with low dose cytosine arabinoside[a]

		Number of patients			
		Total	CR	PR	Failure
ANLL	ANLL > 65 years	48	24	7	17
	ANLL < 65 years	9	1	4	4
No previous treatment	Secondary AL	14	3	4	7
ANLL					
In relapse		13	5	1	7
Unresponsive to previous treatment		15	7	3	5
ALL					
In relapse or unresponsive to previous treatment		7	2	1	4
MDS					
(RAEB, RAEB-T, post-RAEB AL)		38	9	6	23
AT of myeloproliferative disorder		8	1	0	7
Other and unknown		7	1	0	6
		159	53	26	80

[a] ANLL: acute nonlymphoblastic leukemia; ALL: acute lymphoblastic leukemia; MDS: myelodysplastic syndrome; RAEB: refractory anemia with excess blasts; RAEB-T: refractory anemia with excess blasts in transformation; AT: acute transformation; CR: complete remission; PR: partial remission

Table 2. Tolerance

	Number of patients affected (%)		Total number of patients
	+	–	
Cytopenia (platelets < 20 000 mm³ and/or PN < 500 mm³)	81 (77%)	24	105
Bone marrow aplasia determined by bone marrow aspirates	38 (48%)	40	78
Hemorrhage	65 (47%)	69	134
Infection	72 (52%)	65	137
Home care	37 (33%)	73	110

course of treatment per month was given. No response after three courses was considered as failure of the therapy.

C. Results

The results obtained for all the patients and for the subgroup of elderly AL patients are listed in Tables 1–3.

D. Discussion

Since the first report published by Baccarani and Tura [4], followed by those of Moloney and Rosenthal [5] and Housset et al. [2], LD Ara-C has been extensively used of late to treat malignant blood disorders. By grouping together 159 cases treated in France and Germany it is possible to improve our assessment of the results of LD Ara-C therapy.

1. The effectiveness of the treatment was confirmed, since a response was observed in 49% of the cases, with complete remission (CR) occurring in 33% of the cases.

2. The response varied with the type of illness treated: de novo ANLL was more responsive (response = 59%, CR = 40%) than MDS (response = 39%, CR = 23%).

Table 3. LD Ara-C therapy for elderly de novo ANLL patients with no previous treatment[a]

		Mean					
Number		Age (years)	Dose	Duration (days)	Number of courses		
48		74	10 mg/m^2 ×2/day	17	1.7		
CR	PR	Failure	Cytopenia	Aplasia	Infection	Hemorrhage	Home care
24/48	7/48	17/48	34/48	18/34	20/48	20/48	14/48

[a] Maintenance therapy: 10 mg/m^2 Ara-C twice daily for 15 days/month or 15 days/6 weeks (19 patients); mean duration of remission: 8 months; mean survival: 15 months. Correlation: +positive between CR and hypoplasia on aspirates at diagnosis; – no correlation between aplasia following treatment and CR

The good results obtained for the 48 de novo ANLL patients aged over 65 years should be emphasized. CR was achieved in half of the cases and the mean duration of the first remission was 8 months. Mean actuarial survival was 15 months. Fourteen patients were treated entirely at home, nine of whom had CR. These results are worth comparing with those obtained by combination chemotherapy. No comparable series of patients (same age group) treated by combination drug therapy has been reported. Quality of life and cost of treatment must also be taken into account in a comparison between the two types of therapy. The results obtained in secondary leukemias (7/14 responses) or during transformation of MDS (1/8 responses) need to be confirmed by trials with greater numbers of patients.

3. The optimum duration of treatment cannot be established from the data of this study. The best rate of responses was obtained in patients treated for 15–21 days, but the difference was not significant compared with patients treated for shorter (19 patients) or longer periods (48 patients). The need for maintenance therapy and the form it should take could not be determined from this series, as the vast majority of the patients received the same maintenance therapy with LD Ara-C.

4. While extrahematologic tolerance was good, cytopenia was noted in ⅔ cases. It is difficult to assess the toxicity related to the treatment and not to the illness. Nevertheless, when two groups of 52 patients were distinguished on the basis of initial platelet count (platelets < or > 50 000), cytopenia following therapy was equally common in both groups, while severe hemorrhage was more frequent in patients with less than 50 000 platelets/mm^3 before treatment. Thus, the appearance of cytopenia does indeed seem to be related to the treatment. On the other hand, the more effective the treatment, the better was the hematologic tolerance. There was a strongly significant relation between obtaining CR and the absence of hemorrhage after treatment for the 48 elderly de novo ANLL patients. Administering the entire treatment in the homes of 14 of the elderly patients shows that the therapy is well tolerated in certain cases, leading to increased patient comfort and suggesting implications for savings in health expenses.

5. The precise mechanism of action of the treatment cannot be deduced solely from the clinical data. Nevertheless, the following observations may contribute to elucidating the mode of action of LD Ara-C. Bone marrow aplasia was noted in half of the cases. However, no correlation was found between the existence of medullary aplasia and CR. This fact was also noted by another group [6]. For elderly ANLL patients, CR was obtained in 10/18 cases when aplasia was observed and in 7/16 cases when aplasia was absent. Thus, in

40% of the cases, CR was obtained without bone marrow aplasia. The therapy seems to be more effective when it is used to treat AL with hypocellular marrow. This observation is comparable to two studies reported in the literature [7, 8]. However, the cellularity of the bone marrow was judged solely from aspirates. The genuineness of this finding would need to be confirmed by the study of bone marrow biopsies. Finally, the fact that Ara-C is more effective in treating de novo AL than MDS is analogous to the results obtained with conventional combination chemotherapy.

The action of LD Ara-C is probably not based on a single mechanism of cytotoxicity bringing on severe aplasia. By its mutagenic action on oncogenes, it might restrain the proliferative capacity of blast cells and permit their maturation, but also repress the clone of leukemic cells sufficiently to liberate the development of normal clones. This phenomenon may perhaps be facilitated when the tumoral mass is small (hypocellular leukemia). The differentiation hypothesis can be viewed in two ways: either as differentiation of the malignant cell from a normal cell, or as the removal of the obstacle to the development of normal cells. No decision between the two is yet possible.

E. Conclusion

The results of the French and German study demonstrate the efficacy of LD Ara-C in the treatment of malignant blood disorders. The treatment can be ethically prescribed for elderly ANLL patients. A randomized trial is currently in progress, comparing conventional combination drug therapy with LD Ara-C. The results obtained in treating MDS and secondary leukemia require confirmation with a large number of cases. Finally, in the light of recent developments in the molecular mechanisms of oncogenesis, clinical trials using agents of differentiation merit attention.

Acknowledgments. The collaboration of D. Bordessoule (Limoges), J. Briere (Brest), P. Colombat (Tours), D. Donadio (Montpellier), S. Drony (Praz Coutant), H. Guy (Dijon), J. Harousseau (Nantes), V. Leblond (Paris Pitié-Salpétrière). P. Le Prise (Rennes), P. Solal Celigny (Paris Beaujon), and H. Weh (Hamburg) is gratefully acknowledged.

References

1. Lotem J, Sachs L (1974) Different blocks in the differentiation of myeloid leukemic cells. Proc Natl Acad Sci USA 71:3507–3511
2. Housset M, Daniel MT, Degos L (1982) Small doses of ARA-C in the treatment of acute myeloid leukaemia: differentiation of myeloid leukaemia cells? Br J Haematol 51:125–129
3. Castaigne S, Daniel MT, Tilly H, Herait P, Degos L (1983) Does treatment with ARA-C in low dosage cause differentiation of leukemic cells? Blood 62:85–86
4. Baccarani M, Tura S (1979) Differentiation of myeloid leukaemic cells: new possibilities for therapy. Br J Haematol 42:485–590
5. Moloney WC, Rosenthal DS (1981) Treatment of early acute nonlymphatic leukaemia with low dose cytosine arabinoside. In: Neth R, Gallo RC, Graf T, Mannweiler K, Winkler K (eds) Modern trends in human leukemia IV. Springer, Berlin, pp 59–62
6. Winter JN et al. (1983) Low dose ARA-C therapy in myelodysplastic syndromes and acute leukemia. Blood 62:209a (abstract)
7. Mahonoran A (1983) Low-dose cytarabine therapy in hypoplastic acute leukemia. N Engl J Med 309/26:1652 (letter)
8. Mufti GJ, Oscier DG, Mamblin TJ, Bell AJ (1983) Low doses of cytarabine in the treatment of myelodysplastic syndrome and acute leukemia. N Engl J Med 309/26:1653 (letter)

Haematology and Blood Transfusion Vol. 29
Modern Trends in Human Leukemia VI
Edited by Neth, Gallo, Greaves, Janka

Treatment of Acute Myeloid Leukemia and Myelodysplastic Syndrome by Low Dose Cytosine Arabinoside *

H. J. Weh, R. Zschaber, A. von Paleske, and D. K. Hossfeld

A. Introduction

Recent reports by Baccarani and Tura [2], Moloney and Rosenthal [9], and Housset et al. [6] prompted us to treat 12 acute myeloid leukemia (AML) and 4 myelodysplastic syndrome (MDS) patients with low dose cytosine arabinoside (Ara-C). In all patients, conventional chemotherapy was contraindicated because of previous inefficacy, advanced age, or heavy comorbidity. Ara-C was given in a dose of 10 mg/m^2 s.c. every 12 h for 14–28 days. All patients received one or two courses. If bone marrow revealed more than 5% blasts 1 week after the end of therapy, another course was started. Patients who obtained a complete or partial remission received maintenance chemotherapy with low dose Ara-C (10 mg/m^2 s.c. every 12 h) for 8 days every 3 or 4 weeks.

B. Results

Nine patients obtained a complete remission (CR), three a partial remission (PR), and four did not respond. Clinical data of the nine patients with complete remission are summarized in Table 1. The three patients who obtained a partial remission were: a 70-year-old woman in first relapse of M_1 leukemia after TAD chemotherapy; a 31-year-old woman in first relapse of M_4 leukemia after TAD chemotherapy; and a 51-year-old man with RAEB who did not respond to TAD chemotherapy. Karyotype was normal in the two women and abnormal in the man (43,X0,del 2 (p14), −8, −9, +del 12 (p11), 17p+, −20). Duration of PR in the three patients was 1 month (death from unrelated disease), 4+, and 12 months.

Four patients did not respond. The first was a 37-year-old man in first relapse of M_4 leukemia with cutaneous, renal, and myocardial leukemic involvement. Chromosome analysis revealed a near hypotetraploid pattern. The second patient was a 43-year-old woman with M_2 leukemia following RAEB resistant to TAD chemotherapy. She had a normal karyotype. The third patient, a 73-year-old man, had AML following polycythemia vera. His karyotype was abnormal (46, XY, +3p+, −9, 20q−). The fourth patient was a 62-year-old woman with RAEB and the pathologic karyotype 46,XX,5q−.

In all patients, treatment was well tolerated without nausea, vomiting, hair loss, or hepatic toxicity, but in all of them peripheral pancytopenia developed or worsened under therapy, necessitating multiple red cell and platelet transfusions. In spite of pronounced neutropenia and thrombocytopenia, no serious infectious or hemorrhagic problems were encountered. Bone marrow cytology revealed hypoplasia or aplasia in most patients, but in some patients it remained normocellular with signs of differentiation. The first sign of bone marrow recovery was a rapid rise in platelets about 10 days after the end of therapy.

* Department of Oncology and Hematology, University of Hamburg, Martinistr. 52, D-2000 Hamburg 20, FRG

Table 1. Clinical data of the nine patients who obtained a complete remission

Case	Sex, age	FAB classification	Blood leukocytes ($\times 10^9$/l)/ % blasts	Bone marrow % blasts	Karyotype	Pretreatment	Number of courses/ duration (days)	Duration of CR (months)
1	M,66	M_1 post-RAEB?	2.5/0	62	46,XY	None	2/21	2
2	M,70	M_2 post-RAEB	2.3/6	30	46,XY	None	2/28 and 14	4
3	M,81	Acute, megakaryoblastic leukemia	5.4/31	58	46,XY	None	1/21	7
4	F,74	M_2	1.1/37	45	46,XX	None	1/23	1+
5	M,61	M_1	3.5/0	65	46,XY	NR after Pred-Dauno-Onc-Aspar	1/15	9
6	F,69	M_1	11.3/46	73	46,XX	First relapse after TAD	2/21	15+
7	F,50	M_4 Eo	2.4/0	35	46,XX	Second relapse after TAD	1/27	7
8	M,75	RAEB	10.1/9	6	47,XY, +8	None	2/21	12+
9	F,75	RAEB in transformation	1.3/0	22	46,XX	none	1/21	3+

C. Discussion

Stimulated by the in vitro studies of Lotem and Sachs [7] and Sachs [11], who showed the capacity of low dose Ara-C to induce differentiation in certain leukemic cells, Baccarani and Tura [2], Moloney and Rosenthal [9], and Housset et al. [6] were the first to obtain complete and partial remissions with low dose Ara-C in patients with AML and MDS. Later, these results were confirmed by Andrey et al. [1], Baccarani et al. [3], Castaigne et al. [4], Manoharan [8], Mufti et al. [10], Wisch et al. [13], and Solal-Celigny [12], whereas Haagenbeek et al. [5] did not find any favorable effect of this type of treatment.

Our results in 16 patients with 9 CR and 3 PR argue strongly in favor of a convincing effect of low dose Ara-C in certain types of AML and MDS. In addition, compared with conventional chemotherapy, this type of treatment was well tolerated without major complications, in spite of considerable pancytopenia. Further studies must find out which patients are candidates for low dose Ara-C and how results, especially duration of CR, can be improved. Based on our experience during the last few months, we think that patients with rapidly progressive disease are not candidates for this type of treatment whereas patients with slowly progressive disease may benefit from low dose Ara-C. It seems noteworthy that 10/11 patients with a normal karyotype had a response and only 2/5 patients with a pathologic karyotype.

So far, the mechanism of this type of treatment is unclear. Pancytopenia and bone marrow hypoplasia argue in favor of a cytostatic effect. On the other hand, our series included some patients without pronounced bone marrow hypoplasia and with cytologic signs of maturation of blasts. This phenomenon was also observed by Castaigne et al. [4]. The mechanism of low dose Ara-C could be approached by diffusion chamber studies, immunologic markers of differentiation, and cytogenetic studies. Unfortunately, there was only one patient with a chromosomal anomaly (47,XY, +8) who achieved CR. In remission, he had a normal karyotype. In this patient, bone marrow aplasia was severe, suggesting a cytostatic effect of therapy.

Acknowledgments. This work was supported by the Hamburger Krebsgesellschaft.

References

1. Andrey C, Beris P, Plancherel C, de Loes S, Maurice P, Chapuis B (1983) Cytosine-arabinoside à doses réduites pour le traitement des leucémies myéloides aiguës. Schweiz Med Wochenschr 113:980
2. Baccarani M, Tura S (1979) Differentiation of myeloid leukaemic cells: new possibilities for therapy. Br J Haematol 43:485
3. Baccarani M, Zaccaria A, Bandini G, Cavazzini G, Fanin R, Tura S (1983) Low dose arabinosyl cytosine for treatment of myelodysplastic syndromes and subacute myeloid leukemia. Leuk Res 7:539
4. Castaigne S, Daniel MT, Tilly H, Herait P, Degos L (1983) Does treatment with ARA-C in low dosage cause differentiation of leukemic cells? Blood 62:85
5. Hagenbeek A, Sizoo W, Löwenberg B (1983) Treatment of acute myelocytic leukemia with low-dose cytosine-arabinoside: results of a pilot study in four patients. Leuk Res 7:443
6. Housset M, Daniel MT, Degos L (1982) Small dose of ARA-C in the treatment of acute myeloid leukemia: differentiation of myeloid leukaemia cells? Br J Haematol 51:125
7. Lotem J, Sachs J (1974) Different blocks in the differentiation of myeloid leukemic cells. Proc Natl Acad Sci USA 71:3507
8. Manoharan A (1983) Low-dose Cytarabine therapy in hypoplastic acute leukemia. N Engl J Med 309:1652
9. Moloney WC, Rosenthal DS (1981) Treatment of early acute nonlymphatic leukemia with low-dose cytosine arabinoside. In: Neth R, Gallo RC, Graf T, Mannweiler K, Winkler K (eds) Modern trends in human leukemia IV. Springer, Berlin Heidelberg New York, pp 59–62
10. Mufti GJ, Oscier DG, Hamblin TJ, Bell AJ (1983) Low doses of cytarabine in the treatment of myelodysplastic syndrome and acute myeloid leukemia. N Engl J Med 309:1653
11. Sachs L (1978) The differentiation of myeloid leukaemia cells. New possibilities for therapy. Br J Haematol 40:509
12. Solal-Celigny P, Desaint B, Herrera A, Chastang C, Amar M, Vroclans M, Brousse N, Mancilla F, Renoux M, Bernard JF, Boivin P (1984) Chronic myelomonocytic leukemia according to FAB classification: analysis of 35 cases. Blood 53:634
13. Wisch JS, Griffin JD, Kufe DW (1983) Response of preleukemic syndromes to continuous infusion of low-dose cytarabine. N Engl J Med 309:1599

Haematology and Blood Transfusion Vol. 29
Modern Trends in Human Leukemia VI
Edited by Neth, Gallo, Greaves, Janka

The Results of High Risk Acute Lymphoblastic Leukemia and Non-Hodgkin's Lymphoma Total Therapy *

J. Bogusławska-Jaworska, J. Pejcz, J. Armata, M. Ochocka, U. Radwańska, R. Rokicka-Milewska, and M. Sroczyńska

A. Introduction

The study was designed to evaluate the efficacy of seven-drug systemic therapy and three-drug intrathecal treatment in children with high risk acute lymphoblastic leukemia (ALL) and non-Hodgkin's lymphoma (NHL). The modified LSA_2L_2 treatment protocol applied for this study is presented in Fig. 1. The total duration of the treatment was 2.5 years. Estimated distribution of continuous remission and survival were calculated using the product limit method of Kaplan and Meier [3]. The differences in remission and survival were compared according to the nonparametric long rank test [5].

B. Acute Lymphoblastic Leukemia

A group of 92 previously untreated children, diagnosed with ALL from 6 hematologic centers, were eligible for this study. The prognostic stratification of patients was made by BFM score system [2]. The increased risk (IR) group was defined by score numbers 3–10. Overall survival and

* Department of Pediatric Hematology, Faculty of Medicine, Wrocław, Poland

Fig. 1. Modified LSA_2L_2 protocol

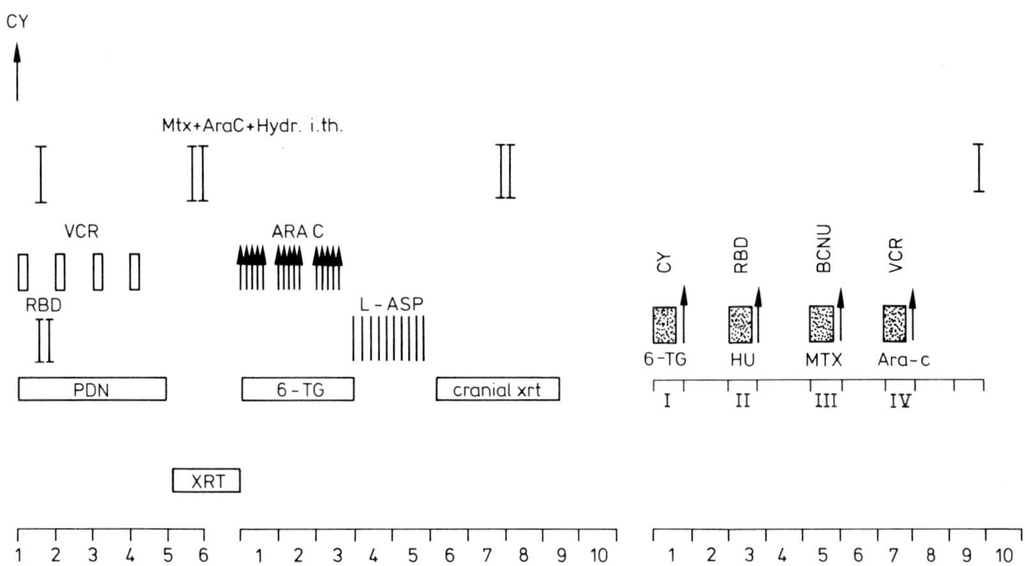

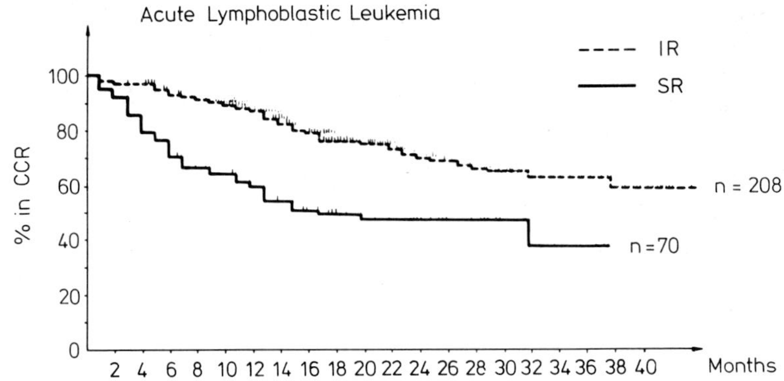

	Admitted to study	Achieved complete remission	%	no remission	%	p
SR	212	208	93	4	2	0.01
IR	92	70	76	22	24	
total	304	278	91	26	9	

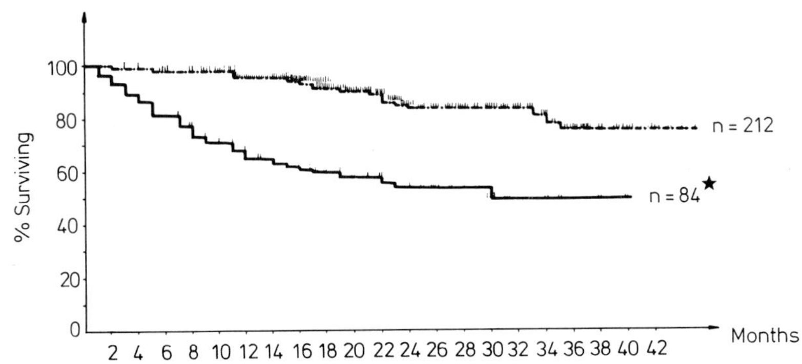

* 8 Dead in first 4 days excluded

Fig. 2. Remission and survival results

CCR duration of IR and SR patient groups are presented in Fig. 2.

Intensification of the induction, preventive CNS treatment, consolidation and maintenance therapy in the high risk ALL patients has resulted in some increase of disease-free and overall survival duration. However, a considerable proportion of induction failure associated with initial CNS leukemia and high WBC count has been observed. In contradiction to some other studies [6], the frequency of CNS relapses remained relatively high, despite intensification of CNS preventive therapy. The high proportion of fatal infectious complications in the maintenance period suggests their relation with immunosuppression caused by the therapy used, despite the intermittent regimen applied. Our data, like others [7], failed to show evident advantage of the modified LSA_2L_2 protocol for the ALL children with score numbers 6–10.

C. Non-Hodgkin's Lymphoma

A total of 97 previously untreated children with NHL were admitted to this study. Staging was done according to the criteria proposed by Murphy [4]. Histologic diagnoses were made according to the Kiel classification. The most common location of tumor was mediastinal mass followed

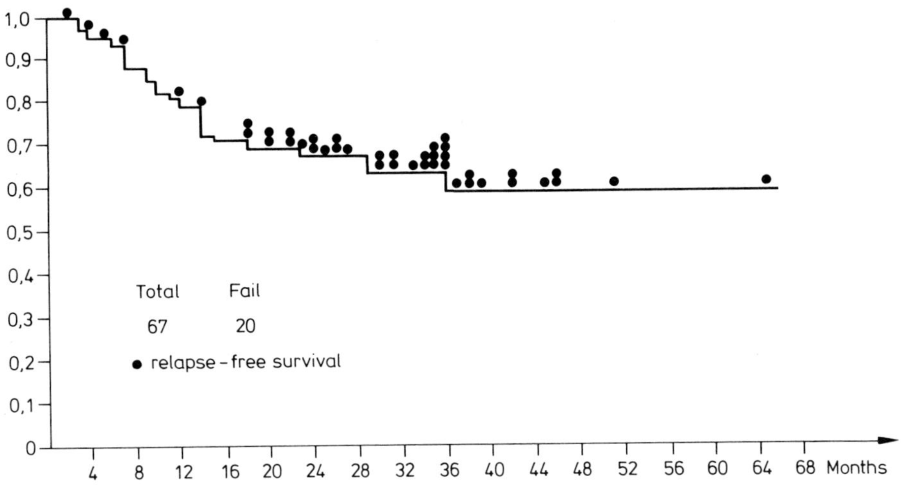

Fig. 3. Relapse-free survival of patients who attained complete remission with LSA_2L_2 treatment

next in frequency by head–neck and abdominal. A total of 22 children received 5 intrathecal doses of methotrexate, cytosine arabinoside, and hydrocortisone, and cranial irradiation, starting at the end of the consolidation phase. After completion of the induction period, radiotherapy (1400–3500 rad) was given to 59 children.

The overall estimate of survival and CCR duration and their relation to histologic type of NHL for complete responders are shown in Figs. 3–5. Of the 67 complete responders, 6 had relapses in the bone marrow, 7 in the CNS, and 7 localized relapses. In only 1 of 22 children with CNS prophylaxis was CNS relapse observed, in comparison with 7 of 39 who were not given cranial irradiation combined with cytostatics.

The overall results of NHL study represent a significant improvement over our historical controls [1]. However, there were evident differences in outcome between lymphoblastic and nonlymphoblastic NHL. These data suggest that the histologic type

Fig. 4. Overall survival of patients treated by the LSA_2L_2 regimen

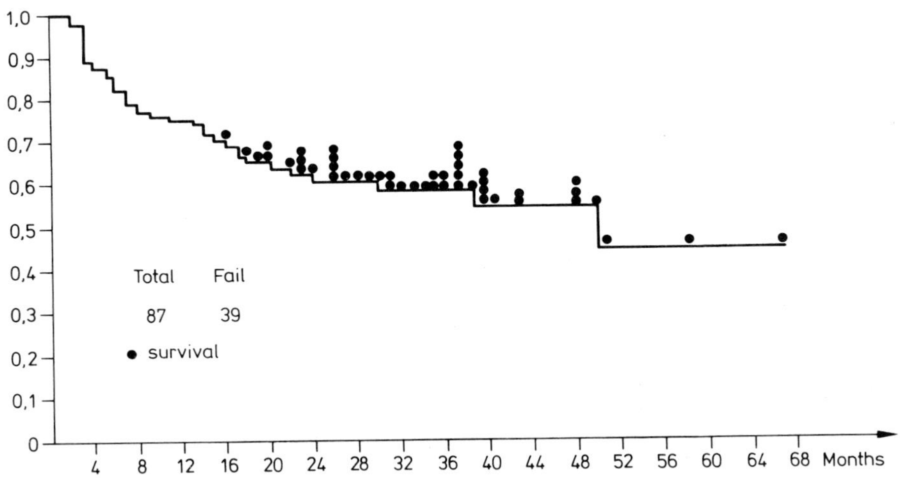

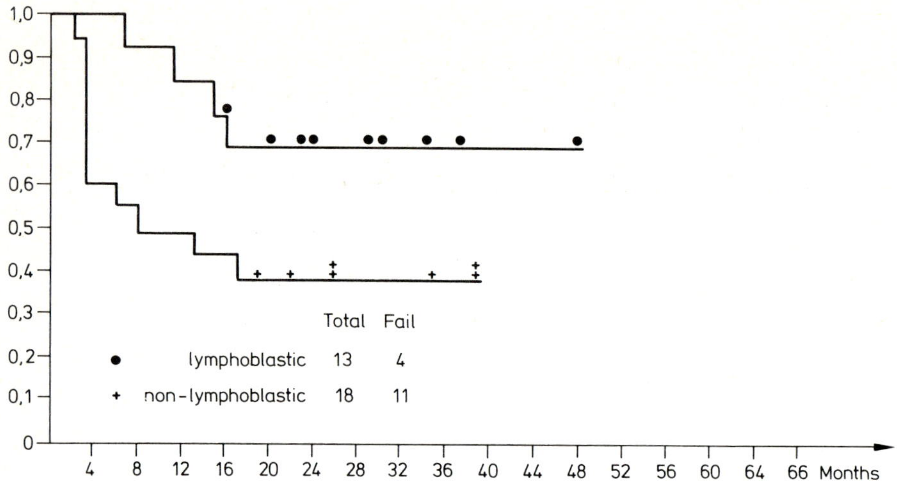

Fig. 5. Survival of patients with nonlocalized disease treated by the LSA_2L_2 regimen according to histologic subtype

of NHL must be taken into account in planning the therapy, and that the LSA_2L_2 protocol is not efficient for non-lymphoblastic subtypes of NHL.

References

1. Bogusławska-Jaworska J, Grześkowiak-Melanowska J, Kaczmarek-Kanold M, Kościelniak E, Legutko L, Sońta-Jakimczyk D, Sroczyńska M, Wójcik Z (1980) Wstępne wyniki leczenia nieziarniczych chłoniaków złośliwych u dzieci według programu BACOP. Ped Pol 55:207–210
2. Henze G, Landermann HJ, Ritter J, Schellong G, Riehm H (1981) Treatment strategy for different risk groups in childhood acute lymphoblastic leukemia: a report from BFM Study Group. Haemat Blood Transf 26:87–93
3. Kaplan EL, Meier P (1958) Nonparametric estimation from incomplete observation. Am Stat Assoc 53:457–480
4. Murphy S (1980) Classification, staging and end results of treatment of childhood non-Hodgkin's lymphomas: dissimilarties from lymphomas in adults. Semin Oncol 73:332–339
5. Peto R, Piko MC, Armitage P, Breslow NE, Sox DR, Howard SV, Muntel N, McPherson K, Peto K, Smith PG (1977) Design and analysis of randomized clinical trials requiring prolonged observation of each patient. II. Analysis and examples. Br J Cancer 35:1–39
6. Pinkel F (1983) Patterns of failure in acute lymphoblastic leukemia. Cancer Treat Symposia 2:259–266
7. Zintl E, Herman J, Katenkamp D, Malke H, Plenert W (1983) Results of LSA_2L_2 therapy in children with high-risk acute lymphoblastic leukemia and non-Hodgkin's lymphoma. In: Neth R, Gallo RC, Greaves MF, Moore AAS, Winkler K (eds) Modern trends in human leukemia. Springer, Berlin Heidelberg New York Tokyo, pp 62–66

Haematology and Blood Transfusion Vol. 29
Modern Trends in Human Leukemia VI
Edited by Neth, Gallo, Greaves, Janka

Adult Acute Lymphoblastic Leukaemia at University Hospital, Malaysia *

J. J. Bosco, R. Cherian, and T. Pang

A. Introduction

Epidemiological studies of lymphoid malignancies show remarkable differences amongst populations of different geographical locations and socioeconomic conditions [1]. An earlier survey by us showed the virtual nonexistence of chronic lymphocytic leukaemia and follicular non-Hodgkin's lymphoma in Malaysians [2]. All patients with acute lymphoblastic leukaemia (ALL) are being studied under an international leukaemia subtyping study organized by Dr. M. Greaves. This is a preliminary review of ALL subtypes.

B. Methods

The study consisted of all patients admitted with a diagnosis of acute leukaemia or lympholeukaemia between January 1980 and February 1984. Routine morphological and cytochemical methods were used in the diagnosis. Cells from bone marrow and peripheral blood of patients with ALL were also characterized for different cell surface antigen expression (see Table 2). The subtypes were defined as follows: common ALL (positive for cALLA and HLA DR antigens), T-ALL (E rosettes and other T cell antigens and HLA DR negative), B-ALL (surface immunoglobulin and HLA DR positive) and Null (cALLA negative, SMIg, ER, T antigens negative, HLA DR antigen positive). Immunofluorescence assays for nuclear TdT were done, but results not included because of technical difficulties.

C. Results

Tables 1 and 2 show the breakdown of ALL in relation to other acute leukaemias and in terms of immunological characterization. The relative proportions of the four ALL subclasses in relation to sex and age are shown in Table 3. The clinical features of the 11 adult cases of T cell leukaemia or leukaemia–lymphoma are shown in Table 4.

D. Discussion

Our study showed "common" acute lymphoblastic leukaemia in approximately 50% of patients. This rate of cALLA positivity may be a reflection of the demographic status of Malaysia where there is a fairly large middle class and a heterogeneous population of Malays, Chinese and Indians [3]. This study also supports the observation of approximately 60% cALLA positivity amongst Asian children in a United Kingdom survey [4]. This is somewhat in contrast to the slightly lower incidence of common ALL in Afro-Caribbean children.

The majority of T cell malignancies were T-ALL lymphoblastic lymphoma–leukaemia with acute onset, marked leu-

* University Hospital, University of Malaysia, Malaysia

Table 1. Acute leukaemia diagnosed at University Hospital, Kuala Lumpur, January 1980 – February 1984

Diagnosis	Total no. of cases	No. of adult cases (> 15 years)
Acute lymphoblastic leukaemia	153	42
Acute myeloid leukaemia	37	26
Acute myelomonocytic leukaemia	21	15
Acute monocytic leukaemia	8	3
Acute promyelocytic leukaemia	12	4
Acute undifferentiated leukaemia	8	5
Total	239	95

Table 2. Acute lymphoblastic leukaemia (ALL) subtypes January 1980 – February 1984

Study	No. of patients tested	Surface marker expression			
		ALL	T	B	Null
1 [a]	18	N.T. [d]	6		12
2 [b, c]	58	27	14	6	5

[a] Limited study carried out before 1982. Only two markers were investigated: sheep erythrocyte (E) rosettes and surface membrane immunoglobulin

[b] Study begun in 1982 as part of the international ALL subgroup survey (coordinated by Dr. M. F. Greaves, London); cells were analysed for E rosettes, CALL antigens and 12 other surface markers using monoclonal antibodies and immunofluorescent visualization

[c] Only 58 of the 79 cases seen since 1982 were studied; 6 cases could not be characterized as any one of the 4 subtypes

[d] N.T. = not tested

Table 3. Acute lymphoblastic leukaemia (ALL) subtypes January 1982 – February 1984

Subtype	No.	Male	Female	M:F ratio	No. of cases < 15 years of age
Common ALL	27	14	13	1:1	17
T-ALL	14	9	5	1.8:1	9
B-ALL	6	4	2	2:1	2
Null	5	4	1		
Undetermined	6	5	1		

cocytosis, hepatosplenomegaly, lymphadenopathy, and mediastinal mass on chest X-ray. This disease was not confined to the adolescent age group alone for it was noted to be fairly uniformly distributed between 2 and 30 years of age. Greaves [5] has indicated that this disease is not confined to adolescence. The approximate 25% incidence of T-ALL is not strikingly different from that observed in Western and industrialized countries.

The recent association of the adult form of T cell malignancy with HTLV is perhaps of great importance in understanding the biology of lymphoid malignancies. Epidemiological surveys such as this to-

Table 4. Clinical features of adult (> 15 years) T cell malignancies

Clinical features	Number[a]
Mediastinal Mass	9
Skin involvement	2
Lymphadenopathy	10
Hepatosplenomegaly	10
CNS involvement	5
Pleural effusion	4
Lytic bone lesions	1
Hypercalcaemia	2
Leucocytosis	8

[a] Number of patients of the total 11 who had the clinical features

gether with virological, molecular and genetic studies of acute T-ALL populations may give further clues to the aetiology of these disorders.

In summary, the subtypes of ALL do not seem to be different from those noted in the West. This is in marked contrast to the situation with non-Hodgkin's lymphoma and CLL. The findings also raise the possibility that with an effective and well-planned treatment programme a large number of the patients may be effectively treated.

Acknowledgments. We would like to thank Dr. M. F. Greaves, Coordinator of the International ALL subgroup survey for providing reagents for immunological studies, Mr. S. Y. Lim for technical assistance, and Puan Rohani for typing the manuscript.

References

1. Magrath IT, O'Connor GT, Ramot B (eds) (1984) Pathogenesis of leukaemias and lymphomas: environmental influences. Raven, New York
2. Bosco J, Cherian R, Lin HP, Pang T (1984) A survey of lymphoid malignancies at University Hospital, Kuala Lumpur, Malaysia. In: Magrath IT, O'Connor GT, Ramot B (eds) Pathogenesis of leukaemias and lymphomas: environmental influences. Raven, New York, pp 61–65
3. Ramot B, Magrath I (1982) Hypothesis: the environment is a major determinant of the immunological subtype of lymphoma and ALL in children. Br J Haematol 50: 183–189
4. Hill FGH, Al Rubei K, Trumpun PA (1984) An epidemiological study of childhood ALL in the West Midlands of the United Kingdom showing seasonal variation in T cell disease. In: Magrath IT, O'Connor GT, Ramot B (eds) Pathogenesis of leukaemias and lymphomas: environmental influences. Raven, New York, pp 147–155
5. Greaves MF (1984) Subtypes of ALL: implications for the pathogenesis and epidemiology of leukaemia. In: Magrath IT, O'Connor GT, Ramot B (eds) Pathogenesis of leukaemias and lymphomas: environmental influences. Raven, New York, pp 129–139

Haematology and Blood Transfusion Vol. 29
Modern Trends in Human Leukemia VI
Edited by Neth, Gallo, Greaves, Janka

The Epipodophyllotoxin VP16-213 in Combination Chemotherapy for Adults with Acute Nonlymphoblastic Leukaemia

P. Jacobs[1]

A. Introduction

Combination chemotherapy programmes that include cytosine arabinoside and an anthracycline antibiotic can cure adult patients with acute nonlymphoblastic leukaemia [1]. Furthermore, clinical trials using these two agents in different schedules [2] and in combination with other active drugs [3] has impressively improved complete remission rates [4]. It is an unfortunate fact that random leukaemic relapse characterises survival curves for most reported treatment programmes so that a major discrepancy persists between improving figures for complete remission and those for survival beyond 5 years [5]. Further improvement in cure rate confronts the clinical scientist with two major challenges. First, remission rates must be improved, and here stratification of patients on the basis of prognostic factors [6] to the most appropriate chemotherapy to balance efficacy against toxicity requires clarification. Second, the durability of complete remission must be improved and therapeutic approaches have included varying maintenance schedules, drug intensification, immunotherapy and the increasing use of bone marrow transplantation [7]. Unfortunately, although results from clinical trials are published [8], there is a striking paucity of well-controlled randomised studies in the scientific literature to provide authoritative statements on these controversial issues [9]. We report the experience with 232 consecutive patients treated at a single institution in four consecutive trials, the last of which is still in progress, examining some of these variables.

B. Materials and Methods

Individuals over the age of 14 years with a confirmed diagnosis of acute leukaemia were eligible for studies approved by the University Ethics Committee, and participated after having given informed consent. Routine haematologic assessment included morphological and cytochemical characterisation of the leukaemic subtype, and following its introduction all patients were classified according to the French–American–British (FAB) recommendations [10]. Plasminogen activator was measured as previously described [11, 12]. Venous access was ensured using a standardised method [13]. All patients received full supportive care, including protocol management with appropriate antibiotics for infectious episodes, granulocyte [14] and platelet [15] support from our own standardised programme.

The four successive studies employed different chemotherapy regimens. In study 1 [16] (80 patients) daunorubicin (55 mg/m^2) was given on day 1 and cytosine arabinoside (70 mg/m^2) by continuous infusion on days 1–5. In study 2 [17] (40 patients) VP16-213 (60 mg/m^2) was given on days 1–5, cytosine arabinoside (75 mg/m^2) by

1 University of Cape Town Leukaemia Centre and the Department of Haematology, Groote Schuur Hospital, Observatory, Cape, South Africa

Table 1. Summary of 232 patients in four consecutive studies at the University of Cape Town. Study 3A is a short intensification (6 months) and 3B is an extended intensification (15 months). In study 4, C represents patients being treated with the Cape Town Regimen (CTRIII) and D those being treated with DAT

Measurement	Study 1	Study 2	Study 3		Study 4	
			A	B	C	D
Patient numbers	80	40	26	26	30	30
Complete remission (%)	30	48.5	44	44	46	46
Duration of complete remission (weeks)	28	48	44	44	>24	>24
Courses						
Number	4	1	1	1	1	2
Range	3–8	1–3	1–3	1–3	1–3	2–4
Survival of responders (weeks)	58	60	95	75	>42	>42
Long survival (%)						
10 years	2					
5 years	2	2.5	8			
2 years	15	2.5	30			

A = short intensification (6 months); B = extended intensification (15 months); C = CTR III; D = DAT

continuous intravenous infusion on days 1–5 and doxorubicin (40 mg/m²) on day 6. In study 3 [18] (52 patients) the identical induction regimen was used and patients in complete remission randomised to short intensification (6 months) or extended intensification (15 months) using 3 months of escalating cyclophosphamide followed by 3 months of vincristine, methotrexate and escalating cytosine arabinoside. In the present study, which is continuing (60 patients to date) the same three-drug induction programme (Cape Town Regimen/CTR III) was directly compared with a combination of doxorubicin (50 mg/m²) on day 1, cytosine arabinoside (200 mg/m²) on days 1–5, and thioguanine (200 mg/m²) on days 1–5 (DAT); the patients in complete remission were randomised to the same short or extended intensification regimens as study 3.

C. Results of the Four Studies are Shown in Table 1.

D. Comments

The complete remission rate in study 1 compared with those described with the same regimen from St. Bartholomew's Hospital [19] is attributed to the late referral of patients resulting in early deaths of type V failure [17, 20]. This pattern has persisted in the ensuing studies, emphasising the inappropriateness of comparing results of studies from different institutions where major variable factors such as nutritional status and clinical condition of patients on admission may differ so widely that valid comparison is impossible. Similarly, this observation emphasises the importance of meticulous demographic description of the patient population being treated and the value of the randomised clinical trial which will control for such factors and without consideration of which the efficacy claimed for different regimens reported from centres having their own characteristic patient populations is very likely to be invalid.

The epipodophyllotoxin VP16-213 included in study 2, where the patient populations are comparable, shows a clear increase in complete remission rate and an anticipated improvement in duration of remission and survival of responders. These benefits are statistically significant and occur with a shorter period of induction since the median number of courses to complete remission is reduced from four to one, and this difference is also significant. These two studies support the conclusion that addition of the epipodophyllotoxin VP16-213, which is known to have activity in adult acute nonlymphoblastic leukaemia as a single agent, represents an advance over the use of cytosine arabinoside–anthracycline antibiotic combination.

The duration of intensification chemotherapy was assessed in study 3, and while there is a trend in favour of a short period of intensification, this difference is not statistically superior to extended treatment. In view of the small numbers involved a β, or type II, effect may obscure significant benefit, and further studies are in progress to accumulate the necessary number of patients to overcome this theoretical objection. These findings are consistent with other available controlled evidence that prolongation of maintenance or intensification therapy is, at best, of limited value once complete remission has been consolidated.

Comparison of DAT and CTR III in a currently active prospective randomised study shows no benefit for replacement of the epipodophyllotoxin VP16-213 by thioguanine in regimens already containing cytosine arabinoside and an anthracycline antibiotic. Furthermore, the greater quantities of cytosine arabinoside used in the DAT programme appear to be without additional benefit and a theoretical explanation may be synergism between epipodophyllotoxin and cytosine arabinoside [21]. In this regard, it remains to be established whether, in the particular population being treated at this institution, further drug escalation, as in a 7-and-3 regimen [22] or the Barts 10 programme, would improve remission rates by decreasing the number of patients with primary drug resistance (type I or type II induction failure) without a commensurate loss due to excessive toxicity (type III or type IV induction failure). Similarly, it is now also necessary to prospectively compare increasing amounts of cytosine and anthracycline in patients randomly receiving the same amount of these two agents in combination with the epipodophyllotoxin; such a study is currently being developed.

Prognostic factors provide the most useful basis for stratification [23]. However, our own studies have failed to show statistical correlation between remission rate or survival with the FAB classification, age, in vitro bone marrow culture [24], initial white cell [25], platelet or blast count [26]. Our experience shows the best correlation to be with patients's achievement of complete remission, and that this appears to correlate closely with the species of plasminogen activator secreted in vitro by leukaemic blasts [11, 12]. Data from study 3 and study 4 have been reanalysed following stratification using this criterion, and to date all individuals secreting the 70 000 daltons or tissue species of plasminogen activator have shown primary drug resistance to regimens containing conventional doses of cytosine arabinoside and an anthracycline antibiotic, whether in combination with thioguanine or the epipodophyllotoxin VP16-213. In contrast, those secreting either the urokinase or a mixed pattern have a complete remission rate in excess of 80% with the same induction chemotherapy. Clearly, biological stratification of previously untreated adults with acute nonlymphoblastic leukaemia on the basis of their plasminogen activator status, at least in our experience, appears to provide a rational means for selecting chemotherapeutic programmes. Support for this concept is found in preliminary experience (P. Jacobs, unpublished work) that high dose cytosine arabinoside [27] is effective salvage therapy in such individuals.

E. Summary

A total of 232 previously untreated adults with acute nonlymphoblastic leukaemia were consecutively entered into four successive studies. In the first, complete remission rates and survival were inferior to a group treated on the same regimen in London, suggesting population differences, possibly on the basis of late referral and poor nutritional status. In the second study the addition of the epipodophyllotoxin VP16-213 to conventional doses of doxorubicin and cytosine arabinoside improved complete remission rate and median duration of survival. In the third study this induction programme was unchanged and short duration of intensification was compared with an extended period, but no statistically significant difference was demonstrated. In the fourth study, which is currently active, the role of the epipodophyllotoxin VP16-213 (Cape Town Regimen/CTR III) was compared with the same two agents in combination with thioguanine (DAT), but to date no difference in remission rate or survival is evident. Four conclusions are supported by data from these studies. First, the addition of VP16-213 to doxorubicin and cytosine arabinoside improves complete remission rate, prolongs median duration of complete remission and survival, with shortening of the time taken to achieve this status in our population. Second, evidence to date shows no advantage for the DAT programme containing thioguanine over CTR III in which this latter agent is replaced by the epipodophyllotoxin VP16-213. Third, there is no statistically significant difference in survival once patients have achieved complete remission following randomisation to receive 6 months in comparison with 15 months of intensification therapy. Finally, of the previously described prognostic factors, only response to initial chemotherapy has proved significant. However, our recent experience indicates that the species of plasminogen activator secreted by the leukaemic blasts allows identification of patients with primary drug resistance to regimens containing conventional doses of cytosine arabinoside and doxorubicin, and may offer a practical approach to initial use of alternative chemotherapy, particularly high dose cytosine arabinoside.

Acknowledgments. This work was supported by the University of Cape Town Leukaemia Centre and Staff Research Fund, the Medical Research Council and the National Cancer Association. I thank Jackie Davies and Keren Edwards for typing and bibliographic assistance, Bristol-Myers for donation of the VP16-213 used in these studies, Dr. E. L. Wilson for plasminogen activator assay and Dr. H.-R. Sanders, Chief Medical Superintendent of Groote Schuur Hospital for permission to publish.

References

1. Preisler HD, Rustum Y, Henderson ES, Bjornsson S, Creaven PJ, Higby DJ, Freeman A, Gailani S, Naeher C (1979) Treatment of acute nonlymphocytic leukemia: use of anthracycline-cytosine arabinoside induction therapy and comparison of two maintenance regimens. Blood 53:455
2. Slevin ML, Rohatiner AZS, Dhaliwal HS, Henry GP, Bell R (1982) A comparison of two schedules of cytosine arabinoside used in combination with adriamycin and 6-thioguanine in the treatment of acute myelogenous leukemia. Med Pediatr Oncol [Suppl] 1:185
3. Armitage JO, Burns CP, Dick FR, Aunan SB, Slymen DJ (1982) Results of aggressive chemotherapy for acute nonlymphoblastic leukemia in adults. Cancer Treat Rep 66:1917
4. Keating MJ, McCredie KB, Bodey GP, Smith TL, Gehan E, Freireich EJ (1982) Improved prospects for long-term survival in adults with acute myelogenous leukemia. JAMA 248:2481
5. Keating MJ (1982) Early identification of potentially cured patients with acute myelogenous leukemia – a recent challenge. In: Bloomfield CJ (ed) Adult leukemias 1. Nijhoff, The Hague, p 237
6. McCredie KB, Bodey GP, Freireich EJ, Gutterman JU, Hester JP, Drewinko B (1976) Adult leukemia. In: Clark RL, Howe CD (eds) Cancer patient care at MD Anderson Hospital and Tumor Institute, University of Texas. Year Book Medical, Chicago, p 165
7. Jacobs P (1981) The changing pattern of therapy in adults with acute myeloblastic leukaemia. Haematologica 66:803
8. Debusscher L, Stryckmans PA (1978) Nonlymphocytic acute leukemia. In: Staquet MJ (ed) Randomized trials in cancer. A critical review by sites. Raven, New York, p 25
9. Jacobs P, Martell R (1985) Controlled trials in therapy of acute nonlymphoblastic leukaemia. In: Staquet MJ, Slevin M (eds) Randomized trials in cancer. A critical review by sites. Raven, New York (in press)
10. Bennett JM, Catovsky D, Daniel MT, Flandrin G, Galton DAG, Gralnick HR, Sultan C (1976) Proposals for the classification of the acute leukaemias. Br J Haematol 33:451
11. Wilson EL, Jacobs P, Dowdle EB (1983) Secretion of plasminogen activators by human myeloid leukemic cells: modulation and therapeutic correlations. In: Neth R, Gallo RC, Greaves MF, Moore M, Winkler K (eds) Modern trends in human leukemia V. Springer, Berlin Heidelberg, p 78
12. Wilson EL, Jacobs P, Dowdle EB (1983) The secretion of plasminogen activators by human myeloid leukemic cells in vitro. Blood 61:568

13. Jacobs P, Jacobson J (1981) Central catheter placement. S Afr Med J 59:3
14. Wood L, Hester JP, Jacobs P (1984) The function and structure of granulocytes collected using the IBM 2997 separator. J Clin Apheresis 2:190
15. Bond R, Wood L, Jacobs P, Kernoff LM (1984) Platelet collection using the IBM 2997 separator. J Clin Apheresis 2:155
16. Jacobs P, Dubovsky D, Hougaard M, Comay S (1975) Epipodophyllotoxin VP16-213 in acute nonlymphoblastic leukaemia. Br Med J 1:396
17. Dubovsky D, Kernoff L, Jacobs P (1978) Rapid remission induction in adult acute nonlymphoblastic leukaemia. Eur J Cancer 14:1179
18. Jacobs P, Dubovsky DW, Wood L (1984) In adult acute nonlymphoblastic leukaemia extended maintenance chemotherapy has no benefit. Am J Hematol 16:255
19. Crowther D, Powles RL, Bateman CJT, Beard ME, Gauci CL, Wrigley PFM, Malpas JS, Hamilton Fairley GH, Scott Sir RB (1973) Management of adult acute myelogenous leukaemia. Br Med J 1:131
20. Preisler HD (1978) Failure of remission induction in acute myelocytic leukemia. Med Pediatr Oncol 4:275
21. Rivera G, Avery T, Roberts D (1975) Response of L1210 to combinations of cytosine arabinoside and VM-26 or VP16-213. Eur J Cancer 11:639
22. Lister RA, Rohatiner AZS (1982) The treatment of acute myelogenous leukemia in adults. Semin Hematol 19:172
23. Brandman J, Bukowski RM, Greenstreet R, Hewlett JS, Hoffmann GC (1979) Prognostic factors affecting remission, remission duration, and survival in adult acute nonlymphocytic leukemia. Cancer 44:1062
24. Preisler HD, Azarnia N, Marinello M (1984) Relationship of the growth of leukemic cells in vitro to the outcome of therapy for acute nonlymphocytic leukemia. Cancer Res 44:1712
25. Hug V, Keating M, McCredie K, Hester J, Bodey GP, Freireich EJ (1983) Clinical course and response to treatment of patients with acute myelogenous leukemia presenting with a high leukocyte count. Cancer 52:773
26. Curtis JE, Till JE, Messner HA, Sousan P, McCulloch EA (1979) Comparison of outcomes and prognostic factors for two groups of patients with acute myeloblastic leukemia. Leuk Res 3:409
27. Herzig RH, Wolff SN, Lazarus HM, Phillips GL, Karanes C, Herzig GP (1983) High-dose cytosine arabinoside therapy for refractory leukemia. Blood 62:361

Haematology and Blood Transfusion Vol. 29
Modern Trends in Human Leukemia VI
Edited by Neth, Gallo, Greaves, Janka

Treatment of Acute Lymphoblastic Leukemia in Childhood: A Report for the ALL 77-02 Group *

R. J. Haas, G. Gaedicke, U. B. Graubner, and G. Meyer

A. Patients and Methods

Since 1 December 1979, 149 children with acute lymphoblastic leukemia (ALL) have been treated according to the prospective study protocol ALL 77-02 [5]. Patients' characteristics are given in Table 1. High risk patients are defined by WBC > 25 $\times 10^3/mm^3$ and/or T cell marker, AUL, or B cell ALL. The treatment protocols for standard risk and high risk patients are given in Figs. 1 and 2. During consolidation therapy, three intermediate dose methotrexate infusions [2] were administered at 10-day intervals; 24 h after the end of MTX infusion, L-asparaginase and citrovorum factor were given [7]. The second part of consolidating consisted, in therapy group B of high dose cyclophosphamide ($\times 2$) and intramuscular Ara- C ($\times 16$) [6].

In both protocols, cranial irradiation was used to treat occult CNS leukemia: standard risk 18 Gy, high risk 24 Gy. All pa-

* Childrens Hospitals of the University of Ulm and Munich, FRG

Table 1. Patient characteristics

Number	149
Age (median)	5 years, 11 months
Age <2 >10 years	36
Boys	82
Mediastinal mass	16
CNS positive	8
Hepatosplenomegaly	87
Leucocytes $<25\,000/mm^3$	102
Leucocytes $>25\,000/mm^3$	47

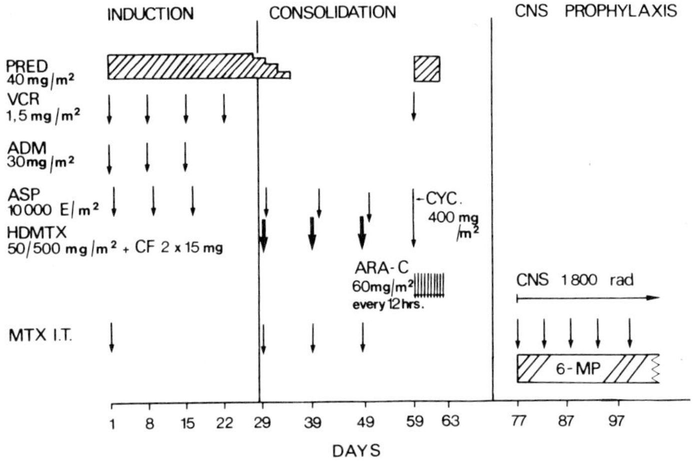

Fig. 1. Treatment protocol, therapy A (standard risk). PRED prednisone; VCR vincristine, ADM adriamycin; ASP L-asparaginase; DMTX high dose methotrexate; CF citrovorum factor; Ara-C cytosine arabinoside; CYC cyclophosphamide; 6-MP 6-mercaptopurine

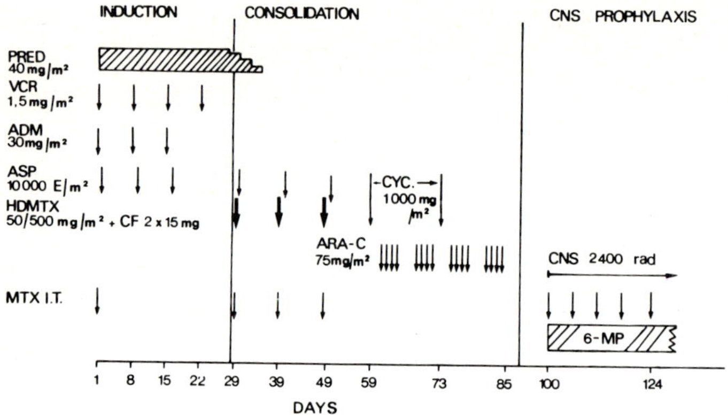

Fig. 2. Treatment protocol, therapy B (high risk). Abbreviations as in Fig. 1

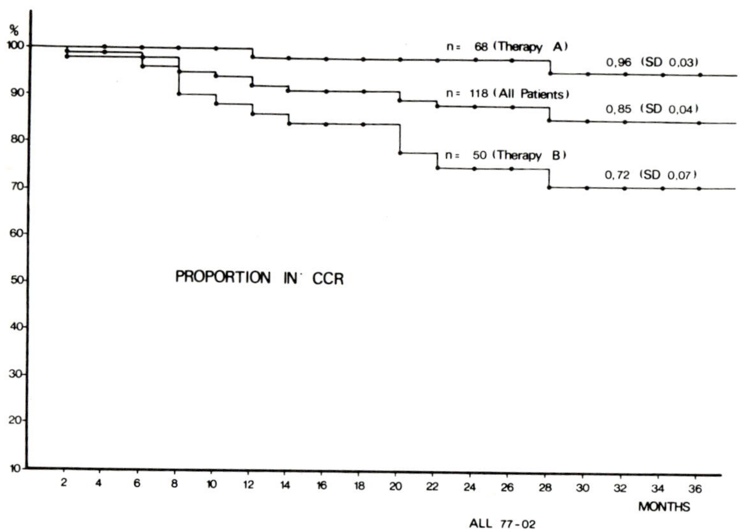

Fig. 3. Life table analysis of probability of continuous complete remission according to therapy

tients received nine doses of intrathecal MTX. Different doses of intrathecal MTX were applied in different age groups [1]: patients less than 1 year of age received 6 mg; patients 1–3 years of age received 8 mg; patients older than 3 years received 12 mg. Maintenance therapy consisted in both groups of daily oral 6-MP (60 mg/m^2) and weekly oral MTX (30 mg/m^2). Treatment was discontinued after 30 months.

B. Results

The clinical course of 81 standard risk and 68 high risk patients is given in Table 2. In Fig. 3, the life table analyses of the entire group, the standard risk group, and the high risk group are given. The 36 months probability of surviving in continuous com-

Table 2. Clinical course

Groups	Total	Standard risk	High risk
Number	149	81	68
Nonresponders	1		1
Early deaths	7	4	3
Deaths during remission	5	1	4
CCR patients	118	68	50
Marrow relapses	12	6	6
CNS relapses	4	1	3
Testes relapses	2	1	1

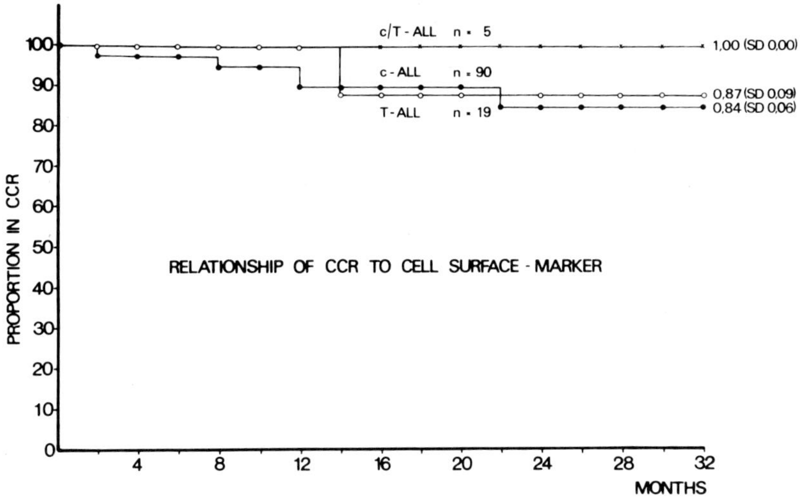

Fig. 4. Life table analysis of probability of continuous complete remission according to cell surface markers

Table 3. Clinical findings and cell surface markers

Groups	c	c/T	T	AUL
Number of patients (124 total)	90	5	19	10
Boys	41	5	15	7
Mediastinal mass	3	0	9	1
Leukocytes $\times 10^3$	38.6	13.6	93.6	73.2
Number $> 25\,000$	27	2	11	4

plete remission is 84% for all patients, 97% for standard risk and 72% for high risk patients. The subtypes of ALL according to surface markers [3, 8] are given in Table 3. In Fig. 4, a comparison of the probability of continuous complete remission for patients with different ALL surface markers is given.

C. Conclusion

As compared with our former study 77-01 [4] these data suggest that the duration of hematologic remission in all patient groups could be improved by intensification of the consolidation therapy by intermediate dose MTX. It could also be shown that the use of MTX and radiation therapy was effective for prevention of CNS leukemia.

References

1. Bleyer WA (1978) Cancer 41:36–43
2. Freeman AI, Brecher ML, Wang JJ, Sinks LF (1979) In: Neth R (ed) Modern trends in human leukemia III. New results in clinical and biologic research. Springer, Berlin Heidelberg New York. Blut [Suppl] 23:115–123
3. Haas RJ, Netzel B, Janka GE, Rodt H, Thiel R, Thierfelder S (1978). Klin Paediatr 191: 446–452
4. Haas RJ, Janka GE, Netzel B, Helmig M (1981) Klin Paediatr 193:137–144
5. Haas RJ, Janka GE, Gaedicke G, Kohne E, Netzel B (1983). Blut 47:321–331
6. Henze G, Langermann HJ, Brämswig J, Breu H, Gadner H, Schellong G, Welte K, Riehm H (1981) Klin Paediatr 193:145–154
7. Lobel JS, O'Brien RT, Mc Intosh S, Aspnes GT, Gapizzi RL (1979) Cancer 43:1089–1094
8. Netzel B, Rodt H, Thiel E, Haas RJ, Thierfelder S (1979) Acta Haematol 61:177–183

Haematology and Blood Transfusion Vol. 29
Modern Trends in Human Leukemia VI
Edited by Neth, Gallo, Greaves, Janka

Recent Results from Total Therapy Study X for Standard and High Risk Acute Lymphoblastic Leukemia in Children: Recognition of New Clinical and Biologic Risk Features*

S. B. Murphy, G. V. Dahl, A. T. Look, J. Ochs, M. Abromowitch, C.-H. Pui, W. P. Bowman, J. V. Simone, D. K. Kalwinsky, W. E. Evans, S. George, J. Mirro, D. Williams, L. Dow, and G. Rivera

A. Introduction

The initiation of Total Therapy Study X in 1979 marked important new directions for leukemia studies at St. Jude, since for the first time treatment for standard and high risk forms of lymphoblastic leukemia differed radically. Furthermore, recognizing the heterogeneity of childhood ALL, the blast cell characteristics of each new patient were prospectively investigated by standard methods [1–3], and the independent impact of various clinical and biologic features on the outcome of therapy was thoroughly investigated. This report will present highlights of our recent results.

B. Total Therapy X: Study Design

For purposes of protocol assignment, children with ALL were defined as high risk if they possessed any of the following features at diagnosis: white blood cell count greater than 100 000/mm^3, a mediastinal mass, lymphoblasts forming spontaneous rosettes with sheep erythrocytes (E+), and/or central nervous system disease. Children lacking these features were standard risk. Using these criteria, approximately 20% of our childhood ALL population is classified as high risk, and the remaining 80% are standard risk.

The background and rationale, specific drug schedules and dosages, and preliminary results of Total Therapy Study X for standard risk (X-S) and high risk patients (X-H) have been presented in detail elsewhere [4, 5]. Briefly, Total Therapy X-S asked the following questions: (a) can the hematologic relapse rate in standard risk ALL be reduced by periodic intravenous (i.v.) infusions of methotrexate or by a sequence of drug pairs during continuation therapy; and (b) can central nervous system relapse be adequately prevented by alternative treatments, rather than the standard 2400 rad cranial irradiation and intrathecal (i.t.) methotrexate early in remission? After remission induction with prednisone, vincristine, and asparaginase, standard risk patients were randomized into two groups: (a) IVIT, i.e., methotrexate (1000 mg/m^2) in 24-h i.v. infusions, plus i.t. methotrexate, weekly ×3, followed by a standard backbone of oral daily mercaptopurine and weekly methotrexate maintenance for 120 weeks, interrupted every 6 weeks for the first year for an i.v. MTX infusion with coordinated intermittent i.t. MTX treatments; and (b) RTSC, i.e., cranial irradiation (1800 rad) plus i.t. methotrexate, followed by rotational sequential combination drug pairs for the first year of maintenance, with methotrexate plus mercaptopurine (weeks 1–36), cyclophosphamide and adriamycin (weeks 36–54), VM-26 and Ara-C (weeks 54–72), followed by an additional standard year of oral mercaptopurine and methotrexate (weeks 72–120).

---

* Leukemia Division, Hematology/Oncology Department and the Pharmacokinetics and Pharmacodynamics Section, Pharmaceutical Division, and the Pathology Department, St. Jude Children's Research Hospital, USA

Study X-H examines the efficacy of early and intermittent treatment with a new drug pair, VM-26 and Ara-C, questioning whether or not the high risk for relapse could be reduced by use of this drug combination, superimposed on an otherwise standard antileukemia regimen. Treatment begins with VM-26 (165 mg/m^2) plus Ara-C (300 mg/m^2) twice weekly for 2 weeks, followed by prednisone, vincristine, and asparaginase at standard doses for 4 weeks. Following this early therapy, an additional 2-week consolidation phase of VM-26 and Ara-C at the same dosages and on the same schedule preceded continuation therapy with daily mercaptopurine and weekly methotrexate, both administered orally for 30 months. In addition, 2-week reinforcement pulses of VM-26 and Ara-C are given every 8 weeks for the first 12 months. Central nervous system prophylaxis is by means of intermittent intrathecal methotrexate during the first year of therapy, following which patients in remission receive cranial irradiation (2400 rad).

C. Results

From June 1979 until the end of 1983, 330 children with standard risk ALL entered Total X-S, and 94% achieved a complete remission in 4 weeks. Subsequently, 154 were randomized to the IVIT methotrexate arm of continuation therapy, and 155 were randomized to receive the rotational combination drug treatment, RTSC. During the same period, 101 children with high risk presentations of ALL entered Total X-H, and 84% achieved remission.

The results to date, as of May 1984, with a median follow-up of 2 years, are statistically superior to our institutional historical experience with comparable standard and high risk patients treated on Total Therapy Studies VIII and IX. The added benefit of the addition of VM-26 and Ara-C to the antileukemic management of high risk ALL patients is particularly apparent, as approximately 50% of patients continue in their first complete remission for 2–3 years following diagnosis. Protection against central nervous system relapse in the group of children on X-S receiving 1800 rad cranial irradiation, plus intrathecal methotrexate (RTSC group) has been adequate and better than the IVIT group, though there is at present a slight superiority in the proportion of patients in continuous complete remission on the IVIT arm of X-S. Whether IVIT methotrexate therapy prevents or merely delays relapse and/or whether it is an acceptable alternative for CNS prevention for children with good prognostic features (for example WBC less than 10 000) will require longer follow-up. Faster rates of systemic methotrexate clearance following i.v. MTX treatment have also been identified as a factor associated with a higher probability of early relapse [6], underscoring a need for further study of interindividual variability in pharmacodynamics as a critical determinant of end results of leukemia trials.

D. Risk Analysis: Recognition of New Factors

In addition to the clinical features of well-established prognostic importance in childhood ALL, such as age and initial circulating white cell count, our studies have revealed new biologic features which have independent prognostic impact on the outcome of therapy in Total X. We have found the most important biologic variables determining the outcome of therapy for ALL to be related to the genetic characteristics of the leukemic clone, as revealed both by the study of the karyotype and by determination of the degree of aneuploidy as measured by the flow cytometric determination of the DNA index ([1, 2, 7] and Williams et al. in preparation). The DNA index (DI), i.e., the ratio of the DNA content of leukemic versus normal G_0/G_1 cells, ranges from 1.06 to 2.0, median 1.2. In our experience, children with a DI > 1.16 have significantly better responses to treatment on Total X-S than do those with either a diploid or pseudodiploid DNA content (DI = 1) or those in the intermediate range, DI = 1.01–1.15. Such cases with DI > 1.16 correspond to those with > 53 chromosomes in the leukemic stem line, a correlation which accounts for the good prognosis associated with this ploidy group,

Table 1. Pretreatment risk assessment for ALL cases assigned to Total Therapy study XI

Risk factor[a]	Unfavorable characteristics
DNA index	≦1.15
Cytogenetics	Pseudodiploid or translocation present
Race	Nonwhite
White blood cell count	≧25 000/mm³
Age	<2 or >10 years

[a] Better risk patients are defined as possessing either none or only one unfavorable characteristic at diagnosis. Worse risk cases are defined as having two or more unfavorable features

as previously reported by us and noted by the Third International Workshop of Chromosomes in Leukemia [8]. Cases with hyperdiploid cellular DNA content (DI > 1.16) are also associated with the favorable age range of 2–9 years and with blast cell surface expression of the common ALL antigen. Though flow cytometry has definite advantages over conventional karyotyping for the detection of hyperdiploid ALL cases, cases with 44–48 chromosomes can not reliably be distinguished from diploid; and, of course, flow cytometric analysis does not detect the presence of structural chromosome abnormalities such as balanced translocations, since the net DNA content is unaffected. Karyotypic translocations are an important and unfavorable prognostic feature with an independent adverse impact on outcome, even after adjustment for white blood cell count, age, and other features of conventional prognostic significance. Translocations have not been observed in our experience in ALL cases with more than 50 chromosomes. The techniques of flow cytometry for analysis of cellular DNA content and karyotype analysis for detection of structural chromosome abnormalities in leukemic cell populations are thus complementary techniques, desirable in the study of every newly diagnosed case of ALL, and helpful for risk assessment in treatment stratification. Indeed, in our new front-line treatment protocol for children with ALL (Total Therapy Study XI), we have incorporated both the cytogenetic analysis and the DNA index, along with initial white blood cell count, age and race, into a newly devised pretreatment risk assignment (Table 1) based on the multivariate analysis of our experience in Total Therapy Study X.

Acknowledgments. The authors gratefully acknowledge the contributions of M. Crone, D. Givens, P. Roberson, C. H. Chen, and J. Harber of the Biostatistics Division, the dedicated assistance of the nursing staff and nurse practitioners, and the expert technical skills of our research technicians. This work was supported by NIH grants CA 20180 and CA 21765, and by ALSAC.

References

1. Williams DL, Tsiatis A, Brodeur GM, Look AT, Melvin SL, Bowman WP, Kalwinsky DK, Rivera G, Dahl GV (1982) Prognostic importance of chromosome number in 136 untreated children with acute lymphoblastic leukemia. Blood 60:864–871
2. Look AT, Melvin SL, Williams DL, Brodeur GM, Dahl GV, Kalwinsky DK, Murphy SB, Mauer AM (1982) Aneuploidy and percentage of S-phase cells determined by flow cytometry correlate with cell phenotype in childhood acute leukemia. Blood 60:959–967
3. Melvin SL (1981) Immunologic definition of leukemic cell surface phenotypes. Cancer Res 41:4790–4793
4. Bowman WP, Ochs J, Pui C-H, Kalwinsky DK, Abromowitch M, Aur RJA, Rivera G, Simone JV (1983) New directions of St. Jude total therapy protocols: study X for standard risk childhood acute lymphoblastic leukemia. In: Murphy SB, Gilbert JR (eds) Leukemia research: advances in cell biology and treatment. Elsevier, Amsterdam, pp 203–211
5. Rivera G, Dahl GV, Murphy SB, Bowman WP, Abromowitch M, Ochs J, Pui C-H, Kalwinsky DK, Avery TL, George SL, Simone JV (1983) The epipodophyllotoxin VM-26 in treatment of high risk acute lymphoblastic leukemia: rationale and early results. In: Murphy SB, Gilbert JR (eds) Leukemia research: advances in cell biology and treatment. Elsevier, Amsterdam, pp 213–220
6. Evans WE, Crom WR, Stewart CS, Bowman WP, Chen C-H, Abromowitch M, Simone JV (1984) Evidence that methotrexate systemic

clearance influences the probability of relapse in children with standard risk acute lymphocytic leukemia. Lancet 1:359–362
7. Look AT, Roberson PK, Williams DL, Rivera G, Bowman WP, Pui C-H, Ochs J, Abromowitch M, Kalwinsky D, Dahl GV, George S, Murphy SB (1985) Prognostic importance of blast cell DNA content in childhood acute lymphoblastic leukemia. Blood, in press
8. Third International Workshop of Chromosomes in Leukemia (1980) Clinical significance of chromosomal abnormalities in acute lymphoblastic leukemia. Cancer Genet Cytogenet 4:96–99

Haematology and Blood Transfusion Vol. 29
Modern Trends in Human Leukemia VI
Edited by Neth, Gallo, Greaves, Janka

Improved Treatment Results in Childhood Acute Myelogenous Leukemia: An Update of the German Cooperative Study AML-BFM-78 *

J. Ritter, U. Creutzig, H. J. Riehm, W. Brandeis, V. Gerein, G. Prindull, M. Rister and G. Schellong

A. Introduction

Major progress in the treatment of children with acute myelogenous leukemia has occurred in the past decade. Advances in chemotherapy and supportive care have been associated with an increase in the complete remission (CR) rate, and more important, an increase in the duration of first remission [1, 5]. In addition, bone marrow transplantation in first remission may provide a new approach for a selected group of patients to improve further on treatment results for AML [3, 4]. In 1978 the AML-BFM-78 chemotherapy protocol was initiated by the German cooperative group with encouraging early results [1, 2]. This report is an update of the trial.

B. Patients and Methods

A total of 151 children with AML from 30 German pediatric centers entered the cooperative study AML-BFM-78 between December 1978 and October 1982. Induction therapy consisted of vincristine, adriamycin, prednisone, cytosine arabinoside (Ara-C) and 6-thioguanine for the first 4 weeks. After a treatment-free interval of 1–2 weeks, a combination of cyclophosphamide, Ara-C, 6-thioguanine, and adriamycin was administered for an additional 4 weeks, together with CNS prophylaxis consisting of four intrathecal methotrexate injections and cranial irradiation. For remission maintenance, daily 6-thioguanine was given together with monthly cycles of subcutaneous Ara-C for 4 days. In the first year, patients also received one dose of adriamycin every 8 weeks. In children with CCR, maintenance was stopped after 2 years [1].

The diagnosis AML was based upon the morphological and cytochemical criteria of the FAB classification. Patients who failed to achieve CR after the induction regimen were classified as nonresponders. Relapse was diagnosed on appearance of more than 5% of blasts in the bone marrow or of leukemic cells at any other site. Methods of statistical analysis were the life table method according to the Kaplan-Meier and Cox regression model. Date of analysis was 1 May 1984.

C. Results

In all, 119 (79%) children achieved CR. After a median follow-up time of 40 (17–62) months, 52 relapses have occurred. Two late relapses occurred after 40 and 58 months, whereas all the other relapses were within the first 30 months. The results for the major morphological subtypes according to the FAB classification are given in Table 1. Life table analysis – influenced by the two late relapses – reveals a probability for remaining in CR of 42% ± 10% at 62 months for patients having achieved CR and of 31 ± 7% for all patients entered into the trial. No risk factors for relapse could be identified so far, whereas early fatal hemorrhage occurred predominantly in

* Univ.-Kinderklinik Münster, Abt. Hämatologie/Onkologie, Albert-Schweitzer-Str. 33, 4400 Münster, FRG

Table 1. AML-BFM-78 results by morphological subtypes

	M1	M2	M3	M4	M5	M6	All patients
Patients	36	34	6	40	32	3	151
Early deaths	3	0	3	4	9	0	19
Nonresponders	4	1	0	5	3	0	13
Complete remission	29 (80%)	33 (97%)	3	31 (77%)	20 (62%)	3	119
Relapses	10	17	0	16	6	3	52

children with the M5 subtype and in children with initially high WBC. An initially high WBC and liver enlargement were unfavorable parameters for achieving CR.

D. Discussion and Conclusions

The update of the German AML-BFM-78 study reveals:

1. A prolonged intensive induction therapy produces a high proportion of remissions in childhood AML and, in combination with maintenance therapy over a period of 2 years, an estimated CCR rate of 42% after more than 5 years.

2. Late relapses may occur after intensive induction therapy, even after 60 months of CR, further follow-up of the trial is needed before definite conclusions can be drawn.

3. The number of children achieving CR is relatively low in the monocytic subtypes M4 and M5; the number of early deaths, mainly because of early fatal hemorrhage was highest in the M5 subgroup.

4. The localization of relapses is markedly different in this study as compared with the VAPA-10 study from Boston: in the BFM study, the CNS was involved in 8/52 relapses, whereas in the VAPA-10 study, where CNS prophylaxis was not included in the treatment, the CNS was a primary site of relapse in 8/19 [6]. In our study most relapses occurred in the bone marrow.

5. Based on these findings, a new trial of the BFM group was started in 1983 with an initial intensive 8-day chemotherapy consisting of Ara-C, VP-16,213, and daunorubicin. After recovery of the bone marrow, a slight modification of the BFM-78 remission induction protocol is given as consolidation therapy. So far, 66 patients have entered this protocol, the CR rate being 85%.

6. The results of the AML-BFM-78 trial emphasize the probability of cure for a significant proportion of children with AML as a consequence of intensive remission induction and postremission multidrug treatment.

References

1. Creutzig U, Ritter J, Langermann HJ, Riehm H, Henze G, Niethammer D, Jürgens H, Stollmann B, Lasson U, Kabisch H, Wahlen W, Löffler H, Schellong G (1983) Akute myeloische Leukämie bei Kindern: Ergebnisse der kooperativen Therapiestudie BFM-78 nach 3¾ Jahren. Klin Paediatr 196:152–160
2. Creutzig U, Schellong G, Ritter J, Sutor AH, Riehm H, Langermann HJ, Jobke A, Kabisch H (1983) Improved results in treatment of acute myelogenous leukemia in children – Report of the German cooperative AML study BFM-78. In: Neth R, Gallo RC, Greaves MF, Moore MAS, Winkler K (eds) Modern trends in human leukaemia 5. Springer, Berlin Heidelberg, p 36 (Haematology and Blood Transfusion, vol 28)
3. Gale RP, Kay HEM, Rimm AA, Bortin MM (1982) Bone marrow transplantation for acute leukaemia in first remission. Lancet 2:1006–1009
4. Thomas ED, Clift RA, Buckner CD (1982) Marrow transplantation for patients with acute nonlymphoblastic leukemia who achieve a first remission. Cancer Treat Rep 66:1463–1466
5. Weinstein HJ, Mayer RJ, Rosenthal DS, Camitta BM, Coral FS, Nathan DG, Frei E III (1980) Treatment of acute myelogenous leukemia in children and adults. N Engl J Med 303:474–478
6. Weinstein HJ, Mayer RJ, Rosenthal DS, Coral FS, Camitta BM, Gelber RD (1983) Chemotherapy for acute myelogenous leukemia in children and adults: VAPA update. Blood 62:315–319

Haematology and Blood Transfusion Vol. 29
Modern Trends in Human Leukemia VI
Edited by Neth, Gallo, Greaves, Janka

Clinical Experiences with a Modified BFM Protocol in Childhood Acute Lymphoblastic Leukemia *

F. Zintl, H. Malke, and W. Plenert

A. Introduction

The most important problem in current therapy of childhood acute lymphoblastic leukemia (ALL) is a failure in over one-half of patients. We were unable to increase the failure-free survival of children with high risk ALL by a ten-drug regimen (modified LSA_2L_2) above 30% at 6 years [1].

The results of the West Berlin therapy study between 1970 and 1976 confirmed the hypothesis that intensification and prolongation of remission induction produce a higher percentage of disease-free long-term survivors [2]. We decided in 1981 to adopt a modified BFM protocol for ALL therapy in our group [3]. This paper presents preliminary results of this multicenter randomized study.

B. Materials and Methods

I. Patients

A total of 208 consecutive, previously untreated children with ALL were entered in-

* Universitäts-Kinderklinik Jena, Abt. Hämatologie/Onkologie/Immunologie, Kochstraße 2, 6900 Jena, GDR

Table 1. Characteristics of patients in the study

Characteristics	Total		SR		MR		HR	
	N	(%)	*N*	(%)	*N*	(%)	*N*	(%)
Patients	208	100	133	100	60	100	15	100
Median age at diagnosis (years)	5	3/12	5	1/12	5	3/12	9	10/12
2 years	13	6	5	4	5	8	3	20
10 years	49	24	31	23	12	20	6	40
Boys	111	53	79	59	23	38	9	60
Median age at diagnosis (years)	5	10/12	5	5/12	5	4/12	11	0/12
Girls	97	47	54	41	37	62	6	40
Medianage at diagnosis (years)	4	9/12	4	10/12	5	2/12	3	10/12
Leukocytes 25 000/mm³	55	26	11	8	34	57	10	67
50 000/mm³	32	15	2	2	20	33	10	67
100 000/mm³	16	8		0	7	12	9	60
CNS involvement	9	4	5	4	2	3	2	14
Mediastinal mass	17	8	10	7	2	3	5	33
Liver 5 cm	67	32	15	11	37	62	15	100
Spleen 5 cm	57	27	9	7	33	55	15	100
Acid phosphatase positive	46	22	26	20	15	25	5	33

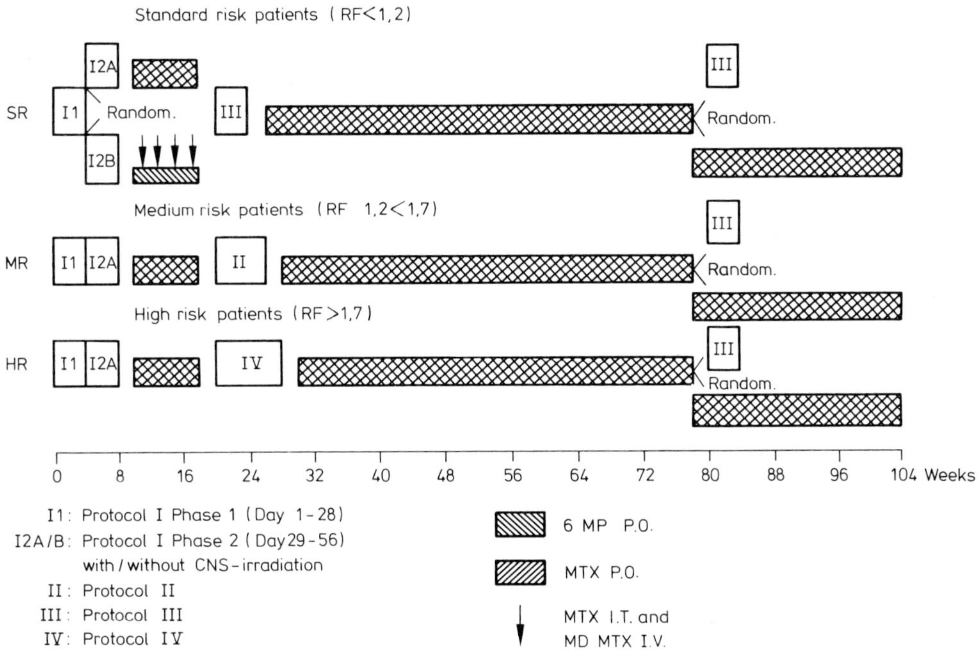

Fig. 1. Schedule for the modified BFM-protocol (ALL study VII/81)

to the study (VII/81) between September 1981 and March 1984. Patients' characteristics are given in Table 1. Patients were divided into three risk groups according to the initial leukocyte count and liver and spleen enlargement: standard (SR), medium (MR), and high risk (HR) groups [4].

II. Treatment

The treatment comprises induction therapy with CNS prophylaxis, reinduction therapy, and continuous maintenance therapy (Figs. 1–5). The induction protocol I, con-

Fig. 2. Outline for the induction protocol

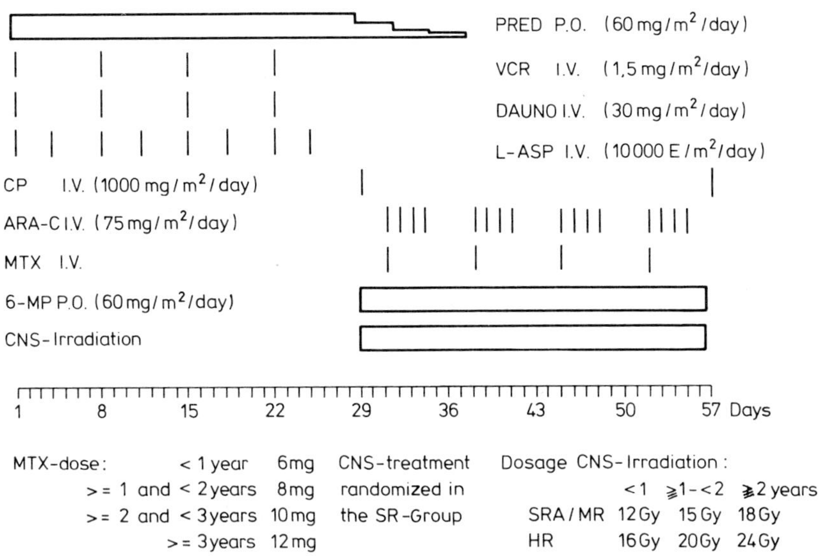

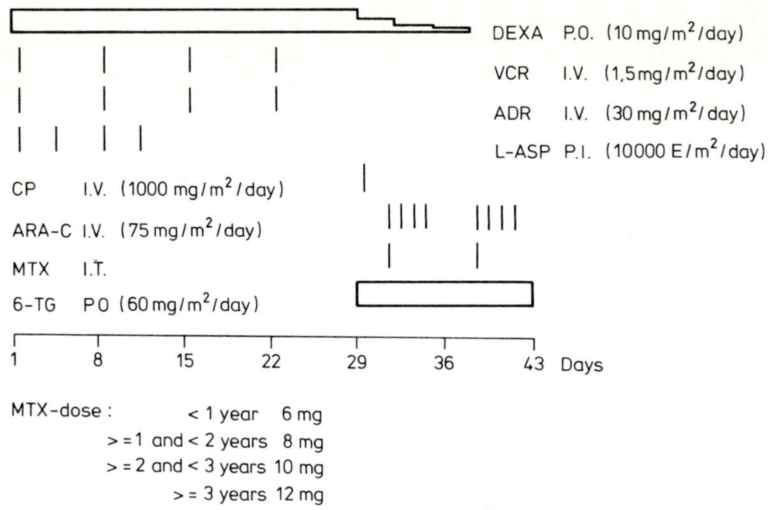

Fig. 3. Outline for the reinduction protocol II (MR patients)

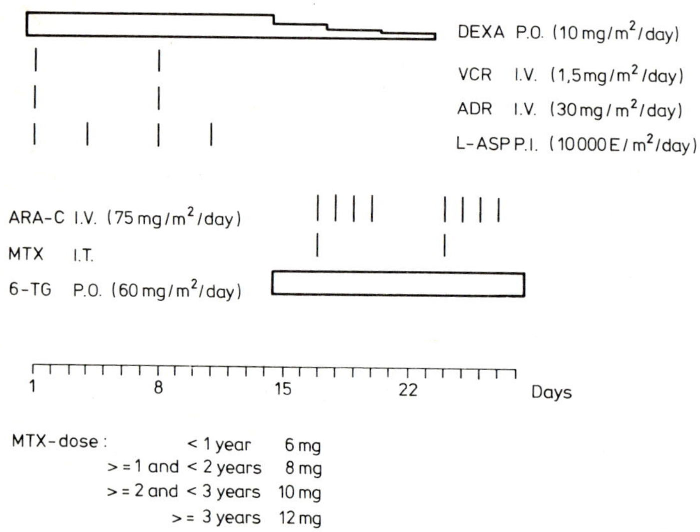

Fig. 4. Outline for the reinduction protocol III (SR patients)

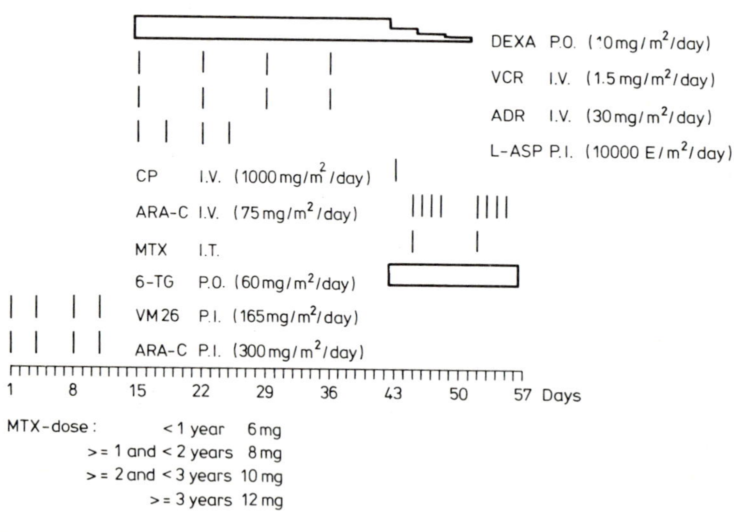

Fig. 5. Outline for the reinduction protocol IV (HR patients)

sisting of two phases, was identical for each risk group. The reinforced reinduction protocols were risk adjusted: protocol III for SR, protocol II for MR, and protocol IV for HR patients. For prophylactic CNS therapy in the SR group, patients were randomized to receive cranial irradiation and intrathecal methotrexate (MTX) or medium dose methotrexate (500 mg/m²) and intrathecal methotrexate (Fig. 1). For the duration of maintenance therapy, patients were randomized after 78 weeks to receive MTX and 6-MP for another 6 months or protocol III. The induction therapy of the BFM scheme was modified by reducing L-asparaginase in dose and duration. The reinduction with protocol III before stopping therapy was the second modification to the BFM protocol.

III. Statistical Analysis

Complete remission (CR) was defined as less than 5% bone marrow and no evidence of extramedullary leukemia. Kaplan-Meier analysis were performed for survival and continuous CR. Failure is defined as induction failure, initial relapse at any site, death during induction, or death during initial CR.

C. Results

Preliminary results are summarized in Table 2. It was found that 93% of patients attained CR after 4 weeks of therapy. The cumulative proportion in continuous CR is 0.77 ± 0.04 for the total group of 195 patients (Fig. 6). No significant difference was found between the treatment groups SR (0.83 ± 0.04) and MR (0.78 ± 0.07) (Fig. 7). Of 14 HR patients, 11 (79%) attained CR. One died in CR and four relapsed (three bone marrow relapses, one CNS relapse). Thus, the proportion in continuous CR was 0.19 ± 0.16. Of the total number of children, 12 relapsed. Eight patients had isolated marrow relapse. Isolated CNS relapses occurred in two children. One patient had a simultaneous marrow and CNS relapse and one patient had an isolated relapse in the eye. Patients with

Table 2. Summary of results

Results of therapy (0–30 months)	Total		SR		MR		HR	
	N	(%)	*N*	(%)	*N*	(%)	*N*	(%)
Patients	195	100	124	100	57	100	14	100
Not yet in remission	13		9		3		1	
Early deaths	9	5	5	4	1	2	3	21
Deaths in initial stage	5	3	3	3	2	4	0	
Complete remission	181	93	116	94	54	95	11	79
Deaths in remission	8	4	5	4	2	4	1	7
Relapses	12	6	4	3	4	7	4	29
BM	8	4	2	2	3	5	3	21
CNS	2	1	1	1	–	–	1	7
BM+CNS	1	1	–	–	1	2	–	–
Testes	–	–	–	–	–	–	–	–
Others (eye)	1	1	1	1	–	–	–	–
In first remission	161	82	107	86	48	84	6	43
Alive	168	86	109	88	50	88	9	64
Proportion in continuous complete remission	0.77±0.04		0.83±0.04		0.78±0.07		0.19±0.16	
Median time of remission (months)	12		12		12		12	

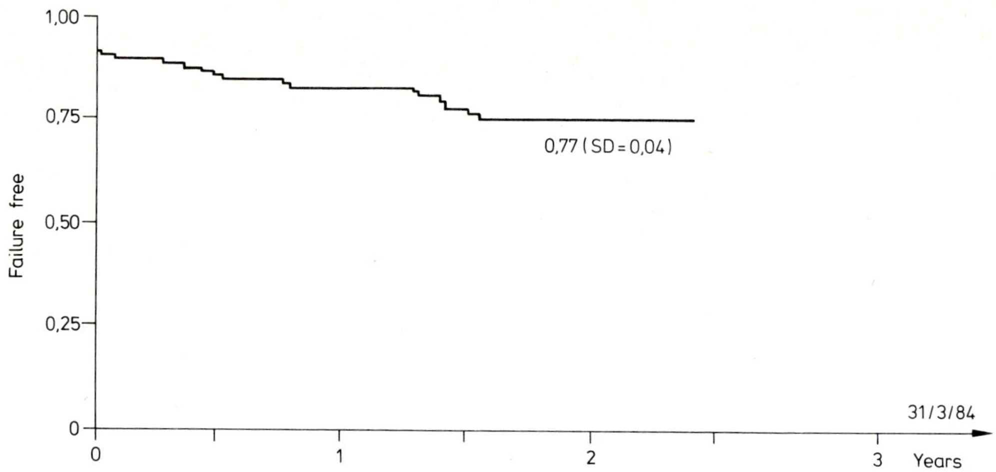

Fig. 6. Probability of continuous complete remission (195 patients, 161 in continous complete remission). Failure = end of remission by relapse or death for any reason

initial WBC above 50 Gpt/l did worse than those who had WBC below 150 Gpt/l (Fig. 8). There were no significant differences in failure-free survival in SR and MR patients with WBC greater or less than 125 Gpt/l. Within the groups of SR and MR patients, mediastinal mass was not significantly related to outcome. The differences over the total group for the parameters thymic involvement and age are closely related to high WBC in HR patients.

Fig. 7. Difference in the duration of continous complete remission (CCR) of the three risk groups. *Dotted line* standard risk (124 patients, 107 in CCR); *full line* medium risk (57 patients, 48 in CCR); *dashed line* high risk (14 patients, 6 in CCR)

D. Discussion

Kaplan-Meier life table analysis of failure-free survival data for 195 patients with ALL of different risk estimates that 77% ± 8% of patients will be in continuous CR 30 months after diagnosis. Although the median time of remission in our study is just 12 months, these results represent a marked improvement compared with former studies. Our results support the hypothesis of

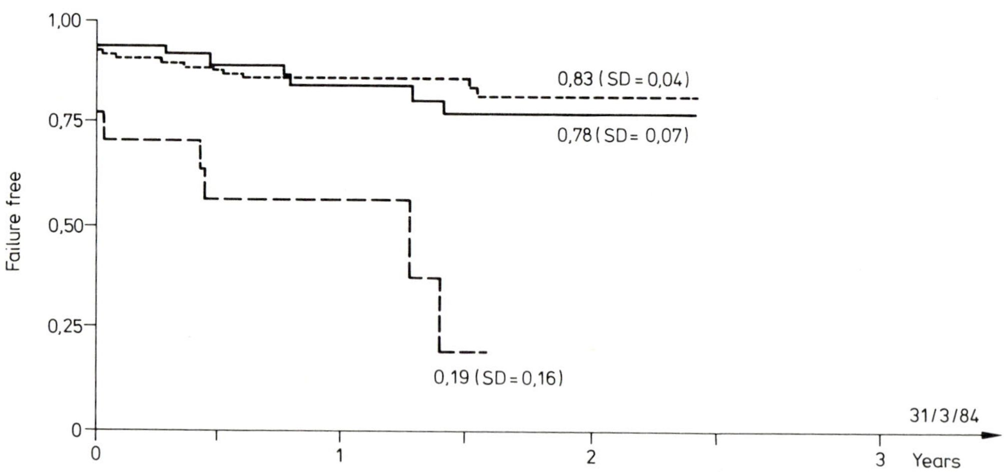

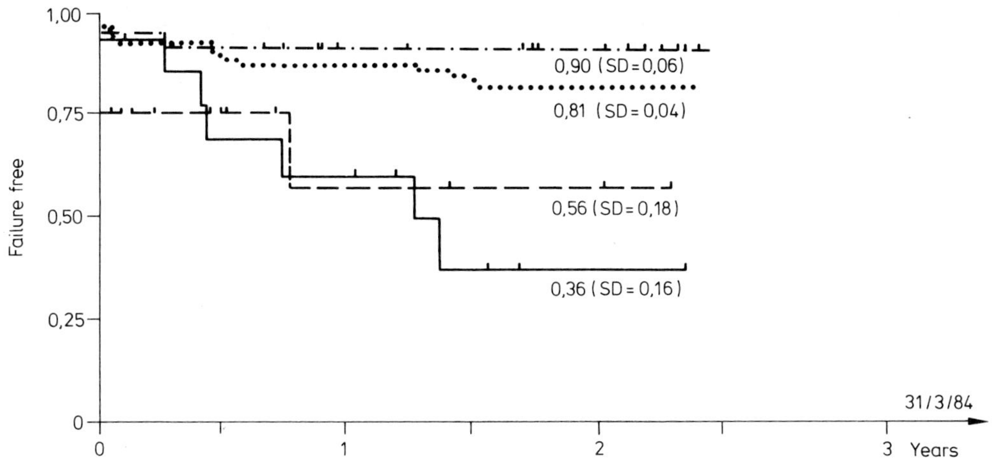

Fig. 8. Probability of continuous complete remission (CCR) in patients with different initial white blood cell counts. *Dotted line* <25 Gpt/l (142 patients, 122 in CCR); *dashed-dotted line* 25–50 Gpt/l (22 patients, 18 in CCR); *dashed line* 50–100 Gpt/l (16 patients, 11 in CCR); *full line* >100 Gpt/l (15 patients, 8 in CCR)

the BFM group that intensification and prolongation of remission induction produce a higher percentage of disease-free long-term survivors [2, 5]. Patients in the HR group (risk factor > 1.7) did worse than those in the SR and MR groups. This is in marked contrast to the results reported by the BFM group [5].

References

1. Zintl F, Hermann J, Katenkamp D, Malke H, Plenert W (1983) Results of LSA_2L_2 therapy in children with high risk acute lymphoblastic leukemia and non-Hodgkin's lymphoma. In: Neth R, Gallo RC, Greaves MF, Moore MAS, Winkler K (eds) Modern trends in human leukemia, vol V. Springer, Berlin Heidelberg New York Tokyo, pp 62–66
2. Riehm H, Gadner H, Henze G, Langermann HJ, Odenwald E (1980) The Berlin childhood acute lymphoblastic leukemia therapy study, 1970–1976. Am J Ped Hematol Oncol 2:299–306
3. Riehm H, Henze G, Langermann HJ (1981) Multizentrische Therapiestudie BFM 81 zur Behandlung der akuten lymphoblastischen Leukämie im Kindes- und Jugendalter. Studienprotokoll, 1981
4. Langermann HJ, Henze G, Wulf M, Riehm H (1982) Abschätzung der Tumorzellmasse bei der akuten lymphoblastischen Leukämie im Kindesalter: prognostische Bedeutung und praktische Anwendung. Klin Pädiatr 194:209–213
5. Henze G, Langermann HJ, Fengler R et al. (1982) Therapiestudie BFM 79/81 zur Behandlung der akuten lymphoblastischen Leukämie bei Kindern und Jugendlichen: intensivierte Reinduktionstherapie für Patientengruppen mit unterschiedlichem Rezidivrisiko. Klin Pädiatr 194: 195–203

Haematology and Blood Transfusion Vol. 29
Modern Trends in Human Leukemia VI
Edited by Neth, Gallo, Greaves, Janka

Mechanisms of Drug Resistance in Human Leukemia *

J. R. Bertino, S. Srimatkandada, M. D. Carman, E. Mini, M. Jastreboff, B. A. Moroson and S. K. Dube

A. Introduction

Drug resistance remains a major obstacle to cure of patients with acute leukemia. At the present time, most centers are reporting 90% complete remission rates in acute lymphatic leukemia (ALL) and 70%–80% complete remission rates in patients with acute nonlymphocytic leukemia (ANLL). However, 5-year disease-free survival rates are only 50% and 10%–15%, respectively, in these diseases. This is almost certainly due to the development of drug resistance even to the combination chemotherapy programs utilized to treat these diseases [1].

In this paper, we review the mechanisms by which cells become resistant to methotrexate (MTX) and strategies to eradicate selectively leukemic cells that have acquired resistance to the drug.

B. Mechanisms of Acquired Resistance to MTX

Methotrexate has been an excellent model drug for the study of acquired drug resistance. There is little metabolism of the drug intracellularly (except for polyglutamylation discussed below), the mechanism of action of the drug is well known [inhibition of the enzyme dihydrofolate reductase (DHFR)], and at least three and possibly four different causes of acquired resistance to this drug have been observed. In addition very sensitive assays for DHFR enzyme activity have been developed, as well as mouse and human cDNA probes to detect gene amplification by sensitive "dot-blot" techniques [2].

When cell lines or transplanted experimental tumors are exposed to MTX, and resistant cells emerge, resistance usually is due to one of two causes. These are either an increase in DHFR or a decreased uptake of MTX. Less commonly observed have been resistant sublines with an altered DHFR (reviewed in [4]) or a decrease in MTX polyglutamate formation [5].

C. Increased Levels of DHFR as a Cause of MTX Resistance Gene Amplification

Mouse, hamster, and human MTX-resistant cell lines have been described in recent years that have increased levels of DHFR (reviewed in [4]). When these lines have been examined with appropriate cDNA probes, in all cases gene amplification has been found to accompany the increase in DHFR level, as well as a corresponding increase in the level of mRNA(s) for this enzyme.

We have recently described three MTX-resistant sublines obtained from human cells propagated in continuous culture with an increased level of DHFR: a lymphoblastic leukemia line (CEM-CCRF) [6], a blast-cell line (K562) [7], and a colon cancer cell line (HCT 8) (J. R. Bertino, unpublished observation). In all of these circum-

* Departments of Pharmacology and Medicine, Yale University School of Medicine, New Haven, CT 06510, USA
Supported by Grants CA 08010 and CA 08341

Table 1. Dihydrofolate reductase activity and gene amplification in human cell lines resistant to MTX

Cell line	DHFR enzyme increase (fold)	DHFR gene copy increase (fold)
CEM-CCRF (R_1)	20	18
K-562/MTX	200	200
HCT-8 (R_1)	50	40

stances, the increased level of DHFR was found to be associated with an increased level of DHFR gene copies (Table 1). Of interest is that two of these lines, CEM-CCRF/R and HCT-8/R, when exposed to continued increased levels of MTX developed an additional transport defect for MTX or an altered DHFR, respectively (see below), presumably as a second mutational event in one of the amplified DHFR genes. When the chromosomes of these sublines with increased levels of DHFR were examined, the K562/MTX line showed a clearly demonstrable abnormal or homogeneous staining region (HSR) [7]. This cell line has three HSRs not found in the parent subline that have been identified as modified chromosomes # 5, 6, and 19. This subline has remained stably resistant even in the absence of MTX for a period of 6 months. In general, this finding is in accord with previous reports that sublines resistant to MTX with a high level of stable resistance demonstrate a HSR, while cell lines with unstable resistance are associated with an increase in "double minute" chromosomes, i.e., small paired chromosomal bodies lacking a centromere [8].

The location of the unique DHFR gene in human cells has been reported to be on the # 5 chromosome [9]: of interest is that another Burkitt's human cell line resistant to MTX was found also to have a large HSR in the # 5 chromosome. However, another report of a KB human cell line also highly resistant to MTX contained an HSR in the # 10 chromosome [10]. In situ hybridization with a human cDNA probe has not yet been reported with any of these cell lines, so it is likely, although unproven, that these HSRs are the site of the amplified DHFR genes.

The human DHFR gene [7, 11, 12] has been reported to be very large (ca. 30 kb), similar to the size reported for the mouse gene [13]. The availability of both mouse and human cDNA probes has allowed us to demonstrate that there is a significant sequence diversity in the noncoding 3′ end of the gene [7]. Chen et al. [12] and Masters et al. [11] have shown the presence in human DNAs of intronless DHFR genes or pseudogenes, which are nonfunctional [12]. Apparently these pseudogenes are not amplified in resistant cells; therefore they are easily missed in Southern blots from resistant-cell lines [12].

D. Gene Amplification as a General Mechanism of Resistance to Anticancer Drugs

Since the initial description of gene amplification as the mechanism by which mammalian cells become resistant to MTX, there have been several examples of gene amplification in cell lines resistant to other drugs (Table 2). Thus, it has become evident that this is a mechanism by which cells can increase the production of a target enzyme or receptor, thus resulting in a drug-resistant phenotype. Although not demonstrated conclusively as yet, the multidrug-resistant phenotype (cross-resistance to several natural product anticancer agents when resistance is developed to only one) may also be due to gene amplification.

E. Gene Amplification in Patients with Leukemia Resistant to MTX

Although gene amplification is commonly observed in MTX-resistant sublines, it was important to demonstrate that this event occurs in patients developing resistance to this drug. It was expected that a low level of amplification would be sufficient to cause MTX resistance, since the dose of MTX that can be safely administered is limited by toxic effects on normal tissues. In the three patients reported (two leukemia [2, 3] and one small-cell lung car-

Table 2. Examples of gene amplification in drug-resistant sublines

Drug	Target enzyme or receptor increased	Gene amplification	Ref.
MTX	Dihydrofolate reductase	Yes	[16]
PALA	Aspartate transcarbamylase	Yes	[17]
Ca^{2+}	Metallothionein	Yes	[18]
Albizzin	Asparaginase synthase	Yes	[19]
5-Fluorodeoxyuridine	Thymidylate synthase	(?)	[20]
Hydroxyurea	Ribonucleotide reductase	(?)	[21]
Deoxycoformycin	Adenosine deaminase	Yes	[22]
Colchicine (actinomycin D, vinblastine, anthracyclines)	Membrane protein (GP-170)	(?)	[23]

cinoma [22]), MTX resistance was found to be due to a low level of gene amplification (two- to fourfold). We are presently examining cells from additional leukemia patients thought to be clinically resistant to MTX in order to determine the frequency of this event as a mechanism of drug resistance to MTX. This will be of importance in regards to alternative treatment strategies (discussed below). We have found a rapid screening test for MTX resistance useful in determining whether resistance to MTX is present ([^{3}H]deoxyuridine incorporation into DNA in the absence and presence of MTX [23]).

F. Altered DHFR as a Mechanism for MTX Resistance

In experimental sublines propagated in vitro or in vivo, alteration of DHFR as a cause of MTX resistance is less commonly observed than is impaired transport or elevated DHFR [24]. Several lines have been reported, however, with altered DHFR enzymes, and one gene has been cloned, and the cDNA sequenced [25]. Table 3 lists the lines that have been described, and the alteration of enzyme activity observed in regards to MTX affinity. It should be pointed out, however, that most of these lines contain normal as well as altered genes, and unless the two enzymes are separated completely, the MTX-binding data may be misleading. We have recently obtained a cell line with an altered DHFR from the HCT-8/R line that also contained an elevated normal DHFR. This line contains an enzyme with a relatively high V_{max} as compared with the 3T6 MTX-resistant line. Thus we believe that a mutation at a different site(s) has occurred, as compared with the 3T6 mutation. Since it is believed that some 13 amino acids are involved in MTX binding to DHFR [26], it is possible that mutations affecting any of these binding sites may produce an altered DHFR.

Table 3. Examples of altered mammalian DHFR enzymes from MTX-resistant cells

Source	Decrease of MTX/binding to MTX (fold)	Ref.
CH0 (hamster)	4	[31]
L1210 (mouse)	10	[30]
W1-L2 (human)	50	[32]
3T6 (mouse)	270	[27]
HCT-8 (human)	100	J. R. Bertino, unpublished observation
L5178Y (mouse)	100,000	[29]

These altered DHFR sublines have been extremely valuable as drug-selectable genes for DNA transfection studies, in particular the cDNA from the 3T6 cell line that has been inserted into plasmid and retrovirus vectors [25, 27, 28].

G. MTX Resistance Due to Impaired Transport

Impaired MTX transport, like increased DHFR enzyme activity, has been noted to be a relatively common mechanism of resistance to this antifolate. In one study of drug resistance produced in vivo to cells in mice, impaired transport was as commonly noted as elevated DHFR as the cause of MTX resistance [24]. Little is known about the molecular nature of this resistance, which involves the carrier transport system present for the active transport for reduced folates (5-methyltetrahydrofolate, 5-formyl tetrahydrofolate). While this could also be an example of gene amplification, there was no cross-resistance to other antitumor agents noted when a CEM-CCRF transport mutant subline was tested [33]. Thus far, the mammalian transport system for reduced folates and MTX has not been isolated or characterized, but these resistant sublines may allow an approach to this problem.

H. Eradication of Drug-Resistant Cells

Although the probability of drug resistance occurring to MTX may be decreased with the use of drug combinations, this possibility is limited for the treatment of many human malignancies because of the lack of useful agents for treatment. Also, the addition of alkylating agents to combination regimens may increase the probability of mutations leading to MTX resistance in surviving cells. Of great potential importance is the recent work of Schimke et al., which suggests that gene amplification may be facilitated by agents that interrupt DNA synthesis early in S-phase [34]. Strategies to eradicate MTX-drug-resistant cells have been suggested by us as well as by others [35–38]. A general approach involves the use of high specific activity $[^3H]$deoxyuridine in the presence of MTX and hypoxanthine and thymidine [35]. This combination would be lethal for MTX-resistant cells, since MTX would not block $[^3H]$deoxyuridine incorporation into DNA, while in sensitive cells it would. This approach works in vitro, but will probably be impractical for in vivo use.

We have recently utilized a new inhibitor of DHFR, trimetrexate (TMQ) [39], to treat MTX-resistant cells [33]. Trimetrexate or other folate antagonists that accumulate in cells to high levels and do not use the folate transport system may be effective agents against MTX-resistant cells with impaired transport or low levels of DHFR gene amplification [33, 34]. Table 4 indicates that trimetrexate is highly effective in a MTX-transport-resistant CCRF-CEM cell line (R3); and more effective than MTX in a CCRF-CEM cell line, with a 20-fold increase in DHFR (R1). In the 3T6 cell line resistant to MTX because of an altered DHFR, trimetrexate also has a markedly decreased affinity for the enzyme and thus would be of no value in the treatment of cells resistant by this mechanism [27]. We are currently attempting to look for inhibitors that would be effective against cells with an altered DHFR; selective inhibition may be possible in this circumstance.

We are testing these strategies by employing combinations of antifolates that presumably would limit the emergence of drug-resistant cells, e.g., concomitant MTX and trimetrexate treatment versus sequential uses of these agents.

Table 4. Effect of MTX and TMQ on the parenteral CCRF-CEM lymphoblastic leukemia cell line and two resistant sublines. The CCRF-CEM/R_1 line has a 20-fold increase in DHFR activity, while the R_3 line has normal DHFR activity, but has a markedly impaired uptake of MTX [33]

Cell line	ED_{50}MTX (n*M*)	ED_{50}TMQ (n*M*)
CCRF-CEM (parent)	15	5
CCRF-CEM/R_1	1500	150
CCRF-CEM/R_3	3400	3

References

1. Gunz FW, Henderson ES (eds) (1983) Leukemia. Grune and Stratton, New York
2. Horns RC, Dower WJ, Schimke RT (1984) Gene amplification in a leukemia patient treated with methotrexate. J Clin Oncol 2:2–7
3. Carman MD, Schornagel JH, Rivest RS, Srimatkandada S, Portlock CS, Bertino JR (1984) Resistance to methotrexate due to gene amplification in a patient with acute leukemia. J Clin Oncol 2:16–20

4. Bertino JR, Srimatkandada S, Carman MD, Schornagel JH, Medina W, Moroson BA, Cashmore AR, Weiner HL, Dube SK (1983) Mechanism of methotrexate in acute leukemia. Normal and neoplastic hematopoiesis. Liss, New York, pp 465–478
5. Cowan KH, Jolivet J (1984) A methotrexate resistant human breast cancer cell line with multiple defects, including diminished formation of methotrexate polyglutamates. J Biol Chem 259:10 798–10 800
6. Mini E, Srimatkandada S, Medina WD, Moroson BA, Carman MD, Bertino JR (1985) Molecular and karyological analysis of methotrexate-resistant and sensitive human leukemic CCRF-CEM cells. Cancer Res. 45, 317–324
7. Srimatkandada S, Medina WD, Cashmore AR, Whyte W, Engel D, Moroson BA, Franco CT, Dube S, Bertino JR (1983) Amplification and organization of dihydrofolate reductase genes in a human leukemic cell line, K562, resistant to methotrexate. Biochemistry 22:5774–5781
8. Kaufman RJ, Brown PC, Schimke RT (1979) Amplified dihydrofolate reductase genes in unstably methotrexate-resistant cells are associated with double minute chromosomes. Proc Nat Acad Sci USA 76:5669–5673
9. Anagou NP, O'Brien SJ, Shimada T, Nash WG, Chen MJ, Nienhuis AW (1984) Chromosomal organization of the human dihydrofolate reductase genes: dispersion, selective amplification, and a novel form of polymorphism. Proc Natl Acad Sci USA 81:5170–5174
10. Wolman SR, Craven ML, Grill SP, Domin BA, Cheng Y-C (1983) Quantitative correlation of homogeneously stained regions on chromosome 10 with dihydrofolate reductase enzyme in human cells. Proc Natl Acad Sci USA 80:807–809
11. Masters JN, Yank JR, Celini A, Attardi GJ (1983) A human dihydrofolate reductase pseudogene and its relationship to the multiple forms of specific messenger RNA
12. Chen MJ, Shimada T, Moneton AD, Cline A, Humphries RK, Maizel J, Nienhuis AW (1984) The functional human dihydrofolate reductase gene. J Biol Chem 259:3933–3943
13. Crouse GF, Simonsen CC, McEwan RN, Schimke RT (1982) Structure of amplified normal and variant dihydrofolate reductase genes in mouse sarcoma S180 cells. J Biol Chem 257:7887–7898
14. Alt FW, Kellems RE, Bertino JR, Schimke RT (1978) Selective multiplication of dihydrofolate reductase genes in methotrexate-resistant variants of cultured murine cells. J Biol Chem 253:1357–1370
15. Wahl GM, Padgett RA, Stark GR (1979) Gene amplification causes overproduction of the first three enzymes of UMP synthesis in PALA *N*-(phosphoroacetyl)-L-asparate-resistant hamster cells. J Biol Chem 254:8679–8869
16. Beach LR, Palmiter RD (1981) Amplification of the metallothionein-I gene in cadmium-resistant mouse cells. Proc Natl Acad Sci USA 78:2110–2114
17. Anarulis IL, Duff C, Evans-Blacker S et al. (1983) Chromosomal alterations associated with overproduction of asparagine synthetase in Albizzin-resistant Chinese hamster ovary cells. Mol Cell Biol 3:391–398
18. Rossana C, Rao LG, Johnson LF (1982) Thymidylate synthetase overproduction in 5-fluorodeoxyuridine-resistant mouse fibroblasts. Mol Cell Biol 2:1031–1037
19. Lewis WH, Wright JA (1979) Isolation of hydroxyurea-resistant CHO cells with altered levels of ribonucleotide reductase. Somatic Cell Genet 5:83–96
20. Yeung C-Y, Ingolia DE, Bobonis C, Dunbar BS, Riser ME, Siciliano MJ, Kellems RE (1983) Selective overproduction of adenosine deaminase in cultured mouse cells. J Biol Chem 258:8338–8345
21. Riordan JR, Ling V (1979) Purification of P. glycoprotein from plasma membrane vesicles of Chinese hamster ovary cell mutants with reduced colchine permeability. J Biol Chem 254:12 701–12 705
22. Curt GA, Carney DN, Cowan KH, Jolivet J, Bailey BD, Drake JC, Kao-shan CS, Minna JD, Chabner BA (1983) N Engl J Med 308:199–202
23. Bertino JR, Skeel RT (1975) On natural and acquired resistance to folate antagonists in man. In: pharmacological basis of cancer chemotherapy. Williams and Wilkins, Baltimore, pp 681–689
24. Sirotnak FM, Moccio DM, Kelleher LE, Goutas LJ (1981) Relative frequency and kinetic properties of transport defective phenotypes among methotrexate-resistant L1210 clonal cells derived in vivo. Cancer Res 41:4447–4452
25. Simonsen CC, Levinson AD (1983) Isolation and expression of an altered mouse dihydrofolate reductase cDNA. Proc Natl Acad Sci USA 80:2495–2499
26. Vol KW, Matthews DA, Alden RA, Freer ST, Hansch C, Kaufman T, Kraut J, Crystal structure of avian dihydrofolate reductase containing phenyltriazine and NADPH. J Biol Chem 257:2528–2536
27. Haber DA, Beverly SM, Kiely ML, Schimke RT (1981) Properties of an altered dihydrofolate reductase encoded by amplified

genes in cultured mouse fibroblasts. J Biol Chem 256:9501–9510
28. Kaufman R, Sharp P (1982) Construction of a modular dihydrofolate reductase cDNA gene: analysis of signals utilized for efficient expression. Mol Cell Biol 2:1304–1309
29. Goldie JH, Krystal G, Hartley D, Gudauskas G, Dedhar S (1980) A methotrexate insensitive variant of folate reductase present in two lines of methotrexate-resistant L5178Y cells. Eur J Cancer 16:1539–1546
30. Duffy TH, Beckman SB, Huennekens FM (1984) Forms of L1210 dihydrofolate reductase differing in affinity for methotrexate. Fed Proc 43:3436 (abstract)
31. Flintoff WF, Essani K (1980) Methotrexate-resistant Chinese hamster ovary cells contain a dihydrofolate reductase with an altered affinity for methotrexate. Biochem J 19:4321–4327
32. Niethammer D, Jackson RC (1975) Changes of molecular properties associated with the development of resistance against methotrexate in human lymphoblastoid cells. Eur J Cancer 4:845–854
33. Mini E, Moroson BA, Franco CT, Bertino JR (1985) Cytotoxic effects of folate antagonists against methotrexate-resistant human leukemia lymphoblast CCRF-CEM cell lines. Cancer Res 45, 325–330
34. Kamen BA, Eibl B, Cashmore AR, Bertino JR (1984) Uptake and efficacy of trimetrexate, a non-classical antifolate in methotrexate-resistant leukemia cells in vitro. Biochem Pharmacol 33:1697–1699
35. Urlaub G, Landzberg M, Chasin LA (1981) Selective killing of methotrexate-resistant cells carrying amplified dihydrofolate reductase genes. Cancer Res 41:1594–1601
36. Bertino JR (1979) Toward improved selectivity in cancer chemotherapy: The Richard and Hinda Rosenthal Foundation Award Lecture. Cancer Res 39:293–304
37. Ryser HJ, Shen WC (1980) Conjugation of methotrexate to poly (l-lysine) as a potential way to overcome drug resistance. Cancer 45:1207–1211
38. Hill BT, Price LA, Harrison SI, Gredi JH (1977) The difference between "selective" folinic acid rescue in 5178Y cell culture. Eur J Cancer 13:861–871
39. Bertino JR, Sawicki WL, Moroson BA, Cashmore AR, Elslager EF (1979) 2,4-diamino-5-methyl-6 [3,4,5-trimethoxyanilino)methyl] quinazoline (TMQ). A potent non-classical folate antagonist inhibitor-I. Biochem Pharmacol 28:1983–1987
40. Schimke RT (1984) Gene amplifacication in cultured animal cells. Cell 37:705–713

Haematology and Blood Transfusion Vol. 29
Modern Trends in Human Leukemia VI
Edited by Neth, Gallo, Greaves, Janka

Summary Overview of Clinical Session

B. Clarkson [1]

It is apparent from the recent work presented at this meeting that great strides have been made in the past few years in our understanding of the biology of leukemia, from the molecular to the clinical levels, but, unfortunately, these advances have not yet been translated into improved methods of treatment. As Hardisty recently pointed out [1], the major advances in the treatment of childhood leukemia took place more than 10 years ago, and there has been relatively little progress since then in developing better treatment for patients presenting with disease features which are associated with a poor prognosis; about half of the children and over half of the adults with acute lymphoblastic leukemia (ALL) are still dying of their disease even with the best modern treatment regimens. The best results yet reported in adults with ALL were achieved with a protocol which was designed over 10 years ago [2], and our own attempts as well as those of other investigators since then to improve further the treatment of adults have been unsuccessful [3, 4].

McCredie presented the combined results of treatment of over 900 adults with acute nonlymphoblastic leukemia (ANLL) at five major centers in the United States. The results in terms of long-term survival are disappointing. Overall, only 14% of the patients survived 5 years, but age had an important influence; 19% of the patients under 50 years of age and only 8% of those over 50 survived 5 years. As in the case of ALL, it is discouraging that despite intensive efforts to develop better treatment protocols, the results have remained almost constant during the past decade.

Except for bone marrow transplantation, which I will discuss shortly, there has also been little progress in improving survival in the chronic leukemias. The recent observations that some of the interferons have therapeutic activity in hairy-cell leukemia [5] and chronic myelogenous leukemia [6] are extremely interesting, but this is certainly not a curative form of treatment, and it is too soon to determine whether survival will be extended.

Patients with leukemia usually have between 10^{12} and 10^{13} leukemic cells at diagnosis. Based on the rapidity of cell kill with modern induction programs [7], it seems possible that some of the current intensive treatment regimens are capable of killing this many leukemic cells (or at least the entire fraction of the population which is capable of serving as stem cells) in highly responsive cases of ALL without producing irreversible damage to normal stem cells. However, it is doubtful if any of the regimens yet devised are capable of entirely eradicating the leukemic cells in the less-responsive types of ANLL without causing lethal injury, and I suspect there must be other factors aside from drug-induced cell kill which come into play to account for the long survivors. As has previously been shown, the human promyelocytic cell line HL-60 is a good target for induction of dif-

1 Memorial Sloan-Kettering Cancer Center, 1275 York Avenue, New York. N.Y. 10021, USA

ferentiation, and fresh promyelocytic leukemia cells can also be forced to differentiate with vitamin A and D analogues and various chemotherapeutic agents employed in leukemic therapy. Induced differentiation may be one reason for the better therapeutic results in acute promyelocytic leukemia (APL); in our experience about 35% of patients with APL survive over 5 years compared with 10%–15% for the other types of ANLL [8], and other groups have had similar results. The observation that enhanced differentiation of leukemic cells can occur using combinations of low doses of cytostatic drugs and differentiation inducers is intriguing, and hopefully these observations will eventually lead to clinical therapeutic advances. A number of investigators are currently trying to define the most effective combinations of agents for different types of leukemia [9], and we can look forward to learning more about the therapeutic potential of this approach during the next few years.

Mixed opinions were expressed concerning the usefulness of low-dose cytosine arabinoside (Ara-C) or high-dose Ara-C, but the general consensus seemed to be that some of the initial highly favorable claims had been overstated. Although occasionally durable responses have been observed with low-dose Ara-C, the responses occurred erratically and most of them were of short duration. High-dose Ara-C of course causes marrow aplasia quite consistently, but although clinical trials in ANLL have been underway for several years now, a substantial effect on survival has not yet been demonstrated. Several interesting new drugs are currently undergoing clinical trials or will be soon, including homoharringtonine, fludarabine, and several new anthracyclines and antifols. While these drugs have potent antileukemic activity, and it is quite possible some of them may prove to have a therapeutic advantage over the present generation of drugs, I am doubtful whether any of them will lead to a major increase in the cure rate. We are still learning how to use the drugs already available more effectively, but so many modifications of intensive treatment programs have already been tried without appreciably altering the end results that it is doubtful if any further minor changes or substitution of new active compounds will be any more successful. Thus, in my opinion, a more radically different approach is needed if we are to see substantial further improvements in curability.

High hopes were held at one time for various forms of immunotherapy, but the results of clinical trials during the past 2 decades have generally been very disappointing, including recent trials with monoclonal antibodies [10–13]. Immunotherapy alone is unlikely to be curative, but it is still quite possible that highly specific monoclonal antibodies will be shown to be useful therapeutically in targeting cytotoxic agents to tumor cells. The current investigations concerning the role of oncogenes in the pathogenesis of leukemia are enormously interesting and important, and while it is not unreasonable to hope that they may eventually lead to the development of more selective forms of treatment, it is not yet possible to predict if or when therapeutically applicable strategies will evolve from this work.

At the present time, probably the most promising approach for the responsive leukemias is high-dose chemotherapy and total body irradiation followed by rescue with bone marrow transplantation. The dose response curves for some of the cytotoxic agents and ionizing irradiation are very steep, and there is abundant evidence from experimental tumor models that responsive tumors which are incurable with conventional doses of active agents can often be cured simply by substantially increasing the dose. I suspect we are coming sufficiently close to curing some of the "high-risk" patients with ALL, who are now still relapsing and dying on conventional chemotherapy, that the incremental dose increases permissible with bone marrow rescue may tip the balance in favor of cure. The challenge is of course more formidable in the less-responsive types of ANLL, but here too it may be possible to cure some patients who are presently dying of their diseases.

Allogeneic BMT is presently limited to the minority of patients who have human leukocyte antigen (HLA)-identical or partially HLA matched donors, usually siblings, although with further advances in transplantation biology better ways may be found to prevent graft rejection and graft versus host disease, and in the future it may be possible to overcome the present restrictions. It is clear that the results are better if the procedure is done early in the course of the disease before drug resistance has developed [14–19]. Because 40%–50% of the patients with ALL are now probably being cured with conventional chemotherapy, to date most of the bone marrow transplantation (BMT) trials in ALL have been done in second or later remissions. However, more recently, with reliable definition of risk factors, selected children at higher risk of early relapse have been transplanted in first remission. Only about 10%–20% of patients transplanted in third or fourth remission survived 2 years, while the results are better for patients transplanted in first or second remission. The relapse rate has been similar for patients transplanted in first or second remission, probably about 30% overall at different centers, but since those transplanted in first remission have almost exclusively been high-risk patients while those in second remission were in varied risk categories, no valid comparison is yet possible. There seems little doubt that patients transplanted in second or later remissions have a better chance of long-term survival than in comparable patients treated with chemotherapy. There is insufficient experience yet to compare the results of BMT and chemotherapy of patients in comparable (high) risk categories in first remission, but because of our inability to improve the treatment results in such patients with chemotherapy alone during the past 10 years, I predict that BMT will soon be shown to produce a higher proportion of long survivors among these high-risk patients than is possible with chemotherapy.

The majority of allogeneic transplants thus far have been performed in children and adolescents and very few patients over the age of 40 have been transplanted. At my own institution, patients over 20 years of age had a significantly higher early mortality [17], but Karl Blume at the City of Hope has also had very good results in adults with ALL [15].

In ANLL, the results of chemotherapy are sufficiently poor that it is justifiable to accept the risks and early mortality associated with BMT and perform the procedure in first remission. Currently there are several ongoing comparative trials of chemotherapy alone versus allogeneic bone marrow transplantation in patients with ANLL in first remission [3], and during the next several years we should be able to get a firm answer to the question of which gives better results. All of the transplant teams are of course working hard to develop more effective ways to prevent the major complications associated with the procedure and to improve the chemotherapeutic and irradiation eradication regimens, and we can anticipate further improvements in the results with fewer complications during the next few years.

Attempts to cure chronic myelogenous leukemia (CML) with intensive treatment programs have so far been unsuccessful [20], and the results with allogeneic BMT performed during the blastic phase have generally been poor with very few long survivors. However, during the past few years over 100 patients throughout the world with CML in the chronic phase or early in the accelerated phase have had allogeneic transplants, with more encouraging early results [21]. While all the results have not yet been compiled and the follow-up is still too short in most cases to determine the long-term results, it appears that approximately 65% of patients transplanted in chronic phase and perhaps half that percentage in accelerated phase are surviving the procedure and that the marrow remains in complete remission (i.e., free of Ph'+ cells) in most of them. Whereas the median survival from diagnosis for patients with chronic-phase disease is 3–4 years, some patients may live 5–10 years and remain in good health for most of this time. Faced with the hazard of a 35% early mortality incidence associated with the transplant procedure, the patients and their physicians are confronted with a serious dilemma of which course of treatment to choose a when. A reliable staging system has long been needed in CML; such a system is presently under development, and once its validity is confirmed, it should prove helpful in advising patients who have suitable donors when to opt for BMT [22]. As in the case of acute leukemia, this option is usually limited to patients under the age of 40, and patients under 25 have a significantly better outcome [21].

The majority of patients with leukemia do not have HLA-identical sibling donors. For younger patients with acute leukemia who lack suitable donors and who are at high risk of failing the best available chemotherapy programs, the most promising approach now available is probably intensive treatment with whole body irradiation and high-dose chemotherapy followed by autologous bone marrow transplantation, using the patient's own remission marrow which has been appropriately treated in vitro to remove residual leukemic cells. The early results in patients with poor-prognosis lymphomas have been encouraging if carried out immediately after primary induction treatment [23]; as expected, heavily pretreated patients do not respond as well. Most of the lymphoma patients successfully treated so far after primary induction therapy had minimal or no marrow involvement with lymphoma prior to treatment, and it is undoubtedly more difficult to eliminate the increased numbers of residual leukemic cells present in the marrows of patients with acute leukemia in first remission. The majority of patients with ANLL as well as the majority of high-risk patients with ALL who achieve remission relapse within the 1st year after doing so [3], and most of these patients probably barely meet the qualifications for complete remission. Using the usual morphological criteria, the marrow can contain between 10^4 and 10^5 leukemic cells/ml and still qualify as a remission [23, 24]; thus, to purge the marrow successfully in patients who are at high risk of early relapse, it is probably necessary to develop purging methods which will kill at least this number of leukemic cells without causing lethal damage to the normal stem cells.

Relatively few patients with acute leukemia have yet been treated with autologous BMT, and, as in the case of the early trials with allogeneic BMT, most of them have been in second or later remissions [25–27]. The results of all the recent trials have not been collected, but it is rumored that the relapse rate has been appreciable in these high-risk patients. However, it is not clear yet whether this is due to failure of the in vitro purging techniques or of failure to eliminate the residual leukemic cells in the patients by the in vivo conditioning programs so far tried. Studies are currently underway at many institutions to develop better purging methods, using physical, immunological, or pharmacological techniques or combined methods [28–33], and it is not unreasonable to expect that improved methods for eradication of leukemic cells both in vitro and in vivo will be forthcoming during the next several years. The maximum tolerable age threshold for autologous BMT is not yet known, but autologous transplants are associated with fewer serious complications than allogeneic transplants, and it may prove possible to treat patients successfully up to the age of 50 years. In the meantime, while these clinically oriented studies are proceeding, the geneticists and molecular biologists will doubtless continue their remarkable advances, and we eagerly anticipate the day when their work will lead to more selective forms of treatment for all types of leukemia.

References

1. Hardisty RM (1983) Acute lymphoblastic leukemia: achievements and prospects. In: Recent results in cancer research, vol 88, Springer, Berlin Heidelberg, pp 37–46
2. Schauer P, Arlin ZA, Mertelsmann R, Cirrincione C, Friedman A, Gee TS, Dowling MD, Kempin S, Straus DJ, Koziner B, Mc Kenzie S, Thaler HT, DuFour P, Little C, Dellaquila C, Ellis S, Clarkson B (1983) Treatment of acute lymphoblastic leukemia in adults. Results of the L-10 and L-10M protocols. J Clin Oncol 1:462
3. Clarkson B, Gee T, Arlin Z, Mertelsmann R, Kempin S, Dinsmore R, O'Reilly R, Andreeff M, Berman E, Higgins C, Little C, Cirrincione C, Ellis S (1984) Current status of treatment of acute leukemia in adults: an overview. In: Büchner T, Urbanitz D, van de Loo (eds) Therapy of acute leukemia. Springer, Berlin Heidelberg New York, pp 1–31

4. Hoelzer D, Thiel E, Loffler H et al. (1984) Intensified therapy in acute lymphoblastic and acute undifferentiated leukemia in adults. Blood 64:38–47
5. Quesada JR, Reuben J, Manning JT, Hersh EM, Gutterman JU (1984) Alpha interferon for induction of remission in hairy cell leukemia. N Engl J Med 310:15–18
6. Talpaz M, McCredie KB, Mavligit GM, Gutterman JU (1983) Concise report. Leukocyte interferon-induced myeloid cytoreduction in chronic myelogenous leukemia. Blood 62: 689–692
7. Hiddemann W, Buchner T, Andreeff M, Wormann B, Melamed MR, Clarkson BD (1982) Cell kinetics in acute leukemia. A critical reevaluation based on new data. Cancer 50:250–258
8. Cunningham I, Gee T, Kempin S, Clarkson B (1984) Acute promyelocytic leukemia (APL): ten years' experience. Proc Am Soc Clin Oncol 3:203, # C-790
9. Bloch A (1984) Induced cell differentiation in cancer therapy. Cancer Treat Rep 68:199 –205
10. Pavlovsky S, Muriel FS, Garay G et al. (1981) Chemoimmunotherapy with levamisole in acute lymphoblastic leukemia. Cancer 48:1500–1507
11. Ritz J, Pesando JM, Sallan SE et al. (1981) Serotherapy of acute lymphoblastic leukemia with monoclonal antibody. Blood 58:141–152
12. Miller RA, Maloney DG, McKillop J, Levy R (1981) In vivo effects of murine hybridoma monoclonal antibody in a patient with T-cell leukemia. Blood 58:78–86
13. Stryckmans PA, Otten J, Delbeke MJ, Suciu S, Fiere D, Bury J, Solbu G, Benoit Y (1983) Comparison of chemotherapy with immunotherapy for maintenance of acute lymphoblastic leukemia in children and adults. Blood 62:606–615
14. Barrett AJ, Kendra JR, Lucas CF, Joss DV, Joshi R, Desai M, Jones KH, Phillips RH, Rogers TR, Tabara Z, Williamson S, Hobbs JR (1982) Bone marrow transplantation for acute lymphoblastic leukemia. Br J Haematol 52:181
15. Blume KG, Spruce WE, Krance RA et al. (1982) Bone-marrow transplantation for acute lymphoblastic leukemia (letter to the Editor). N Engl J Med 306:610
16. Thomas ED, Sanders JE, Flournoy N et al. (1983) Marrow transplantation for patients with acute lymphoblastic leukemia: a long-term follow-up. Blood 62:1139
17. Dinsmore R, Kirkpatrick D, Flomenberg N, Gulati S, Kapoor N, Shank B, Reid A, Groshen S, O'Reilly RJ (1983) Allogeneic bone marrow transplantation for patients with acute lymphoblastic leukemia. Blood 62:381
18. Gale RP, Kersey JH, Bortin MM et al. (1983) Bone marrow transplantation for acute lymphoblastic leukemia. Lancet 2:663–666
19. Woods WG, Nesbit ME, Ramsay NKC et al. (1983) Improved disease-free survival and determination of prognostic factors for patients with acute lymphocytic leukemia (ALL) in remission receiving intensive therapy followed by bone marrow transplantation (BMT). Blood 61:1182–1189
20. Goto T, Nishikori M, Arlin Z, Gee T, Kempin S, Burchenal J, Strife A, Wisniewski D, Lambek C, Little C, Jhanwar S, Chaganti R, Clarkson B (1982) Growth characteristics of leukemic and normal hematopoietic cells in PH′+ chronic myelogenous leukemia and effects of intensive treatment. Blood 59:793 –808
21. Speck B, Bortin MM, Champlin R, Goldman JM, Herzig RH, McGlave PB, Messner HA, Weiner RS, Rimm AA (1984) Allogeneic bone-marrow transplantation for chronic myelogenous leukemia. Lancet 665–668
22. Sokal JE, Cox EB, Baccarani M, Tura S, Gomez GA, Robertson JE, Braun TJ, Clarkson BD, Cervantes F, Rozman C and The Italian Cooperative CML Study Group (1984) Prognostic discrimination in "good-risk" chronic granulocytic leukemia. Blood 63:789–799
23. Gulati S, Shank B, Straus D, Koziner B, Lee B, Mertelsmann R, Dinsmore R, Gee T, Yopp J, O'Reilly R, Clarkson B (to be published) Autologous stem cell transplant for poor prognosis lymphoma. Proc Second Int Conf on Malignant Lymphomas, Nijhoff
24. Blumenreich MS, Strife A, Clarkson BD (1983) A technique to quantify cytoreduction in the bone marrow induced by cytotoxic chemotherapy. J Clin Oncol 1:552–558
25. Ritz J, Sallan SE, Bast RC Jr et al. (1982) Autologous bone marrow transplantation in CALLA-positive acute lymphoblastic leukemia after in vitro treatment with J5 monoclonal antibody and complement. Lancet 2:60
26. Dicke KA, Spitzer G, Peters L et al. (1979) Autologous bone marrow transplantation in relapsed adult acute leukemia. Lancet I: 514–517
27. Kaizer H, Stuart RK, Brookmeyer R, Colvin M, Santos GW (1983) Autologous bone marrow transplantation (BMT) in acute leukemia: a phase I study of in vitro treatment of marrow with 4-hydroperoxycyclophosphamide (4-HC) to purge tumor cells. Blood 62:224a

28. Dicke KA (1983) Purging of marrow cell suspensions. In: Crale RP (ed) Recent advances in bone marrow transplantation. Liss, New York, pp 689–702
29. Rizzoli V, Carmatti C, Mangoni L (1983) The effect of 4-hydroperoxycyclophosphamide (4-HC) and VP-16-213 on leukemia and normal myeloid progenitor cells. Exp Hematol 11 [Suppl 14]:9
30. Gulati S, Gandola L, Vega R, Yopp J, Chang TT, Ibrahim S, Siena S, Castro-Malaspina H, Colvin M, Clarkson B (1984) Chemopurification of bone marrow in vitro and its clinical applications. Proc Am Assoc Cancer Res 25:201
31. Muirhead M, Martin RJ, Torok-Storb B, Uhr JW, Vitella ES (1983) Use of an antibody Ricin A-chain conjugate to delete neoplastic B cells from human bone marrow. Blood 62: 327–332
32. Mitsuyasu R, Champlin R, Ho W et al. (1983) Autologous bone marrow transplantation after in vitro marrow treatment with anti-CALLA heteroantiserum and complement for adult acute lymphoblastic leukemia. In: Crale RP (ed) Recent advances in bone marrow transplantation. Liss, New York, pp 678–687
33. Poynton CH, Dicke KA, Culbert S et al. (1983) Immunomagnetic removal of CALLA positive cells from human bone marrow. Lancet I:524

Haematology and Blood Transfusion Vol. 29
Modern Trends in Human Leukemia VI
Edited by Neth, Gallo, Greaves, Janka

Red Cell Transfusions for Polytransfused Patients

S. F. Goldmann[1]

Patients with chronic anemia tolerate much lower levels of hemoglobin than those experiencing acute blood loss or acute hemolysis. The compensating mechanism is the increase of red cell 2,3-diphosphoglycerate (DPG), causing increased release of oxygen to the tissues. For this and further clinical and epidemiologic reasons, it is unnecessary to transfuse patients with chronic anemia unless symptoms of anoxia are expressed. This rarely occurs at hemoglobin levels higher than 8 g/dl. Many patients tolerate lower levels of hemoglobin and, therefore, do not require RBC transfusions.

In leukemia, lymphoma, and iatrogenically induced anemia, there is decreased or absent production of erythrocytes. Such patients will respond well to transfusion of red blood cells (RBC) as long as increased organ-specific or peripheral destruction of erythrocytes does not occur. However, current RBC preparations also contain leukocytes and platelets. The nonerythrocytic cells possess alloimmunogenic specific antigens different from known blood groups. Thus, substitution of chronic anemia patients with RBC preparations may result in sensitization to leukocyte- and/or platelet-specific antigens [1–5]. Patients previously sensitized to leukocytes and platelets are subject to febrile nonhemolytic transfusion reactions and may be resistant to a later required leukocyte and/or platelet transfusion [6–8]. This is a further reason why transfusion of patients with chronic anemia should be restricted to absolute clinical necessity.

If red cells are needed, HLA-compatible blood is the best solution. Owing to the extreme polymorphism of the HLA system, however, this is seldom practicable. Since the occurrence of leukocyte and platelet antibodies is correlated to frequency and volume of whole blood transfusion [5, 9–11], only leukocyte- and platelet-depleted erythrocytes should be transfused.

Packed RBC are partially plasma depleted and contain 100% of the original leukocytes and platelets. The sensitizing capacity of these preparations is similar to whole blood units. But even buffy-coat-free or washed RBC preparations demonstrate the same alloimmunization pattern as whole blood, although they contain only 41% of original leukocytes and 11% of platelets (Tables 1, 2). The transfusion reaction incidence using these preparations is lower than in whole blood transfusion, but it remains impossible to predict the clinical outcome in individual patients.

I have analyzed published [12–17] and my own data [5] and calculated the minimal leukocyte alloimmunogenic leukocyte dose: 10×10^8 leukocytes transfused in 1 day (whole blood, washed buffy-coat-free RBC) or small cumulating quantities, independent of transfusion frequency and interval or donor, will cause sensitization to leukocyte antigens (Table 3; [5, 12–17]). Only leukocyte- and platelet-free preparations [5, 18–21] contain less than 4% of

1 Abteilung Transplantationsimmunologie, DRK-Blutspendezentrale Ulm, und Abteilung Transfusionsmedizin, Universität Ulm, D-7900 Ulm, FRG

Table 1. RBC-enriched blood units

RBC Preparation[a]		N	Leukocytes × 10^8		Platelets × 10^{10}		Hemoglobin (gramm)	
			Initial	After Preparation	Initial	After preparation	Initial	After preparation
1	Buffy-coat-free	50	25.1	10.2 (41%)	10.7	1.2 (12%)	62	50 (81%)
2	Washed	30	23.0	9.0 (42%)	9.0	1.0 (11%)	64	51 (80%)
3	Filtered	30	24.0	0.9 (4%)	10.2	0.2 (2%)	63	51 (81%)
4	Incubated (37 °C), followed by buffy-coat-free preparation	30	27.3	1.0 (3.6%)	13.2	0.03 (0.3%)	77	60 (78%)
5	Frozen	30	28.0	0.5 (2%)	11.0	0.15 (1%)	72	56 (78%)

[a] Techniques: 1, 2 leukocyte- and platelet-poor blood; 3–5 leukocyte- and platelet-free blood

Table 2. Alloimmunization patterns

	Units per patient	Patients	Alloimmunized patients	Alloimmunization rate (%)
Whole blood	16 ± 6 (2 – 34)	27	17	63
Washed RBC	14 ± 7 (2 – 68)	60	32	53
Filtered RBC	22 ± 9 (2 – 76)	44	2	4

Table 3. Alloimmunization to leukocyte antigens in RBC transfusion[a]

First immunized recipient after:	Leukocytes	Ref.
1 One whole blood unit (400–500 ml)	25 × 10^8	[13], [14]
2 Repeating transfusion of 80–100 ml whole blood from the same donor, after 5 weekly transfusions (5 × 80–100 = 400–500 ml)	25 × 10^8	[22], [16]
3 As in 2, but 20 ml weekly after 9 weekly transfusions (9 × 20 = 180 ml)	10 × 10^8	[17]
4 One unit washed buffy-coat-free RBC	10 × 10^8	[12]
5 Filtered leukocyte-free RBC; after 13 transfusions from different donors with clinically dependent intervals	13 × 10^8	[5]

[a] Conclusion: Minimal leukocyte immunizing dose = 10 × 10^8 = 1 unit

the initial value (Table 1); they contain fewer leukocytes than the minimal immunogenic dose (Table 4). These preparations contain only 0.1 dose compared with 1.0 in buffy-coat-free blood and washed RBC, and 2.5 doses in whole blood and packed RBC. This explains why these preparations very seldom sensitize to leukocyte antigens (Table 2); [5, 12]).

Brittingham and Chaplin [15, 22] and Perkins et al. [23] described the minimal leukocyte dose causing nonhemolytic trans-

Table 4. RBC-containing blood units

	Leukocytes × 10^8 (% of initial)	Minimal leukocyte immunizing dose (10×10^8 leukocytes = 1 unit)	Leukocyte dose causing transfusion reaction (2.5×10^8 leukocytes = 1 unit)
1 Whole blood	25 (100%)	2.5	10 Leukocyte-rich
2 warm blood	25 (100%)	2.5	10 Leukocyte-rich
3 Packed RBC	25 (100%)	2.5	10 Leukocyte-rich
4 Buffy-coat-free	10 (41%)	1.0	4 Leukocyte-poor
5 Washed buffy-coat-free	10 (42%)	1.0	4 Leukocyte-poor
6 Filtered	0.9 (4%)	0.1	0.4 Leukocyte-free
7 Incubated	1.0 (4%)	0.1	0.4 Leukocyte-free
8 Frozen	0.5 (2%)	0.05	0.2 Leukocyte-free

Table 5. Recommendation for administration of RBC-containing blood units[a]

	Content (%)				Alloimmunization to leukocyte and platelet antigens	Transfusion reaction to leukocytes and platelets	Indication
	RBC	Leukocytes	Platelets	Plasma			
Whole blood	100	100	100	100	+ + + +	+ + + +	None!
Warm blood (<6 h)	100	100	100	100	+ + + +	+ + + +	1 Acute life-threatening blood loss 2 Bleeding not manageable with clotting factors and platelets 3 Massive transfusion
Packed RBC	100	100	10	30	+ + + +	+ + + +	None!
Buffy-coat-free RBC	81	41	12	15	+ + + +	+ +	Acute life-threatening anemia without presensitization to leukocyte and platelet antigens
Washed RBC	80	41	11	0	+ + + +	+ +	Hyperkalemia, allergic reaction, IGA deficiency
Leukocyte- and platelet-free blood							
Filtered	81	4	2	10	(+)	0	Transfusion-dependent chronic anemia: prevention of alloimmunization and transfusion reaction to nonerythrocytic blood cells
Incubated	78	3.6	0.3	20	(+)	0	
Frozen	78	2	1	0	(+)	0	

+ + + + Very often; + + sometimes – often; (+) seldom = cumulating doses due to polytransfusion

fusion reaction (2.5×10^8 leukocytes). Whole blood and packed RBC contain 10 such doses, buffy-coat-free and washed RBC 4 doses, and leukocyte-free preparations only 0.2–0.4 dose (Tables 1, 4). Consequently, nonhemolytic transfusion reactions to leukocyte antigens have not been described with leukocyte- and platelet-free RBC units [5, 21].

These data indicate that only leukocyte- and platelet-free RBC minimize sensitization to leukocyte and platelet antigens, avoid nonhemolytic febrile transfusion reactions to nonerythrocytic cells of the donor, and may guarantee an efficient granulocyte and platelet substitution in RBC polytransfused patients. Recommendations for administration of RBC preparations are summarized in Table 5.

Patients with severe aplastic anemia transfused prior to bone marrow transplantation reject allogeneic grafts more frequently than untransfused patients. The mechanism for this reaction is unknown. It should be stressed, however, that even leukocyte- and platelet-free RBC contribute to graft rejection. Thus, patients with severe aplastic anemia should not be transfused prior to bone marrow transplantation. The low number of lymphocytes in leukocyte-free RBC preparations is able to cause graft-versus-host reactions. Consequently, these preparations should be irradiated before transfusion to immunodeficient patients, e.g., patients with Hodgkin's disease, patients conditioned for bone marrow transplantation, and patients with severe combined immunodeficiency.

References

1. Doan CA (1926) The recognition of biologic differentiation in the white blood cells with especial reference to blood transfusion. J Am Med Assoc 86:1593
2. Dausset J (1954) Leuco-agglutinins. IV. Leuco-agglutinins and blood transfusion. Vox Sang 4:190
3. André R, Dreyfus B, Salmen C (1956) Isoanticorps immune antileucocytes après transfusion. Etude de son activité agglutinate lysante et opsonisante. Rev Haematol 11:390
4. Van Loghem JJ, von der Hart M, Hijmans W, Schuit HRE (1958) The incidence and significance of complete and incomplete white cell antibodies with special reference to the use of the Coombs consumption test. Vox Sang 3:203
5. Goldmann SF (1980) Hämotherapie nach Maß: Untersuchungen zur Vermeidung der transfusionsbedingten Alloimmunisierung gegen Leukozyten- und Thrombozytenantigene. Thesis, University of Ulm
6. Ahrons S, Kissmeyer-Nielsen F (1968) Serological investigation of 1358 transfusion reactions in 74 000 transfusions. Dan Med Bull 15:259
7. Kissmeyer-Nielsen F (1966) Der Zwischenfall bei Bluttransfusion und seine Beherrschung. Ärztl Fortb 16:78
8. Milner LV, Butcher K (1978) Transfusion reactions reported after transfusions of red blood cells and whole blood. Transfusion 18:493
9. Caseley J, Moses VK, Lichter EA, Jonasson O (1971) Isoimmunization of hemodialysis patients. Leukocyte-poor versus whole blood transfusions. Transplant Proc 3:365
10. Beutler E, West C, Blume KG (1976) The removal of leukocytes and platelets from whole blood. J Lab Clin Med 88:328
11. Jensen KG (1962) The significance of leucoagglutinins for development of transfusion reactions. Dan Med Bull 9:198
12. Goldmann SF, Schmidt-Wiederkehr P, Spiess H (1976) Leukozytenantikörper nach Transfusion von leukozytenarmem Blut bei Dialysepatienten. Forschungsergebnisse der Transfusionsmedizin und Immunhämatologie. Medicus, Berlin, pp 225–228
13. Payne R (1957) Leukocyte agglutinins in human sera. Arch Intern Med 99:587
14. Killmann SA (1958) Febrile transfusion reactions in patients with leukocyten agglutinins. Dan Med Bull 5:178
15. Brittingham TE, Chaplin H Jr (1957) Febrile transfusion reactions caused by sensitivity to donor leukocytes and platelets. J Am Med Assoc 165:819
16. Ceppelini R, Celada F, Mattinez P, Zanalda A (1964) Study of the possible correlation between blood antigens and histocompatibility in man. I. Production of leukoagglutinins by repeated transfusions from one donor. Ann NY Acad Sci 120:335
17. Ferrara GB, Tosi RM, Azzolino G, Carminate G, Kissmeyer-Nielsen F (1972) The production of anti HL-A cytotoxic antisera through planned immunization by intravenous injection of small aliquots of whole blood. I. Immunization of unrelated recipients. Tissue Antigens 2:359
18. Goldmann SF, Heiss F (1971) A method for preparing buffy-coat-poor blood for transfusion. Vox Sang 21:540

19. Diepenhorst P, Sprokholt R, Prins K (1972) Removal of leukocytes from whole blood and erythrocyte suspension by filtration through cotton wool. I. Filtration technique. Vox Sang 23:308
20. Schneider W, Stützle G (1979) Neues Verfahren zur Herstellung von leukozyten-/thrombozytenarmen Erythrozytensedimenten. Med Welt 30:1597
21. Huggins CE, Russel PS, Winn HJ, Fuller TC, Beck CH Jr (1973) Frozen blood in transplant patients: Hepatitis and HL-A isosensitization. Transplant Proc 5:809
22. Brittingham TE, Chaplin H Jr (1961) The antigenicity of normal and leukemic human leukocytes. Blood 17:139
23. Perkins HA, Payne R, Ferguson J, Wood M (1966) Nonhemolytic febrile transfusion reactions. Quantitative effects of blood components with emphasis on isoantigenic incompatibility of leukocytes. Vox Sang 11:578

Haematology and Blood Transfusion Vol. 29
Modern Trends in Human Leukemia VI
Edited by Neth, Gallo, Greaves, Janka

Gram-Negative Bacteraemia: New Therapeutic Possibilities with Anti-Endotoxin Antibodies

S. L. Gaffin[1]

A. Introduction

Gram-negative bacteria are coated by highly toxic and chemically stable lipopolysaccharide (LPS, endotoxin) which is partially shed when the bacteria are destroyed [1], e.g. by antibiotics in the blood of the patient. Since antibiotics have no effect on the LPS [2], this toxic LPS persists in the circulation of affected patients and causes much of the mortality and morbidity in gram-negative bacteraemia. Moreover, LPS is also present in the gut in large amounts and it may enter the circulation and cause toxic reactions when the gut is damaged by almost any mechanism, including radiotherapy of cancer patients [3, 4]. Normally small amounts of LPS leaving the gut are cleared by the reticuloendothelial system (RES), but in the case of damage to the gut lining the massive amounts of LPS involved may overwhelm the capacity of the RES. In addition, the immunosuppressive effect of ionizing radiation may deplete the body of anti-LPS antibodies, which are involved in part, in LPS detoxification.

A number of studies have shown that passive administration of anti-LPS antibodies into an animal or patient can reduce mortality and morbidity of endotoxaemia [5–7]. For clinical exploitation however, the development of a source of adequate amounts of human anti-LPS is a fundamental problem. Active LPS is so toxic it cannot be used directly as an immunogen in humans. McCutchan, Ziegler, Braude and colleagues actively immunized volunteers with an Escherichia coli preparation containing an LPS mutant to produce an anti-"core" LPS hyperimmune serum in a most important study [8]. This serum significantly reduced the mortality of patients suffering from shock and bacteraemia. However, this serum is not at present available for general use, in part because of problems associated with the active immunization route. Moreover, there may be therapeutic benefit in using a different type of anti-LPS which is a mixture of antibodies, some directed to the core and others to the surface regions of LPS [9]. In order to overcome these problems we found that some plasma units donated to blood banks contained high concentrations of "natural" anti-LPS IgG [10]. We developed an ELISA for efficient screening of all blood units donated to a blood bank [11] in order to isolate them and have used such anti-LPS antibodies therapeutically.

In this paper I review our animal and human experiments which led to the present conclusion that anti-LPS produced by our simple blood bank screening procedure can significantly reduce morbidity and mortality in septic shock. Such anti-LPS might be expected to beneficially augment an immuno-suppressed patient's antibody stores.

1 Department of Physiology, University of Natal Medical School, Durban, South Africa

B. Human and Equine Anti-LPS Preparations

I. Human Anti-LPS

Plasma units donated to a blood bank (Natal Blood Transfusion Service, Pinetown, South Africa) were screened by an ELISA for the presence of high concentrations (> 40 μg/ml) of anti-LPS IgG [11]. Approximately 7% of donations had such antibodies in South Africa and Israel [12]. One full-time technician using semiautomated apparatus can process 200 samples per day with a yield of 14/day × 300 days/year = 4200 high titer plasma units (anti-LPS) per year. We found that adult patients in septic shock require 2–10 units (mean = 5–6) anti-LPS as a therapeutic dose [13]. Therefore 760 adult unit doses per year can be produced. We have pooled several hundred high titer units and fractionated them to produce an LPS-specific immunoglobulin with standardized properties. However, this was an intramuscular globulin preparation. We expect shortly to produce an intravenous form of this LPS-specific globulin. As an alternative anti-LPS source for i.v. administration, individual high titer plasma units have been freeze-dried (FDP) [13]. These have the added advantage of causing no licensing problems since this FDP is produced entirely by the routine licensed methods. Merely an additional test was done to determine whether the plasma contained LPS-specific IgG. There was no correlation between the presence of high concentrations of specific IgM and IgG in these plasma units. Since the IgG antibody is easier to prepare and has a longer half-life, we selected it rather than the IgM. While the anti-LPS FDP is more convenient and faster to prepare than the immunoglobulin, it has the disadvantage of not being standardized since each plasma unit contains a somewhat different distribution of anti-LPS antibodies from other units. In one unit they may be directed to LPS from *Shigella,* in another to *E. coli* and *Salmonella typhosa,* and still another mainly to *Klebsiella* and *Pseudomonas.* A pooled preparation containing mixtures of antibodies to a wide range of LPS sources is desirable. Practically, we found in our pooled LPS-specific globulin the following relative anti-LPS binding activities in decreasing order [12]: *Shigella flexneri, Salmonella abortus equi, Salmonella typhimurium, Klebsiella pneumoniae, Salmonella enteritidis, E. coli* 026 : B6, *Salmonella typhosa, E. coli* 055 : B5, *E. coli* 0111 : B4, *E. coli* 0128 : B12, *Salmonella minnesota, Salmonella marcescens, E. coli* 0127 : B8. Significantly almost the same *order* of anti-LPS binding activities was found in blood samples obtained from Australia, Papua New Guinea and England, but at much lower levels of activity[2].

It was expected that prior exposure of the donor to subclinical gram-negative bacterial infections led to the distribution of anti-LPS antibodies in any particular plasma sample. However, no correlation was seen in our pooled anti-LPS between the antibody level to LPS from a particular bacterial strain and the frequency of this strain's being isolated by the hospitals serving the same area in which the donors live. As an example, *Shigella flexneri* was isolated only rarely in King Edward VIII Hospital, Durban, but pooled anti-LPS from donors in the Durban region had its highest activity against *Shigella flexneri* LPS.

II. Animal Anti-LPS

Equine anti-LPS hyperimmune plasma is currently produced on a large scale by the plasmapheresis of suitably immunized horses (ATOX Pharmaceutical Company, 14 Old Main Road, Gillitts, 3600 South Africa). The original minimum concentrations were 150 μg/ml [14], i.e. almost four times that acceptable for humans. Owing to improvements in methods, it is now produced at a concentration of 1500 μg/ml. Currently it is produced as a frozen solution and thawed just prior to administration. Specific IgG in it also bind to a wide range of gram-negative bacteria.

---

2 Courtesy of Dr. Brian Feery, Commonwealth Serum Laboratories, Parkville, Australia

C. Summary of Animal Studies Using Human and Equine Anti-LPS

I. SMAO Shock

Experimental rabbits received 2 ml/kg equine anti-LPS s.c.; 2 days later a laparotomy was performed on these rabbits and in untreated controls. The superior mesenteric arteries were occluded (SMAO) for 1 h and then released. The incisions were then closed. The ischaemia damaged the gut and led to endotoxaemia and shock. After 10 days survivors were observed. Survivors in the controls were 2/12 (17.7%), but in those receiving anti-LPS prophylaxis 7/8 (87.5%; $P < 0.001$) [15]. This has important implications in the field of abdominal surgery. Prophylactic anti-LPS appears useful whenever intestinal ischaemia may occur. This is becoming routine practice in South African equine veterinary medical practice.

II. Haemorrhagic Shock

Cats were bled via femoral arterial catheter into a reservoir and held at a MAP of 40 mmHg. After 4 h the shed blood was returned to the cat via femoral venous catheter. During the shock period the cats were infused with either high titer anti-LPS human plasma or normal human plasma. Survivors at 24 h were noted. Survivors in the controls were 1/8 (12.5%) compared with 7/8 (87.5%) in the anti-LPS group [10]. That is, haemorrhagic shock became "irreversible" unless anti-LPS was present to bind the LPS leaving the ischaemic bowel.

III. Radiation Sickness

Mice (more than 200 animals) were irradiated with 630 rads in a hospital radiotherapy facility, 6 days later they received either normal equine plasma or anti-LPS equine plasma. Survival at 30 days post-radiation was observed. Survivors among the serum controls were 10%, but in the anti-LPS group survivors were 50% ($P < 0.025$) [16]. That is, radiation damage to the gut and plasma cells led to a high mortality. Anti-LPS inactivated LPS and "bought time" for the partially denuded gut to repair itself.

IV. Topical Infections

Pseudomonas keratitis of rabbit eyes led to inflammation, scarring and blindness. Such eyes were treated by equine anti-LPS as drops for 8 days. The infections were controlled, partial healing of the eye occurred and sight returned to some rabbits [17].

V. *Pseudomonas* Infection

Mice received 0.1 ml human anti-LPS and 1 h later received 0.1 ml *Pseudomonas aeruginosa* broth culture. Only 15% of controls survived compared with 85% of those receiving anti-LPS [12].

VI. Septic Abortion

Pregnant rats received anti-LPS or saline followed by low doses of *E. coli;* 2 weeks later fetuses were examined. Control fetuses were small and partially resorbed. Fetuses from anti-LPS-treated infected rats were of normal size. Placentas of control rats were inflamed and necrotic with viable *E. coli* present. Placentas in the anti-LPS-treated group were all normal [18]. Anti-LPS may have a potential value in preventing abortion of infected pregnant women.

VII. Veterinary Use

Equine anti-LPS is used in the veterinary medical industry of South Africa to treat a wide variety of diseases mediated in part by endotoxins. It is used parenterally, orally or topically. It has proved effective in treating the following cases: septic arthritis in Thoroughbred horses, septicaemia, peritonitis, diarrhoea, shock secondary to parvovirus infection, *Klebsiella* intrauterine infections, mastitis and *Pseudomonas* ear infections [14].

D. Summary of Human Studies Using Human Anti-LPS

I. Multicentre Septic Shock Study

In a multicentre study, consecutive cases of septic shock or imminent septic shock were treated with anti-LPS FDP or specific globulin; 20/22 improved [19].

II. Neonatal Septicaemia Study

Among severely septicaemic low birth weight infants no difference in survival was seen between those who received anti-LPS immunoglobulin and placebo, but anti-LPS-treated survivors had a much reduced period of hospitalization compared with the placebo-treated controls [20]. The slow rate of absorption of the intramuscular immunoglobulin may have caused the poor results in this trial. In addition this group of babies were of low birth weight and hence many had underdeveloped RES which might have been poorly responsive to any therapy. Because of the need for a rapid response in critically ill patients, an *intravenous* anti-LPS preparation is to be preferred. On the other hand there may be a place for the slowly absorbed immunoglobulin as a prophylaxis.

III. Single Centre Septic Shock Study

Women in a department of obstetrics and gynaecology who developed septic shock were admitted to the trials [13]. They received conventional antibiotic and supportive therapy and surgery where indicated. On a random basis some also received anti-LPS FDP. Mortality of controls was 9/19 (47.4%) and of the anti-LPS-treated group was 1/14 (7.1%). The anti-LPS group also developed fewer complications of shock and had a much reduced period of hospitalization.

IV. Current Studies

In essentially a continuation of the study on women in septic shock (sect C. III) the following results were obtained: mortality in controls = 11/27 (40.7%); mortality in anti-LPS-treated group = 1/23 (4.3%) [21].

E. Discussion

Human anti-LPS prepared by two different methods has been shown to protect patients therapeutically against septic shock. A wide variety of animal studies have previously shown similar results. The main problem had been to obtain reasonable amounts of human anti-LPS. In part, this has been solved by the use of our ELISA screening procedure which is appropriate to any medium to large-sized blood bank.

Some one-third of all cancer patients and two-thirds of leukaemia patients die of gram-negative bacteraemia. It is to be expected that radiotherapy or chemotherapy contribute to this bacteraemia by causing the partial denudation of the gut lining which permits an increased leakage of LPS into the circulation. At the same time this therapy reduces the rate of production of the natural protective anti-LPS antibodies and leucocytes. There appears to be a potential benefit in using anti-LPS in addition to conventional antibiotic therapy for treating septicaemia in immunosuppressed patients, particularly leukaemic patients. It must now be verified in clinical trials.

Acknowledgments. This work was supported by the SA MRC. Excellent technical work in these studies was carried out by Ms. Michelle Wells.

References

1. Goto H, Nakamura S (1980) Liberation of endotoxin from E. coli by addition of antibiotics. Jpn J Exp Med 50:35
2. Spink W, Braude AI, Castaneda MR, Goytia R (1948) Aureomycin therapy in human brucellosis due to Brucella militensis. JAMA 138:1145
3. Cuevas P, Ishiyama N, Koizumi S, Woodruff P, Kaufmann A, Fine J (1974) Role of endotoxemia of intestinal origin due to large burns. Surg Gynecol Obstet 138:725
4. Quastler H (1956) The nature of intestinal radiation death. Radiat Res 4:303–320

5. Davis D, Brown K, Douglas H, Take W, Braude AI (1969) Prevention of death from endotoxin with antiserum. Immunology 102:563
6. Milner KC (1973) Patterns of tolerance to endotoxin. J Infect Dis 128 [Suppl]: S237
7. Pollack M (1983) Antibody against Pseudomonas aeruginosa in immune globulins prepared for intravenous use. J Infect Dis 147:1090
8. Ziegler E, McCutchan J, Fierer J et al. (1982) Treatment of gram negative bacteremia and shock with human antiserum to a mutant E. coli. N Engl J Med 307:1226–1230
9. Gaffin SL (1983) Large scale production of antigram negative bacterial antibodies. Lancet 2:1420
10. Gaffin SL, Grinberg Z, Abraham C, Shechter Y, Birkhan J (1981) Protection against hemorrhagic shock in the cat by human plasma rich in endotoxin specific antibodies. J Surg Res 31:18–21
11. Gaffin SL, Badsha N, Brock-Utne J, Vorster B, Conradie J (1982) An ELISA procedure for detecting human anti-endotoxin antibodies in serum. Ann Clin Biochem 19:191–194
12. Badsha N, Vorster B, Gaffin SL (1985) Production and properties of human lipopolysaccharide specific globulin. Vox Sang (in press)
13. Lachman E, Pitsoe SB, Gaffin SL (1984) Anti-lipopolysaccharide immunotherapy in management of septic shock of obstetric and gynaecological origin. Lancet 1:981–983
14. Gaffin SL, Baker B, Du Preez J, Katzwinkel R, Fleming J (1982) Prophylaxis and therapy with antiendotoxin hyperimmune serum against gastroenteritis and endotoxemia in horses. Proc Am Assoc Eq Pract (Atlanta) 28:335–340
15. Zanotti A, Gaffin SL (1985) Protection against superior mesenteric artery occlusion shock by anti-lipopolysaccharide antibodies. J Surg Res (in press)
16. Gaffin SL, Zanotti A et al. (1984) Anti-LPS antibodies successfully treated shock, radiation sickness, surface infections and septic abortion in animals. S Afr J Sci 80:130
17. Welsh NH, Rauch A, Gaffin SL (1985) Topical immunotherapy for Pseudomonas keratitis in rabbits: Use of Anti-LPS plasma. Br J Ophthalmol (in press)
18. Lachman E, Gaffin SL, Sanker D, Pitsoe SB (1982) Prevention of septic abortion in rats by antiendotoxin antibodies. Abstract of the 3rd British Congress for Obstetrics and Gynaecology, July 1982, Birmingham, p 132
19. Gaffin SL, Lachman E (1984) The use of anti-lipopolysaccharide antibodies in the manegement of septic shock. S Afr Med J 65:158
20. Adhikari M, Coovadia H, Brock-Utne J, Pudifin D, Gaffin SL (to be published)
21. Lachman E, Pitsoe S, Gaffin SL (1984) Antilipopolysaccharide antibodies: Update. Lancet 2:875–876

Haematology and Blood Transfusion Vol. 29
Modern Trends in Human Leukemia VI
Edited by Neth, Gallo, Greaves, Janka

Empiric Antimicrobial Therapy in Cancer Patients*

M. T. Browne and P. A. Pizzo

A. Introduction

The majority of fevers which occur in granulocytopenic cancer patients appear to have an infectious etiology [1]. The practice of initiating empiric antibiotic therapy when the granulocytopenic cancer patient becomes febrile is now well established and has markedly reduced the early morbidity and mortality of infections in these patients. Nonetheless, infections still remain the leading cause of death in neutropenic cancer patients, necessitating refinements in the diagnosis and management of the complications in high risk patients.

The impetus for empiric antibiotic therapy in febrile granulocytopenic patients was the early death due to untreated infection (particularly *Pseudomonas* septicemia) when the granulocytopenic patient became febrile. Indeed, during the late 1960s and early 1970s, 50% of patients with *Pseudomonas* bacteremia died within 72 hours of their initially positive blood culture [2]. The early initiation of antibiotics significantly reduced this early mortality. Nonetheless, a number of questions regarding the role of empiric antimicrobial therapy for cancer patients in the 1980s can still be asked, including: Who should receive empiric therapy and when should it be started? What constitutes appropriate initial empiric therapy? How should the initial therapy be modified for patients who remain graulocytopenic or who fail to respond to the initial regimen? How long should empiric antibiotics be continued?

In dealing with the first question, who should receive empiric therapy and when should it begin, it appears that granulocytopenia is probably the single most important risk factor for infection in cancer patients [3, 4]. Whether or not all granulocytopenic patients require prompt empiric antibiotic management when they become febrile (i.e., patients with solid tumors as well as patients with hematologic malignancies) has been addressed in a number of recent studies. In a survey of 1001 consecutive episodes of fever in 324 pediatric and young adult cancer patients at the NCI, Bethesda, Maryland, there was no apparent difference in the incidence, pattern, or severity of infectious complications that occurred, regardless of the patients' underlying malignancy, once they became granulocytopenic. There were comparable numbers of episodes of fever and granulocytopenia and of documented infections such as sepsis and pneumonia in patients with solid tumors as in those with hematologic malignancies [1]. Similarly, Markmann and Abeloff observed that in adults with solid tumors, early empiric antibiotics were useful in reducing infectious morbidity and mortality [5]. Thus, all granulocytopenic patients, regardless of their underlying cancer, should be considered to be at risk for infection and, once febrile, are candidates for early empiric therapy. The level of granulocytopenia that should prompt empiric ther-

* Pediatric Branch Clinical Oncology Program, Division of Cancer Treatment, National Cancer Institute, National Institutes of Health, Bethesda, Maryland, USA

apy varies in different studies, with some recommending beginning antibiotics when the neutrophil count falls below 1000/mm³, while most would wait until the neutrophil count is less than 500/mm³. The rate at which the counts are falling may be as important as the absolute neutrophil number [6].

The degree of fever that should prompt therapy is defined differently at various centers. At the NCI, three oral temperatures above 38 °C or one oral temperature over 38.5 °C with a granulocyte count less than 500/mm³ is sufficient to begin empiric therapy. What is most important is for each center to adhere rigidly to predetermined criteria for defining high risk patients. This is particularly important since the diminished inflammatory capability of the granulocytopenic patient can mask the usual signs and symptoms of infection.

B. Preantibiotic Evaluation

Because untreated infections can be rapidly fatal, it is important that a thorough preantibiotic evaluation be carried out expeditiously. This should include a history and physical examination, at least two sets of preantibiotic blood cultures (if an indwelling line is present, peripheral vein cultures must also be obtained), chest X-ray, urinalysis, urine culture, and aspirate or biopsy cultures from accessible sites suggestive of infection. In spite of such an evaluation, it was not possible to differentiate patients with bacteremia from those with unexplained fever [1] in a recent prospective evaluation of 140 febrile granulocytopenic patients. More than half of the patients with bacteremia in this study lacked any specific physical findings.

C. Initial Empiric Antibiotic Combinations

Since approximately 85% of the initial pathogens are bacterial, the initial therapy is focused on bacterial pathogens. The original targets of empiric antibiotics were gram-negative bacteria, particularly *Pseudomonas aeruginosa,* and although gram-negative organisms still predominate, infections due to *Pseudomonas* have inexplicably declined. In contrast, infections due to gram-positive cocci (i.e., *Staphylococcus aureus* and *Staphylococcus epidermis*) have increased in recent years, in part due to the more widespread use of indwelling intravenous catheters [7, 8]. In order to give empiric cover for both gram-negative and gram-positive bacteria, broad-spectrum antibiotic therapy is essential. Thus, drug combinations are usually necessary and ideally should be bactericidal and synergistic, with a low potential for organ toxicity. In general, this has usually necessitated a combination of two or three antibiotics.

The importance of combination antibiotic therapy has been suggested since patients with gram-negative bacteremia have a greater than 80% survival when their isolate is sensitive to and treated with two antibiotics compared with a survival of 59% when the isolate is sensitive to only one of the two antibiotics [9–11]. In spite of the advantages of combined therapy, drug toxicity (particularly nephrotoxicity) is a concern in the cancer patient who is being exposed to many other toxic drugs.

The properties of some of the newer antibiotics raise the possibility of using them as single agents for the empiric management of febrile granulocytopenic patients. For example, in an ongoing study at the NCI, we are comparing monotherapy with ceftazidime (CTZ), a third generation cephalosporin, with our standard three-drug regimen of cephalothin (Keflin), gentamicin, and carbenicillin (KGC). To date, 349 episodes in 212 patients have been randomized to receive either combination therapy with KGC or monotherapy with CTZ when they became febrile and neutropenic (< 500 polys). The patients have been analyzed according to whether they had a documented infection or whether the etiology of their fever was unexplained. In addition, since the goal of empiric therapy is to protect the patient until results of the preantibiotic cultures are known, it is important to evaluate the efficacy of empiric antibiotic regimens both early in treatment – during the first 72 hours of therapy (i.e., prior to the time that the cause of the fever is known), as well as for the entire duration of neutropenia. The success rate in the first 72 hours for both the CTZ- and KGC-treated patients with fevers of unknown origin (FUO) or documented infections was over 97%. In addition, the overall outcome (i.e., at the time of resolution of granulocytopenia) for patients with FUO was over 98% for both the KGC and CTZ arm, and was comparable for both antibiotic regimens for patients with documented infections. Thus, it would appear that with future advances in antitiotic development, it may be possible to provide effective initial empiric antibiotic management with a single antibiotic in the febrile neutropenic cancer patient. Continued study of this approach is, however, necessary.

D. Empiric Antifungal Therapy

A second problem is related to patients who remain neutropenic for extended periods and who may be at risk for second infections and superinfections, particularly due to fungi. Because even invasive fungal disease is so difficult to diagnose and because these infections are particularly difficult to treat, especially if the infection has already advanced at the time of diagnosis, an empiric approach to antifungal therapy has also been investigated in high risk patients. Currently, evidence for invasive fungal disease is present in 8%–69% of granulocytopenic patients dying with cancer [12–14].

Persistent fever is often the only indication of an early fungal infection. The major fungal organisms of concern in neutropenic patients are *Candida, Aspergillus,* Phycomycetes, and *Cryptococcus* [15]. Blood cultures are rarely of diagnostic help (being positive in fewer than 25% of cases of disseminated candidiasis and virtually never positive in aspergillosis or mucormycosis) [16].

It is notable that successful therapy of *Candida* and even *Aspergillus* has been accomplished when amphotericin B has been instituted very early in the course of the infection [17]. Thus, early empiric antifungal therapy has a rational basis for high risk patients. Several issues are relevant: Who are the patients at high risk? Which antifungal agent should be used? When should it be started and how long should it be continued?

Several studies suggest that patients who are persistently neutropenic and febrile in spite of a week or more of antibiotic therapy are at particular risk for developing a fungal infection. Burke et al. utilized empiric amphotericin B in acute leukemia patients experiencing recrudescent fever during empiric therapy with gentamicin and carbenicillin. The incidence of serious fungal infection was found to decrease from 33% to 10% when early empiric antifungal therapy was utilized [18].

In a study at NCI, we addressed the value of empiric antifungal therapy for patients with proven infections who remained febrile and granulocytopenic after 1 week of appropriate antibiotic therapy and who had alimentary tract colonization with *Candida.* Gastrointestinal colonization was associated with a heightened frequency of disseminated fungal invasion in the postmortem analysis by Young et al. Of the 329 episodes of proven infections we treated between November 1975 and December 1979, 22 (6.7%) had gastrointestinal colonization with fungi while febrile and neutropenic and had amphotericin B added empirically to their antibiotic schedule. It was notable that half of these patients actually defervesced within a median of 3 days after starting amphotericin B, despite remaining markedly granulocytopenic. Of the 22 patients, 20 began the amphotericin within 2 weeks after starting antibiotics and continued therapy until the resolution of granulocytopenia. All of these patients recovered, none with evidence of fungal infections [19].

A second study [19] prospectively addressed the issue of using empiric amphotericin B in the granulocytopenic patient with persistent unexplained fever. The question being addressed in this study was whether the persistent fever represented an undiagnosed bacterial infection for which the antibiotic regimen should be modified or whether it represented a secondary infection, perhaps due to fungi. The usual approach in the patient with persistent unexplained fever is either to discontinue antibiotics and reevaluate the patient or to continue the antibiotics in spite of the persistent febrile course. We compared these two approaches with one in which the antibiotics were continued and empiric antifungal therapy was added with amphotericin B.

Patients were randomized to one of three groups: I to have their broad spectrum antibiotics (Keflin, gentamicin, carbenicillin) discontinued after 7 days of therapy; II to continue antibiotics until resolution of fever and neutropenia; and III to continue antibiotics along with empiric amphotericin B until the resolution of fever and granulocytopenia. We observed that stopping antibiotics resulted in early complications, predominantly due to bacterial organisms, with 56% of the patients developing complications within a median of 3 days of stopping antibiotics. Continuing antibiotics seemed to prevent early bacterial infection, but 31% of the patients randomized to this group developed fungal infections. The patients randomized both to continue antibiotics and to receive empiric antifungal therapy appeared to do best in this study. While 1 of the 18 patients in this group did develop a fungal infection, this was with Petriellidium boydii, an organism resistant to amphotericin. Thus, it seems appropriate both to continue antibiotics and to give empiric amphotericin B in the persistently febrile granulocytopenic patient. We have chosen 7 days of persistent fever while the patient is on appropriate antibiotics as the criteria for initiating antifungal therapy, although this decision is somewhat arbitrary. Amphotericin B is the present drug of choice, although we are presently comparing empiric amphotericin B with high dose oral ketoconazole in patients who are persistently febrile and granulocytopenic after 1 week of antibiotics. If no evidence for a fungal infection is found, the empiric antifungal therapy can be discontinued when the patient's granulocyte count recovers. On the other hand, if a fungal infection is documented, a more extended course of therapy is indicated. The dose of amphotericin ranges from 500 mg for an uncomplicated fungemia to 2 g or more when there is evidence of organ involvement or a disseminated infection.

Antifungal therapy may also be administered empirically to patients with progressive mucositis and symptomatic esophagitis. Although other organisms, e.g., bacteria, herpes simplex, can cause symptoms of mucositis or esophagitis, patients with *Candida* lesions will generally improve within a 48 hour trial of empiric amphotericin.

E. Duration of Therapy

A third problem relates to the duration that empiric treatment with antibiotics and antifungals should be continued, particularly when the initial evaluation has not revealed a documented infection and yet the patient remains granulocytopenic for more than 1 week. In patients with a documented infection who have defervesced on therapy and who do not have a persistent site of infection, our practice has been to continue antibiotics for 10–14 days. The more difficult situation arises in patients who have no documented source of infection and who remain persistently granulocytopenic for over 1 week. Simply continuing empiric antibiotics in these patients without a source of infection must be balanced against superinfections and the risk for organ toxicity. A series of prospective trials at the NCI has addressed this problem by randomizing patients with a FUO either to discontinue their antibiotics or to continue them until the resolution of the granulocytopenia. The patients in these trials were stratified according to whether they had defervesced or remained febrile after the initiation of antibiotics. Within 3 days of discontinuing antibiotics, 41% of the FUO patients who had initially defervesced became febrile again and the organisms obtained on reevaluation were sensitive to the antibiotics they had previously received. Similarly, 56% of the FUO patients who had remained febrile in spite of antibiotics developed complications (including hypotension in 38%) within 3 days of stopping their therapy [20].

Although patients with persistent fever and granulocytopenia did best when empiric antibiotics were continued and empiric amphotericin was added, nearly half of these patients did well even when antibiotics were stopped. This has led some investigators to suggest that stopping antibiotics may be appropriate, providing the patient can be closely monitored and the antibiotics promptly reinstituted if necessary. However, because reliable end points for reinstituting therapy are vague and because these patients can deteriorate quite rapidly, it is our opinion that it is prudent to continue antibiotics, especially in the persistently febrile patient.

Other modifications of therapy may also be required in light of preantibiotic culture results and the patient's clinical response. Common modifications include the addition of vancomycin for *S. epidermidis* bacteremias and line site infections and the addition of clindamycin for anaerobic coverage in a patient with either perirectal tenderness, necrotizing gingivitis, or a possible abdominal source. The issue of narrowing the patient to pathogen-specific therapy versus continuing the broad spectrum therapy in patients who have microbiologically documented bacteremias and for whom the antibiotic sensitivities are known is also currently being addressed in a prospective randomized trial at the NCI. Thus far, no clear advantage has emerged to either strategem, but this study is ongoing.

F. Antiviral Therapy

In addition to antibiotics and antifungal drugs, antiviral agents have recently been added to the empiric therapeutic armamentarium. For example, acycloguanosine (Acyclovir) has been shown to reduce the incidence of herpes simplex stomatitis when administered prophylactically to patients undergoing bone marrow transplantation or to patients receiving intensive courses of chemotherapy [21]. Similar protection, however, has not been observed with other important viruses in the immunocompromised host, such as cytomegalovirus (CMV) although the recent observation that CMV pneumonitis may be prevented when patients receive passive immunization with high titer CMV antisera is intriguing [21–24].

G. Diffuse Pulmonary Infiltrates

Yet another situation in which empiric therapy may be advantageous is in the cancer patient with a diffuse interstitial pulmonary infiltrate. In the non-neutropenic cancer patient, the protozoan *Pneumocystis carinii* is a frequent etiologic agent, carrying a 100% mortality if untreated. Because of the nonspecific signs and symptoms, *P. carinii* pneumonia is virtually indistinguishable from other etiologic agents causing diffuse interstitial pulmonary infiltrates, including CMV, bacteria (e.g., *Legionella, Mycoplasma*), fungi (*Candida, Aspergillus, Cryptococcus*) and viruses (influenza, RSV, adenoviruses, rhinoviruses, and measles). Prior to the availability of trimethoprim–sulfamethoxazole (TMP/SMX), most clinicians agreed that biopsy confirmation of *P. carinii* was essential to justify the administration of potentially toxic treatment with pentamidine isothionate. Presently, there is considerable debate as to whether it is preferable to proceed directly to some invasive diagnostic procedure in the patient with a diffuse infiltrate or simply to begin antibiotics empirically and monitor the patient's response to this therapy [25, 26]. However, the appropriate "empiric therapy" can quickly become complicated and can include broad spectrum antibiotics and even antifungal agents in patients who are neutropenic and already on antibiotics when the infiltrate appears. The balance between the potential side effects of broad spectrum therapy and the risks of an invasive diagnostic procedure must be carefully weighed. Presently, at the NCI, we are addressing this issue in a study which randomizes patients with a diffuse interstitial pulmonary infiltrate to either appropriate initial empiric therapy or to an open-lung biopsy and pathogen-specific therapy. If the patient randomized to the empiric therapy arm does not stabilize or improve within 4 days, an open-lung biopsy is then performed as a further guide to therapy. The major question, of course, is whether an invasive procedure can be avoided. To date, 53 patients with diffuse pulmonary infiltrates have been evaluated and 29 have been eligible and randomized. 12 were randomized to immediate open-lung biopsy, of whom 8 improved and 4 (33%) died and 17 to empiric therapy, of whom 15 improved and 2 (11.7%) died. Of the 15 patients who had an open-lung biopsy, 12 immediately and 3 after 4 days of therapy, 10 had *P. carinii* pneumonia, and 5 had nonspecific pneumonitis. Cutaneous T cell lymphoma and *Hemophilus influenzae* were diagnosed in addition to *P. carinii* pneumonia in two patients. Only one patient (with *H. influenzae*) had therapy changed as a result of the open-lung biopsy. Therefore, it appears that appropriate empiric therapy may also have a role in cancer patients with diffuse pulmonary infiltrates. Whether new procedures, such as pulmonary lavage, may provide an alternative diagnostic approach is presently being evaluated.

In conclusion, major advances have been made in decreasing the morbidity and mortality due to infectious complications in immunocompromised cancer patients with the use of empiric antimicrobial therapy, but refinements of management continue to be necessary. Clinical studies addressing these problems will be extremely helpful in defining appropriate empiric management of these patients.

References

1. Pizzo PA, Robichaud KJ, Wesley R, Commers JR (1982) Fever in the pediatric and young adult patient with cancer. Medicine 61:153
2. Schimpff SC, Saterlee W, Young VM (1971) Empiric therapy with carbenicillin and gentamicin for febrile patients with cancer and granulocytopenia. N Engl J Med 284:1061
3. Love TJ, Schimpff SC, Schiffer CA et al. (1980) Improved prognosis for granulocytopenic patients with gram-negative bacteremia. Am J Med 68:643
4. Pizzo PA (1984) Empiric therapy and prevention of infection in the immunocompromised host. In: Mandell G, Douglas G, Bennett J (eds) Principles and practice of infectious diseases, chap 276. Wiley, New York
5. Markman M, Abeloff MD (1983) Management of hematologic and infectious complications of intensive induction therapy for small cell carcinoma of the lung. Am J Med 74:741
6. Pizzo PA (1985) Management of infections in cancer patients. In: De Vita VT, Hellman S, Rosenberg SA (eds) Principles and practice of oncology, 2nd edn, chap 55. Lippincott, Philadelphia
7. Wade JL, Schimpff SC, Newman KA et al. (1982) Staphylococcus epidermidis: an increasing cause of infection in patients with granulocytopenia. Ann Intern Med 97:503
8. Pizzo PA, Ladisch S, Simon R et al. (1978) Increasing incidence of gram-positive sepsis in cancer patients. Med Pediatr Oncol 5:241
9. Davis DB (1982) Bactericidal synergism between B-lactams and aminoglycosides: mechanisms and possible therapeutic implications. Rev Infect Dis 4:237–245
10. Klastersky J, Zinner SH (1982) Synergistic combinations of antibiotics in gram-negative bacillary infections. Rev Infect Dis 4:294–301
11. Young LS (1982) Combination or single drug therapy for gram-negative sepsis. In: Remington JS, Swartz MN (eds) Current clinical topics in infectious diseases, vol 3. McGraw-Hill, New York, p 77
12. Cho SY, Chol HY (1979) Opportunistic fungal infection among cancer patients. Am J Clin Pathol 72:617–621
13. Krick JA, Remington JS (1976) Opportunistic fungal infections in patients with leukemia and lymphoma. Clin Haemotol 5:249–310
14. Singer C, Kaplan MH, Armstrong D (1977) Bacteremia and fungemia complicating neoplastic disease. Am J Med 62:731–742
15. Commers JR, Pizzo PA (1982) The role of empiric antifungal therapy for granulocytopenic cancer patients with persistent fever. In: Klastersky S (ed) Infections in cancer patients. Raven, New York, p 157
16. Commers JR, Pizzo PA (1983) Empiric antifungal therapy in the management of the febrile-granulocytopenic cancer patient. Pediatr Infect Dis 2:56
17. Pennington JE (1972) Aspergillus pneumonia in hematologic malignancy. Arch Intern Med 137:769
18. Burke PJ, Braine HG et al.. The clinical significance and management of fever in acute myelocytic leukemia. Johns Hopkins Med J 139:1–12
19. Pizzo PA, Robichaud KJ, Gill FA et al. (1982) Empiric antibiotic and antifungal therapy for cancer patients with prolonged fever and granulocytopenia. Am J Med 72:101
20. Pizzo PA, Robichaud KJ, Gill FA et al. (1979) Duration of empiric antibiotic therapy in granulocytopenic cancer patients. Am J Med 67:194

21. Wade JC, Newton B et al. (1982) Intravenous acyclovir to treat mucocutaneous herpes simplex virus infection after marrow transplantation: a double blind trial. Ann Intern Med 96:265–269
22. Winston DJ, Pollard RB (1982) Cytomegalovirus immune plasma in bone marrow transplant recipients. Ann Intern Med 97:11–18
23. Meyers JD, Zaia JA et al. (1983) Prevention of cytomegalovirus infection by cytomegalovirus immune globulin after bone marrow transplantation. Ann Intern Med 98:442–446
24. Hiemenz J, Pizzo PA (to be published) New developments in the etiology, diagnosis, treatment and prevention of infectious complications in patients with leukemia
25. Haverkos HW, Dowling JW, Hakale TR et al. (1983) Diagnosis of pneumonitis in immunocompromised patients by open-lung biopsy. Cancer 52:1093–1097
26. Hiatt JR, Ramaning KP (1982) The value of open-lung biopsy in the immunosuppressed patient. Surgery 92:285

Haematology and Blood Transfusion Vol. 29
Modern Trends in Human Leukemia VI
Edited by Neth, Gallo, Greaves, Janka

Prophylaxis of Infection in Granulocytopenic Patients

L. S. Young[1]

Most reviews of infectious complications in granulocytopenic patients stress the critical role of infection as a primary cause of death, and in influencing the outcome of therapy of the underlying disease. Aside from documented infections, fever almost invariably occurs in neutropenic patients when their functioning neutrophil count plunges below 500/mm^3 and this usually prompts the initiation of systemic antimicrobial therapy, in spite of the fact that the microbial cause of fever often remains undocumented.

In this review, I shall briefly document the efforts that have been expended toward the prophylaxis of infection in neutropenic subjects [1–4]. Each of the broad categories of intervention is listed in Table 1, along with those microorganisms that appear to be affected by such measures. The bulk of work in recent years has been primarily addressed to antimicrobial prophylaxis with or without isolation procedures. Nonetheless, it must be acknowledged that there have been some studies in the area of antifungal prophylaxis, active or passive immunization, chemoprophylaxis of fungal infection, and attempts to prevent viral infection with drugs, antiserum, and biologic response modifiers like interferon and transfer factor. Other well studied, but still controversial approaches involve the use of measures aimed at augmenting host defenses such as the transfusion of exogenous leukocytes. The recognition that patients with neoplastic diseases become colonized and subsequently infected by organisms that are present in the environment or commonly contaminate food has led to measures aimed at limiting the access of specific infecting microbes. More than 15 years ago "total protective isolation" facilities such as the "Life Island" with laminar airflow filtration were used to hospitalize the highly susceptible patients (on an experimental basis). While some evidence exists that these isolation facilities are effective, these units are too expensive and cumbersome for routine use. Laminar airflow units have been difficult to justify on a cost/efficacy basis and presently the sheer demands on nursing time have virtually precluded their widespread use outside the investigative setting.

In 1975, Schimpff and colleagues published a landmark study in which they compared isolation within the environment of the laminar airflow room with conventional ward care. The most important part of their study was the recognition that patients managed in a laminar airflow room were also given prophylactic oral nonabsorbable antimicrobials. Therefore, one of the control groups not only received routine ward care, but received the same prophylactic oral antimicrobial regimen of gentamicin, vancomycin, and nystatin given to patients in the isolation facility. A third arm of the study consisted of patients who received general ward care. Both in terms of infection rates and of survival, the patients who were managed on the open

1 M.D., Department of Medicine, Division of Infectious Diseases, UCLA Medical Center, Los Angeles, California, 90024, USA

Table 1. Intervention against infection

Intervention	Against			
	Bacteria	Fungi	Viruses	Parasites
Environmental control	GNB	Aspergillus	Varicella zoster	
Antimicrobial prophylaxis	GNB ? G+C	*? Candida*	Herpes	PCP Toxo
Prophylactic antibody (active, passive)	? GNB ? Pneumococci		V/Z Hep CMV	
Prophylactic granulocytes	GNB		↑ CMV	
Biologic response modifiers			TF–V/Z IF	

GNB = gram-negative bacilli; G + C = gram-positive cocci; PCP = *Pneumocystis carinii*; Toxo = *Toxoplasma gondii*; V/Z = varicella zoster; Hep = hepatitis; CMV = cytomegalovirus; TF = transfer factor; IF = interferon

ward with prophylactic oral antimicrobials did almost as well as the patients managed in the laminar airflow rooms. This is consistent with the experience of a number of investigators. True airborne infection, even in the highly neutropenic patient, is rare. Perhaps the best accepted example is that of pulmonary aspergillosis. Other so-called true airborne pathogens, such as varicella zoster, tuberculosis, and perhaps the Legionnaire's bacillus are rather infrequently encountered in most cancer treatment centers. The expensive part of laminar airflow is the air filtration equipment and the requirement for supportive services for the patient in total isolation. Single-room isolation with antimicrobial prophylaxis seems to be a more cost-effective compromise.

Oral nonabsorbable antimicrobial suppression regimens (or as some investigators have called them, "total decontamination regiments") are quite expensive and may be poorly tolerated. Anyone who has ingested oral gentamicin and/or polymyxin B is immediately aware of the unpalatability of such prophylactic agents. The suggestion that trimethoprim/sulfamethoxazole might be an alternative prophylactic regimen came from the work of Hughes and associates. They found the routine use of co- trimoxazole prevented pneumocystis infections in leukemic children and resulted in a generalized reduction in all bacterial infections in this patient population (the notable exception was an increase in oral candidiasis). Soon thereafter, other investigators began exploring the routine prophylactic use of trimethoprim/sulfamethoxazole to prevent sepsis originating from the gastrointestinal tract. While the majority of published studies seem to suggest a beneficial role for trimethoprim/sulfamethoxazole in this setting, major reservations have also been expressed. First, both trimethoprim and sulfamethoxazole are not oral, nonabsorbable agents, but are systemically absorbed. The sulfonamide component may be quite sensitizing. Second, while some studies have demonstrated an overall reduction in infection rates, resistance to either agent may emerge. Third, folate antagonism may result in the prolongation of neutropenia in recipients of trimethoprim. Fourth, other side effects like gastrointestinal intolerance may develop. Fifth and perhaps most important, trimethoprim/sulfamethoxazole is inactive against *Pseudomonas aeruginosa* and these bacteria are a major cause of serious infection in neutropenic patients.

At present, there is considerable interest and enthusiasm about the potential prophylactic role of the new quinoline agents. Several agents of this class have antipseudomonal, antistaphylococcal, and antienterococcal activity with minimal impact upon the anerobic gastrointestinal flora. These would appear to be most attractive properties for prophylactic use. Only well-executed clinical trials, however, will be able to demonstrate their advantages over other regimens. A central issue in whether they will truly prevent serious systemic infections, not just "mask" infection by making bacterial cultures negative.

For nonbacterial infections, there has been some progress in certain areas. There is no doubt that herpes simplex infections can be prevented by the use of a acyclovir. The protection, however, seems to last only for the duration of prophylaxis. Infection rates quickly rebound as soon as the medication is discontinued. Varicella zoster immunoglobin is thought to have a definite use in the prophylaxis of chickenpox in exposed juvenile patients. The use of immunoglobulins or vaccines for hepatitis may have an indication in some immunocompromised patients. As mentioned previously, the routine use of trimethoprim/sulfamethoxazole is effective in preventing *Pneumocystis carinii* pneumonia. Such regimens may also be effective in preventing nocardial and toxoplasmal infection, but definitive proof is not available from controlled studies.

Perhaps the greatest area of need for effective prophylactic measures is the field of fungal infections. Nystatin and amphotericin B have been available for many years; more recently, ketoconazole has been introduced as an oral prophylactic agent. There has been a paucity of real evidence that these measures actually reduce the incidence of systemic candidiasis.

In view of the likelihood that many pharmacologic agents will be used in an attempt to prevent infection, I would like to comment on the nature of study design. The desirable characteristics of a prophylactic antimicrobial study are summarized in Table 2. Relatively few published studies have incorporated the majority of these desirable features. One of the major problems that I perceive in the published literature is not only a lack of well-designed double-blind trials, but the failure to exclude from study any patient who has evidence of fever or infection at the point of entry into the study. Many trials fail to assess patient compliance and use objective end points for microbiologic documentation of infection. In the final analysis, we are interested in not only the reduction of infection, but evidence that the use of prophylactic agents reduces systemic antibiotic usage, shortens the duration of febrility or clinically suspected infection, and improves survival. We must be concerned that prophylaxis can mask infection and predispose to emergence of resistant organisms. It is possible that prophylaxis will result in an overall reduction in the incidence of infections, but those that do occur are more severe and possibly more resistant to antimicrobials. Therefore, effective prophylaxis could still result in the same costs,

Table 2. Desirable characteristics of prophylactic antimicrobial studies

Randomized, double-blind study designs
Inclusion of patients who are free of infection and fever at randomization
Objective measurement of patient compliance with the prophylactic regimen
Inclusion of large numbers of patients with similar diseases and at the same stage of disease
Uniform treatment of underlying diseases
Minimization or elimination of variables that could affect infection rates (e.g., protected environments and prophylactic granulocyte transfusions)
Comparison of regimens according to the onset of fever, the first documented infection, and the start of antimicrobial therapy
Adequate intervals for prophylactic regimens to have taken effect before the beginning of the observation period
Objective end points of microbiologically documented infection for analysis
Evaluation of complications, including side effects and emergence of resistance
Analysis to include survival of treatment and control groups by life-table analysis

measured in terms of hospital charges for prolonged hospitalization, to say nothing of infection morbidity.

Augmentation of host defenses as a prophylactic measure is theoretically a highly appealing approach. It does not risk selection for antibiotic resistance, nor will drug toxicity ensue. It does not place the patient at risk of the psychiatric complications of management within a laminar air flow unit. However appealing these approaches may be, their implementation has met with only limited success. Augmentation of host defenses through active immunization has led to only limited gains against organisms such as the pneumococci or *Pseudomonas aeruginosa.* While my personal feeling is that such approaches can do no harm, the real impact upon disease incidence has yet to be well demonstrated. In the case of *Pseudomonas* immunization, one vaccine that I have used has been quite toxic in itself. Routine use of exogenous immunoglobulins to prevent infection, particularly with some of the newer preparations that can be more easily delivered intravenously is attractive, but expensive. Convincing evidence of prophylactic efficacy in neutropenic subjects is not yet available.

Finally, we have been through a period during the last 10 years when there was considerable initial enthusiasm for the use of transfused granulocytes to prevent infection. While such approaches may result in a reduction of some infections, complication rates associated with granulocyte transfusions are high, including a large number of pulmonary infiltrates. Several studies have now shown that granulocyte transfusions predispose to cytomegalovirus infection in the previously seronegative patient. The routine use of prophylactic granulocytes cannot be justified based on our current perception of the high risk of complications, not only from the physical infusion of granulocytes, but from transfusion-associated viral infections.

References

1. Young LS (1981) Nosocomial infections in the immunocompromised adult. Am J Med 70:398–404
2. Young LS (1981) Management of infections in leukemia and lymphoma. In: Rubin RH, Young LS (eds) Clinical approach to infection in the compromised host. Plenum, New York, pp 461–506
3. Young LS (1983) Role of granulocyte transfusions in treating and preventing infection. Cancer Treat Rep 67:109–111
4. Young LS (1983) Antimicrobial prophylaxis against infection in neutropenic patients. J Infect Dis 147:611–614

Haematology and Blood Transfusion Vol. 29
Modern Trends in Human Leukemia VI
Edited by Neth, Gallo, Greaves, Janka

Are Granulocyte Transfusions Helpful in Treating and Preventing Infections?

R. G. Strauss [1]

A. Introduction

"Can granulocyte transfusions (GTX) treat and prevent infections?" Clearly, the answer is "yes"! Should all patients, then, with severe neutropenia (< 500 neutrophils/μl blood) receive therapeutic GTX to treat bacterial infections – or if free of infections, receive prophylactic GTX to prevent infections? Most emphatically, the answer is "no"! In this report, the literature will be reviewed as it pertains to the use of therapeutic and prophylactic GTX as supportive care for severely neutropenic patients. Conclusions of the review are:

1. Therapeutic GTX definitely should be used to treat episodes of gram-negative septicemia that have failed to respond to optimal, combination antibiotics.
2. Therapeutic GTX probably should be used to treat documented bacterial or fungal infections of other types under similar circumstances.
3. Prophylactic GTX should not be used except in investigational settings. However, renewed considerations might be given to conducting studies of prophylactic GTX in certain clinical settings.

B. Therapeutic Granulocyte Transfusions

A total of 24 papers pertaining to the use of therapeutic GTX in neutropenic patients were analyzed [1–24]. The role of therapeutic GTX has been extensively reviewed recently [25–30], and this paper will not reiterate an exhaustive discussion. Instead, data will be combined and analyzed collectively. Patients from all 24 papers who were treated with GTX for specific types of infections are displayed in Table 1 together with the results of therapy. When drawing conclusions, several limiting factors must be kept in mind: (a) except for patients with culture-proven septicemia, diagnostic criteria for each type of infection varied; (b) only the index infections which prompted GTX are listed (additional infections recognized during therapy or postmortem were not tabulated); (c) with the exception of septicemia, it was impossible to study the response of individual categories of infections caused by specific types of organisms; and (d) criteria to judge clinical response varied and eventual outcome could not always be ascribed to the course of the index infection. All patients who received therapeutic GTX were tabulated in the "treated" column (Table 1), but only those whose course and mortality could be clearly documented were included in the "evaluable" column. Criteria for "favorable response" included absence of fever, sterile blood cultures, clearing of chest roentgenograms, disappearance of skin inflammation, and survival.

Many patients with septicemia have been reported (Table 1). Important information has been learned from the study of gram-negative sepsis in recipients of therapeutic GTX. Investigators agree that most septic patients will recover with antibiotics alone

1 M.D., Professor of Pathology and Pediatrics, Medical Director, Elmer L. DeGowin Memorial Blood Center, University of Iowa Hospitals and Clinics, Iowa City, Iowa 52242, USA

Table 1. Pooled results of 24 studies of therapeutic GTX

Types of infections	Treat-ed	Evalu-able	Favorable response[a]
Total septicemias[b]	435	247	146/247 (59)
Gram-negative sepsis	238	172	103/172 (60)
Gram-positive sepsis	44	18	16/18 (89)
Polymicrobial sepsis	15	15	7/15 (47)
Fungemia	6	3	–
Sepsis organism unspecified	132	39	18/39 (46)
Total pneumonias	130	45	23/45 (51)
Gram-negative	3	–	–
Gram-positive	1	–	–
Polymicrobial pneumonia	1	–	–
Fungal pneumonia	10	9	1/9 (11)
Pneumonia organism unspecified	115	11	7/11 (64)
Total localized infections[c]	142	48	–
Cellulitis-abscess	76	38	32/38 (84
Genitourinary	11	8	6/8 (75)
Total fever of unknown origin	184	85	64/85 (75)

[a] Number with favorable response/total number evaluable (percentage)
[b] All septic patients included (patients with septicemia plus a localized infection are listed here, not under the localized infection)
[c] Infections of skin, pharynx, genitourinary and gastrointestinal systems. Detailed data tabulated only for cellulitis–abscess and genitourinary categories

if they experience bone marrow recovery during the early days of infection [1, 10, 11, 23, 24]. Such patients do not require GTX. In contrast, patients with persistent, severe neutropenia due to continuing marrow failure may [11] or may not [24] benefit when GTX are added to antibiotics. It should be noted that only 36% of nontransfused, control patients (antibiotics only) in the first study [11] survived, whereas, 72% of controls survived in the last [24]. Thus, it was fairly easy in the first [11], and impossible in the last [24], to demonstrate a significant benefit from the added effects of therapeutic GTX. The greatest benefit of therapeutic GTX is apparent in patients with persistent marrow failure [1, 11, 23].

Regarding other types of septicemia and other kinds of infection (Table 1), information published to date is insufficient to determine whether therapeutic GTX offer advantages over antibiotics alone. Patients with pneumonia, localized infections, and fever of unknown origin responded well to GTX. However, comparable responses have been reported using antibiotics alone.

Because of the clinical complexity of these heterogeneous patients, seven controlled studies were performed (Table 2). The response of infected, neutropenic patients to treatment with GTX plus antibiotics was compared with that of nontransfused, control patients given antibiotics alone and evaluated concurrently. Three of the seven studies found a significant overall benefit for GTX [11, 12, 23]. A fourth study [1] found a significant improvement in survival only for the subgroup of GTX recipients who did not have early endogenous marrow recovery. It must be emphasized, however, that patients in these reports were selected by study design to be unusually ill. Thus, information provided may not be directly applicable to many neutropenic patients encountered in practice. For example, in three studies [7, 12, 23] patients were eligible to receive GTX only after failing 48–72 h of antibiotic

Table 2. Seven controlled therapeutic granulocyte transfusion trials

Reference	Randomized	Patients entered		Percentage septic	Percentage survival	
		Transfused	Controls		Transfused	Controls
[8]	No	39	37	100	46	30
[11]	Yes	13	14	100	75[a]	36
[12]	Yes	17	19	31	76[a]	26
[7]	No	17	22	34	78	80
[23]	Yes	17	13	67	59[a]	15
[1]	Yes	12	19	39	82[b]	62
[24]	Yes	48	47	80	63	72

[a] Survival of transfused patients significantly ($P < 0.05$) greater than controls
[b] Survival was improved in the subgroup of patients who did not have endogenous marrow recovery

therapy. As another factor, many patients had cancer resistant to therapy and, as expected, GTX were able to prolong life in these terminal patients with persistent marrow failure. In practice, however, it is difficult to justify therapeutic GTX as a routine part of palliative therapy offered to terminal patients for whom there is no effective anticancer therapy. Finally, antibiotic therapy in the controlled studies may not have been optimal by current standards. Antibiotics chosen and doses employed were recorded, but in only one study [24] was there an indication that proper precautions (antibiotic blood levels, serum bacteriostatic/bactericidal activity, or sensitivity testing designed to detect antibiotic synergism) were employed to ensure adequate antibiotic therapy. As reviewed in references [25] and [26], the survival of cancer patients with sepsis is significantly better in patients receiving antibiotics deemed appropriate than it is in those given ineffective therapy. Perhaps GTX are most likely to benefit patients whose infecting bacteria are being inadequately treated by antibiotics [31, 32]. Certainly (Table 2), survival of the nontransfused controls was inferior in the studies showing an overall benefit for GTX [11, 12, 23] when compared with the better survival of controls in the studies unable to demonstrate an advantage for GTX.

Despite these reservations, a number of conclusions can be drawn from the therapeutic GTX trials published to date. Clearly, some neutropenic patients die from bacterial infections, despite the most skilled use of combination antibiotics. Among these patients, therapeutic GTX have improved the survival of those with persistent, severe neutropenia who have gram-negative sepsis that fails to respond to antibiotics. It is likely that similar patients with other types of documented bacterial infections will also benefit from GTX, but efficacy has not been proven. On the other hand, therapeutic GTX have never been shown to be efficacious for treating nonbacterial infections or for fever of unknown origin. Unquestionably, the return of bone marrow function early in the course of a bacterial infection is usually associated with resolution of that infection, whether or not GTX are added to appropriate antibiotics. However, nearly all patients with persistent marrow disease eventually die, either from the index infection or from a later one.

C. Prophylactic Granulocyte Transfusions

Eleven studies that pertain to prophylactic GTX were reviewed (Table 3). Five were randomized studies attempting to prevent infections in leukemic patients [33–37]; three additional studies of leukemic patients were controlled, but not randomized [5, 38, 39]. Three reports were randomized studies of bone marrow transplant recipients [40–42]. One published report [43] was not included because it was presumed to include the same patients reported by Clift et al. [40]; abstracts and letters were not included.

Data from the 11 studies are presented in Tables 3 and 4. Several qualifying statements are required for proper interpretation. The precise number of subjects in each group was difficult to determine in some studies because: (a) patients occasionally failed to complete the trial; (b) some "nontransfused" controls received therapeutic GTX; (c) patients may have been counted more than once if they experienced more than one course of remission induction therapy; (d) tabulation of infections varied considerably among investigators; and (e) authors' judgments regarding overall benefit were not always based on statistical significance, and contrasting results were sometimes noted when subpopulations of patients were analyzed separately.

Prophylactic GTX are considered by nearly all investigators to be of marginal value because the benefits are few while the risks and expenses are substantial (reviewed in references [26–30]). However, in two studies [34, 40], prophylactic GTX undeniably decreased the incidence of infections in severely neutropenic patients (Table 4). Of note, fairly large doses of granulocytes were infused daily in these studies, and efforts were made to optimize donor–recipient compatibility by HLA typing and/or leukocyte cross-matching (donors were excluded if recipient sera reacted with donor lymphocytes). Although

Table 3. Eleven studies of prophylactic granulocyte transfusions

Reference	Patients entered	GTX recipients	No GTX
Randomized leukemia			
[33]	18	9	9
[34]	50	22	28
[35]	92	49	43
[36]	65	29	36
[37]	24	13	11
Not randomized leukemia			
[38]	63	38	25
[5]	27	7	20
[39]	45	18	27
Randomized bone marrow transplants			
[40]	69	29	40
[41]	38	19	19
[42]	182	92	90
Total patients	673	325	348

Table 4. The success of prophylactic granulocyte transfusions

Reference	Dose	Matching
Definite success		
[34]	2.1 × 10 daily	LCT-negative [a]
[40]	1.5 – 2.2 × 10 daily	LCT-negative, HLA [b]
Partial success		
[35]	0.7 × 10 daily	None
[5]	0.07 × 10 ?	HLA
[39]	1.6 × 10 daily	HLA
[42]	? daily	HLA
Lack of success		
[33]	1.2 × 10 alternate day	None
[37]	1.5 × 10 alternate day	None
[36]	0.9 × 10 daily	None
[38]	2.6 × 10 twice weekly	LCT-negative, HLA
[41]	1.2 × 10 daily	None

[a] LCT-negative = Recipient sera negative for lymphocytotoxic antibody

[b] HLA = Donor and recipient at least haploidentical for HLA-A and HLA-B

Table 5. Incidence of immediate, nonhemolytic, febrile transfusion reactions

Reference	HLA matching	Reactions/course	Reactions/ individual GTX
[35]	No	39/53 (72%)	158/987 =(16%)
[45]	No	Not reported	1233/6020=(18%)
[37]	No	12/13 (92%)	Not reported
[33]	No	7/10 (70%)	Not reported
[36]	No	23/31 (74%)	Not reported
[41]	No	19/48 (40%)	Not reported
[23]	Yes[a]	0/17 (0%)	Not reported

[a] Donor-recipient compatible by leukocyte cross-match; recipients premedicated with diphenhydramine and acetaminophen

overall success could not be documented in four reports [5, 35, 39, 42], partial success was demonstrated when certain groups of patients were examined separately. Prophylactic GTX were found to decrease the incidence of bacterial sepsis [35], clinical infections (but not those proven by culture) [5], and pneumonia [39]. Success was implied in another study [42] since prophylactic GTX were equally effective as a comprehensive program of protected environment (laminar flow, etc.) in decreasing infections in bone marrow transplant recipients.

Five studies [33, 36–38, 41] failed to show benefit (Table 4). None of these studies provided both large numbers of granulocytes and granulocytes from matched donors. Among the nine studies that found only partial or no success, only one [39] provided at least 10^{10} granulocytes daily from donors selected by leukocyte matching (Table 4). Thus, the failure of prophylactic GTX trials published to date might be explained, at least in part, by transfusion of suboptimal granulocyte concentrates.

The other major deterrent to the widespread use of prophylactic GTX is concern for the risks involved. The use of GTX exposes both granulocyte donors and recipients to potential risks. The majority of granulocyte donors do not experience adverse effects, and even when they occur, they usually are of little consequence [44]. Despite their importance, hazards to donors will not be discussed further in this paper. Instead, the adverse effects of GTX experienced by recipients will be reviewed.

Immediate, nonhemolytic, febrile transfusion reactions occur during or within a few hours after transfusion, and are characterized by fever and chills. Other findings include cyanosis, dyspnea, wheezing, nausea, vomiting, itching, urticaria, anxiety, and fluctuations in blood pressure. The majority of patients can be expected to experience a reaction if they receive a course of several GTX from random donors (Table 5). The chance that an individual GTX will provoke a reaction is fairly small. Alloimmunization to leukocyte antigens is the most likely causative mechanism with transfused leukocytes interacting with anti-leukocyte antibodies in recipient sera. The lack of reactions in Table 23 of reference [23] supports this mechanism since donors were selected by HLA typing and by compatibility with leukocyte cross-match. However, reactions may have been masked as recipients were premediated prior to each GTX.

The incidence of alloimmunization following GTX, and the importance of emerging antibodies are only partly defined. Reports indicating the detection of anti-leukocyte antibodies in patients following GTX are listed in Table 6. At the present time, it is impossible to predict accurately the likelihood that an individual patient might become immunized during a course of GTX, or whether the antibody would have clinical importance. Several methods exist to detect anti-leukocyte antibodies and difficulties arise in comparing data from different laboratories. For example (Table 6), none of the patients of Cooper et al. [38]

Table 6. Prevalence of anti-leukocyte antibodies following GTX

Reference	HLA-matched donors	Antibodies detected [a]	(%)
[34]	No	7/23	(30)
[33]	No	7/10	(70)
[38]	Yes	0/14	(0)
[46]	No	23/26	(88)
[54]	No	13/22	(59)

[a] Subjects with antibody/total subjects studied (percentage)

were alloimmunized after receiving GTX from HLA-matched donors when antibodies were measured only by lymphocytotoxicity – a technique detecting primarily anti-HLA antibodies. In contrast, nearly all patients evaluated by Thompson et al. [46] produced anti-leukocyte antibodies in response to random donor GTX when studied by a battery of assays that were designed to detect antibodies directed against multiple lymphocyte and granulocyte antigens. Based on current knowledge, it seems likely that the majority of patients receiving a series of GTX from random donors will develop anti-leukocyte antibodies if their sera are evaluated by a battery of tests.

The importance of such antibodies is unclear. In animals [47, 48], immunization with blood products decreases the effectiveness of subsequent GTX. Post-transfusion increments of blood leukocyte counts were diminished, granulocyte function was impaired, thrombocytopenia was induced, and survival of immunized animals was decreased. Studies in humans are not as definitive, but data suggest that anti-leukocyte antibodies mediate transfusion reactions, adversely affect post-transfusion increments of blood leukocyte counts, alter the circulating kinetics of infused granulocytes, and decrease the antimicrobial effects of GTX. For example, Goldstein et al. [49] observed transfusion reactions following 90% of GTX administered to immunized recipients, while only 11% of GTX given to patients without anti-leukocytic antibodies evoked reactions. In contrast, Ungerleider et al. [50] studied 187 donor–recipient pairs with a battery of anti-leukocyte antibody assays. They were unable to establish a significant relationship between the presence of antibodies and either transfusion reactions or postinfusion neutrophil recovery. McCullough et al. [50] found the intravascular kinetics of transfused granulocytes to be altered adversely (decreased recovery, half-life, and migration to sites of infection with increased liver sequestration) by granulocyte agglutinating antibodies, but not by granulocytotoxic or lymphocytotoxic antibodies. Dutcher et al. [52] found transfused neutrophils to be sequestered in the lungs of alloimmunized patients. In additional studies, this same group [53] observed that radiolabeled leukocytes obtained from random donors failed to reach sites of infection in alloimmunized patients (defined by refractoriness to random donor platelets and the presence of lymphocytotoxic antibodies reacting against more than 20% of a lymphocyte panel). Dahlke et al. [6] noted decreased survival of patients with gram-negative septicemia, who received therapeutic GTX deemed to be incompatible by a granulocyte indirect immunofluorescence antibody assay, when compared with similar patients given more compatible GTX. Finally, pulmonary infiltrates are a serious complication that may be related to alloimmunization [3, 24, 35]. However, they can occur in patients not receiving GTX [24], and the exact mechanisms involved in individual patients are often unclear. Whether immediate, nonhemolytic, febrile transfusion reactions and pulmonary reactions can be consistently eliminated in individual recipients by HLA matching and leukocyte compatibility testing remains to be shown.

Other potential hazards of GTX do not pose major barriers to prophylactic GTX. The concern over fatal pulmonary reactions due to the interaction of GTX and amphotericin B [55] simply has not been confirmed by several other investigators (reviewed in reference [27]). However, it may be a useful practice to infuse amphotericin B during the morning and GTX during the late afternoon in patients receiving both agents. Graft-versus-host disease can be eliminated by irradiating granulocyte concentrates with 1500–5000 rads prior to transfusion. Finally, transfusion-associated cytomegalovirus infections that arise in seronegative patients can be avoided by selecting donors who are likewise seronegative for anti-cytomegalovirus antibodies.

The following recommendations can be made. Based on current evidence, prophylactic GTX cannot be recommended for treating neutropenic cancer patients (except on an investigational basis) because the benefits are few and the risks and costs are substantial. Although still investigational because of the multiple complex issues involved, an argument can be made to support bone marrow transplant recipients with prophylactic GTX when granulocyte concentrates are obtained from HLA closely matched donors. Since many earlier prophylactic GTX trials can be criticized for transfusing small numbers of neutrophils, too infrequently, and without regard for leukocyte compatibility, consideration probably should be given to renewed investigations in this area using HLA-matched donors who produce good *platelet* increments (as a sign of compatibility). In such trials, prophylactic GTX should be discontinued if anti-leukocyte antibodies appear and/or if immediate, febrile transfusion reactions occur that cannot be eliminated with premedications. Granulocyte concentrates should contain $\geqq 1.5 \times 10^{10}$ and be given daily. Patients seronegative for anti-cytomegalovirus antibody should receive GTX from seronegative donors, and granulocyte concentrates should be irradiated. Obviously, careful comparisons of the costs of prophylactic GTX versus alternative therapies (e.g., protected environments) must be made, in addition to observations of efficacy and toxicity.

Note added in proof: Gomez-Villagran et al. (Cancer 54:734–738, 1984) reported prophylactic GTX to successfully decrease infections in leukemic patients when given as 1.24×10^{10} per day.

References

1. Alavi JB, Root RK, Djerassi I et al. (1977) A randomized clinical trial of granulocyte transfusions for infection in acute leukemia. N Engl J Med 296:706–711
2. Ambinder EP, Button GR, Cheung T et al. (1981) Filtration versus gravity leukapheresis in febrile granulocytopenic patients: a randomized prospective trial. Blood 57:826–840
3. Bow EJ, Schroeder ML, Louie TJ (1984) Pulmonary complications in patients receiving granulocyte transfusions and amphotericin B. Can Med Assoc J 130:593–597
4. Buchholz DH, Blumberg N, Bove JR (1979) Long-term granulocyte transfusion in patients with malignant neoplasms. Arch Intern Med 139:317–320
5. Curtis JE, Hasselback R, Bergsagel DE (1977) Leukocyte transfusions for the prophylaxis and treatment of infections associated with granulocytopenia. Can Med Assoc J 117:341–345
6. Dahlke MB, Keashen M, Alavi JB et al. (1982) Granulocyte transfusions and outcome of alloimmunized patients with gram-negative sepsis. Transfusion 22:347–378
7. Fortuny IE, Bloomfield CD, Hadlock DC et al. (1975) Granulocyte transfusion: a controlled study in patients with acute non-lymphocytic leukemia. Transfusion 15:548–558
8. Graw RG Jr, Herzig G, Perry S, Henderson IS (1972) Normal granulocyte transfusion therapy. N Engl J Med 287:367–371
9. Hahn DM, Schimpff SC, Young VM et al. (1977) Amikaein and cephalothin: empure regimen for granulocytopenic cancer patients. Antimicrob Agents Chemother 12:618–624
10. Hershko C, Naparstck I, Eldor A, Izak G (1978) Granulocyte transfusion therapy. Vox Sang 34:129–135
11. Herzig RH, Herzig GP, Graw RG Jr et al. (1977) Successful granulocyte transfusion therapy for gram-negative septicemia. N Engl J Med 296:702–705
12. Higby DJ, Yates JW, Henderson ES, Holland JF (1975) Filtration leukapheresis for granulocytic transfusion therapy. N Engl J Med 292:761–766
13. Higby DJ, Freman A, Henderson ES et al. (1976) Granulocyte transfusions in children using filter-collected cells. Cancer 38:1407–1413
14. Love LJ, Schimpff SC, Schiffer CA, Wiernik PH (1980) Improved prognosis for granulocytopenic patients with gram-negative bacteria. Am J Med 68:643–648
15. Maybe DA, Milan AP, Ruymann FB (1977) Granulocyte transfusion therapy in children. South Med J 70:320–324
16. McCredie KB, Freireich EJ, Hester JP, Vallejos C (1973) Leukocyte transfusion therapy for patients with host-defense failure. Transplant Proc 5:1285–1289

17. Morse EE, Katz AJ, Buchholz DH, Houx J (1981) Clinical effectiveness of transfusion of granulocytes obtained by filtration or intermittent flow centrifugation. Cancer 47:974–977
18. Pflieger H, Arnold R, Bhaduri S et al. (1981) Granulocyte transfusions in acute leukemia: regeneration of granulopoiesis as determining factor of survival. Scand J Haematol 26:215–220
19. Pole JG, Davie M, Kershaw I et al. (1976) Granulocyte transfusions in acute leukemia: regeneration of granulopoiesis as determining factor of survival. Scand J Haematol 26:215–220
20. Schiffer CA, Buchholz DA, Aisner J et al. (1975) Clinical experience with transfusion of granulocytes obtained by continuous flow filtration leukapheresis. Am J Med 58:373–381
21. Steinherz PG, Reich IM (1979) Granulocyte transfusions in infected neutropenic children with malignancies. Med Pediatr Oncol 6:67–76
22. Strauss RG, Goedken MM, Maguire LC et al. (1980a) Gram-negative sepsis treated with neutrophils collected exclusively by intermittent flow centrifugation leukapheresis. Transfusion 20:79–81
23. Vogler WR, Winton EF (1977) A controlled study of the efficacy of granulocyte transfusions in patients with neutropenia. Am J Med 63:548–555
24. Winston DJ, Ho WG, Gale RP (1982) Therapeutic granulocyte transfusions for documented infections: a controlled trial in 95 infectious granulocytopenic episodes. Ann Intern Med 97:509–515
25. Strauss RG (1978) Therapeutic neutrophil transfusions: are controlled trials no longer appropriate? Am J Med 65:1001–1006
26. Strauss RG, Connett JE (1982) The role of prophylactic and therapeutic granulocyte transfusions in adult leukemia. In: Bloomfield CD (ed) Adult leukemia, vol 1. Martinus Nijhoff, Boston, pp 351–380
27. Strauss RG (1983) Granulocyte transfusion therapy. Clin Oncol 2:635–655
28. Schiffer CA (1983) Granulocyte transfusion therapy. Cancer Treat Rep 67:113–119
29. Clift RA, Buckner CD (1984) Granulocyte transfusions. Am J Med 76:631–636
30. Wright DG (1984) Leukocyte transfusions: thinking twice. Am J Med 76:637–645
31. Anderson ET, Young LS, Hewitt WL (1976) Simultaneous antibiotic levels "breakthrough" gram-negative bacteremia. Am J Med 61:493–498
32. Laurenti F, Ferro R, Giancarlo I et al. (1981) Polymorphonuclear leukocyte transfusion for the treatment of sepsis of the newborn infant. J Pediatr 98:118–123
33. Schiffer CA, Aisner J, Daly PA et al. (1979) Alloimmunization following prophylactic granulocyte transfusion. Blood 54:766–774
34. Mannoni P, Rodet M, Vernant JP et al. (1979) Efficiency of prophylactic granulocyte transfusions in preventing infections in acute leukaemia. Blood Transfusion Immunohaematol 22:503–518
35. Strauss RG, Connett JE, Gael RP et al. (1981) A controlled trial of prophylactic granulocyte transfusions during initial induction chemotherapy for acute myelogenous leukemia. N Engl J Med 305:597–603
36. Sutton DMC, Shumak KH, Baker MA (1982) Prophylactic granulocyte transfusions in acute leukemia. Plasma Therapy 3:45–50
37. Ford JM, Cullen MH, Roberts MM et al. (1982) Prophylactic granulocyte transfusions: results of a randomized controlled trial in patients with acute myelogenous leukemia. Transfusion 22:311–316
38. Cooper MR (1981) Personal communication update of earlier study, Cooper MR, Heise E, Richards F et al. (1975) A prospective study of histocompatible leukocyte and platelet transfusions during chemotherapeutic induction of acute myeloblastic leukemia. In: Goldman JM, Lowenthal RM (eds) Leukocytes: separation, collection and transfusion. Academic, New York, pp 436–449
39. Hester JP, McCredie KB, Freireich EJ (1979) Advances in supportive care: blood component transfusions. In: Care of the Child with Cancer. American Cancer Society, pp 93–100
40. Clift RA, Sanders JE, Thomas ED et al. (1978) Granulocyte transfusions for the prevention of infection in patients receiving bone-marrow transplants. N Engl J Med 298:1052–1057
41. Winston DJ, Ho WG, Young LS, Gale RP (1982) Prophylactic granulocyte transfusions during human bone marrow transplantation. Am J Med 68:893–897
42. Buckner CD, Clift RA, Thomas ED et al. (1983) Early infections complications in allogenic marrow transplant recipients with acute leukemia: effects of prophylactic measures. Infection 11:243–250
43. Buckner CD, Clift RA, Sanders JE, Thomas ED (1978) The role of a protective environment and prophylactic granulocyte transfusions in marrow transplantation. Transplant Proc 10:255–257
44. Strauss RG, Koepke JA, Maguire LC, Thompson JS (1980b) Clinical laboratory ef-

fects on donors of intermittent-flow centrifugation platelet-leucapheresis performed with hydroxyethyl starch and citrate. Clin Lab Haematol 2:1–11
45. Buchholz DH, Houx JL (1979) A survey of the current use of filtration leukapheresis. Exp Hematol 7:1–10
46. Thompson JS, Herbick JM, Burns CP et al. (1978) Granulocyte antigens detected by cytotoxicity (GCY) and capillary agglutination (CAN). Transplant Proc 10:885–888
47. Appelbaum FR, Hapani RJ, Graw RG (1977) Consequences of prior alloimmunization during granulocyte transfusion. Transfusion 17:460–464
48. Westrick MA, Debelak-Fehir KM, Epstein RB (1977) The effect of prior whole blood transfusion on subsequent granulocyte support in leukopenic dogs. Transfusion 17:611–614
49. Goldstein IM, Eyre JH, Terasaki PI et al. (1971) Leukocyte transfusions: role of leukocyte alloantibodies in determining transfusion response. Transfusion 11:19–24
50. Ungerleider RS, Appelbaum FR, Trapani RJ, Deisseroth AB (1979) Lack of predictive value of antileukocyte antibody screening in granulocyte transfusion therapy. Transfusion 19:90–94
51. McCullough JJ, Weiblen BJ, Clay ME, Forstrom L (1981) Effect of leukocyte antibodies on the fate, in vivo, of Indium-111-labelled granulocytes. Blood 58:164–170
52. Dutcher JP, Fox JJ, Riggs C et al. (1982) Pulmonary retention of indium-111-labelled granulocytes in alloimmunized patients (Abstract). Blood 60:177 a
53. Dutcher JP, Schiffer CA, Johnston GS et al. (1983) Alloimmunization prevents the migration of transfused ^{111}Indium-labeled granulocytes to sites of infection. Blood 62
54. Arnold R, Goldmann SF, Pflieger H (1980) Lymphocytotoxic antibodies in patients receiving granulocyte transfusions. Vox Sanguinis 38:250–258
55. Wright DG, Robichaud KJ, Pizzo PA, Deisscroth AB (1981) Lethal pulmonary reactions associated with the combined use of amphotericin B and leukocyte transfusions. N Engl J Med 304:1185–1189

Haematology and Blood Transfusion Vol. 29
Modern Trends in Human Leukemia VI
Edited by Neth, Gallo, Greaves, Janka

Single Donor Platelet Transfusion

C. A. Schiffer [1]

Cytopheresis equipment from a number of manufacturers now permits the rapid, safe, and efficient procurement of functionally normal platelets from single donors. There has been an extensive proliferation of these blood cell separators and virtually all large blood collection centers and most large hospitals have at least one blood cell separator in operation. Transfusions from single donors selected by HLA typing are a well-accepted feature of the management of alloimmunized patients [1, 2]. In addition, occasional centers located at a distance from regional blood transfusion centers utilize nonmatched transfusions from single donors as a major part of their "regular" platelet supply. Because most single donor transfusions are not obtained from "closed systems" however, these collections cannot be stored for more than 24 h, making it more difficult to utilize such products rationally as a form of long-term platelet inventory. Furthermore, the availability of newer plastic bags now allows storage of platelet concentrates at ambient temperatures with preservation of normal post-transfusion recovery after 7 days of storage [3]. Thus, there should be few such "geographic peculiarities" which necessitate the widespread use of single donor platelets as "random donor platelets" in the future.

Alloimmunization with refractoriness to random donor platelet transfusions remains the major complication of any type of platelet transfusion therapy. There has been considerable interest in the last 5 years in the use of single donor platelets as a means of preventing or delaying immunization in transfusion recipients. There are a number of scientific, theoretic, and practical considerations which are implicit in such an approach. These will be discussed in detail with evidence presented which on balance will support the approach of reserving single donor platelet transfusion for alloimmunized patients.

The "scientific" evidence is perhaps the simplest of the issues to deal with. There has only been a single evaluable study done comparing the use of single donor with pooled random donor platelets performed in a prospectively randomized fashion in a homogeneous patient population. This was a small study performed in Zurich by Gmur and colleagues in which patients with acute leukemia were randomized to receive either platelets prepared solely from single donors or pooled random donor platelet concentrates [4]. A total of 54 patients were studied and life table analysis suggested that alloimmunization was significantly delayed in the group of patients receiving single donor platelets. Both serologic and clinical criteria were used to document alloimmunization and in this study, as in previous observations from our institution, lymphocytotoxic (anti- HLA) antibody served as an excellent marker for the presence of alloimmunization [5, 6]. All patients re-

1 M.D., Professor of Medicine and Oncology, Chief, Division of Hematologic Malignancies, University of Maryland Cancer Center, University of Maryland School of Medicine, 22 South Greene Street, Baltimore, Maryland 21201, USA

ceived leukocyte-poor red blood cells (RBC). Although the study was very carefully performed and analyzed, there are a number of questions about the interpretation of the data, including: (a) the inclusion of patients who had received granulocyte transfusions; (b) the failure to censor patients who had early deaths; (c) and the possibility that a genetically more homogeneous Swiss population might not be representative of the donor gene pool in a country with more racial heterogeneity such as the United States. Only a small number of patients were studied and statistically significant benefit was most prominent in women who had had prior exposure to histocompatibility antigens through pregnancy, a somewhat surprising finding. In addition, entry to the study was limited to patients with no past or recent transfusions. This is not necessarily representative of the leukemia patient population, however. In a recent study at our referral center, 10/56 evaluable leukemia patients had received packed RBC transfusion immediately prior to transfer from other hospitals with an additional 8 patients having received RBC for other illnesses in the past [7]. Whether such patients would benefit from single donor platelets is unknown.

Nonetheless, this is an important and provocative study which represents the only observation of its kind in humans to satisfy these important study guideline criteria:

1. Prospective randomization
2. Serologic criteria for alloimmunization
3. Homogeneous patient group in terms of diagnosis and chemotherapy received
4. Use of leukocyte-poor RBC
5. Analysis over the entire course of induction therapy
6. Minimal number of protocol violations

Other studies which have attempted to address this issue fail to meet most if any of these criteria. Thus, although Sintnicolaas et al. [8] purport to demonstrate a benefit for single donor platelets in a randomized study, the results must be viewed with care because of: (a) the relatively small number of patients (34) with a variety of diagnoses; (b) the absence of serologic data in many patients; (c) the inclusion of patients with prior random donor transfusions in the single donor group; and (d) perhaps most critically, only the first two random or single donor transfusions received by the patient were compared rather than the entire transfusion history.

There are a number of theoretic considerations which must also be kept in mind about which there are relatively few data available. One could conceive of different strategies of using either multiple "random" single donors, repeated transfusions from small numbers of single donors, or repeated transfusions from small numbers of HLA-matched single donors. Because of the relatively small number of HLA-matched donors available per patient, even in centers with large numbers of typed donors [9], the latter approach would be extremely difficult to implement and furthermore could reduce the number of donors available for patients who are already alloimmunized. Furthermore, if only closely HLA-matched donors are utilized, it is possible that one could select for the development of antibody against platelet-specific antigens which are extremely difficult to detect reliably at this time. Despite the proliferation of an enormous number of different techniques for detection of anti-platelet antibody, none of these are reliably applicable to donor cross-matching at this time [10, 11]. Experiments in dogs by O'Donnell and Slichter have indicated that platelet transfusions from DLA-matched littermates can result in a high incidence of refractoriness, probably due to platelet-specific antigens [12]. Although platelet-specific antigens tend to be found in the overwhelming majority of the population in humans (greater than 95%–99% for most antigens), there are no comparable post-transfusion data available in humans and one must be cognizant of this theoretical concern when utilizing HLA-matched platelets alone.

The repeated use of a small number of single donors is predicated on the theorem that should refractoriness develop to one donor, it should be relatively simple to switch to another donor of a totally different HLA type. There is however considerable serologic cross-reactivity within the HLA system [1] and it is probable that recipients exposed to even a few HLA antigens would also develop antibody directed against the large number of HLA antigens that may be antigenically similar. The development of multispecific antibody of this pattern was noted in a small study performed at our institution many years ago [13]. Similar observations were also noted in the canine studies already mentioned [12]. Overall, the alloimmunization rate was similar using either pooled random donor platelets or a sequence of transfusions from single donor dogs.

It is perhaps the practical problems which represent the most compelling barrier to the exclusive use of single donor platelet transfusions. Obviously, cost features are an important factor. All patients with leukemia and thrombocytopenia also require RBC transfusions. It would be illogical to utilize a "clean" platelet product while providing large amounts of antigenic material from leukocytes and platelets contaminating packed RBC obtained from "random" RBC donors. Leukocyte-poor blood or perhaps more ideally frozen RBC will increase the cost of RBC transfusions by a factor of 2–3. Such a program would also markedly increase the procedural burdens on any blood center involved in the supportive care of large numbers of such patients. Furthermore, platelet concentrates are a relatively inexpensive by-product of RBC donations which are constantly occurring in large blood centers. The charge to the patient for single donor platelets is greater in most hospitals and does not include the "cost" to society of donors missing work for at least half a day because of travel and donation time. Lastly, donor morbidity must be considered. Although available blood cell separators have an excellent safety record, there are side effects associated with platelet pheresis which include the frequent occurrence of reactions to the citrate anticoagulant, the annoyance of multiple venipunctures and the possible immunologic consequences of removing circulating lymphocytes with long-term immunologic "memory" which can occur with frequent donations processed through the cytopheresis machines. Newer equipment [14, 15] and modification to older equipment [16] will make this less of an issue in the future, however.

An additional problem is that it would be difficult if not impossible for most blood centers to adhere to the rigorous requirements of supplying only single donor platelets on weekends and during emergencies. The study by Gmur et al. [4] was performed in a small pheresis center in which the blood bank physicians were also primarily responsible for the patient care. This is similar to the arrangement in our own center and in studies that we have carried out in the past, it has often been extremely difficult to coordinate the scheduling of single donors with the patient's requirements for transfusion. I am aware of at least two studies in large centers in which the investigators found it impossible to provide either the single donor platelets or the leukocyte-poor blood cells at all times for the patients randomized to these products. "Protocol violations" occurred in up to 50% of the patients on study. It would obviously be inappropriate to utilize an expensive modality such as single donor platelets only part of the time. Thus, implementation of any approach to modify or prevent alloimmunization will require much greater coordination between blood transfusion services and clinicians than exists at most centers at this time. Indeed, it could be suggested that the energy required for improving such coordination could be best directed at improving the quality control and clinical usage of the random donor platelet concentrates provided in many blood banks.

Lastly, there is a misconception in many centers that alloimmunization is an inevitable consequence of the administration of repeated platelet transfusions. On the contrary, data from a number of centers indicate that in cancer patients receiving cytotoxic and immunosuppressive therapy, alloimmunization develops in a minority of patients [4, 6, 17, 18]. In large studies of more than 200 leukemia patients treated with standard, intensive induction chemotherapy at our institution, only about 40%–50% of patients became immunized as documented by the development of lymphocytotoxic antibody [6]. In most of these patients, alloimmunization did not develop until 3–5 weeks after initial antigenic exposure (i.e., at a time when patients would be entering remission) so that alloimmunization is even less common in patients undergoing remission induction therapy. In a recent study completed at the University of Maryland Cancer Center, only 19% of 100 platelet transfusion recipients actually required HLA-matched platelet transfusions during their initial induction therapy [7]. Similar findings were noted by Gmur et al. [4]. Additional data from our center demonstrate that patients who become alloimmunized develop antibody within 3–8 weeks after their initial platelet transfusion. If antibody does not develop at this time, then it is quite unusual for such patients to become alloimmunized in the future despite the administration of further platelet transfusions [18].

With this background in mind it is of interest to consider exactly how many patients with leukemia might be benefited from any approach by which alloimmunization may be reduced. If one begins with 100 newly diagnosed patients with acute leukemia, approximately 10% of such patients will be alloimmunized on admission or become alloimmunized following their first transfusion as a result of an anamnestic antibody response due to prior transfusions or pregnancies. This would leave a total of 90 patients who might benefit from any approach to modify alloimmunization. If one assumes a final alloimmunization rate of approximately 50%, then the number of patients is reduced to 45. All patients receiving therapy do not achieve complete remission. Assuming a remission rate of 70%, the figure is reduced to approximately 30 patients. Not all patients who achieve complete remission are candidates for aggressive subsequent therapy. If one assumes (perhaps somewhat liberally) that 80% of such patients would receive repeated intensive therapy, the number of patients is further reduced to 24. In our experience, approximately 10%–20% of patients receive granulocyte transfusions because of infections not responsive to antibiotic therapy alone, reducing the number of potential "beneficiaries" to approximately 20 patients. Lastly, it is unlikely that any approach to modify alloimmunization would be 100% effective. If one generously assumes a halving of the immunization rate, then one is left with a figure of approximately 10–15 patients who might benefit from any such approach. Short-term benefit is even lower because, as noted, only 20% of patients require HLA-matched platelets during induction. Unfortunately, it has been impossible to distinguish prospectively between patients who are more or less likely to become immunized. Thus, it would be necessary to "treat" 100 patients for what at this time remains the theoretic possibility of benefiting only some 10%–15% of such patients. Furthermore, most of these alloimmunized patients can be managed successfully with HLA-matched volunteer donors or family members.

In summary, it is likely that the exclusive use of single donor platelets would strain the apheresis capabilities of most centers so that it would be more difficult to supply histocompatible platelets and granulocytes for patients who clearly need and could benefit from them. In addition, because the number of HLA-typed donors available for patients is usually limited, one has to question if this is the appropriate use of this valuable resource compared with saving these donors for alloimmunized patients. It is also unlikely, because of the issues raised, that such an approach could even be carried out at most blood centers. Thus, the current practice of administering random donor platelets followed by single donor platelets should alloimmunization develop is justified by both economic and scientific reasoning at this time [19]. Further scientific documentation of the potential effectiveness of the use of single donor platelets alone is required before this therapeutic modality is utilized, even in specialized transfusion centers.

References

1. Duquesnoy RJ, Filip DJ, Rodey GE, Rimm AA, Aster RH (1977) Successful transfusion of platelets "mismatched" for HLA antigens to alloimmunized thrombocytopenic patients. Am J Hematol 2:219–226
2. Yankee RA, Grumet FC, Rogentine GN (1969) Platelet transfusion therapy – the se-

lection of compatible platelet donors for refractory patients by lymphocyte HL-A typing. N Engl J Med 281:1208–1212
3. Hogge DE, Thompson B, Schiffer CA (1985) Platelet storage for seven days in second generation CLX blood bags. Transfusion (In press)
4. Gmur J, Von Felten A, Osterwalder B, Honegger H, Hormann A, Sauter C, Deubelbeiss K, Berchtold W, Metaxas M, Scali G, Frick PG (1983) Delayed alloimmunization using random single donor platelet transfusion: A prospective study in thrombocytopenic patients with acute leukemia. Blood 62:473–479
5. Daly PA, Schiffer CA, Aisner J, Wiernik PH (1980) Platelet transfusion therapy – One-hour posttransfusion increments are valuable in predicing the need for HLA-matched preparations. JAMA 243:435–438
6. Hogge DE, Dutcher JP, Aisner J, Schiffer CA (1983) Lymphocytotoxic antibody is a predictor of response to random donor platelet transfusion. Am J Hematol 14:363–369
7. Schiffer CA, Dutcher JP, Aisner J, Hogge D, Wiernik PH, Reilly JP (1983) A randomized trial of leukocyte-depleted platelet transfusion to modify alloimmunization in patients with leukemia. Blood 62:815–820
8. Sintinicolaas K, Sizoo W, Haije WG, Abels J, Vriesendorp HM, Stenfert Kroese WF, Hop WCJ, Lowenberg B (1981) Delayed alloimmunisation by random single donor platelet transfusions – A randomised study to compare single donor and multiple donor platelet transfusions in cancer patients with severe thrombocytopenia. Lancet 1:750–754
9. Schiffer CA, Keller C, Dutcher JP, Aisner J, Hogge D, Wiernik PH (1983) Potential HLA-matched platelet donor availability for alloimmunized patients. Transfusion 23:286–288
10. Aster RH (1978) Matching of blood platelets for transfusion. Am J Hematol 5:373–378
11. Schiffer CA (1980) Clinical importance of antiplatelet antibody testing for the blood bank. In: Bell CA (ed) A seminar on antigens on blood cells and body fluids. American Association of Blood Banks, Washington, DC, pp 189–208
12. O'Donnell MR, Slichter SJ (1979) Platelet alloimmunization: correlation with donor source. Clin Res 27:390
13. Schiffer CA, Aisner J, Daly PA, Schimpff SC, Wiernik PH (1979) Alloimmunization following prophylactic granulocyte transfusion. Blood 54:766–774
14. Katz AJ, Genco PV, Blumberg N, Snyder EL, Camp B, Morse EE (1981) Platelet collection and transfusion using the Fenwal CS-3000 cell sorter. Transfusion 21:560–563
15. Hester JP, Kellogg RM, Mulzet AP (1982) Platelet collection in the dual stage channel. In: Vogler WR (ed) Cytapheresis and plasma exchange: clinical indications. Liss, New York, pp 143–151
16. Hogge DE, Schiffer CA (1983) Collection of platelets depleted of red and white cells with the "surge pump" adaptation of a blood cell separator. Transfusion 23:177–181
17. Holohan TV, Terasaki PI, Deisseroth AB (1981) Suppression of transfusion-related alloimmunization in intensively treated cancer patients. Blood 58:122–128
18. Dutcher JP, Schiffer CA, Aisner J, Wiernik PH (1981) Long-term follow-up of patients with leukemia receiving platelet transfusions: Identification of a large group of patients who do not become alloimmunized. Blood 58:1007–1011
19. Schiffer CA, Slichter SJ (1982) Platelet transfusion from single donors. N Engl J Med 307:245–248

Haematology and Blood Transfusion Vol. 29
Modern Trends in Human Leukemia VI
Edited by Neth, Gallo, Greaves, Janka

Advances in Parenteral Nutrition Support of Children with Neoplastic Diseases *

K. A. Rickard, J. L. Grosfeld, T. D. Coates, R. M. Weetman, A. J. Provisor and R. L. Baehner

A. Introduction

In the last decade, advances were made in understanding the significance of protein energy malnutrition (PEM), in recognizing PEM in specific subpopulations of children with malignancies, in staging and assessment of nutritional status, and in understanding the efficacy and limitations of various options for nutrition support. This report describes our experience in providing nutrition support for over a 100 children with newly diagnosed malignancies who have been monitored carefully on study protocols and treated at a single pediatric cancer facility. This work was possible because of the close collaboration between the Departments of Pediatric Hematology Oncology, Pediatric Surgery, Radiation Oncology, and Pediatric Nutrition and Dietetics at James Whitcomb Riley Hospital for Children.

B. Significance of PEM

PEM is associated with impaired immunocompetence, increased susceptibility to infections, major organ dysfunctions, and, when severe, increased morbidity and mortality. The organ systems most readily affected by PEM, i.e., the hematopoietic, gastrointestinal, and immunologic systems, are also those which are the most sensitive to oncologic treatment. Improvement in these systems may be one of the goals for either reversing or preventing PEM.

In an initial study [9] of children with newly diagnosed advanced solid tumors and relapsed leukemia–lymphoma, anergy (as defined by the inability to respond to any one of four recall skin test antigens) was documented in 17 of 18 patients considered malnourished. Anergy was reversed with 28 days of central parenteral nutrition support in approximately two-thirds of the patients (7/11 retested), despite continuing oncologic treatment. Van Eys et al. [17] documented significantly higher rates of infectious complications in malnourished compared with well-nourished children with metastatic disease involving bone who received parenteral nutrition support. Current data suggest that bone marrow suppression may be attenuated by parenteral nutrition support, at least in patients with stages III and IV neuroblastoma [12, 15], patients with acute nonlymphocytic leukemia (ANLL [7]), and patients with metastatic disease involving bone [17]. Nutritional status at the time of diagnosis of neoplastic disease has been clearly associated with outcome in adults [2] as well as children [3, 12].

C. Childhood Neoplasms with High Risk for PEM

PEM is a common occurrence in certain high risk populations of children with neo-

* Departments of Pediatric Nutrition and Dietetics, Pediatric Hematology Oncology and Pediatric Surgery. James Whitcomb Riley Hospital for Children, Indiana University School of Medicine, 702 Barnhill Drive, Indianapolis, Indiana 46223, USA

plastic diseases. The incidence of PEM at diagnosis of childhood neoplasms and during treatment of childhood cancer varies from 6% (children with newly diagnosed leukemia) to as high as 50% (children with newly diagnosed stage IV neuroblastoma), depending upon tumor type, stage of disease, and criteria for PEM [11]. We sequentially monitored the nutritional status (energy intakes, weights, weight for height proportionality, skinfold measurements, albumin, and transferrin) of more than 100 children with newly diagnosed neoplastic diseases during initial phases of therapy. These data formed the basis for determination of the factors that place a patient at a higher risk for the development of PEM (Table 1). The tumor types usually associated with high and low nutritional risk are listed in Table 2.

D. Staging and Assessment of Nutritional Status

In the past, states of malnutrition may have been overlooked because of lack of tangible criteria for establishing the nutritional status of these patients, or, possibly owing to an insensitivity to the significance of PEM. We developed a system for nutrition staging patients not only at diagnosis, but also during ongoing oncologic treatment because changes in nutritional status are dynamic.

Table 1. Common risk factors for the development of PEM

Advanced disease
Lack of tumor response
Abdominal and pelvic irradiation
Intense frequent courses of chemotherapy ($\leqq 3$ weeks) in the absence of corticosteroids or appetite stimulants
Major operative procedures of the abdomen
Psychologic factors, removal from familiar surroundings, separation from parents and siblings
Absence of supportive health care team

I. Identification of PEM (Staging) at Diagnosis

Criteria for staging patients as malnourished at diagnosis include: > 5% weight loss, weight for height < 5th percentile, or serum albumin < 3.2 g/dl. A patient who does not meet any of these criteria is staged as well-nourished. The significance of nutrition staging at diagnosis has been emphasized in a recent study [12] of 18 of our children with newly diagnosed stage IV neuroblastoma. In an equal number of malnourished and well-nourished patients at diagnosis, significantly more malnourished patients had relapsed or died by 180 days after treatment was initiated ($P < 0.05$). The differences in survival between the two groups of patients approached significance ($P = 0.08$) at 1 year into treatment. The median survival of the malnourished group was 5 months compared with 12 months for the well-nourished group. It remains to be determined whether the patients considered to be malnourished at diagnosis have a more aggressive or advanced form of neuroblastoma, or, whether the nutritional status influenced the outcome.

II. Ongoing Nutritional Assessment

Dramatic changes in nutritional status have occurred over as short a period as 1 week

Table 2. Types of neoplastic disease associated with high and low nutritional risk

High nutritional risk	*Low nutritional risk*
Stage III and IV Wilms' tumor	Acute lymphocytic leukemia
Advanced neuroblastoma	Nonmetastatic diseases
Acute nonlymphocytic leukemia	Advanced diseases during maintenance treatment and when in remission
Pelvic rhabdomyosarcoma	
Brain tumor	
Some non-Hodgkin's lymphomas	

because of the almost immediate adverse impact of oncologic treatment upon the gastrointestinal system and upon nutrient intake. The current criteria used for staging patients at diagnosis may not be sensitive enough to detect ongoing nutritional depletion.

Some pitfalls may be associated with the monitoring of weight changes as the only index of nutritional status. Children who are < 5th percentile weight for height have relatively small losses in weight compared with well-nourished children with equally low energy intakes. Malnourished children have fluid changes which mask some of the tissue wasting. Edema and dehydration may alter weight so that accurate interpretation is difficult. Furthermore, monitoring only absolute weight changes may provide a false sense of security. Weights need to be plotted sequentially on growth grids and expressed as a percentage of weight loss. For example, a 2 kg weight loss for a 60 kg teenager (3% weight loss) may not seem impressive, however, the same 2 kg loss in a 20 kg toddler represents a 10% weight loss.

Changes in weight, weight for height, and subscapular skinfold thickness are particularly useful indicators of real or impending nutrition depletion. Low energy intakes and decreases in skinfold measurements were the first indicators of nutrition depletion and occurred despite weight maintenance or a slight weight gain in several children who had no evidence of edema. Fomon and associates [5] reported a similar phenomenon in normal infants fed skim milk formula (67% of energy requirement). This group of babies experienced approximately 25% decreases in triceps and subscapular skinfold measurements even though they gained weight, albeit at a slower rate than normal.

Skinfold calipers are valuable in detecting more subtle, subclinical changes in nutritional status during early phases of treatment. Subscapular skinfold decreases > 0.3 mm correlated with low energy intakes (more than 2 standard deviations below the mean of Beal's data [1] for healthy children) in patients who initially had skinfold measurements in the normal range. Changes > 0.3 mm are twice the coefficient of variation which was determined from 265 data sets for each subscapular skinfold measurement.

For ongoing nutritional assessment, albumin concentrations in relation to energy intake are monitored. Albumin is a useful indicator of mild to moderate PEM in some patients, i.e., decreases are seen which correspond to very low protein or energy intakes and may be observed before significant weight loss. However, albumin concentrations may be preserved at marginal or low ranges of normal (2.9–3.2 g/dl) in some children with obvious tissue wasting. Transferrin, prealbumin, and retinol binding proteins are serum proteins which may indicate subclinical PEM. They have shorter half-lives and different synthetic rates than albumin. In a current study [14] of these biochemical indicators, preliminary data strongly support the use of these serum proteins as early indicators of successful repletion.

E. Options for Nutritional Support

I. Enteral Nutrition

Several modes of nutrition support are available for the pediatric patient. For most children with cancer, provision of nutrients by the enteral route with oral feeding is the preferred method because treatment may last several years. An individualized feeding program which uses favorite, nutritious foods of the child during treatment-free periods has numerous practical and psychologic advantages over parenteral nutrition. These include a lower risk of infection and other catheter-related complications, more normal play activities and life-style, and a positive way for parent and child to be involved in their own care. In addition, enteral feeding is more economic. In our experience, however, this type of enteral feeding program has not been effective in either preventing or reversing PEM in most of the patients at high nutritional risk during initial intense treatment. In a study [9] of 21 children with advanced cancer who were enterally nourished, energy intake was very low, averaging 48% ± 24% of the Recommended Dietary Allowances (RDA) for kilocalories, and weight loss averaged 16% in less than 1 month of treatment. Similarly, in a recent study of 32 children with stages III and IV neuroblastoma [15] significant loss of fat reserves and weight occurred during the initial 28 days of treatment when enteral nutrition alone was provided. The children who became malnourished were unable to make nutritional gains thereafter, despite numerous delays in treatment.

We feel that the use of nasogastric tubes to provide nutrition is contraindicated in the older infant, toddler, and preschool age groups of children because of psychologic trauma associated with the insertion and maintenance of tubes. Nausea and vomiting in addition to decreased intestinal motility and absorption from oncologic therapy make this modality less favorable and less effective. Gastrostomy feedings also seem to be of limited value for similar reasons. In a few older schoolage and teenage children, continuous nasogastric nighttime feedings have been beneficial.

II. Parenteral Nutrition

1. Nutritional and Immunologic Benefits

Parenteral nutrition is both safe [18, 13] and efficacious in children with neoplastic diseases. In a group of 28 patients who had stage III or IV solid tumors or second relapse leukemia–lymphoma, the effectiveness of central parenteral nutrition (CPN) in reversing PEM and restoring immunity was documented [9]. Of the 28 patients who were malnourished, 20 received CPN for a mean of 24 days (average caloric intake of 90% of the RDA during weight gain). Initially, patients were randomized to either 10 or 28 days of CPN. The 10-day randomization was abandoned after the initial three patients rapidly returned to their initial malnourished state because of continuing oncologic treatment. Review of data from 20 patients who received longer intervals ($\geqq$ 28 days) of parenteral nutrition indicated that shorter intervals (9–14 days) did not restore an appropriate weight for height (though weight gains were significant) nor fat reserves, and, did not return serum albumin concentrations to $\geqq$ 3.2 g/dl. Despite the failure of shorter intervals of parenteral nutrition to reverse PEM, an improvement in transferrin concentration occurred, suggesting that transferrin was more responsive than albumin. Another short-term benefit was a significant improvement in the child's general state of well-being. A period of 28 days CPN restored weight for height percentiles, subscapular skinfold percentiles, albumin, and transferrin concentrations to normal values. Curtailment of parenteral nutrition support before reversal of PEM and completion of intensive oncologic support reduced the benefits of previous nutrition support. Therefore, we recommend continuing the parenteral nutrition support for several days beyond cessation of chemotherapy or irradiation treatment which induce anorexia, nausea, and vomiting. Nutritional benefits from effective parenteral nutrition support are maintained after completion of the intense treatment, unless complicating factors in the patient's clinical course such as relapse, sepsis, or major abdominal procedures occur [10, 15].

In a recent study [13] comparing the effectiveness of parenteral nutrition provided by either central or peripheral veins, the central line allowed provision of greater concentrations of glucose and obviated problems with subcutaneous peripheral infiltrations. In 19 children with advanced neuroblastoma or Wilms' tumor, both routes of administration were effective in reversing PEM when adequate energy and protein were provided over a 21- to 28-day period. Significant increases in anthropometric measurements and albumin were similar for the two groups. Both groups had a similar incidence of anemia, fever episodes (with and without documented sepsis), and mildly elevated SGOT concentrations. The peripheral parenteral nutrition (PPN) group, however, had a high incidence of line changes associated with peripheral infiltrations and related psychologic trauma. In this study, the effectiveness of PPN was dependent upon an oral intake which provided an average of 30% additional energy to meet the RDA. Based upon these results, a central line is used for our standard parenteral nutrition support program and a peripheral line for periods when the central line is interrupted.

2. *Treatment Tolerance Benefits*

Treatment tolerance benefits from parenteral nutrition compared with oral nutrition have been documented in several recent prospective randomized studies of children with specific tumors. In an initial report of a randomized study [12] of 17 patients with stage IV neuroblastoma, those who had a favorable nutrition course during the first 21 days of therapy had significantly fewer treatment delays (secondary to absolute granulocyte counts ≧ 1000/μl or platelets ≧ 75 000/μl) and fewer drug dose reductions throughout the first 10 weeks of treatment. Treatment consisted of 5-day cycles of DTIC, vincristine, and cyclophosphamide given at 3-week intervals. The treatment tolerance benefits from effective reversal or prevention of PEM were further documented in 32 patients with stages III and IV neuroblastoma [15].

Three other prospective randomized studies of children with cancer have also documented treatment benefits from CPN compared with oral nutrition in improving tolerance to chemotherapy [17], in improving adherence to chemotherapy schedules [6], or in accelerating recovery of normal marrow function [7]. In contrast to these findings, Shamberger et al. [16] failed to document benefit from CPN compared with oral nutrition in improving recovery from bone marrow suppression in a series of 27 young patients who received extremely aggressive treatment for poor prognosis sarcomas. In a multi-institutional study [4] of 25 patients who received abdominal irradiation, the CPN and oral nutrition groups of patients did not differ in ability to adhere to the radiotherapy schedule. Thus, the value of CPN in improving treatment tolerance probably relates to certain types and stages of tumors as well as specific treatment.

3. *Complications and Limitations*

Complications can be minimized or safely controlled with careful patient management and strict adherence to a parenteral nutrition protocol. In a multi-institutional study of complications of adults with cancer randomized to either CPN (125 patients) or control groups (126 patients), Mullen [8] reported that CPN adds little serious morbidity and mortality. An increased incidence of fever ($P < 0.003$), anemia ($P < 0.09$), and pulmonary dysfunction ($P < 0.12$) was documented in the CPN group, however, incidence of documented infections (25%) at distant sites was similar for both groups.

The possibility that CPN stimulates tumor growth in excess of host repletion needs to be considered, although clinically this has not been observed when aggressive oncologic treatment is given simultaneously. In fact, it is conceivable that CPN may beneficially stimulate cell replications and increase effectiveness of cell-cycle-specific drugs. Certainly, tumor response may be improved when effective oncologic treatment is completed on schedule.

Acknowledgments. This work was supported in part by grants RO1-CA 28531 and RO1-CA 28005 from the National Cancer Institute, Bethesda, Maryland 20205.

References

1. Beal VA (1970) Nutritional intake. In: McCammon RW (ed) Human growth and development. Thomas, Springfield, Ill, pp 63–100
2. DeWys WD, Begg C, Lavin PT, Band PR, Bennett JM, Bertino JR, Cohen MH, Douglass HO, Engstrom PF, Ezdinli EZ, Horton J, Johnson GJ, Moertel CG, Oken MM, Perlia C, Rosenbaum C, Silverstein MN, Skeel RT, Sponzo RW, Tormey DC (1980) Prognostic effect of weight loss prior to chemotherapy in cancer patients. Am J Med 60:491–497
3. Donaldson SS, Wesley MN, DeWys WD, Suskind RM, Jaffee N, Van Eys J (1981) A study of the nutritional status of pediatric cancer patients. Am J Dis Child 135: 1107–1112
4. Donaldson SS, Wesley MN, Ghavimi F, Shils ME, Suskind RM, DeWys WD (1982) A prospective randomized clinical trial of total parenteral nutrition in children with cancer. Med Pediatr Oncol 10:129–139
5. Fomon SJ, Filer LJ, Ziegler EE, Bergmann KE, Bergmann RL (1977) Skim milk in infant feeding. Acta Pediatr Scand 66:17–30
6. Ghavimi R, Shils ME, Scott BF, Brown M, Tamaroff M (1982) Comparison of morbidity in children requiring abdominal radiation

and chemotherapy with and without total parenteral nutrition. J Pediatr 101:4: 530–537
7. Hays DM, Merritt RJ, Ashley J, White L, Siegel SE (1983) Effect of total parenteral nutrition on marrow recovery during induction therapy for acute nonlymphocytic leukemia in childhood. Med Pediatr Oncol 11:134–140
8. Mullen J (1981) Complications of total parenteral nutrition in the cancer patient. Cancer Treat Rep 65 [Suppl 5]:107–113
9. Rickard KA, Grosfeld JL, Kirksey A, Ballantine TVN, Baehner RL (1979) Reversal of protein-energy malnutrition in children with advanced neoplastic disease. Ann Surg 190: 771–781
10. Rickard KA, Kirksey A, Baehner RL, Provisor AJ, Weetman RM, Ballantine TVN, Grosfeld JL (1980) Effectiveness of enteral and parenteral nutrition in the nutritional management of children with Wilm's tumor. Am J Clin Nutr 33:2622–2629
11. Rickard KA, Baehner RL, Coates TD, Weetman RM, Provisor AJ, Grosfeld JL (1982) Supportive nutritional intervention. Cancer Res 42 [Suppl]:766–773
12. Rickard KA, Detamore DM, Coates TD, Grosfeld JL, Weetman RM, White NM, Provisor AJ, Boxer LA, Loghmani ES, Oei TO, Yu P, Baehner RL (1983a) Effect of nutrition staging on treatment delays and outcome in stage IV neuroblastoma. Cancer 52: 587–598
13. Rickard KA, Foland BB, Detamore CM, Coates TD, Grosfeld JL, White NM, Weetman RM, Provisor AJ, Loghmani ES, Oei TO, Yu P, Baehner RL (1983b) Effectiveness of central parenteral nutrition vs peripheral parenteral nutrition plus enteral nutrition in reversing PEM in children with advanced neuroblastoma and Wilms' tumor: a prospective randomized study. Am J Clin Nutr 38:445–456
14. Rickard KA, Foland BB, Grosfeld JL, Loghmani ES, Yu P, Detamore CM, Coates TD, Weetman RM, Provisor AJ, Oei TO, Baehner RL (1984a) Prealbumin and retional binding protein: Early biochemical indicators of nutritional repletion in children with neuroblastoma or Wilms' tumor. Fed Proc 43:468 (Abstract 1070)
15. Rickard KA, Loghmani ES, Grosfeld JL, Detamore CM, White NM, Foland BB, Coates TD, Yu P, Weetman RM, Provisor AJ, Oei TO, Baehner RL (1984b) Effectiveness of enteral and parenteral nutrition in preventing and/or reversing PEM in children with advanced neuroblastoma. Am Soc Clin Oncol Proc 3:109 (Abstract C-423)
16. Shamberger RC, Pizzo PA, Goodgame JT, Lowry SF, Maher MM, Wesley RA, Brennan MF (1983) The effect of total parenteral nutrition on chemotherapy-induced myelosuppression. Am J Med 74:40–48
17. Van Eys J, Copeland EM, Cangir A, Taylor G, Teitell-Cohen B, Carter P, Ortiz C (1980) A clinical trial of hyperalimentation in children with metastatic malignancies. Med Pediatr Oncol 8:63–73
18. Van Eys J, Wesley MN, Cangir A, Copeland EM, Donaldson SS, Ghavimi F, Shils M, Suskind R, Jaffe N, Filler R (1982) Safety of intravenous hyperalimentation in children with malignancies: A cooperative group trial. JPEN 6:291–294

Haematology and Blood Transfusion Vol. 29
Modern Trends in Human Leukemia VI
Edited by Neth, Gallo, Greaves, Janka

Antiemetics in Cancer Chemotherapy

M. Higi[1]

A. Introduction

Nausea and vomiting induced by several cancer chemotherapy agents is often the most distressing side effect of treatment. The mechanisms are quite complex. The vomiting center in the reticular formation can be stimulated by either afferent stimuli from the gastrointestinal tract or by the chemoreceptor trigger zone (CTZ). The latter is probably the primary site for emetic activity of most cancer chemotherapeutic agents and is accessible to drugs that do not cross the blood–brain barrier. It is quite possible that several agents have different receptors. The wide spectrum of antiemetics is in contrast to the often observed lack of effectiveness. The more successful trials have concentrated on agents, doses, schedules, or routes of administration that were not generally used prior to 1980. An effective study design has reduced methodological difficulties and reproducible data have been reported.

For most chemotherapeutic agents with emetic properties, the onset of emesis occurs 2–3 h after administration in previously untreated patients. In most instances, the drug dose and the route of administration are important variables affecting the incidence of nausea and vomiting. Many patients manifest prechemotherapy emesis; the anticipatory vomiting overlaps continuously with the drug-induced symptoms.

1 Klinik Dr. Schedel, 8391 Kellberg-Passau, FRG

Therefore, successful antiemetic treatment needs prophylactic pharmaceutical intervention, starting 1–12 h before administration of emetic cancer chemotherapy to prevent or lessen the initial occurrence of vomiting.

B. Antiemetic Agents

I. Phenothiazines

Phenothiazines can prevent apomorphine-induced vomiting. The antiemetic effectiveness in various chemotherapeutic regimens has been examined under randomized conditions. Phenothiazine derivatives are therefore the most frequently used agents to prevent emesis in cancer chemotherapy. Toxicity usually consists of sedation, with occasional extrapyramidal and "paradoxical" reactions.

II. Butyrophenones

Droperidol and haloperidol are also effective antiemetics. Like the other agents, the antiemetic activity probably acts on the CTZ of the area postrema. Several clinical studies have shown, in addition to the high antiemetic qualities, a very low incidence of side effects, including sedation and extrapyramidal reactions.

III. Cannabinoids

Tetrahydrocannabinol (THC), the psychoactive substance of cannabis, has antiemetic properties. THC and synthetic cannabinoids (nabilone, levonantradol) have been studied in randomized trials. Some authors reported a higher antiemetic activity than conventional agents, but toxicity has been frequent. The side effects include sedation, hypotension, dizziness, and a psychotropic "high". The psychogenic reactions have caused a decreased acceptance of cannabinoids.

IV. Benzamides

Metoclopramide, alizapride, and benzquinamide are also widely used as antiemetics. It has been postulated that these agents exert their antiemetic potency by blocking dopamine receptors in the CTZ and the gastrointestinal tract. Low doses of metoclopramide failed to show antiemetic activity in chemotherapeutic-induced vomiting. Given in high doses (1–2 mg/kg every 2 h) to patients receiving Cisplatin chemotherapy, metoclopramide demonstrated antiemetic efficacy. Sedation is the most frequent side effect. Occasionally dystonic reactions and akathisia have been reported.

V. Corticosteroids

In most clinical trials, dexamethasone or methylprednisolone have been used. Useful antiemetic results have been reported. The mechanisms are unknown. Toxicity with short-course regimens of steroids has been mild. Interactions with the antitumor efficacy of the chemotherapeutic drugs were not noted. Corticosteroids are effective antiemetics with a low degree of toxicity.

C. Conclusions

Successful antiemetic treatment needs prophylactic pharmaceutical intervention starting before administration of emetic cancer chemotherapy to prevent or lessen the initial occurrence of vomiting. Phenothiazines, butyrophenones, cannabinoids, benzamides, and corticosteroids given in high doses have demonstrated antiemetic efficacy and represent to date the most active agents. It is possible that the chemotherapeutic drugs exert their emetic effects through different pathways. Therefore, combination regimens may be expected to produce an improvement in patient care.

Haematology and Blood Transfusion Vol. 29
Modern Trends in Human Leukemia VI
Edited by Neth, Gallo, Greaves, Janka

Chromosome Abnormalities in Malignant Lymphoma: Biologic and Clinical Correlations*

C. D. Bloomfield, D. C. Arthur, E. G. Levine, G. Frizzera, K. J. Gajl-Peczalska, T. W. LeBien, D. D. Hurd, and B. A. Peterson

A. Introduction

Among the hematologic malignancies, the clinical and biologic significance of chromosome abnormalities have been most extensively studied in the acute leukemias and chronic myelogenous leukemia (CML). Clonal chromosome abnormalities are now identified in essentially all cases of CML and in most cases of acute nonlymphoblastic leukemia (ANLL) and acute lymphoblastic leukemia (ALL). In the acute leukemias, specific chromosome abnormalities have now been correlated with morphology (ANLL), immunologic phenotype (ALL), and various clinical features. In both ANLL and ALL, they have been found to be clinically important as independent risk factors for predicting response to treatment, remission duration, and survival [1–4].

Limited data are available regarding chromosomal abnormalities in malignant lymphoma, other than Burkitt's. The few reported studies of banded chromosomes have generally included small numbers of cases, and primary tumor masses have rarely been the major source of tissue studied. Moreover, for a given lymph node, chromosome findings have rarely been correlated with histology and immunologic phenotype. Since July 1978, we have been prospectively studying chromosomes in lymph nodes from patients with lymphoma and correlating them with histology, immunologic phenotype, and clinical findings [5, 6]. This report briefly summarizes our findings in the first 115 patients.

B. Materials and Methods

Chromosomes from involved lymph nodes or other tumor masses from 115 patients (ages 8–85 years; median 55 years) with non-Hodgkin's malignant lymphoma were studied. In 73 patients, neoplastic tissue was analyzed at diagnosis prior to any treatment; in 42 patients, tissue was first studied at relapse. In all instances, the tumor was simultaneously studied for histology, immunologic markers, and G-banded chromosomes. Histologic classification was done using the International Working Formulation for Clinical Usage [7].

Immunologic phenotyping, as described previously, was based on study of both single cell suspensions and tissue frozen sections in all cases [8]. All cases were studied for surface (SIg) and cytoplasmic (CIg) immunoglobulin, and receptors for complement (C′), Fc, and unsensitized sheep erythrocytes (E); 79 cases were also studied with a panel of monoclonal antibodies including BA-1, BA-2, and BA-3 [9].

For cytogenetic studies, a portion of the same tumor mass biopsied for histology and immunologic phenotyping was obtained directly from the surgical pathology laboratory and processed within 1 h of bi-

* Section of Medical Oncology, Department of Medicine and Department of Laboratory Medicine and Pathology, University of Minnesota Health Sciences Center, Minneapolis, MN 55455, USA

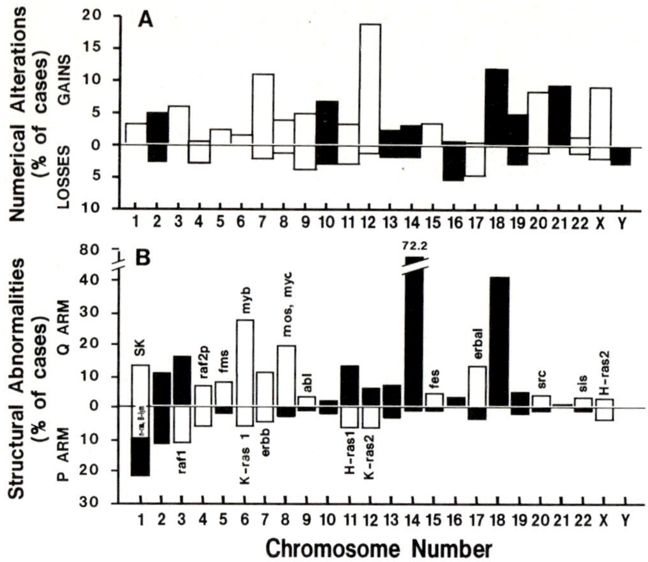

Fig. 1 A, B. Histogram of **A** gains and losses of whole chromosomes and **B** structural abnormalities involving each chromosome arm in 115 cases of lymphoma. Chromosomes **A** or the percentage of cases with rearranged chromosome arms **B** involving areas to which cellular oncogenes have been mapped are indicated by *open bars*

opsy. Metaphase chromosomes were harvested from direct preparations and unstimulated or methotrexate-synchronized short-term (24- and 48-h) cultures using methods described previously [6]. G-banding was done using the Wright's technique of Sanchez et al. [10]. Photographs of metaphases were taken on high contrast SO115 film, and multiple karyotypes were constructed in each case.

Chromosomes have been designated according to the ISCN (1978, 1981), and the karyotypes are expressed as recommended under this system [11, 12]. Chromosome abnormalities were designated as clonal if two or more metaphase cells had identical structural anomalies or extra chromosomes, or if three or more metaphase cells had identical missing chromosomes.

C. Results

Clonal chromosome abnormalities were identified in 96% of the 115 patients. Two clones were identified in 12% of patients. Most clones had multiple abnormalities. The abnormal karyotypes included gains of one or more whole chromosomes (without apparent structural abnormalities) in 58% of patients and losses of one or more whole chromosomes in 27%. Chromosomes most commonly gained were 12 (19% of patients), 18 (12%), and 7 (11%). Chromosomes most frequently lost were 16 (5%) and 17 (4%).

Structural abnormalities were more frequent than numerical alterations, occurring in 90% of patients. All chromosomes were affected, but with considerable variation in frequency. The chromosome regions (by arm) most frequently rearranged were 14q (72% of patients), 18q (41%), 6q (28%), 1p (21%), 8q (19%), 3q (16%), 1q, 11q, and 17q (14% each), 2p, 2q, and 7q (11% each), and 3p (10%).

Translocations were the most common type of structural abnormality; 84 different translocations were identified, but only the t(14; 18)(q32; q21) and t(8; 14)(q24; q32) occurred in three or more different patients. Other common types of structural abnormalities included deletions, duplications, and isochromosomes. Specific chromosome regions most commonly rearranged were 14q32 (67%) of patients, 18q21 (31%), 6q21 (15%), 8q24 (13%), 11q21–25 (11%), and 1p36 (10%).

An analysis was performed to determine if the chromosome abnormalities seen in lymphoma were preferentially in regions to which oncogenes have been mapped. In Fig. 1, the frequency of abnormalities involving individual chromosomes for nu-

Table 1. Karyotype findings which differed significantly among histologies[a]

	International Working Formulation groups[b]									
	A	B	C	D	F	G	H	I	J	
Cases	19	28	8	9	13	23	4	3	5	
	Median value									*P*
Normal cells (%)	18	22	7	15	20	0	12	45	0	0.002
Modal number	46	47	48	49	47	49	48	46	46	<0.001
Chromosome or region altered	Frequency of specific abnormality in each histology (%)									
6q21	21	29	25	22	23	39	75	0	20	0.0085
+7	0	4	25	33	0	30	0	0	0	0.0071
+8	0	4	38	11	0	0	0	0	0	0.0018
8q	16	14	25	0	0	30	25	0	100	0.0003
8q24	16	0	0	0	0	30	0	0	100	0.0000
t (8;14) (q24;q32)	5	0	0	0	0	22	0	0	80	0.0000
13p13	0	0	38	0	0	4	0	0	0	0.0002
14q32	42	89	100	67	46	74	0	33	100	0.0001
17q21-25	0	0	0	44	8	9	0	0	0	0.0007
18q	16	68	63	44	15	52	0	0	20	0.0013
18q21	5	64	63	44	0	26	0	0	20	0.0000
t (14;18) (q32;q21)	0	61	63	44	0	26	0	0	20	0.0000

[a] Only abnormalities with a $P<0.009$ are listed. This conservative P value has been chosen because of the large number of possibilities tested

[b] A small lymphocytic; B follicular, predominantly small cleaved; C follicular, mixed, small cleaved and large cell; D follicular, predominantly large cell; F diffuse, mixed small and large cell; G diffuse, large cell; H diffuse large cell immunoblastic; I lymphoblastic; J small noncleaved

merical alterations and each chromosome arm for structural abnormalities are indicated. Chromosomes or chromosome regions to which cellular oncogenes have so far been localized are indicated as open bars. As can be seen, many chromosome abnormalities involved regions to which oncogenes have been mapped. Chromosomes to which oncogenes have so far been mapped which were frequently involved in numerical changes were 12 (K-*ras* 2), and 7 (*erb* b) (Fig. 1 a). Among chromosomes commonly involved in numerical changes, only number 18 contains no known oncogene. Among structural abnormalities, the two most commonly involved regions (14q, 18q) are not ones to which oncogenes have been mapped; however, more than 10% of the patients had structural rearrangements in regions to which the following oncogenes have been mapped: *myb* (6q22–24), *myc* (8q24), *sk* (1q12→qter), *raf* 1 (3p23→pter), and *erb* a1 (17p11→q22) (Fig. 1 b). Overall, 91 (79%) of the 115 patients demonstrated clonal chromosome abnormalities involving regions to which oncogenes have been mapped. These data, of course, represent a high estimate of the possible number of patients in whom oncogenes may be rearranged since many oncogenes have not been precisely localized and patients with any abnormality of the broad area to which the oncogene might be mapped are included, as are patients with losses and gains to whole chromosomes.

The results of cytogenetic analysis were compared among histologic groups. Several features appeared to differ significantly in their distribution among histologies. These included the median percentage of normal cells, the median modal number of the clonal chromosome abnormalities, and the frequency of certain specific chromosome abnormalities (Table 1). No chromosome region or specific chromosome abnormality was restricted to a single histology, but sev-

Table 2. Chromosome abnormalities which differed significantly among B cell monoclonal groups

	Expression of BA-1, BA-2, BA-3							BA-1[a]		
	+−−	−−−	++−	−+−	+++	+−+		+	−	
Cases	28	5	13	5	6	4	*P*	51	12	*P*
	Chromosome abnormalities in each immunologic group (%)									
1p abnl	4	40	46	20	0	50	0.0085			
5q abnl	0	60	0	40	0	0	0.0000	0	42	0.0000
6q15	0	0	0	40	17	0	0.0036			
6q21	18	60	8	60	0	0	0.0157	12	50	0.0086
+7	7	0	8	60	0	0	0.0065			
16q abnl	0	0	0	0	0	50	0.0000			

[a] Two additional cases were studied for BA-1 which were not studied for BA-2 and BA-3

eral were frequent in only one or two groups. These included an extra 7 in follicular center cell lymphomas with large cells (groups C, D, and G), an extra 8 in the follicular lymphomas, mixed small cleaved and large cell (C), t(8;14)(q24;q32) in large and small noncleaved malignant lymphoma (G and J), 13p13 in C, 17q21–25 in D, and t(14;18)(q32;q21) in follicular lymphomas (B–D) and diffuse large (follicular center) cell lymphoma (G). Rearrangements of specific chromosome regions, but not specific abnormalities, were occasionally found in 100% of a given histologic group.

When the results of cytogenetic analysis were compared among broad immunologic groups (B, T, C′, null), only abnormalities involving 18q differed significantly among the groups, occurring in all three cases of C′ lymphoma, 44% of B lymphomas, but no T lymphomas ($P=0.003$). Since most cases studied were B cell (98), a detailed analysis of the distribution of chromosome abnormalities among lymphomas expressing different heavy and light chains was possible. No highly significant differences (all P values > 0.03) in distribution were found. However, when the B cell lymphomas were classified according to expression of the antigens identified by the monoclonal antibodies BA-1, BA-2, and BA-3, the distribution of certain chromosome abnormalities varied significantly (Table 2). Most interesting was the frequent absence of BA-1 expression in lymphomas with chromosome rearrangements involving 5q and 6q.

To determine if cytogenetic analysis had clinical use as a prognostic factor, the 73 patients studied at diagnosis prior to treatment were evaluated. Median follow-up of the surviving patients in this group is 32 months (minimum of 9 months). Various aspects of karyotype were correlated with response to treatment and survival. It was found that 65% of patients achieved a complete remission. No significant correlations with cytogenetic findings were identified. Length of survival varied significantly according to a number of aspects of karyotype analysis. In particular, patients whose lymphomas had more than 20% normal metaphases survived significantly longer than those with fewer than 20% normal cells (Fig. 2a). Similarly, patients whose lymphoma had a modal number of 46 survived longer than those with a modal number of $\geqq 47$ or $\leqq 45$ (Fig. 2b). Too few patients have been studied to determine if these various features of karyotype are independent prognostic factors.

D. Discussion

In this large study of G-banded chromosomes in lymphoma, clonal chromosome abnormalities have been found in 110 of 115 cases. Multiple recurring abnormalities were noted, some of which are associated with specific histologies or immunologic phenotypes. Certain aspects of cytogenetic analysis also seemed to correlate with patient survival. However, analysis is com-

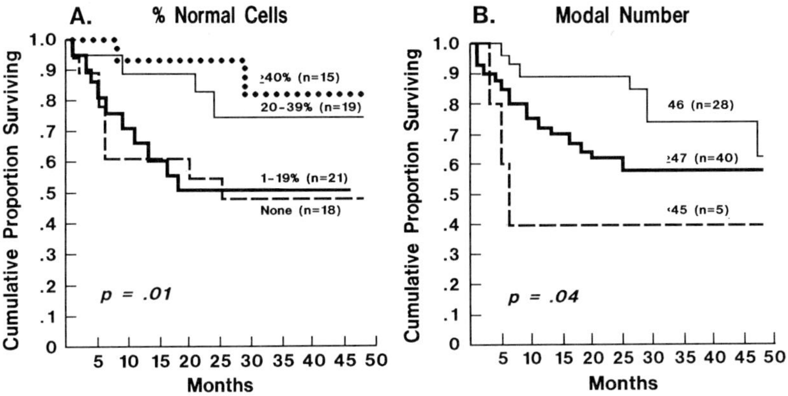

Fig. 2A, B. Survival of 73 patients with lymphoma according to **A** the frequency of normal metaphases identified cytogenetically in a neoplastic lymph node studied before treatment and **B** the modal number of the primary clonal chromosome abnormality identified in a pretreatment neoplastic lymph node

plicated by the multiple abnormalities found in most patients and the relatively small numbers of patients with each recurring abnormality studied. The clinical relevance of cytogenetic analysis for diagnosis, classification, and prognosis in non-Hodgkin's lymphoma obviously requires further study.

The biologic significance of these recurring clonal chromosome abnormalities is also unknown. However, that 79% of patients had numerical or structural rearrangements involving chromosomes or chromosome regions to which oncogenes have been mapped is of interest. Detailed study of the role of oncogenes in lymphoma would appear to be a profitable endeavor.

Acknowledgments. This work was supported in part by the Coleman Leukemia Research Fund. E.G.L. is a Fellow and T.W.L. a Scholar of the Leukemia Society of America.

References

1. Bloomfield CD (in press) The clinical usefulness of chromosome abnormalities in acute leukemia. In: Büchner T, Hiddemann W, Hossfeld D et al. (eds) Tumor aneuploidy. Springer, Berlin
2. de la Chapelle A, Berger R (1984) Report of the committee on chromosome rearrangements in neoplasia and on fragile sites. Cytogenet Cell Genet 37:274–311
3. The Third International Workshop on Chromosomes in Leukemia (1983) Cancer Res 43:868–873
4. Fourth International Workshop on Chromosomes in Leukemia (1984) Cancer Genet Cytogenet 11:332–350
5. Bloomfield CD, Arthur DC, Frizzera G et al. (1982) Chromosomal abnormalities in non-Hodgkin's malignant lymphoma. In: Vitetta E (ed) B and T cell tumors. Academic, New York, pp 227–231
6. Bloomfield CD, Arthur DC, Frizzera G, Levine EG et al. (1983) Nonrandom chromosome abnormalities in lymphoma. Cancer Res 43:2975–2984
7. National Cancer Institute-sponsored study of classifications of non-Hodgkin's lymphoma: summary and description of a working formulation for clinical usage (1982) Cancer 49:2112–2135
8. Gajl-Peczalska KJ, Bloomfield CD, Frizzera G et al. (1982) Diversity of phenotypes of non-Hodgkin's malignant lymphoma. In: Vitetta E (ed) B and T cell tumors. Academic, New York, pp 63–67
9. Bloomfield CD, Gajl-Peczalska KJ, Frizzera G et al. (1984) The clinical utility of cell surface markers in malignant lymphoma. In: Ford RJ, Fuller LM, Hagemeister FB (eds) New perspectives in human lymphoma. Raven, New York, pp 263–276
10. Sanchez O, Escobar JJ, Yunis JJ (1973) A simple G-banding technique. Lancet 11:269
11. An international system for human cytogenetic nomenclature (1978). Cytogenet Cell Genet 21:309–404
12. An international system for human cytogenetic nomenclature in high-resolution banding (1981). Cytogenet Cell Genet 31:1–23

Haematology and Blood Transfusion Vol. 29
Modern Trends in Human Leukemia VI
Edited by Neth, Gallo, Greaves, Janka

Oncogenetic Aspects of Chronic Myelocytic Leukemia

C. R. Bartram [1], A. de Klein, and G. Grosveld [2]

A. Introduction

Over the last several years, evidence has been accumulating that cellular oncogenes are involved in carcinogenesis, whatever its proximal cause. These genes constitute a functionally heterogeneous group that may cooperate with one another during tumorigenesis. The localization of oncogenes near breakpoints involved in specific chromosomal aberrations occurring in various neoplasms emphasizes their possible role in the development of those tumors [1, 4, 12, 15].

The cytogenetic hallmark of chronic myelocytic leukemia (CML) is the Philadelphia chromosome (Ph^1) in leukemic cells of 94% of cases. Recently, we demonstrated the consistent, reciprocal translocation of the human c-*abl* oncogene from chromosome 9 to the Ph^1 chromosome in standard (t (9; 22)), complex, variant, and masked cytogenetic subtypes of Ph^1-positive CML [2, 6, 10, unpublished work].

Moreover we have molecularly cloned sequences from chromosome 9 and 22 involved in the Ph^1 translocation, immediately adjacent to the chromosomal breakpoints [7, 9]. The sites of these breakpoints are individual in different patients and distributed over a relatively large region on chromosome 9, 5′ of human v-*abl* sequences. The breakpoints on chromosome 22, however, are clustered within a very limited region of yet unknown function [7], termed the breakpoint cluster region (*bcr*).

1 Universitätskinderklinik Ulm, Prittwitzstraße 43, 7900 Ulm, FRG
2 Department of Cell Biology and Genetics, Erasmus University Rotterdam

B. Results

DNA samples isolated from peripheral blood of nine Ph^1-positive CML patients were subjected to Southern blot analysis and hybridized to a *bcr*-specific Hind III/ Bgl II probe [7]. As is evident from Fig. 1, this probe detects, apart from a 4.8 kilobases fragment hybridizing to normal chromosome 22 sequences, variable rearranged fragments in Ph^1-positive patients. Since abnormalities were not seen in fibroblasts from Ph^1-positive CML patients (e.g., lane *J**), leukemic cells of Ph^1-negative patients (e.g., *K*) or in DNA isolated from other neoplasms, including acute myelocytic or myelomonocytic leukemia, lymphoma, glioblastoma, melanoma, and teratocarcinoma [7], we believe these rearrangements to be highly specific for leukemic cells in Ph^1-positive CML.

To investigate the possibility that the breakpoint cluster region exhibits additional rearrangements during progression of the chronic to the final acute state of CML, we studied DNA from leukemic cells of two Ph^1-positive CML patients in chronic phase and blast crises, respectively (Fig. 2). Obviously, there occur no further rearrangements within this limited region associated with blast crisis; this result is in agreement with the observation of specific, additional, secondary chromosomal aberrations during that terminal state of disease in the majority of patients.

Strong support for the hypothesis that an activation of the c-*abl* oncogene represents an important step during the development of Ph^1-positive CML results from the de-

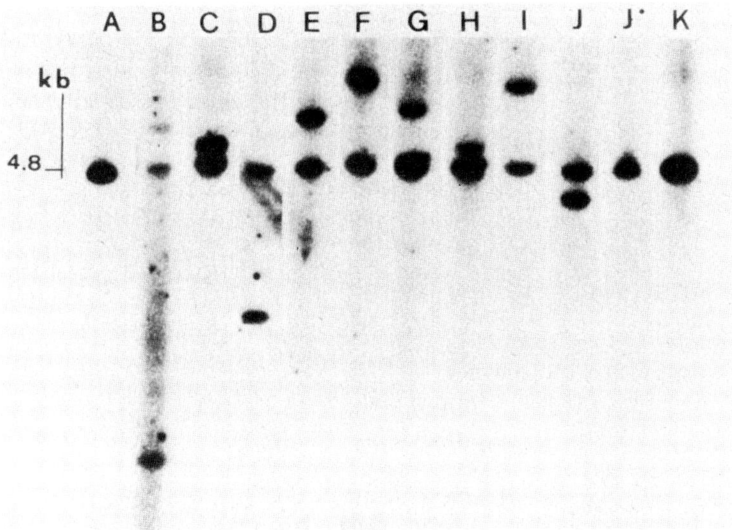

Fig. 1. Analysis of DNA samples from CML patients. DNA was isolated from human placenta (control, *lane A*), peripheral blood cells of Ph[1]-positive CML patients (*B–J*) and a Ph[1]-negative CML patient (*K*) as well as from fibroblasts of patient *J* (*J**); 10 μg DNA was digested with BGl II, electrophoresed on agarose gel, blotted, and hybridized to a *bcr*-specific 1.0 kilobases Hind III/Bgl II probe from chromosome 22 [7]. This probe detects abnormal Bgl II fragments in Ph[1]-positive CML patients in addition to a 4.8 kilobases fragment representing normal, unrearranged chromosome 22 sequences. Patient B apparently has a breakpoint in a region encompassing the probe; therefore the 1.0 kilobases Hind III/ Bgl II probe detects both the 22q- and 9q+ breakpoint fragments

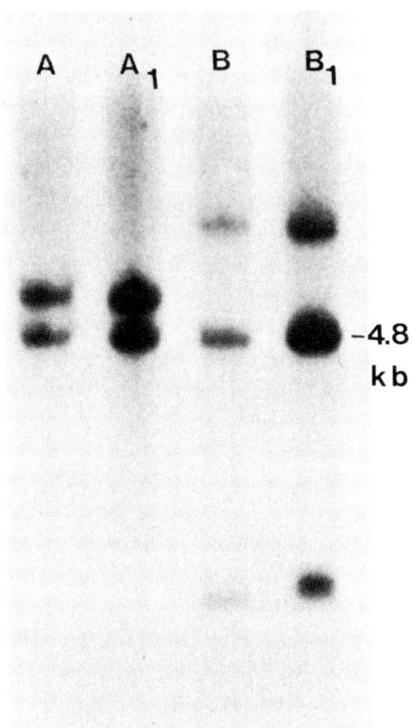

Fig. 2. Analysis of DNA samples isolated from peripheral blood cells of two CML patients during chronic phase (*lanes A, B*) and final blast crisis (A_1, B_1), respectively. DNA was digested, blotted, and hybridized as described in Fig. 1

tection of a new *abl* RNA transcript in leukemic cells (Fig. 3). HeLa and normal human hemopoietic cells (data not shown) contain major *abl* transcripts of 6.0 and 7.0 kilobases, as demonstrated by us and others [5, 14]. However, in CML cell line K562 and leukemic cells of Ph[1]-positive CML patients obtained during both chronic and acute phase (data not shown), a novel *abl* RNA species of 8.5 kilobases is apparent; we thus confirm similar results recently published by Canaani et al. [5]. It appears to be of particular importance that exactly the same novel RNA transcript is identified using *bcr*-specific probes instead of c-*abl* fragments. On the other hand,

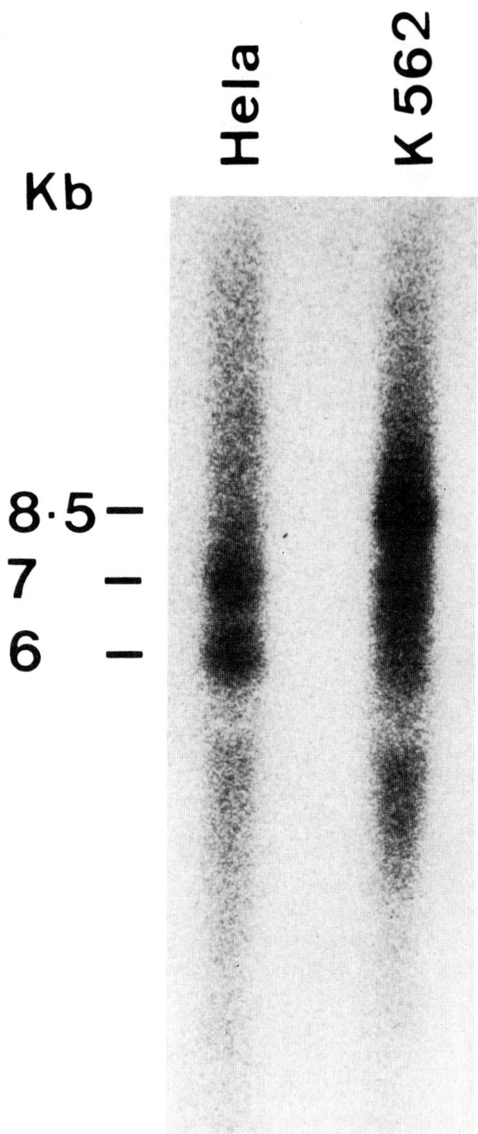

Fig. 3. Analysis of c-*abl*-related RNA in HeLa cells and CML cell line K562; 20 μg poly-A-selected RNA was blotted after gel electrophoresis and hybridized to a 0.6 kilobases BamH I 5′ c-*abl* probe [6]. HeLa cells contain two major *abl* transcripts of 6 and 7 kilobases; in contrast, K562 exhibits a new *abl* RNA species of 8.5 kilobases

there is no significant increase in *abl* expression in leukemic cells, with the known exception of cell line K562 containing amplified c-*abl* sequences [9].

C. Discussion

The consistent translocation of the human c-*abl* gene to the Ph^1 chromosome in all cytogenetic subtypes of Ph^1-positive CML, together with the detection of a novel *abl* RNA species in leukemic cells, suggests the involvement of this oncogene in the development of CML; it seems tempting to speculate that the *abl*-encoded protein in leukemic cells likewise has a higher molecular weight as compared with its counterpart in normal tissues.

A second molecular hallmark of Ph^1-positive CML is the clustering of all Ph^1 breakpoints within *bcr,* a region on chromosome 22 of approximately 5 kilobases length and yet unknown function. Although the λ light chain genes have been localized to the same band 22q11, no cross-homology was observed between *bcr* and λ clones. The detection of a new 8.5 kilobases RNA species in leukemic cells by c-*abl* and *bcr* probes further supports the view that sequences residing on both chromosomes 9 and 22, may be associated with Ph^1-positive CML. However, mechanisms responsible for the recombination of the two gene transcripts have still to be elucidated and one has particularly to take into account that the breakpoints on chromosome 9 are distributed over a relatively large region of several hundred kilobases.

Apparently, additional genes are essential for the generation of Ph^1-positive CML, as suggested by DNA transfection assays [11, 13]. The c-*sis* oncogene, however, appears to be an unlikely candidate (Fig. 4). This gene is localized on region 22q12.3-q13.1, far away from the breakpoint region, and segregates with the translocated part of chromosome 22 to different chromosomes in Ph^1-positive patients [3]. Moreover, *sis*-related transcripts have not been detected in CML cells or other hematopoietic malignancies.

The minority (6%) of CML patients without a Ph^1 chromosome exhibit neither c-*abl* translocation, novel *abl* transcripts, nor rearrangements within *bcr* on chromosome 22. Therefore, this disease appears to be a distinct subclass of myelocytic leukemia with an altogether different origin; this view is supported by clinical observations,

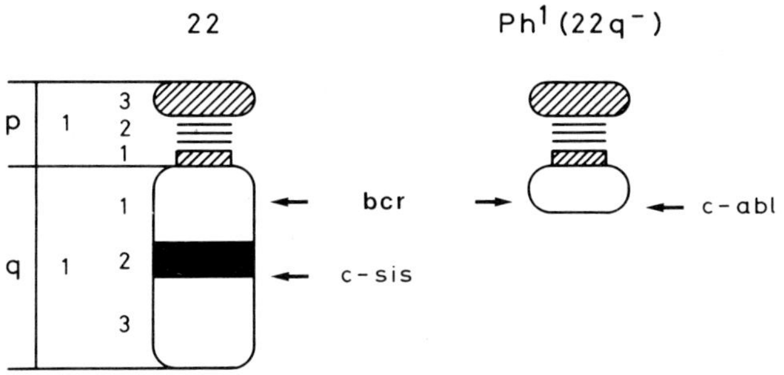

Fig. 4. Ph¹-positive CML is molecularly characterized by translocation of c-*abl* sequences from chromosome 9 to the Ph¹-chromosome and by a limited region on chromosome 22, termed *bcr,* that contains the Ph¹ breakpoints. However, c-*sis* is localized far away from the breakpoint region 22q11 and seems not to be important for the generation of CML

including correlations which reveal a poorer prognosis.

Acknowledgments. We thank T. Verwoard for expert technical assistance and Dr. N. Heisterkamp, Dr. G. Groffen, and Professor D. Bootsma for helpful discussions. The work was supported by the Deutsche Forschungsgemeinschaft and the Netherlands Cancer Society (Koningin Wilhelmina Fonds).

References

1. Bartram CR (1984) Eur J Pediatr 14:134
2. Bartram CR, de Klein A, Hagemeijer A, van Agthoven T, Geurts van Kessel A, Bootsma D, Grosveld G, Ferguson-Smith MA, Davies T, Stone M, Heisterkamp N, Stephenson JR, Groffen J (1983) Nature 306:277
3. Bartram CR, de Klein A, Hagemeijer A, Grosveld G, Heisterkamp N, Groffen J (1984) Blood 63:223
4. Bishop JM (1983) Ann Rev Biochem 52:301
5. Canaani E, Steiner-Saltz D, Aghai E, Gale RP, Berrebi A, Januszewicz E (1984) Lancet I:593
6. de Klein A, Geurts van Kessel A, Grosveld G, Bartram CR, Hagemeijer A, Bootsma D, Spurr NK, Heisterkamp N, Groffen J, Stephenson JR (1982) Nature 300:765
7. Groffen J, Stephenson JR, Heisterkamp N, de Klein A, Bartram CR, Grosveld G (1984) Cell 36:93
8. Heisterkamp N, Groffen G, Stephenson JR (1983) J Mol Appl Genet 2:57
9. Heisterkamp N, Stephenson JR, Groffen G, Hansen PE, de Klein A, Bartram CR, Grosveld G (1983) Nature 306:239
10. Hagemeijer A, Bartram CR, Smit EME, van Agthoven AJ, Bootsma D (1984) Cancer Genet Cytogenet 13:1
11. Lane MA, Neary D, Cooper GM (1982) Nature 300:659
12. Land H, Parada LF, Weinberg RA (1983) Science 222:771
13. Ozanne B, Wheeler T, Zack J, Smith G, Dale B (1982) Nature 299:74
14. Wang JY, Baltimore D (1983) Mol Cell Biol 3:773
15. Yunis JJ (1983) Science 221:227

Haematology and Blood Transfusion Vol. 29
Modern Trends in Human Leukemia VI
Edited by Neth, Gallo, Greaves, Janka

Association Between the Philadelphia Chromosome and a Unique *abl* Transcript *

E. Canaani and R. P. Gale

A. Introduction

Chronic myeloid leukemia (CML) is a myeloproliferative disorder in which the neoplastic transformation of a stem cell results in the proliferation and accumulation of granulocytes and their progenitors. The disease, which accounts in western countries for 20%–25% of all leukemias, is divided clinically into a chronic phase of 3–4 years duration followed by a terminal acute phase of 3–6 months. During the chronic phase, the neoplastic clone is already established and represents the majority of replicating cells. The cells mature normally and the principal abnormality during this phase appears to be an increase in the stem cell compartment committed to granulopoiesis. In contrast, during the acute phase, cells from the leukemic clone lose their ability to differentiate and mature normally [1]. Perhaps the hallmark of CML is that a specific chromosomal abnormality, the Ph[1] (Philadelphia) chromosome is present in over 90% of cases [2]. The Ph[1] chromosome, also termed $22q^-$, results in most instances from a balanced reciprocal translocation between chromosomes 22 and 9 with very specific breakpoints [3–5]. Recently, the oncogenes *abl* and *sis* were mapped to chromosomes 9 and 22, respectively [6–8]. Moreover, *abl* was shown to reside on the translocated segment of chromosome 9 [9] and *sis* on the corresponding portion of chromosome 22 [10]. Finally, in one case of CML, the translocation breakpoint was localized to the 5′ region of the *abl* gene [11]. We asked whether one or both of these oncogenes is activated and altered in its expression because of the translocation. To answer this we used the RNA transfer technique (Northern blotting) to analyze transcription of *abl* and *sis* in leukemic cells from the peripheral blood or bone marrow of CML patients.

* Department of Chemical Immunology, The Weizmann Institute of Science, Rehovot, 76100, Israel, and Department of Medicine (Hematology and Oncology) UCLA School of Medicine, Los Angeles, California 90024, USA

B. Results

We examined transcription of the *sis* gene in CML. RNA samples from four patients with CML and t(9;22), three patients with AML without t(9;22), and HeLa cells were tested by the Northern technique for hybridization to a v-*sis* probe composed of sequences of simian sarcoma viral genome homologous to *sis*. No discret species of *sis* RNA could be detected in any of the samples (Fig. 1, lanes *a–h*). Preparation of RNA from normal rat kidney (NRK) cells infected with simian sarcoma virus served as a positive control and showed multiple size transcripts of v-*sis* (Fig. 1, lane *i*).

We next analyzed expression of the *abl* oncogene in samples from 13 CML patients, 22 patients with other leukemias, and 2 normal bone marrows. Representative data are shown in Fig. 2. Human cells contain two major *abl* transcripts of 6 and 7 kilobases, as well as a few other minor species [12–14] and the non-CML samples

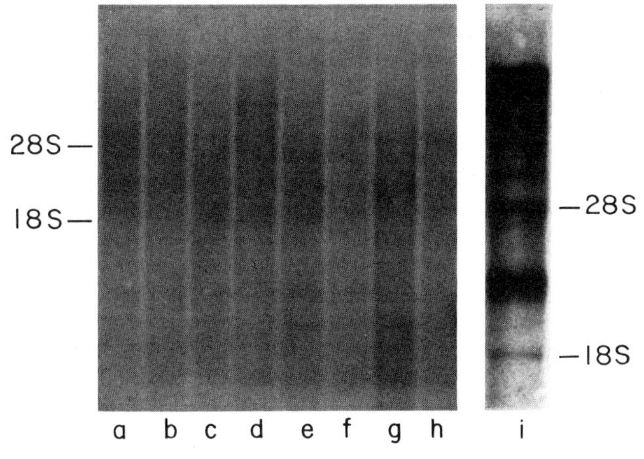

Fig. 1. Absence of *sis* RNA in CML, AML, and HeLa cells; 15-μg samples of RNA from CML (*lanes b, d, f, h*), AML (*lanes a, e, g*), HeLa cells (*lane c*), and NRK cells infected with simian sarcoma virus (*lane i*) were screened for *sis* RNA. Data from [20]

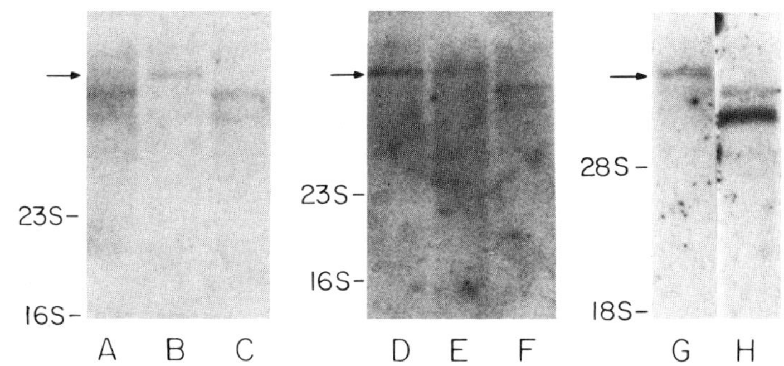

Fig. 2. Gel electrophoresis of *abl* RNA from normal bone marrow, HeLa cells, CML, and AML. *Lane A* normal bone marrow; *lanes B, E* bone marrow from CML patients in chronic phase; *lanes C, F* peripheral blood of AML patients; *lane D* peripheral blood of CML patient in chronic phase; *lane G* peripheral blood of CML patient in blast crisis; *lane H* HeLa cells. Bacterial 23 and 16 *S* ribosomal RNA and human 28 and 18 *S* ribosomal RNA were used as molecular weight standards. *Arrows* correspond to new 8 kilobases *abl* RNA species. Samples of 10 μg RNA were analyzed in *A–G* and a sample of 3 μg was analyzed in *H*. Data from [28]

we analyzed showed the major two RNA (Fig. 2, lanes *A, C, F, H*). CML patients with the Ph[1] chromosome and the 9;22 translocation showed a new *abl* RNA species of 8 kilobases (Fig. 2, lanes *B, D, E, G*). This transcript either replaced the 6 and 7 kilobases species or appeared with them, it was present in samples obtained during both the chronic and acute phases of the disease.

Results of the 37 samples analyzed are summarized in Table 1. The 8 kilobases *abl* RNA transcript was detected in 11 of 12 patients with CML and the t(9;22) translocation, but not in one patient with juvenile CML without t(9;22). The 8 kilobases *abl* transcript was also detected in 1 of 12 patients with AML. Approximately 5% of individuals with AML have the t(9;22) translocation. Unfortunately, chromosome analysis was not performed in this patient so we are unable to determine if he had the t(9;22). The 8 kilobases transcript was absent in the remaining 11 patients with AML and in 10 patients with a variety of other leukemias, including chronic lymphocytic leukemia, acute lymphocytic leukemia, prolymphocytic leukemia, chronic monocytic leukemia, and acute undifferentiated leukemia. The 8 kilobases species was also lacking in cells from two normal bone marrows. A novel 9 kilobases *abl* RNA was detected together with the 8 kilobases species in 2 of 11 samples from patients with CML and t(9;22).

Table 1. The 8 kilobases *abl* RNA in CML and other leukemias (data from [20])

Diagnosis[a]	Ph^1	Number tested	8 kilobases *abl* RNA
CML	+	12	11
CML[b]	–	1	0
AML	–	11	0
AML	?	1	1
CLL	–	4	0
ALL	–	3	0
AProL	–	1	0
CMoL	–	1	0
AUL	–	1	0
Normal BM	–	2	0

[a] CML chronic myelogenous leukemia; AML acute myelogenous leukemia; ALL acute lymphoblastic leukemia; AProL acute prolymphocytic leukemia; CMoL chronic monocytic leukemia; AUL acute undifferentiated leukemia; BM bone marrow

[b] "Juvenile" CML

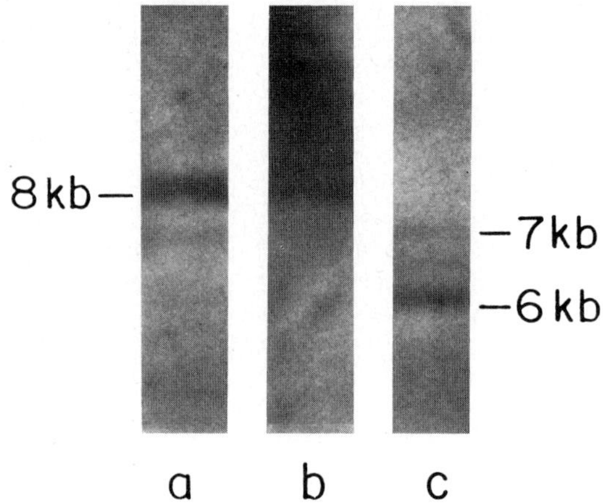

Fig. 3. The 8 kilobases *abl* RNA in two Ph^1-positive cell lines; 8-μg aliquots of RNA from lines K562 (*lane a*), EM2 (*lane b*), and SMS-SB (Ph^1-negative line) (*lane c*), were examined for presence of 8 kilobases *abl* RNA. Data from [20]

Next, we investigated whether human cell lines containing the Ph^1 chromosome synthesized the altered *abl* transcript. These included five hematopoietic cell lines with and without t(9;22) and four nonhematopoietic cell lines without t(9;22). The K562 cell line [15] is an erythroid–myeloid precursor line derived from a patient with CML. K562 has a Ph^1 chromosome [16] or an altered form of it [17]. Analysis of RNA from K562 indicated a major band corresponding to 8 kilobases *abl* RNA and minor bands of the normal species of 6 and 7 kilobases (Fig. 3, lane *a*). Similar analyses of the human myeloid precursor line EM-2 derived from a CML patient and containing one or more Ph^1 chromosomes [18] showed a single *abl* transcript of 8 kilobases (Fig. 3, lane *b*). We performed a similar analysis on the human cell line SMS-SB derived from the leukemic lymphoblasts of a patient with pre-B cell acute lymphoblastic leukemia [19]. This cell line is Ph^1 negative and was recently shown [13] to contain the normal *abl* transcripts as well as additional species of *abl* RNA. Our analysis (Fig. 3, lane *c*) demonstrated the normal 6 and 7 kilobases *abl* transcripts as well as additional 6.5 kilobases *abl* species. No 8 kilobases *abl* RNA was observed. Two other hematopoietic cell lines (HL-60 and Molt-4) which lack the Ph^1 chromosome and four Ph^1 negative nonhematopoietic cell lines demonstrated the normal 6 and 7 kilobases *abl* transcripts, but lacked the novel 8 kilobases *abl* transcript. EM-2, K562, Molt-4, HL-60, and HeLa cells contain substantially more polyadenylated *abl* RNA than fresh hematopoietic cells, both normal and leukemic.

C. Discussion

The absence of *sis* transcripts in leukemic cells from patients with CML indicates that this oncogene is probably not activated by the t(9;22) translocation. These and other data, including the variability of the reciprocal chromosome to which *sis* is translocated, suggest that *sis* does not play a role in CML. The important finding of this work is that a new *abl* transcript of 8 kilobases is found in 11 of 12 patients with CML with the t(9;22) translocation. The 8 kilobases *abl* transcript was also found in two hematopoietic cell lines containing the Ph^1 chromosome. A single patient with AML also had this transcript, but it is unknown whether his cells had a Ph[1] chromosome. This novel RNA was not observed in cells from 22 leukemias unassociated with t(9;22), including a case of Ph[1] negative CML, nor in seven human hematopoietic and nonhematopoietic cell lines which lacked the Ph[1] chromosome. Two samples of normal bone marrow also lacked to 8 kilobases RNA. The association between the t(9;22) translocation and presence of the 8 kilobases *abl* transcript is highly significant.

The strong correlation between the synthesis of the new 8 kilobases transcript and the translocation of *abl* to chromosome 22 suggests a causal association. The new transcript, as well as the normal *abl* species, are homologous to probes from the 5′, central, and 3′ regions of v-*abl* [20]. Therefore, it is likely that the new transcript contains much of the information of normal *abl* RNA. It is possible that the new *abl* RNA is due to a modified splicing pattern of a normal precursor, however, two lines of evidence suggest a possibility that the extra information in the 8 kilobases *abl* RNA originates from a region 5′ to the gene. First, in one case of CML it was shown that the translocation placed the *abl* gene into a position adjacent to the breakpoint, with the 5′ region of the oncogene facing sequences of chromosome 22 [11]. Second, the detection in cells from two CML patients of an additional new *abl* species of 9 kilobases might suggest that the 8 and 9 kilobases *abl* RNA are related to the 6 and 7 kilobases normal species, respectively, and that the former were derived by acquisition of the same sequence. Since the 6 and 7 kilobases human *abl* RNA (by analogy with the corresponding mouse species [14]) presumably initiate at the same promoter, but terminate at different poly (A) signals 1000 base pairs apart, the 8 and 9 kilobases RNA might terminate at the same sites as the normal species, but initiate at a new transcriptional promoter upstream of the normal promoter. Such a new promoter could reside in chromosome 9 sequences or in chromosome 22 information behind the breakpoint [21]. The initiation at a new promoter would be probably associated with a modified splicing pattern.

The formation of the new *abl* transcript might be the critical factor in the increased committed myeloid stem cell compartment typical of the chronic phase of CML and/or the loss of differentiative capacity found in the acute phase of CML. The transcript might be translated into an altered protein, perhaps modified at the NH_2 terminus region. This region has been previously shown to be critical for the transforming activity of the v-*abl*-encoded protein [22]. Moreover, if the 8 kilobases *abl* RNA represents a fusion transcript, then it is also possible that it encodes a novel fused protein. Finally, the possibility raised by this study and others that the *abl* gene is directly involved in generation of CML is consistent with the well-documented capacity of Abelson murine leukemia virus, which carries within its genome the viral homolog of mouse cellular *abl,* to transform hematopoietic cells, including lymphocytes, plasma cells, macrophages, and promyelocytes [23–27].

References

1. Koeffler P, Golde DW (1981) N Engl J Med 304:1201–1209, 1269–1274
2. Nowel PC, Hungerford DA (1960) J Natl Cancer Inst 25:85–109
3. Rowley JD (1973) Nature 243:290–293
4. Rowley JD, Testa JR (1982) Adv Cancer Res 36:103–148
5. Yunis JJ (1983) Science 221:227–236
6. Heisterkamp NY, Groffen J, Stephenson JR, Spurr NK, Goodfellow PN, Solomon E, Carritt B, Bodmer WF (1982) Nature 299: 747–750
7. Swan DC, McBride OW, Robbins KC, Keithley DA, Reddy EP, Aaronson SA (1982) Proc Natl Acad USA 79:4691–4695
8. Dalla-Favera R, Gallo RC, Giallongo A, Croce CM (1982) Science 218:686–688
9. de Klein A, Geurts van Kessel A, Grosveld G, Bartrarn CR, Hagemeyer A, Bootsma D, Spurr NK, Heisterkamp N, Groffin J, Stephenson JR (1982) Nature 300:765–767
10. Groffen J, Heisterkamp N, Stephenson JR, Guerts van Kessel AG, de Klein A, Grosveld G, Bootsma D (1983) J Exp Med 158:9–15
11. Heisterkamp N, Stephenson JR, Groffen J, Hansen PF, de Klein A, Bartram CR, Grosveld G (1983) Nature 306:239–242

12. Westin EH, Wong-Staal F, Gelmann EP, Dalla-Favera R, Papas TS, Lautenberger JA, Eva A, Reddy EP, Tronick SR, Aaronson SA, Gallo RC (1982) Proc Natl Acad Sci USA 79:2490–2499
13. Ozanne B, Wheeler T, Zack J, Smith G, Dale B (1982) Nature 299:744–747
14. Wang JYJ, Baltimore D (1983) Molec Cell Biol 3:773–779
15. Lozzio CB, Lozzio BB (1975) Blood 45: 321–334
16. Collins SJ, Groudine MT (1983) Proc Natl Acad Sci USA 80:4813–4817
17. Selden JR, Emannuel BS, Wang E, Cannizaro L, Palumbo A, Erikson J, Nowell PC, Rovera G, Croce CM (1983) Proc Natl Acad Sci USA 80:7289–7292
18. Keating A, Martin P, Bernstein I, Papayannopoulou T, Raskind W, Singer JW (1983) In: Golde DW, Marks PM (eds) Normal and neoplastic hematopoiesis. Liss, New York, pp 513–520
19. Smith RG, Dev VG, Shannon WA Jr (1981) J Immunol 126:596–602
20. Gale RP, Canaani E (1984) Proc Natl Acad Sci USA 81:5648–5652
21. Groffen J, Stephenson JR, Heisterkamp N, de Klein A, Bartram CR, Grosveld G (1984) Cell 36:97–99
22. Prywes R, Foukes JG, Rosenberg N, Baltimore D (1983) Cell 34:569–579
23. Abelson HT, Rabstein LS (1970) Cancer Research 30:2213–2222
24. Potter M, Sklar MD, Rowe WP (1976) Science 182:592–594
25. Raschke WC, Bairds S, Ralph P, Nakoinz I (1978) Cell 15:261–267
26. Rosenberg N, Baltimore D, Scher CD (1975) Proc Natl Acad Sci USA 72:1932–1936
27. Greenberger JS, Davisson PB, Gans PJ, Moloney WC (1979) Blood 53:987–1001
28. Canaani E, Gale RP, Steiner-Saltz D, Berrebi A, Aghai E, Januszewicz E (1984) Lancet 1:593–595

Haematology and Blood Transfusion Vol. 29
Modern Trends in Human Leukemia VI
Edited by Neth, Gallo, Greaves, Janka

Somatic N-*ras* Oncogene Activation in a Patient with Acute Myeloblastic Leukemia *

C. Moroni, C. Gambke, E. Signer, and J. Jiricny

A. Introduction

The recognition that retroviral oncogenes (v-*onc*) are derived from normal cellular sequences termed proto-oncogenes or c-*onc*, has led to a search to see whether human proto-oncogenes present in human tumors show alterations in structure or expression. Of particular interest are the activated forms of *ras* proto-oncogenes; these can be assayed in a biologic test system, since activated *ras* genes from tumor tissue, but not normal alleles have the ability to transform NIH 3T3 cells in tissue culture [1–4]. The role, if any, of this transforming activity in the natural history of the human tumor is still unknown. The human genome contains three functional *ras* genes, localized on different chromosomes: H-*ras* (related to v-*ras* of Harvey sarcoma virus), K-*ras* (related to v-*ras* of Kirsten sarcoma virus), and N-*ras*, a *ras* family member identified by nucleic acid hybridization through its relatedness to the former *ras* genes [5–8]. Activation of *ras* genes was found to be the result of point mutations altering amino acid 12 of the H-*ras* or K-*ras* [11–18] or amino acid 61 of the H-*ras* or N-*ras* genes [9, 10, 19].

We have initiated a study to see whether human leukemias, prior to treatment, contain activated *ras*-genes, and if so, whether and how the presence of the activated gene correlates with the course of the disease. In this report, we summarize our analysis of a patient with acute myeloblastic leukemia (AML) with an activated N-*ras* gene.

* Friedrich Miescher-Institut, P.O. Box 2543, CH-4002 Basel, and Children's Hospital, University of Basel, Basel, Switzerland

B. Materials and Methods

I. NIH 3T3 Transfection Test

High molecular weight DNA was isolated by phenol and subsequent chloroform extraction as described [20]. DNA was precipitated by the calcium phosphate method on NIH 3T3 cells, seeded one day before at 5×10^5 cells per 10-cm plate, and foci of transformed cells were enumerated after 2 weeks. Details of the procedure are given in [20].

II. Oligonucleotide Synthesis

The oligonucleotides were synthesized by the modified phosphotriester approach described by Sproat and Bannwarth [21], using a semiautomated continuous-flow benchtop synthesizer of our own design. The synthesis were carried out starting with 40 mg controlled-pore glass support, corresponding to approximately 4 μmol nucleoside functionality; 40 mg mononucleotide building blocks and 60 mg condensing agent (mesitylenesulfonylnitrotriazolide, MSNT) were used for each addition. The cycle time was 24 min.

The products were fully deprotected and purified by ion exchange HPLC, using a Partisil 10/SAX 25 analytic column, eluted with a linear gradient of 0.001–0.4 *M* potassium phosphate buffer pH 6.5, containing 60% formamide. Desalting was achieved by means of a Biogel P2 column (2.5 × 50 cm), eluted with a mixture of ethanol and water (2:8 v/v). The pure oligonucleotides were 5'-labeled with ^{32}P following the method of Smith and Zoller [22].

III. Southern Blot Analysis of Cloned N-*ras* Fragments

Plasmids containing the transforming, "activated gene", and the nontransforming, "normal gene", N-*ras*, respectively, were electrophoresed on 0.8% agarose gels. After transfer of DNA to nitrocellulose, hybridization was done in the presence of 10% dextran sulfate for 18 h at 40 °C using 1.4×10^6 cpm/ml labeled "normal probe" (see Fig. 2a) or 0.8×10^6 cpm/ml "activated probe" (see Fig. 2b). Filters were washed 3 × 15 min at 8 °C with 2 × SSC, 3 min at 40 °C with 2 × SSC in 0.1% SDS, and 4 min at 54 °C with 2 × SSC in 0.1% SDS, and autoradiographed for 6 days at – 70 °C.

C. Results and Discussion

We have recently described a patient with AML where a NIH 3T3 transfection test performed with bone marrow-derived DNA was positive [20]. The salient laboratory data of this patient together with transfection data are summarized in Table 1. The focus-forming activity of this DNA (0.056 foci per microgram DNA), which is derived from a marrow with 68% atypical blasts is comparable to values obtained by other workers with DNA from cloned cell lines. This suggests that the transforming gene may be represented clonally in all atypical myeloblasts and thus might have been present early in the history of this malignant clone, perhaps at the time of the leukemogenic transformation. The transforming gene was not present in the germ line of this patient, as DNA from cultured fibroblast cells did not have transforming activity. Thus, the generation of the transforming gene must have been a somatic

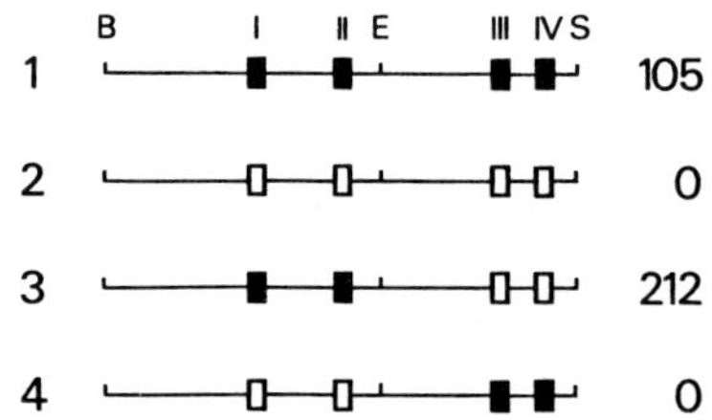

Fig. 1. Transforming activity of chimeric N-*ras* molecules. The four exons of the N-*ras* gene reside on a 12.5 kilobases Bam HI-Sac I fragment [10]. An Eco RI site separates exons I and II from exons III and IV. From cloned normal and transforming N-*ras* genes, Bam HI-Eco RI and Eco RI-Sac I fragments were isolated, ligated to construct chimeric molecules (3, 4) and to reconstruct transforming (1) and normal (2) molecules for control. The ligation mixture was assayed on NIH 3T3 cells for transforming activity. The numbers on the right indicate the number of foci obtained after 2 weeks. *Full boxes* exons of transforming N-*ras* allele; *open boxes* exons of normal N-*ras* allele; B Bam HI; E Eco RI; S Sac I

Table 1. Hematologic data and transforming activity of AML bone marrow DNA[a]

NIH 3T3 transfection test	Bone marrow DNA: 0.056 foci/μg DNA Fibroblast DNA: 0.002 foci/μg DNA
Bone marrow	Hypercellular 68% Atypical myeloblasts (peroxidase + ve, Sudan black + ve, PAS – ve, nonspecific esterase – ve) Karyotype: no abnormal findings
Blood	WBC: $62 \times 10^9\ l^{-1}$ (mostly atypical myeloblasts) Platelets: $55 \times 10^9\ l^{-1}$ Hemoglobin: 91 g l^{-1}

[a] At time of diagnosis and before chemotherapy administration

Table 2. Mutations affecting amino acid 12 of the *ras* genes

Gene	Codon	Amino acid	Origin	References
N-*ras*	GGT	Gly	Normal DNA	[9, 10]
	GAT	ASP	AML	This study; [23]
H-*ras*	GGC	Gly	Normal DNA	[11]
	GTC	Val	Bladder carcinoma EJ, T24	[11, 12, 13, 14]
K-*ras*	GGT	Gly	Normal DNA	[14]
	TGT	Cys	Lung carcinoma Calu-1	[15, 16]
	TGT	Cys	Lung carcinoma PR371	[17]
	GTT	Val	Colon carcinoma SW480	[16]
	CGT	Arg	Bladder carcinoma A1698	[18]
	CGT	Arg	Lung carcinoma A2182	[18]
	CGT	Arg	Lung carcinoma LC-10	[18]

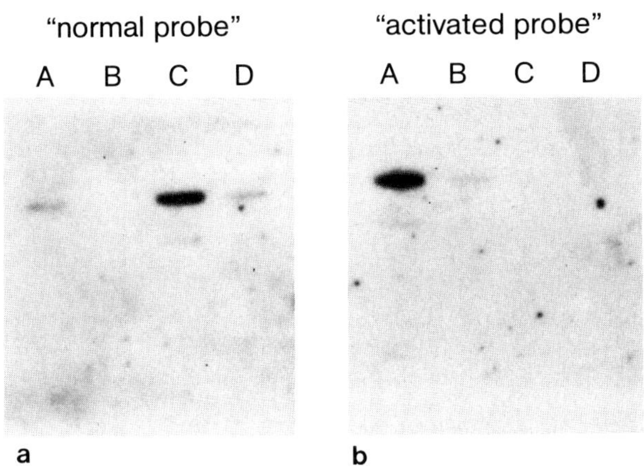

Fig. 2a, b. Southern blot analysis of cloned transforming, "activated gene" and nontransforming "normal gene" N-*ras* genes using synthetic ^{32}P-labeled heptadeca-nucleotides as probes. **a** "normal probe" complementary to normal N-*ras* gene, **b** "activated probe" complementary to mutated N-*ras* gene. The sequence of the normal probe is TGGAGCA<u>GGT</u>GGTGTTG. The sequence of the activated probe is TGGAGCAGATGGTGGTG. The triplet coding for amino acid 12 is *underlined.* A activated gene 1.0 ng; B activated gene 0.1 ng; C normal gene 1.0 ng; D normal gene 0.1 ng

event. This gene was identified as N-*ras* by analyzing primary and secondary transfection foci [20]. Both the transforming N-*ras* gene (derived from a secondary locus) and the nontransforming N-*ras* gene (derived from the patient's fibroblasts) were cloned in phage L47.1 as described elsewhere [23]. The four exons of the N-*ras* gene are localized on a Bam HI-Sac I fragment (Fig. 1), where an Eco RI site separates exons I and II from exons III and IV. The chimeric N-*ras* molecules between the transforming and nontransforming gene fragments were constructed from subfragments (Fig. 1), and analyzed for transforming activity. As shown in Fig. 1, focus formation was only seen when exons I/II from the transforming gene were present, which suggested that a mutation occurred in exons I/II. These exons were therefore sequenced. While the sequence of the nontransforming N-*ras* gene was identical to the published N-*ras* sequence [9, 10], the transforming gene differed in one nucleotide. The GGT triplet coding for amino acid 12 was altered to GAT which changes the coding from Gly to Asp. The two formerly known N-*ras* activations seen in a neuroblastoma line and a fibrosarcoma line both affect amino acid 61 [9, 10]. However, as already mentioned, alterations at positions 12 have been observed with H-*ras* and K-*ras* genes. Table 2 summarizes the codon 12 nucleotide changes of all *ras* genes observed so far. Both the first and second G can be altered, 7/8 cases involve G → T or

G → C transversions, while our case involves a G → A transition.

Since, in all appropriately analyzed cases of *ras* activation, one finds an alteration of amino acid 12 or 61, one may, using suitable oligonucleotide probes, diagnose a mutational event by Southern blot analysis. This would circumvent the time-consuming and cumbersome NIH 3T3 transfection test. To approach this possibility we have synthetized two heptadecanucleotides corresponding to the normal and the mutated N-*ras* gene (Fig. 2). In preliminary experiments using cloned normal and mutated N-*ras* genes, we found hybridization conditions under which each probe specifically hybridized with its homologous allele. Thus, a G → A transition can be positively or negatively detected by either probe (compare for example lanes A and C in both examples shown). We are presently trying to establish this methodology to genomic DNA. It should be particularly interesting to use these probes to assay for the presence of the N-*ras* mutation in DNA isolated from bone marrow during clinical remission. Such probes should be generally useful for studying the role of *ras* genes in leukemias and other malignancies.

References

1. Parada LF, Tabin CJ, Shih C, Weinberg RA (1982) Nature 297:474–478
2. Der CJ, Krontiris TG, Cooper GM (1982) Proc Natl Acad Sci USA 79:3637–3640
3. Pulciani S et al. (1982) Nature 300:539–541
4. Santos E, Tronick SR, Aaronson SA, Pulciani S, Barbacid M (1982) Nature 298:343–347
5. Ellis RW, DeFeo D, Shih TY, Gonda MA, Young HA, Tsuchida N, Lowy DR, Scolnick EM (1981) Nature 292:506–511
6. Taparowski E, Shimizu K, Goldfarb M, Wigler M (1983) Cell 34:581–586
7. Marshall CJ, Hall A, Weiss RA (1982) Nature 299:171–173
8. Murray MJ, Cunningham JM, Parada LF, Dautry F, Lebowitz P, Weinberg RA (1983) Cell 33:749–757
9. Wigler M, Pellicer A, Silverstein S, Axel R, Urlab G, Chasin L (1979) Proc Natl Acad Sci USA
10. Brown R, Marshall CJ, Pennie SG, Hall A (1984) EMBO J 3:1321–1326
11. Tabin CJ, Bradley SM, Bargmann CI, Weinberg RA, Papageorge AG, Scolnick EM, Dhar R, Lowy DR, Chang EH (1982) Nature 300:143–149
12. Reddy EP, Reynold RK, Santos E, Barbacid M (1982) Nature 300:149–152
13. Taparowski E, Suard Y, Fasano O, Shimizu K, Goldfarb M, Wigler M (1982) Nature 300:762–765
14. McGrath JP, Capon DJ, Smith DH, Chen EY, Seeburg PH, Goeddel DV, Levinson AD (1983) Nature 300:501–506
15. Shimizu K, Birnbaum D, Ruley MA, Fasano O, Suard Y, Edlund L, Taparowsky E, Goldfarb M, Wigler M (1983) Nature 304: 497–500
16. Capon DJ, Seeburg PH, McGrath JP, Hayflick JS, Edmann U, Levinson AD, Goeddel DV (1983) Nature 304:507–513
17. Nakano H, Yamamoto F, Neville C, Evans D, Mizuno T, Perucho M (1984) Proc Natl Acad Sci USA 81:71–75
18. Santos E, Martin-Zanca D, Reddy EP, Pierotti MA, Della Porta G, Barbacid M (1984) Science 223:661–664
19. Yuasa Y, Srivastava SK, Dunn CY, Rhim JS, Reddy EP, Aaronson SA (1983) Nature 303: 775–779
20. Gambke C, Signer E, Moroni C (1984) Nature 307:476–478
21. Sproat BS, Bannwarth W (1983) Tetrahedron Letters 24:5771–5774
22. Zoller MJ, Smith M (1983) Methods Enzymol 100:468–500
23. Gambke C, Hall A, Moroni Ch (1984) Proc Natl Acad Sci USA 82:879–882

Haematology and Blood Transfusion Vol. 29
Modern Trends in Human Leukemia VI
Edited by Neth, Gallo, Greaves, Janka

Behavior of Human Leukemic Progenitor Populations in Long-Term Marrow Culture *

C. Eaves, L. Coulombel, I. Dubé, D. Kalousek, J. Cashman, and A. Eaves

A. Introduction

An analysis of mechanisms that underlie abnormal hemopoiesis requires methods that allow the cell populations involved to be characterized and quantitated under conditions that can be defined, and ideally manipulated. Although such methodologies are not yet fully developed, the past 2 decades have seen major advances in several areas relevant to this need. Of major importance has been the establishment of semisolid culture systems capable of supporting the short-term clonal growth and differentiation of individual primitive human hemopoietic progenitor cells of various types. These include pluripotent progenitors [1] as well as different classes of lineage-restricted progenitors [2–4]. Also noteworthy has been the successful exploitation of various genetic markers to examine the cell of origin of the abnormal clone in rare patients who are constitutional mosaics and in whom a clonal hemopoietic neoplasm [5, 6] has subsequently developed. The fact that in many such patients the clone responsible for the disease may continue to produce some cells that are able to differentiate relatively normally has allowed some inference to be made about the cell type initially transformed. For example, in some patients with acute myoblastic leukemia (AML) all of the circulating red cells or their precursors have been found at presentation to belong to the same clone as the circulating myeloid blasts, suggesting a common derivation from a neoplastic pluripotent stem cell. On the basis of such arguments it is now generally accepted that the myeloproliferative disorders as a group as well as some cases of AML and preleukemia arise from altered pluripotent stem cells.

These latter findings have focussed attention on the need for culture systems that allow the most primitive pluripotent stem-cell types to be maintained for extensive periods, ideally under conditions similar to those prevailing in the marrow of the patient so that the mechanisms controlling normal and leukemic stem-cell behavior in vivo might be accessible to study. For the initial definition of these it would be anticipated that colony assay systems might be relatively unsuitable since direct cell–cell interactions are minimized and regulation of growth and differentiation is dependent on the addition of suitable diffusible factors. Of particular interest in the case of patients with clonal neoplasms is the question not only of how leukemic stem-cell proliferation is supported, but also that of how normal hemopoiesis usually comes to be suppressed. In this latter regard the anticipated inadequacy of colony assay systems has already been demonstrated, as shown by the finding that residual normal (i.e., nonclonal) progenitors from patients with chronic myelocytic leukemia (CML) or polycythemia vera (PV) can successfully

* Terry Fox Laboratory, B.C. Cancer Research Centre, 601 West 10th Avenue, Vancouver, B.C. V5Z 1L3, Canada, and Departments of Medical Genetics, Pathology and Medicine, University of British Columbia, Vancouver, B.C. Canada

generate colonies of mature red cells and granulocytes in vitro, even though they fail to produce detectable numbers of mature progeny in vivo [7, 8]. The long-term marrow culture system was thus an obvious alternative to consider.

B. Long-Term Human Marrow Cultures: Present State of the Art

In long-term marrow cultures primitive hemopoietic cells are maintained for many weeks in a confluent adherent layer composed of a variety of hemopoietic and nonhemopoietic cell types (e.g., fibroblasts) of marrow origin [9–12]. Exogenous provision of specific growth factors is not required and there is some evidence that the nonhemopoietic elements of the adherent layer substitute in this role as they may do in vivo [9].

However, in spite of the now widespread success in establishing long-term cultures from mouse bone marrow, the reproducible development and characterization of analogous cultures using human marrow has only recently been achieved [10–12]. This is due in part to the recognition that long-term maintenance of hemopoiesis in human marrow cultures depends on their initiation with specimens of adequate cellularity (i.e., aspirates containing at least $2–3 \times 10^7$ nucleated cells/ml), the inclusion of horse serum as well as fetal calf serum in the growth medium [10, 11], and the retention of half of the old growth medium at each weekly medium change [12, 13]. In addition, it was not until detailed studies of the adherent layer were undertaken that the greater tendency of the most primitive progenitor cell types to remain in this layer in the human system was appreciated [12]. In long-term mouse marrow cultures, relatively large numbers of stem cells are released into the nonadherent fraction every week from the time the cultures are first initiated [14, 15]. As a result the accumulated output over several weeks commonly exceeds the number initially added [15]. This is not the case in human cultures.

Evidence of stem-cell turnover can, however, be found by assessment of the proportion of progenitors that are in S-phase at any given time. Such evidence is obtained from a comparison of the relative numbers of colonies produced from two aliquots of a culture harvest, one of which is exposed for 20 min at 37 °C to high-specific-activity tritiated thymidine, the other serving as a control. Progenitors in S-phase are inactivated by this treatment and inactivation levels of up to approximately 50% can be reproducibly demonstrated in actively cycling progenitor populations [16]. In normal marrow very few of the most primitive erythropoietic [17] and pluripotent [18] progenitor cells detectable by colony assays (i.e., primitive BFU-E and CFU-G/E, respectively) are killed by this treatment, suggesting a low level of cycling activity in these compartments. In contrast, the later erythropoietic progenitor compartments in the marrow (i.e., mature BFU-E and CFU-E) and the marrow granulopoietic colony-forming progenitor compartment (CFU-C) looked at as a whole are found to have significant S-phase components [17, 19].

In long-term marrow cultures where granulocyte and macrophage production takes place continuously, the same broadly defined granulopoietic progenitor population also shows a significant S-phase component irrespective of the age of the culture or the time since the previous medium change. Erythropoiesis is blocked at a relatively early stage of erythropoietic progenitor development so that after 4 weeks CFU-Es are rarely detected and mature BFU-E numbers are also too low [15] to allow cycling data to be readily obtained. Primitive BFU-Es which, like CFU-G/Es, are almost exclusively confined to the adherent layer, show a cyclic pattern of turnover. A significant S-phase component appears transiently 2 days after each medium change but is no longer detectable 7 days later. A similar pattern of regulated cycling changes in the pluripotent stem-cell compartment with continuous cycling of the granulopoietic progenitor compartment has also been found to occur in long-term mouse marrow cultures [9]. This suggests that similar control mechanisms are operative in both systems in spite of the differences in primitive progenitor output.

C. Long-Term CML Marrow Cultures

For our first experiment to compare the separate behavior of normal and leukemic progenitors in long-term marrow culture, we chose a patient with Philadelphia chromosome (Ph^1)-positive disease who presented with 5% normal metaphases in his initial direct marrow preparation. Cytogenetic analysis of the erythroid and granulopoietic colonies cultured from the same marrow sample confirmed the presence of detectable Ph^1-negative cells in these early hemopoietic compartments. Because of his low WBC count he remained untreated. A second marrow was obtained 1 month later. Part of this specimen was used to reassess the frequency of proliferating Ph^1-negative cells and Ph^1-negative progenitors in his marrow at that time. The remainder was used to initiate long-term cultures. These were maintained in the usual way [12] and 4 weeks later the adherent layers were then harvested and assayed for erythropoietic, granulopoietic, and pluripotent progenitors in standard methylcellulose assays. Cytogenetic analysis of the larger colonies obtained showed that the proportion of these that were Ph^1-negative had increased from 11% (before culture) to 55% (by 4 weeks) [20]. Thus the conditions prevailing in these cultures had clearly either favored the growth of Ph^1-negative cells or had selected against the initially dominant Ph^1-positive population.

We have now studied another 16 Ph^1-positive CML patients with the same experimental protocol. Nine of these were recently diagnosed and untreated at the time when their marrows were obtained for culture. The other seven had been previously treated for various periods (ranging from 5 months to 7 years). Twelve of the 16 have given the same result as our first experiment, i.e., a switch from an initially predominantly Ph^1-positive progenitor population that rapidly declined in long-term culture to a progenitor population that within 4 weeks was predominantly Ph^1-negative. In long-term cultures from three of the other four patients the Ph^1-positive progenitor population also underwent a precipitous decline, but Ph^1-negative progenitors did not become detectable. Presumably in these cases either there were no Ph^1-negative stem cells present initially or the cultures obtained from these marrow aspirates were inadequate to support the maintenance of even a normal hemopoietic population.

In one patient's long-term cultures Ph^1-positive progenitors did not rapidly disappear. Rather, they showed kinetics typical of their normal counterparts in control cultures [21]. This exceptional behavior was also associated with an unusually cellular adherent layer. Because of this finding and because of the results of another experiment which showed that only Ph^1-negative progenitors had adhered to the bottom of the culture at the end of the 1st week of incubation [21], we formulated the following hypothesis. It seemed that the typical failure of Ph^1-positive progenitors to be maintained might simply reflect the natural death of a population critically disadvantaged by a reduced or delayed ability to become part of the adherent layer during the initial development of the culture. To test this idea we added Ph^1-positive marrow or peripheral blood cells (the latter containing similar or larger numbers of primitive Ph^1-positive progenitors) to preestablished marrow adherent layers derived from normal marrow. These adherent feeders had been initiated with cells from a donor of the opposite sex and kept at 37 °C (rather than 33 °C) with complete removal of all nonadherent cells after 3, 7, and 14 days to reduce the hemopoietic progenitor content to undetectable levels (as shown by assays of replicate adherent layers) at the time when CML cells were added. Following the addition of the Ph^1-positive CML cells, these cultures with and without feeders were handled in the usual way. Although only a limited number of such experiments have been completed, thus far the number of hemopoietic progenitors found in the cultures initiated on preestablished feeders has been consistently higher than the number measured in the matching control cultures without feeders, regardless of the genotype of the progenitors present. However, overall this enhancing effect has appeared to be more pronounced on the Ph^1-positive population with one exception, where the Ph^1-negative cells still became dominant. In spite of the preliminary nature of these findings, they clearly indicate that the numbers of both Ph[1]-positive and Ph[1]-negative progenitors maintained in the long-term culture system can be enhanced. Whether such manipulations will be useful for analyzing factors that favor the selective growth of one genotype over the other still remains to be determined.

Finally, we have also recently addressed the question of whether the Ph[1]-negative progenitors usually detectable in 4-week-old long-term CML marrow cultures are neoplastic (i.e., members of the neoplastic clone). This was tested by examining the karyotype of progenitors obtained from long-term marrow cultures established from a patient with a fertile mosaic Turner syndrome and whose Ph[1]-positive CML clone was known to have arisen in the minor (10%) 45,X lineage [5]. All colonies analyzed from this patient's 4- to 6-week-old adherent layer assays were found to be 46,XX; i.e., they were both Ph[1]-negative and nonclonal [22].

D. Long-Term AML Marrow Cultures

Our initial observations with long-term CML marrow cultures prompted us to examine other hemopoietic malignancies to establish whether failure of neoplastic progenitor maintenance might prove to be a phenomenon of more general significance. Marrow cells from 13 newly diagnosed AML patients have been used to initiate long-term cultures and the progenitors in these cultures evaluated for 6–8 weeks. The majority showed a rapid disappearance of progenitors of abnormal (blast) colony- and cluster-forming cells to undetectable levels within 4 weeks in both nonadherent and adherent fractions. Concomitantly hemopoietic progenitors capable of producing large granulocyte colonies became readily detectable, typically for the first time. Similarly primitive erythroid progenitors frequently attained higher levels than those anticipated simply from the numbers of this type of progenitor initially detectable. In two cases cytogenetic studies were also undertaken. These confirmed that the progenitors of phenotypically normal colonies detected after 4–6 weeks were cytogenetically normal and not members of the initially prevalent chromosomally abnormal population.

As found for the long-term CML marrow cultures, this was the predominant, although not exclusive, pattern exhibited by the progenitor populations present in long-term AML marrow cultures. In fact, the maintenance of abnormal (blast) colony- and cluster-forming cells was consistently observed for 6–8 weeks in two of the AML experiments. In both of these and the other two experiments, progenitors of normal granulocyte colonies were not detectable, and only the occasional erythroid progenitor was found.

E. Conclusion

The most striking finding from these studies is the apparent incompatibility of leukemic cell growth and normal hemopoiesis both in vivo and in the long-term marrow culture system. Particularly noteworthy is the rapidity with which normal hemopoietic progenitors often become detectable as the leukemic cells and their precursors disappear. This suggests that terminal maturation may be more sensitive to the suppressive effects of a large neoplastic cell population than is the maintenance of more primitive normal hemopoietic progenitor cell types. However, preliminary evidence that the long-term culture system may be manipulated to alter favorably the ability of neoplastic cells to be maintained is also of considerable importance, since it should then be possible to delineate those factors that promote or alternatively diminish clonal dominance in vivo.

Acknowledgments. This work was supported in part by the National Cancer Institute of Canada, the British Columbia Health Care and Research Foundation, and the Ligue Nationale Contre le Cancer, France, with core support from the Cancer Control Agency of British Columbia and the British Columbia Cancer Foundation. C. Eaves is a Research Associate of the National Cancer Institute of Canada and I. Dubé was a recipient of a National Cancer Institute of Canada Studentship.

References

1. Fauser AA, Messner HA (1978) Granuloerythropoietic colonies in human bone marrow, peripheral blood, and cord blood. Blood 52:1243–1248
2. Senn JS, McCulloch EA, Till JE (1967) Comparison of colony-forming ability of normal and leukemic human marrow in cell culture. Lancet II:597–598
3. Eaves CJ, Eaves AC (1977) Human marrow cells capable of erythropoietic differentiation in vitro: definition of three erythroid colony responses. Blood 49:855–864
4. Messner HA, Jamal N, Izaguirre C (1982) The growth of large megakaryocyte colonies from human bone marrow. J Cell Physiol [Suppl 1]:45–51
5. Fialkow PJ (1982) Cell lineages in hematopoietic neoplasia studied with glucose-6-phosphate dehydrogenase cell markers. J Cell Physiol [Suppl 1]:37–43
6. Chaganti RSK, Bailey RB, Jhanwar SC, Arlin ZA, Clarkson BD (1982) Chronic myelogenous leukemia in the monosomic cell line of a fertile Turner syndrome mosaic. Cancer Genet Cytogenet 5:215–221
7. Prchal JF, Adamson JW (1978) Polycythemia vera – the in vitro response of normal and abnormal stem cell lines to erythropoietin. J Clin Invest 61:1044–1047
8. Dubé ID, Gupta CM, Kalousek DK, Eaves CJ, Eaves AC (1984) Cytogenetic studies of early myeloid progenitor compartments in Ph[1]-positive chronic myeloid leukaemia (CML). Br J Haematol 56:633–644
9. Dexter TM, Spooncer E, Toksoz D, Lajtha LG (1980) The role of cells and their products in the regulation of in vitro stem cell proliferation and granulocyte development. J Supramol Struct 13:513–524
10. Gartner S, Kaplan HS (1980) Long-term culture of human bone marrow cells. Proc Natl Acad Sci USA 77:4756–4759
11. Greenberg HM, Newburger PE, Parker LM, Novak T, Greenberger JS (1981) Human granulocytes generated in continuous bone marrow culture are physiologically normal. Blood 58:724–732
12. Coulombel L, Eaves AC, Eaves CJ (1983) Enzymatic treatment of long-term human marrow cultures reveals the preferential location of primitive hemopoietic progenitors in the adherent layer. Blood 62:291–297
13. Coulombel L, Eaves CJ, Dubé ID, Kalousek DK, Eaves AC (1984) Variable persistence of leukemic progenitor cells in long-term CML and AML marrow cultures. In: Wright DG, Greenberger JS (eds) Longterm bone marrow culture. Liss, New York, pp 243–254
14. Mauch P, Greenberger JS, Botnick L, Hannon E, Hellman S (1980) Evidence for structured variation in self-renewal capacity within long-term bone marrow cultures. Proc Natl Acad Sci USA 77:2927–2930
15. Eaves C, Coulombel L, Eaves A (1983) Analysis of hemopoiesis in long-term human marrow cultures. In: Killmann S-A, Cronkite EP, Muller-Berat CN (eds) Haemopoietic Stem Cells. Munksgaard, Copenhagen, pp 287–302
16. Becker AJ, McCulloch EA, Siminovitch L, Till JE (1965) The effect of differing demands for blood cell production on DNA synthesis by hemopoietic colony-forming cells of mice. Blood 26:296–308
17. Eaves CJ, Humphries RK, Eaves AC (1979) In vitro characterization of erythroid precursor cells and the erythropoietic differentiation process. In: Stamatoyannopoulos G, Nienhuis AW (eds) Cellular and molecular regulation of hemoglobin switching. Grune and Stratton, New York, pp 251–278
18. Fauser AA, Messner HA (1979) Proliferative state of human pluripotent hemopoietic progenitors (CFU-GEMM) in normal individuals and under regenerative conditions after bone marrow transplantation. Blood 54:1197–1200
19. Morardet N, Parmentier C (1977) Description of a suicide technique in vitro for granulocytic stem cells (CFU_c) by hydroxyurea on normal human bone marrow. Biomedicine 27:349–353
20. Coulombel L, Kalousek DK, Eaves CJ, Gupta CM, Eaves AC (1983) Long-term marrow culture reveals chromosomally normal hematopoietic progenitor cells in patients with Philadelphia chromosome-positive chronic myelogenous leukemia. N Engl J Med 308: 1493–1498
21. Dubé ID, Kalousek DK, Coulombel L, Gupta CM, Eaves CJ, Eaves AC (1984a) Cytogenetic studies of early myeloid progenitor compartments in Ph[1]-positive chronic myeloid leukemia. II. Long-term culture reveals the persistence of Ph[1]-negative progenitors in treated as well as newly diagnosed patients. Blood 63:1172–1177
22. Dubé ID, Arlin ZA, Kalousek DK, Eaves CJ, Eaves AC (1984b) Nonclonal hemopoietic progenitor cells detected in long-term marrow cultures from a Turner syndrome mosaic with chronic myeloid leukemia. Blood 64: 1284–1287

Haematology and Blood Transfusion Vol. 29
Modern Trends in Human Leukemia VI
Edited by Neth, Gallo, Greaves, Janka

Stromal Progenitor Cells in Bone Marrow of Patients with Aplastic Anemia *

E. Elstner, E. Schulze, R. Ihle, H. Stobbe, and S. Grunze

A. Introduction

The pathogenesis of aplastic anemia (AA), which is defined by pancytopenia and hypocellularity of the bone marrow (BM), is still an unsolved problem and is most probably heterogeneous. Hemopoietic stromal defects have been suggested as one of the possible pathophysiologic mechanisms for AA. Up to now, in all investigations on stromal cells of patients with AA, the fibroblast colony assay (CFU-F) has been used [4, 12, 13]. Fibroblasts, however, are only one component of the hemopoietic stroma; they are not capable of maintaining hemopoiesis in vitro alone.

For our study we used the Dexter culture [1] modified for human BM [3], because in this system a complex adherent cell layer develops after 2 weeks, containing, in addition to fibroblasts, other stromal elements (macrophages, adipocytes, endothelial cells) and which is known to maintain hemopoiesis in this system for several weeks. The aim of these investigations was to find out if there are differences in the ability to form stromal elements between normal and AA BM cells in vitro.

B. Material and Methods

BM of nine normal volunteers and six patients with idiopathically acquired AA (Table 1) were investigated in a liquid system [3] with slight modifications (Fig. 1). The BM cells were obtained by iliac crest puncture (2 ml) and immediately diluted with the same volume of McCoy's 5A medium (Serva) containing heparin without preservative (Gedeon Richter, Hungary). After spontaneous sedimentation of erythrocytes, the supernatant, including the fat droplets floating on the surface (the lipid substance can be utilized as a source of energy in rapidly proliferating cell systems) [11], was added to the culture medium (McCoy's 5A supplemented with 10% fetal calf serum, SIFIN, GDR) and 10% horse serum (Flow, Manchester) in order to get a cell concentration of 5×10^5 cells per milliliter suspension. The cells were cultivated in Petri dishes at 37 °C in 7.5% CO_2 for 14 days without feeding. After 14 days, the liquid fraction was removed. The air-dried adherent layer was stained according to Pappenheim. GM-CFC of 18 AA patients was performed in a double-layer culture (Pike and Robinson) [10].

Table 1. Criteria for diagnosis of aplastic anemia

Aplastic anemia is defined by:
Pancytopenia
Hypocellularity of the hemopoietic bone marrow, with absence of neoplastic infiltration or significant fibrosis

It is distinct from:
Aplasia induced by cytostatics or irradiation
Primary pancytopenia with hyperplastic marrow or myelodysplasia

* University Hospital (Charité), Department of Internal Medicine, Division of Hematology, Berlin, GDR, and Central Institute of Molecular Biology of the Academy of Sciences of the GDR, Berlin, GDR

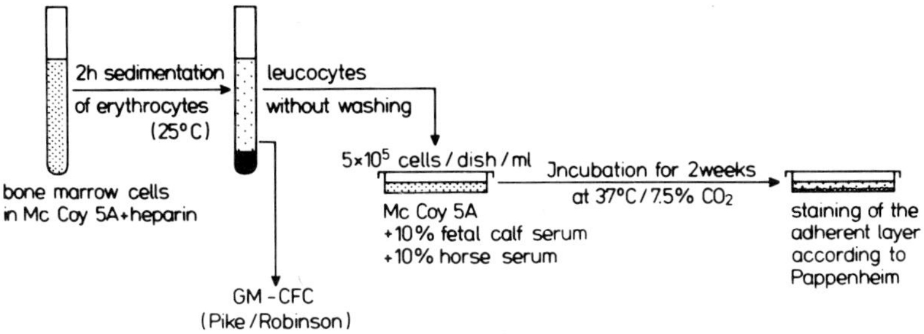

Fig. 1. Schematic representation of the method

C. Results

Figure 2 shows the growth pattern of GM-CFC of BM from patients with AA in agar culture. The number of colonies (> 40 cells) was decreased in most cases. The results of the stromal cultures are represented in Fig. 3. After 1 week of cultivation, there was a very poor adherent layer in both normal and aplastic BM cultures, and no difference between them could be detected. After 14 days, however, an adherent layer was established, which was distinctly more compact in the BM cultures of normal subjects compared with those of patients with AA (Figs. 4, 5). In addition to these quantitative differences, qualitative differences were also apparent. Thus, in normal BM cultures well-established "cobblestone" areas were formed (Fig. 4). In cultures of AA BM, such areas were rare.

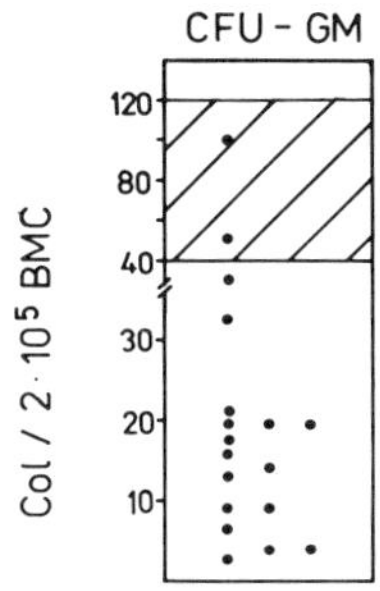

Fig. 2. Growth pattern of bone marrow from patients with aplastic anemia in agar culture (*hatched area* shows range of 20 normal volunteers)

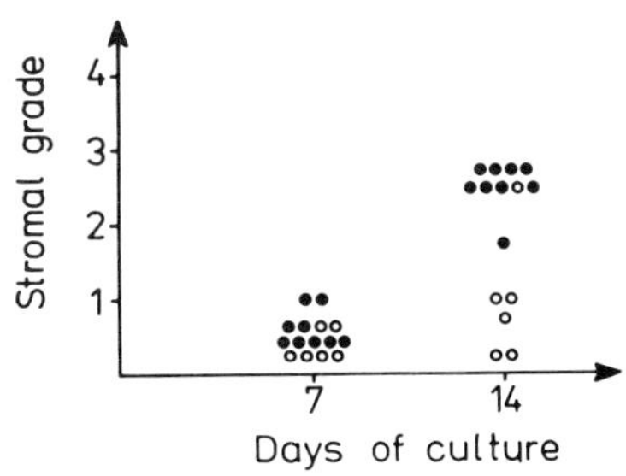

Fig. 3. Stromal layer in liquid culture from bone marrow cells. *Full circles* normal volunteers; *open circles* patients with aplastic anemia. Each dish was assigned a score from 1 to 4, corresponding to a stromal layer covering from 25% to 100% of the area of the culture dish

D. Discussion

The pancytopenia and hypocellularity of the hemopoietic BM in AA patients is the final outcome of functional failure in the hemopoietic stem cells (HSC). In most AA patients, the number of GM-CFC, BFU-E, CFU-E, CFU-D, and CFU-mix is decreased [2, 5, 7, 9]. For effective hemopoiesis it is essential to have an intact microenvironment (stroma cells), on which HSC renew and differentiate. Therefore, the failure of the HSC in AA can also be caused secondarily by damage of the stromal cells, as was shown in experimentally induced aplasia in animals [6, 8]. The pathogenetic role of stromal cells in the development of AA in vitro has been investigated up to now only with CFU-F assay, which gives evidence for only one component of stromal cells, i.e. fibroblasts, and no information about the interplay of stromal cells and HSC. For our investi-

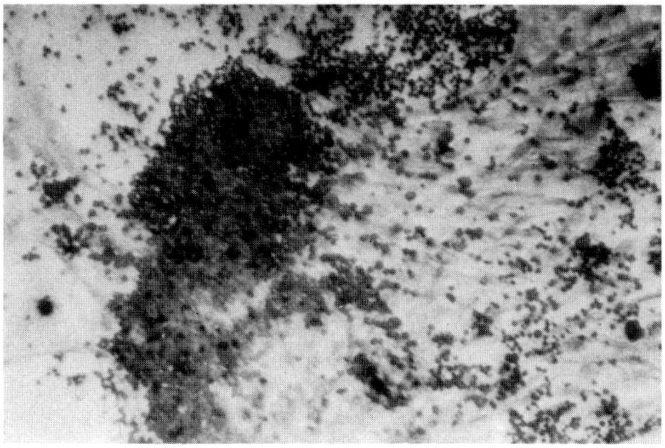

Fig. 4. Pappenheim-stained adherent layer with hemopoietic islands formed by normal bone marrow after 14 days cultivation (×32)

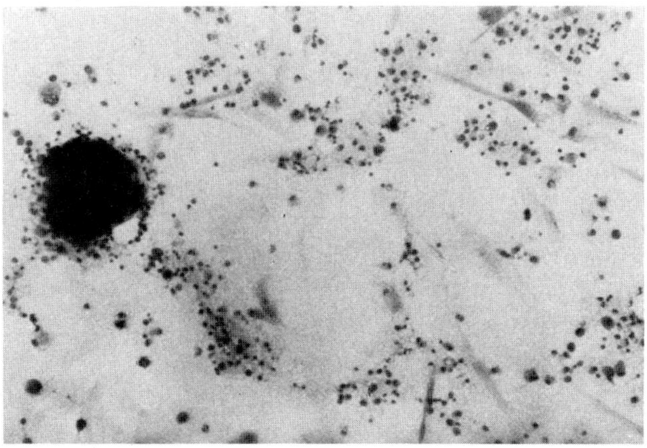

Fig. 5. Pappenheim-stained adherent layer formed by aplastic anemia bone marrow after 14 days cultivation (×32)

gations we have used the Dexter culture [3] which allows study of the interaction between the complex stroma and hemopoiesis.

Our findings indicate that in AA not only is hemopoiesis insufficient, but the stromal cells are affected also. It is not clear whether these two phenomena are independent of each other, or if the decreased number of HSC is caused by a disturbed microenvironment. Since for our experiments we used unwashed cells, including the patients' sera, autoimmunologic processes (humoral and cellular) cannot be excluded.

References

1. Dexter TM, Allen TD, Lajtha LG (1977) Conditions controlling the proliferation of haemopoietic stem cells in vitro. J Cell Physiol 91:335–344
2. Elstner E, Schulze E, Ihle R, Schütt M, Stobbe H (1983) Proliferation and maturation of hemopoietic cells from patients with preleukemia and aplastic anemia in agar and diffusion chamber cultures. In: Neth, Gallo, Greves, Moore, Winkler (eds) Haematology and blood transfusion, vol 28, Modern trends of human leukemia V. Springer, Berlin Heidelberg, pp 358–361
3. Gartner S, Kaplan HS (1980) Long-term culture of human bone marrow cells. Proc Natl Acad Sci USA 77:4756–4759
4. Gordon MY, Gordon-Smith EC (1981) Bone marrow fibroblastoid colony-forming cells (P-CFC) in aplastic anaemia: colony growth and stimulation of granulocyte-macrophage colony-forming cells (GM-CFC). Br J Haematol 49:465–477
5. Hara H, Kai S, Fushimi M, Taniwaki S, Okomoto T, Ohe Y, Fujita S, Noguchi K,

Senba M, Hamane M, Kanamaru A, Nagai K (1980) Pluripotent hemopoietic precursors in vitro (CFU_{mix}) in aplastic anemia. Exp Hematol 8:1165–1171
6. Hays E, Hale L, Villarreal B, Fitchen JM (1982) "Stromal" and hemopoietic stem cell abnormalities in long-term cultures of marrow from busulfan-treated mice. Exp Hematol 10:383–392
7. Heimpel H, Heit W (1983) Panmyelophthisis and other bone marrow disorders. Verh Dtsch Ges Pathol 67:276–285
8. Knospe WH, Blom J, Crosby WH (1968) Regeneration of locally irradiated bone marrow I. Dose dependent long-term changes in the rat with particular emphasis upon vascular and stromal reactions. Blood 28:398
9. Kurnick JE, Robinson WA, Dickey CA (1971) In vitro granulocytic colony forming potential of bone marrow from patients with granulocytopenia and aplastic anemia. Proc Soc Exp Biol Med 137:917–920
10. Pike BL, Robinson WA (1970) Human bone marrow colony growth in agar-gel. J Cell Physiol 76:77–84
11. Tavassoli M (1984) Marrow adipose cells and hemopoiesis: an interpretative review. Exp Hematol 12:139–146
12. Wiktor-Jedrzejczak W, Siekierzynski M, Szczylik C, Gornas P, Dryjanski T (1982) Aplastic anemia with marrow defective information of fibroblastoid cell colonies in vitro. Scand J Haematol 28:82–90
13. Zaritsky AY, Kulik MA, Kazhdan IJ, Lisovskaya VA, Ivasenko IN, Arkadyeva GE (1983) Colony-forming capacity of fibroblast precursor cells of the bone marrow in patients with different neutropenic conditions. Ter Arkh 8:110–114

Haematology and Blood Transfusion Vol. 29
Modern Trends in Human Leukemia VI
Edited by Neth, Gallo, Greaves, Janka

Dyserythropoiesis in Acute Lymphoblastic Leukemia of Childhood*

O. Hrodek, I. Stará, and J. Šrajer

A. Introduction

The purpose of this study was to review bone marrow appearances of erythroid cells in children with acute lymphoblastic leukemia (ALL) in order to assess the extent of dyserythropoiesis at two phases of disease: at diagnosis and after multidrug induction treatment at the beginning of complete remission.

B. Materials and Methods

A total of 15 morphological abnormalities characteristic of dyserythropoiesis were evaluated in bone marrow smears stained with May-Grünwald–Giemsa stain. Abnormalities were classified as: (a) anomalies of the nucleus (binuclearity, multinuclearity, nuclear lobulation, budding, fragmentation, chromatin lumping and pyknosis, intranuclear bridging, extrusion of the nucleus); and (b) anomalies of the cytoplasm (cytoplasmic connections, basophilic stippling, Howell–Jolly bodies, atypical mitotic figures, asynchrony of nuclear cytoplasmic maturation, megaloblastic changes).

A group of 23 children with ALL of different immunologic subtypes were investigated at diagnosis and after successful induction of first complete remission. According to multidrug induction regimen two groups of patients were compared: 8 patients with a two- or three-drug regimen (2 children with prednisone and vincristine, 6 children with prednisone, vincristine, and rubidomycin), and 15 patients with a four- or five-drug regimen (prednisone, vincristine, rubidomycin or adriamycin, plus cytosine arabinoside, L-asparaginase, or cyclophosphamide). The mean frequency of all anomalies per 100 erythroid cells and the absolute frequency of the individual anomalies (number of signs observed in all cases) were statistically tested. A logarithmic normal distribution of data was found and, therefore, a logarithmic transformation was used in comparison of means.

C. Results

The percentage of erythroblasts in the bone marrow at diagnosis was greatly reduced (Fig. 1). The mean of all cases investigated was 3.1% and reflected a quantitative decrease of erythropoiesis. After complete remission, it was significantly increased to 26% ($P < 0.01$). The mean frequency of dyserythropoietic signs per 100 erythroblasts was 12.5 at diagnosis and 60.9 at the beginning of complete remission ($P < 0.01$).

The most significant increase ($P < 0.001$) was found in megaloblastosis (from 89 to 524), then in cytoplasmic connections (from 15 to 144) and in basophilic stippling (from 39 to 195). Other significant increases ($P < 0.01$) occurred in Howell–Jolly bodies, asynchrony of nuclear cytoplasmic maturation, blurred structures of nucleus,

* 2nd Dept. of Paediatrics, Charles University, Prague, Czechoslovakia

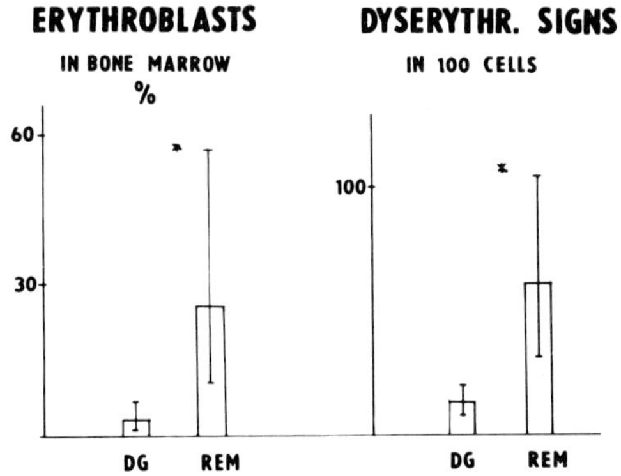

Fig. 1. Proportion of erythroblasts and frequency of dyserythropoietic signs in the bone marrow at diagnosis (DG) and after achieving complete remission (REM)

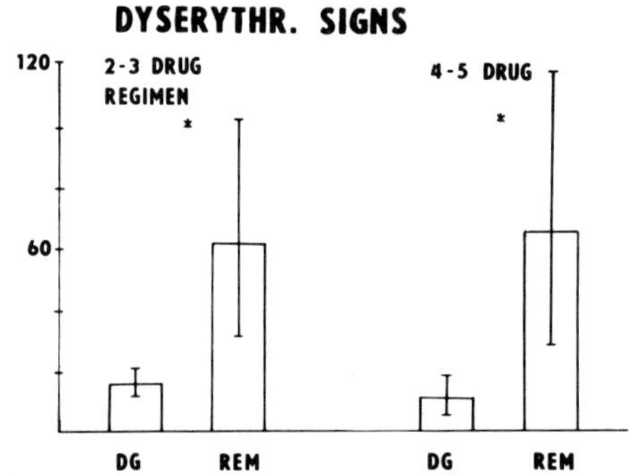

Fig. 2. Frequency of dyserythropoietic signs in the bone marrow at diagnosis (DG) and after achieving complete remission (REM) with less intensive and more intensive induction therapy

binuclearity, nuclear lobulation, budding, fragmentation, and chromatin lumping or pyknosis. The increase of all remaining abnormalities, such as multinuclearity, nuclear bridges, premature extrusion of nucleus, and atypical mitotic figures, was less significant ($P < 0.05$).

Dyserythropoietic changes in 8 children with less intensive induction therapy (two- or three-drug regimen) were compared with 15 children with more intensive regimens (four- or five-drug regimen). The mean frequency of abnormalities at diagnosis and the increase at the beginning of complete remission were the same (Fig. 2). There was no significant difference between the two groups investigated.

D. Discussion and Conclusions

The present study has shown the extent to which morphological abnormalities in erythroid cells occur as part of hematologic pattern in ALL and as a consequence of multidrug induction chemotherapy. Many of the morphological manifestations occur as a result of disturbances of mechanisms which regulate the cell cycle and normal mitosis, normal hemoglobin synthesis, and other protein synthesis. Other manifestations are probably degenerative or due to increased cell fragility. From the static pictures of cells as seen in marrow aspirates, however, it is difficult to deduce dynamic processes involved in the abnormal, functionally inefficient erythropoiesis. More complex studies are necessary to elucidate the connections between morphological and functional defects of erythroid marrow cells and their clinical significance in children with ALL. The effect of more or less aggressive drug regimens can be established after collecting data from larger series of patients treated with the same protocol.

Haematology and Blood Transfusion Vol. 29
Modern Trends in Human Leukemia VI
Edited by Neth, Gallo, Greaves, Janka

Ultrastructural Analysis of Normal and Leukaemic Cells by the Immunogold Method and Monoclonal Antibodies *

E. Matutes and D. Catovsky

A. Introduction

Morphological and membrane marker analysis of the leukaemic cells are useful for the diagnosis and classification of human leukaemias. A combination of immunological and electron microscope (EM) techniques can now be carried out by using electron-dense tracers such as colloidal gold particles to visualise the reaction with a monoclonal antibody (MoAb)–immunogold method (IGM) [1]. Application of this technique has allowed the characterisation of distinct T lymphocyte subpopulations in normal blood [2, 3]. In this study we analyse by this method the expression of various lineage-specific membrane antigens in normal haemopoietic precursor cells and in blast cells from patients with acute leukaemia and blast crisis from chronic granulocytic leukaemia (CGL) and myelofibrosis (MF) to see if a more precise characterisation of the immature cells can be made.

B. Materials and Methods

Peripheral blood and bone marrow samples from healthy donors and 16 leukaemic patients: 9 acute leukaemias and 7 blast crisis from CGL [3] and MF [4] were studied. Mononuclear cells were isolated by centrifugation on Lymphoprep (Nyegaard) and washed twice in phosphate-buffered saline (PBS).

I. Monoclonal Antibodies

The following MoAb were used: LICR LON/R10 (anti-glycophorin A) against erythroid precursors [4]; AN51, C15, C17 and J15 against platelet glycoproteins Ib, IIIa and the complex IIb/IIIa [5, 6, 7]; My9 against myeloid precursors [8]; J5, anti-cALL antigen, to identify lymphoblasts [9] and 3C5 against myeloid and lymphoid precursors [10].

II. Immunogold Staining

A 200-μl (5×10^6 cells) volume was resuspended in PBS, 1% bovine serum albumin (BSA), 0.2% sodium azide. 2% human AB serum (pH 7.4) and incubated with the relevant MoAb for 30 min at room temperature (RT). Cells were washed twice and incubated for 1 h at RT with 40 μl goat anti-mouse IgG conjugated to 30-nm colloidal gold particles (Janssen Life Sciences, Beerse, Belgium). After three washes, samples were processed for EM analysis following standard techniques. Controls were carried out by omitting the first layer MoAb or by using an irrelevant anti-mouse immunoglobulin. In several instances the following cytochemical reactions: myeloperoxidase (MPO), acid phosphatase (AP) and platelet peroxidase (PPO) were performed.

* MRC Leukaemia Unit, Royal Postgraduate Medical School, London W12 OHS, England

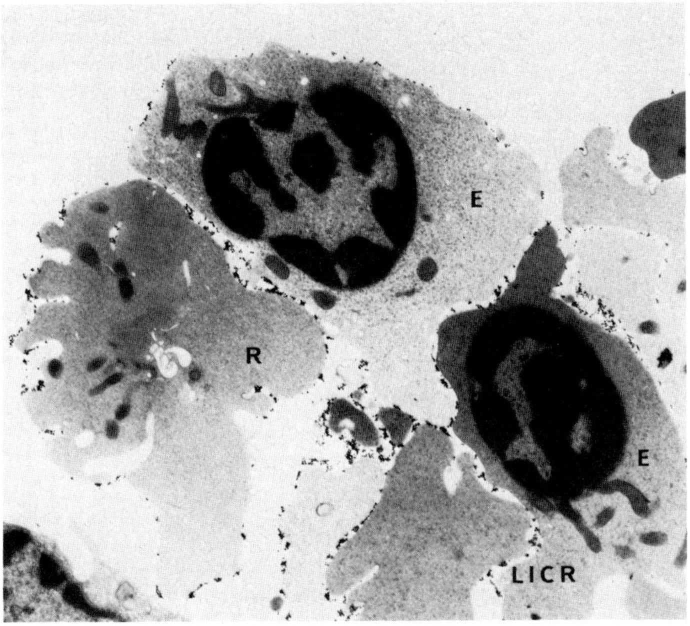

Fig. 1. Normal bone marrow erythroblasts (E) reactive with LICR anti-glycophorin A and heavily labelled with colloidal gold particles. Note the presence of a reactive reticulocyte (R) (uranyl acetate and lead citrate stain, × 16 000)

C. Results

I. Erythroid

A proportion of cells (22% and 23%) from two patients (one with erythroid blast crisis of CGL and one with erythroleukaemia) were seen gold labelled with LICR anti-glycophorin A. According to the morphological features, various stages of cell differentiation were identified in the reactive cells. Undifferentiated blasts were seen together with more mature cells which had specific features (e.g. siderosomes) of the erythroid lineage. AP activity when present, was localised in large lysosomal granules and/or endoplasmic reticulum (ER) in both immature and mature erythroid cells. In normal bone marrow, the expression of LICR was demonstrated from proerythroblasts to reticulocytes and red blood cells (Fig. 1)[1]. The degree of reactivity as judged by the number of gold particles in the cell membrane increased with cell maturation, both in normal and leukaemic samples.

1 In Figs. 1–6, unless otherwise stated, 30-nm colloidal gold particles conjugated to goat anti-mouse IgG were used

II. Megakaryocytic

Reactivity with the various anti-platelet MoAb was seen in cells from patients with CGL and MF in megakaryoblastic transformation. Blast cells having a "lymphoid" appearance (Fig. 2) in addition to cells with features of megakaryocytic differentiation (e.g. α-granules) and giant platelets were identified by the gold labelling with the several MoAb used. In the differentiated cells, gold particles were distributed on the cell membrane and in the open canalicular system. The number of antigenic sites differed from one case to another, but a stronger staining was more frequently seen in the more mature cells and platelets.

III. Myeloid

Myeloblasts from four cases of acute leukaemia (three acute myeloid leukaemia and one mixed leukaemia–lymphoid and myeloid) displayed a different pattern of reactivity with the MoAb 3C5 and My9 when studied in combination with the MPO reaction. Myeloblasts that were MPO negative or with little MPO activity showed strong reaction with 3C5 (Figs. 3 and 4)

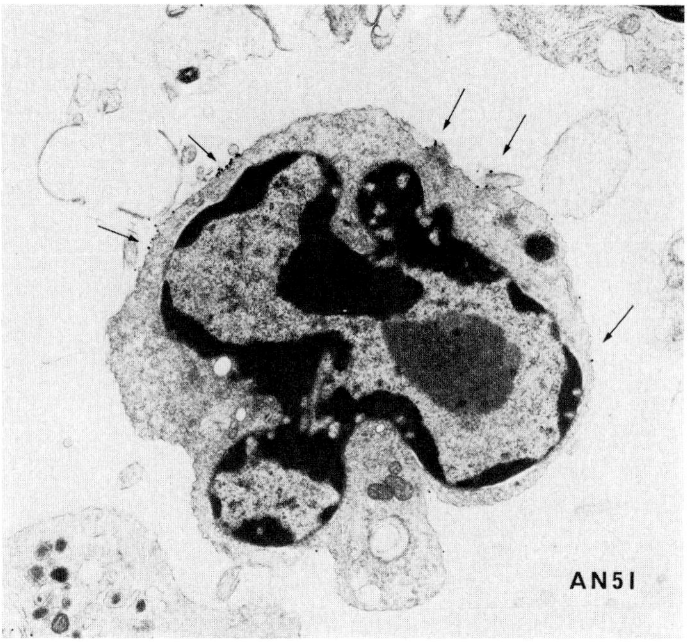

Fig. 2. AN51 gold-labelled (*arrows*) megakaryoblast from a patient with MF in megakaryoblastic transformation. The cell shows a "lymphoid" appearance without identifiable features of megakaryocytic differentiation (uranyl acetate and lead citrate stain, × 18 000)

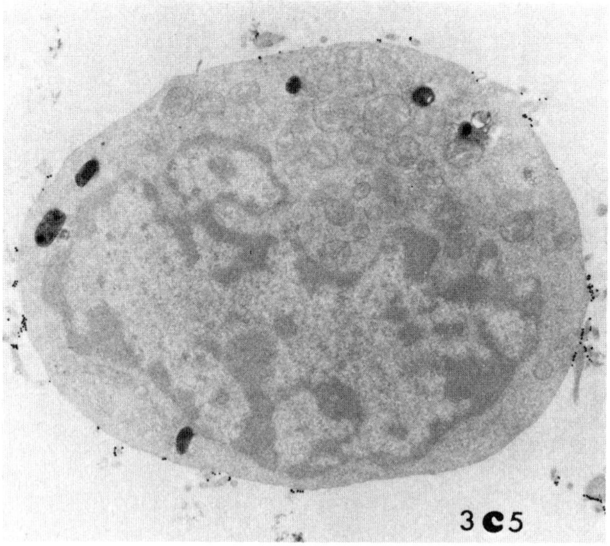

Fig. 3. 3C5 reactive blast from a patient with acute myeloid leukaemia, showing MPO activity localised in various granules (unstained section, × 16 000)

and were either My9 positive or My9 negative, whereas the reactivity with My9 increased in parallel to the MPO content of the cells. Promyelocytes and myelocytes were also seen labelled with My9. This pattern was also observed in normal bone marrow although the degree of reactivity was lower in normal cells when compared with the leukaemic cells.

IV. Lymphoid

Leukaemic cells from two patients with ALL and two CGL in lymphoid blast crisis

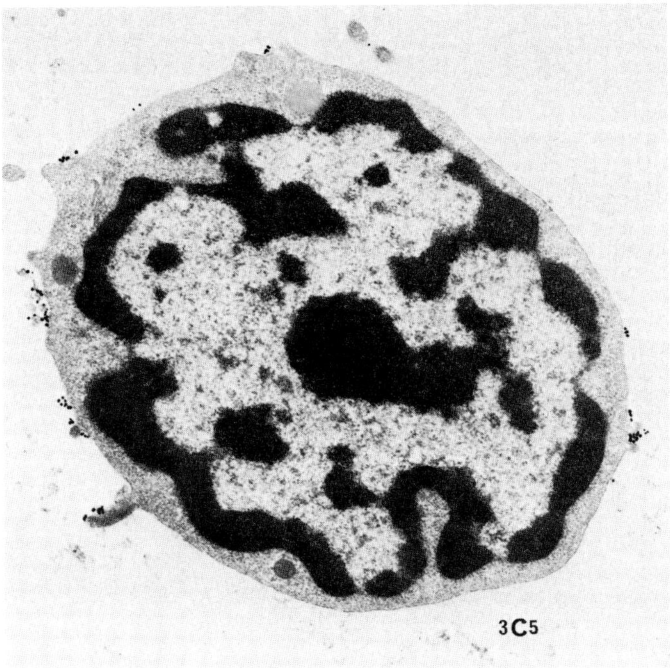

Fig. 4. 3C5-positive (gold labelled), MPO-negative blast from a patient with mixed acute leukaemia (My + Ly) showing a lymphoid morphology (uranyl acetate and lead citrate stain, × 18 000)

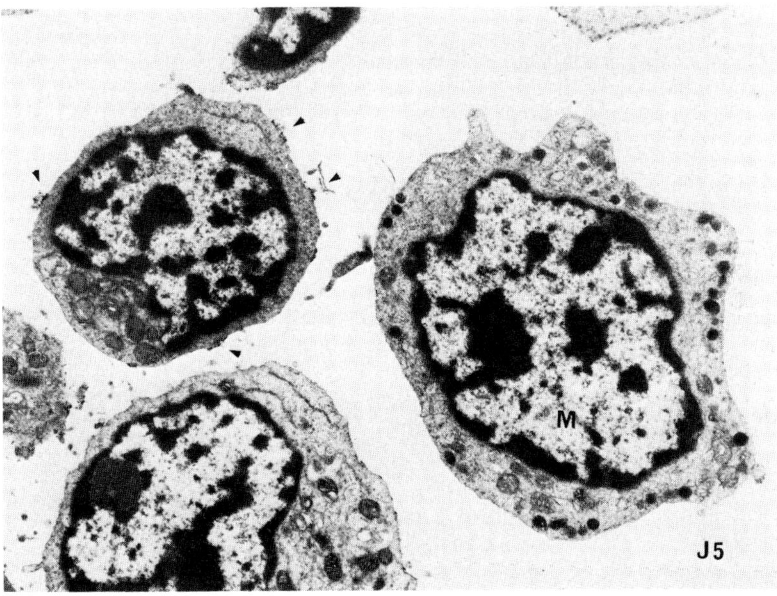

Fig. 5. J5-positive (labelled with 20-nm gold particles) (*arrows*) cell from a CGL-lymphoid blast crisis. Note the presence of a J5-negative (gold-unlabelled) myeloid cell (M) (uranyl acetate and lead citrate stain, × 10 200)

were J5 positive. The specificity of the labelling could be assessed in the latter disease in which the remaining myeloid cells from the chronic phase were clearly J5 negative (Fig. 5). In normal bone marrow, a minority of small cells having a high

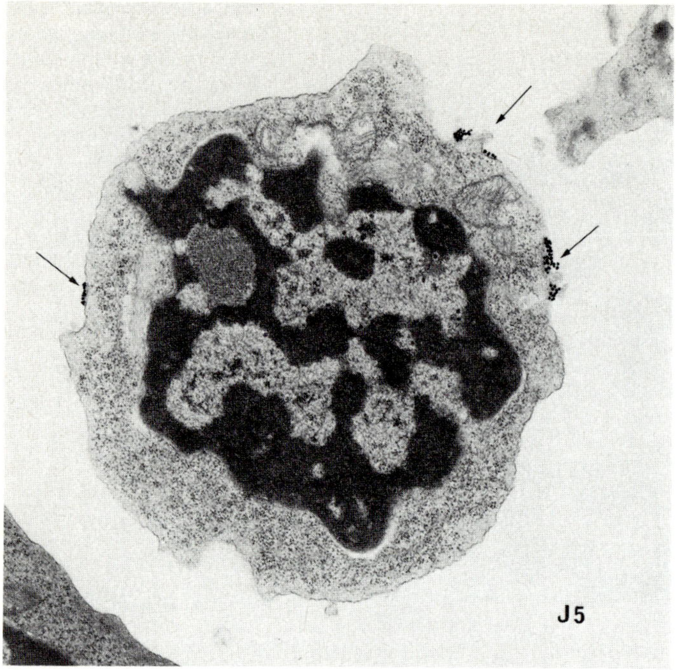

Fig. 6. Normal bone marrow cell reactive with J5 (*arrows*). A small nucleolus and abundant ribosomes in the cytoplasm can be seen (uranyl acetate and lead citrate stain, × 18 000)

nucleocytoplasmic ratio, a small nucleolus and scattered ribosomes in the cytoplasm were identified as gold labelled with the MoAb J5 (Fig. 6).

Acknowledgment: EM was supported by the Leukaemia Research Fund of Great Britain.

D. Conclusions

This study shows that the application of the IGM in the analysis of normal and leukaemic haemopoietic precursors is useful:

1. To establish the specificity of a particular MoAb.
2. To determine in single cells the presence of two specific markers of differentiation: immunological and ultrastructural and/or cytochemical.
3. To recognise the various stages of cell maturation present in some acute leukaemias on the basis of their membrane phenotype and enzyme activity.
4. To characterise the different cell populations that proliferate in mixed leukaemias.
5. To identify normal bone marrow lymphoid and megakaryocytic precursors which appear to have "lymphoid" ultrastructural morphology similar to that observed in their leukaemic counterparts.

References

1. De Mey J (1983) Colloidal gold probes in immunocytochemistry. In: Polak JM, Van Noorden S (eds) Immunocytochemistry: practical applications in pathology and biology. Wright, Bristol, pp 82–112
2. Matutes E, Catovsky D (1982) The fine structure of normal lymphocyte subpopulations – a study with monoclonal antibodies and the immunogold technique. Clin Exp Immunol 50:416–425
3. Matutes E, Robinson D, O'Brien M, Haynes BF, Zola H, Catovsky D (1983) Candidate counterparts of Sézary cells and adult T-cell lymphoma leukaemia cells in normal peripheral blood: an ultrastructural study with the immunogold method and monoclonal antibodies. Leuk Res 7:878–892
4. Edwards PAW (1980) Monoclonal antibodies that bind to the human erythrocyte membrane glycoproteins glycophorin A and band 3. Biochem Soc Trans 8:334
5. McMichael AJ, Rust NA, Pilch J, Sochynsky R, Morton J, Mason DY, Ruan C, Tabelem

G, Caen J (1981) Monoclonal antibody to human platelet glycoprotein I. I. Immunological studies. Br J Haematol 49:501–509
6. Tetteroo PA, Lansdorp PM, Leeksma OC, Kr von dem Borne AEG (1983) Monoclonal antibodies against human platelet glycoprotein IIIa. Br J Haematol 55:509–522
7. Vainchenker W, Deschamps, J, Bastin J, Guichard J, Titeux M, Breton-Gorius J, McMichael A (1982) Two monoclonal antibodies as markers of human megakaryocyte maturation. Immunofluorescent staining and platelet peroxidase detection in megakaryocyte colonies and in vivo cells from normal and leukaemic patients. Blood 59:514–521
8. Griffin JD (1984) Expression of myeloid differentiation antigens in acute myeloblastic leukaemia. In: Bernard A, Boumsell L, Dausset J, Milstein C, Schlossman SF (eds) Leucocyte typing. Human leucocyte differentiation antigens detected by monoclonal antibodies. Springer, Berlin Heidelberg New York
9. Ritz J, Pesando J, Notis-McConarty J, Lazarus H, Schlossman SF (1980) A monoclonal antibody to human lymphoblastic leukaemic antigen. Nature 283:583–585
10. Tindle RW, Nichols RAB, Chan LC, Campana D, Catousky D, Birnie GD (1985) A novel monoclonal antibody BI-3C5 recognises myeloblasts and non-B non-T lymphoblasts in acute leukaemias and CGL blast crises and reacts with immature cells in normal bone marrow. Leuk Res (in press)

Haematology and Blood Transfusion Vol. 29
Modern Trends in Human Leukemia VI
Edited by Neth, Gallo, Greaves, Janka

Immunocytochemical Labelling of Haematological Samples Using Monoclonal Antibodies *

W. N. Erber, A. K. Ghosh, and D. Y. Mason

A. Introduction

Monoclonal antibodies have become increasingly important in the diagnosis and classification of neoplastic blood disorders. Immunofluorescent labelling of cell surface antigens has been the conventional method used for this purpose. However, this method of antigen detection presents a number of drawbacks when used in a routine hospital haematology laboratory: namely that blood or bone marrow samples must be processed within a short time of collection; antigen labelling is not permanent; and cell morphology cannot be visualised.

The present paper describes the method for labelling routine haematological samples by an immunoalkaline phosphatase technique which is used routinely in this laboratory for leukaemia phenotyping. This approach has several practical advantages over conventional immunofluorescent labelling, i.e. staining can be performed on routinely prepared bone marrow and blood smears, samples can be stored for long periods before labelling, cell morphology can be visualised simultaneously with the antigen label and the staining reaction is permanent. As detailed below a wide range of cellular antigens can be detected in marrow and blood smears using this technique.

* University of Oxford, Department of Haematology, John Radcliffe Hospital, Oxford OX3 9DU, UK

B. Methods

Immunoalkaline Phosphatase Labelling

Antigen labelling is performed by the APAAP immunoalkaline phosphatase technique as described elsewhere [1, 2]. The method (shown schematically in Fig. 1) involves primary incubation of blood or bone marrow samples with monoclonal antibody, followed by unlabelled sheep anti-mouse Ig and then monoclonal alkaline phosphatase : anti-alkaline phosphatase (APAAP) complexes. Each incubation step lasts 30 min and is followed by a brief wash in Tris-buffered saline (for 1–5 min). Amplification of the staining is possible by repeating the anti-mouse Ig and APAAP stages (for 10 min each). The alkaline phosphatase reaction is then developed (by incubation for 15 min) in a naphthol-AS-MX/fast red substrate. Slides are washed, counterstained with haematoxylin and mounted in an aqueous medium.

C. Results

Staining of blood and marrow smears using the APAAP technique yields a vivid red reaction on antigen-positive cells. The staining reaction contrasts clearly with the haematoxylin counterstain and there is no background staining of antigen-negative cells. The labelling reactions are equally strong whether they are performed on freshly prepared smears or on smears that have been stored at – 20 °C. The nature of

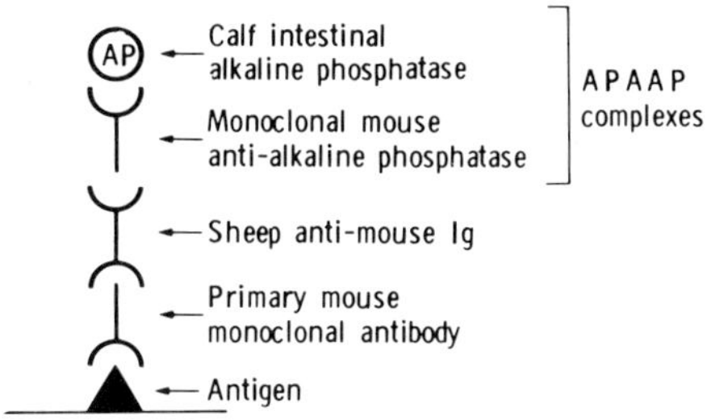

Fig. 1. Schematic representation of the APAAP immunoalkaline phosphatase procedure

the labelled cells can easily be determined because of the preservation of morphological detail.

D. Discussion

Cytological examination of peripheral blood and bone marrow plays a major role in the diagnosis of neoplastic blood disorders. The introduction of monoclonal antibodies in the late 1970s greatly aided the objective identification of cell types. Cellular antigens are conventionally detected by immunofluorescent staining of cells in suspension, however, this method does not enable antigen labelling and cell morphology to be visualised simultaneously.

Immunoalkaline phosphatase labelling of cell smears combines labelling of cellular antigens with visualisation of morphological detail. Preliminary mononuclear-cell separation and washing is unnecessary as staining can be performed on routinely prepared blood and bone marrow smears. Background labelling of the smears (as occurs with peroxidase labelling) is avoided, and the intense red reaction product is easy to visualise. Blood and marrow smears can be stored for long periods (at $-20\,°C$) prior to labelling. This enables samples to be analysed in batches and also facilitates retrospective analysis of stored cases (e.g. when it is necessary to test a new monoclonal antibody against a panel of different leukaemia cases). Smears sent by post from other hospitals also give staining reactions identical to those of samples processed fresh in this laboratory. Finally, the labelling reaction is permanent, allowing slides to be reviewed after a period of time.

Using these labelling procedures a wide range of cellular antigens, both surface and intracellular, can be detected (as noted in Table 1) in routinely prepared blood and bone marrow smears. APAAP labelling may thus be used to enumerate lymphocyte populations in peripheral blood smears and to detect abnormal T-helper/suppressor ratios [3]. This lends itself to mass screening, e.g. of blood donors. The technique is also very convenient for phenotyping cases of leukaemia and lymphoma. The markers used for this purpose include terminal transferase, HLA-DR, B- and T-cell antigens, and common ALL antigen.

Finally, the APAAP procedure is valuable for detecting metastatic malignant cells in bone marrow smears, since malignant cells can often be demonstrated which are not identifiable on routine haematological examination [4].

Table 1. Cell surface antigens detectable in cell smears by the APAAP technique

T-cell markers[a]	B-cell markers[b]
CD1 (T6)	p95
CD2 (T11)	IgM
CD3 (T3)	IgD
CD4 (T4)	HLA-DR
CD5 (T1)	p135
CD7	
CD8 (T8)	
Miscellaneous	
CALLA	
MY906 (Myeloid)	
IL2-receptor (Tac)	
HC1, HC2 (hairy cells[c])	
Glycophorin	
p150,95 (macrophages, hairy cells[d])	
gp Ib, IIb-IIIa, IIIa (platelet/megakaryocytes)	
Terminal transferase	

[a] The T-cell markers are indicated according to the "CD" system introduced at the 1st Workshop on Leucocyte Differentiation Antigens (Paris 1982), with their alternative nomenclature in the OKT series shown in parenthesis

[b] p95 (CD19) and p135 (CD22) are B-cell-associated markers detected by, respectively, antibody B4 [5] and Tol5 (DAKO PAN-B)

[c] [6]

[d] [7]

Acknowledgments. This work is supported by grants from the Leukaemia Research Fund and the Cancer Research Campaign. W. N. Erber holds a Rhodes Scholarship.

References

1. Cordell JL, Falini B, Erber WN, Ghosh AK, Abdulaziz A, MacDonald S, Pulford KAF, Stein H, Mason DY (1984) Immunoenzymatic labelling of monoclonal antibodies using immune complexes of alkaline phosphatase and monoclonal anti-alkaline phosphatase (APAAP complexes). J Histochem Cytochem 32:219–229
2. Moir DJ, Ghosh AK, Abdulaziz A, Knight P, Mason DY (1983) Immunoenzymatic staining of haematological samples with monoclonal antibodies. Br J Haematol 55:395–410
3. Erber WN, Pinching AJ, Mason DY (1984) Immunocytochemical detection of T and B cell populations in routine blood smears. Lancet I: 1042–1045
4. Ghosh AK, Erber WN, Hatton C, Falini B, O'Connor NJ, Osborn M, Mason DY (1985) Detection of metastatic tumour cells in routine bone marrow smears by immuno-alkaline phosphatase labelling with monoclonal antibodies. Br J Haematol (in press)
5. Nadler LM, Anderson KC, Marti G, Bates M, Park E, Daley JF, Schlossman SF (1983) B4, a human B lymphocyte-associated antigen expressed on normal, mitogen-activated, and malignant B lymphocytes. J Immunol 131: 244–250
6. Posnett DN, Chiorazzi N, Kunkel HG (1982) Monoclonal antibodies with specificity for hairy cell leukaemia cells. J Clin Invest 70:254–261
7. Falini B, Schwarting R, Erber WN, Posnett DN, Martelli MF, Grignani F, Zuccaccia M, Gatter KC, Cernetti C, Stein H, Mason DY (1985) The differential diagnosis of hairy cell leukaemia with a panel of monoclonal antibodies. Am J Clin Pathol (in press)

Haematology and Blood Transfusion Vol. 29
Modern Trends in Human Leukemia VI
Edited by Neth, Gallo, Greaves, Janka

Myelolactoferrin Index (MLF) and Myelopoiesis During Bacterial Infections and Malignant Diseases*

R. Neth, J. Nowrath, M. Thomsen, C. Wiggers, M. Gabrecht, W. Rehpenning, K. Winkler, U. Krause, H. Soltau, and H. Kraemer-Hansen

Abstract

The myelolactoferrin index (MLF) is significantly lowered in patients with bacterial infections and with malignant diseases. In both cases it can be assumed that the alteration of the granulopoietic storage pool is followed by a decrease in lactoferrin. Therefore, it seems advisable to study (a) to what extent the immunocytochemical quantitative evaluation of lactoferrin content of mature neutrophil granulocytes can be used to recognize any toxic damage caused to bone marrow cells by long-term therapies or environmental toxins and (b) whether this method is more sensitive than the conventional counting of granulocytes and thrombocytes.

A. Introduction

Myelopoiesis is regulated by cell-derived molecules that stimulate or inhibit proliferation and differentiation of granulocyte-macrophage progenitor cells. The interactions of positive and negative feedback mechanisms regulate the production of granulocytes and macrophages and probably keep granulocytes and monocytes within the tightly controlled limits noted in vivo. Lactoferrin located in the secondary granules of mature neutrophil granulocytes has been implicated as a negative feedback regulator of myelopoiesis [1]. Lactoferrin acts in vitro as an inhibitor of granulocyte and macrophage colony formation, and in vivo mouse granulopoiesis is decreased by lactoferrin [1]. However, there is no information available on a possible physiological role of lactoferrin on the regulation of myelopoiesis in humans. A correlation between the lactoferrin content of granulocytes and the bone marrow pool of these cells seems to indicate that lactoferrin may also function as a negative feedback regulator substance of myelopoiesis in the human. A reduction of the granulopoietic storage pool is known to occur during bacterial infections by way of increased cell turnover and during treatment of malignant diseases by way of drug-induced inhibition of myelopoiesis. We have, therefore, studied the lactoferrin content of mature granulocytes in conjunction with the myeloperoxidase and the usual hematological parameters in these two disease classes.

B. Materials and Methods

In all, 40 normal persons and 54 patients with bacterial infections and 94 with malignant diseases were chosen. Myeloperoxydase was cytochemically determined [2] with o-Tolidin. Lactoferrin was determined by the immunoperoxidase technique according to Stein [3] with Dako reagents purchased from Boehringer Ingelheim Diagnostica. The quantitative evaluation of

* Universitätskliniken D-2000 Hamburg 20, Martinistrasse 52, FRG
Supported by the Deutsche Forschungsgemeinschaft and the Deutsche Krebshilfe

date	MLF - Index
29.9.	248
30.9.	239
4.10.	261
5.10.	232
6.10.	242
7.10.	254
8.10.	254
9.10.	260
12.10.	269
13.10.	271
	$\bar{x}$ 253
	$2_s \pm 26$

Fig. 1. Individual biological variation of MLF

variation in myeloperoxidase and lactoferrin content was performed as in the case of ALP, using a score of 0–3. The 2s range of multiple determinations in one blood sample was found to be ± 11.4, and the biological variation among blood specimens taken daily over 14 days, to be ± 26 (Fig. 1) index points.

Fig. 2. MLF index in *A* normal persons; *B* patients with bacterial infections; *C* patients with malignant diseases and receiving chemotherapy; *D* patients with kidney transplants and receiving long-term chemotherapy

C. Results

The normal persons ($n = 40$) showed a normal distribution with a mean of 231 and a 2s range of ± 34. In contrast, the two groups of patients did not show a normal distribution, more than 50% of their lactoferrin values lying below the 2s range of the normal group with mean values of 158, 189 and 153 for patients with bacterial infections and malignant diseases (Fig. 2), respectively. In patients with bacterial infections, 2–4 days after granulocytosis and left shift a decrease of lactoferrin was noted, which was followed by an increase to the normal values 2 days after normalization of the granulocyte kinetics (Fig. 3). In addition, in patients chronically treated with cytostatic drugs chronically subnormed lactoferrin values were found (Fig. 4).

D. Discussion

Our data demonstrate a close correlation between the lactoferrin content of mature granulocytes and the reactive changes with the granulocytic system during bacterial infections. The low lactoferrin values in patients with malignant diseases could be due

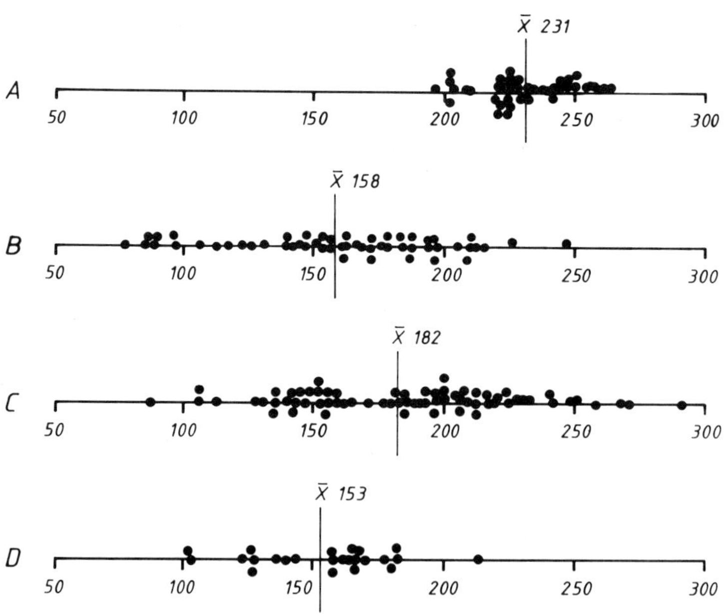

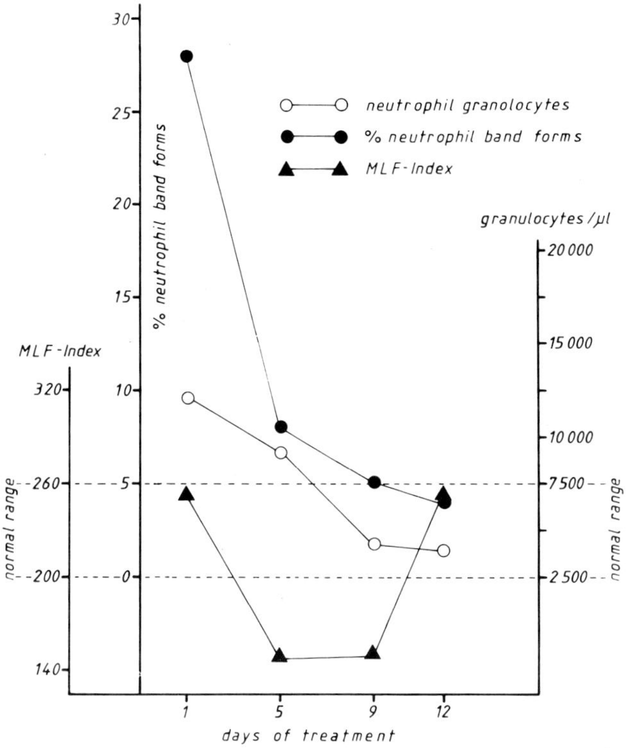

Fig. 3. Follow-up study of a patient with urinary tract infection

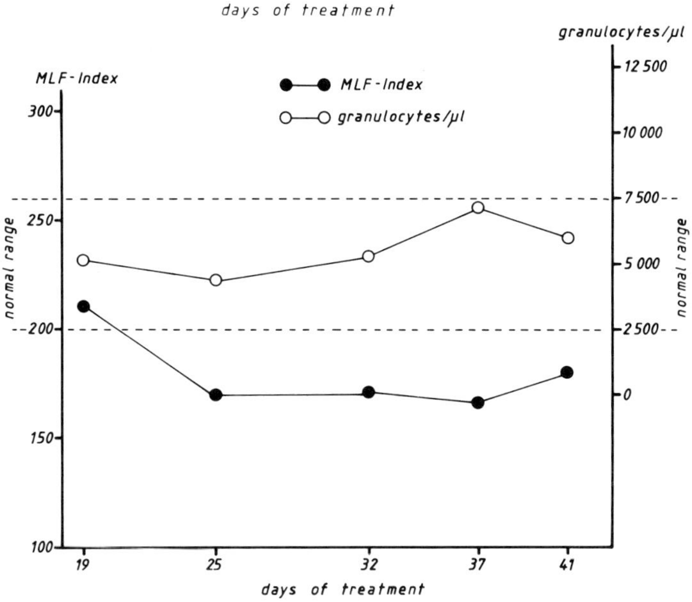

Fig. 4. Follow up study of a patient with a kidney transplant and receiving long-term chemotherapy

to inefficiency of the granulopoietic differentiation. Our data, however, do not support this possibility: Decreased myeloperoxidase levels are known to occur in leukemia and indicate a disturbance of granulopoietic differentiation [4]. In our group of patients with malignant diseases, however, normal myeloperoxidase values were found, and no correlation could be determined between myeloperoxidase and lactoferrin (correlation coefficient below 0.1). A disturbance of granulopoietic differ-

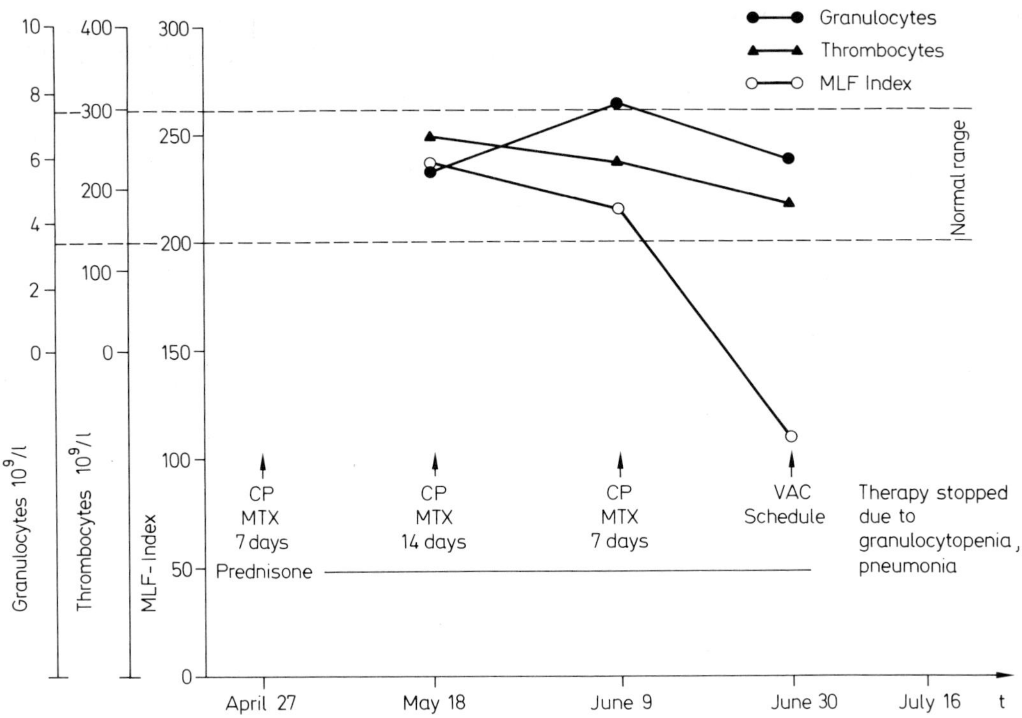

Fig. 5. Follow-up study of a patient with metastatic breast cancer. *CP* cyclophosphamide; *MTX* methotrexate; *VAC* vincristine/adriblastine/cyclophosphamide

entiation as a cause of the lower lactoferrin values can therefore be excluded in these patients. In both groups of patients it can be assumed that the alteration of the granulopoietic storage pool is followed by a decrease in the lactoferrin content of mature neutrophil granulocytes. Therefore, it seems advisable to study (a) to what extent the immunocytochemical quantitative evaluation of lactoferrin can be used to recognize any toxic damage caused to bone marrow cells by long-term therapies or environmental toxins and (b) whether this would be more sensitive than conventional counting of granulocytes and thrombocytes (Fig. 5).

References

1. Broxmeyer HE, DeSousa M, Smithyman A, Ralph P, Hamilton J, Kurland JI, Bognacki J (1980) Specifity and modulation of the action of lactoferrin, a negative feedback regulator of myelopoiesis. Blood 55:324
2. Undritz E (1952) Hämatologische Tafeln. Sandoz, Basel, p 28
3. Stein H, Gerdes J, Schwab U, Lemke H, Mason DY, Ziegler A, Schienle W, Diehl V (1982) Identification of Hodgkin and Sternberg-Reed cells as a unique cell type derived from a newly detected small-cell population. Int J Cancer 30:445
4. Rabe K, Rehpenning W, Winkler K, Heinisch B, Krause U, Soltau H, Neth R (1983) Persistent deficiency of myeloperoxidase and lactoferrin in granulopoietic cells of patients with acute leukemia. Springer, Berlin Heidelberg New York Tokio, p 362 (Modern trends in human leukemia, vol 5)

Haematology and Blood Transfusion Vol. 29
Modern Trends in Human Leukemia VI
Edited by Neth, Gallo, Greaves, Janka

β-Hexosaminidase Isoenzyme I: An Early Marker of Hematopoietic Malignancy *

G. Gaedicke [1], J. Novotny [1], A. Raghavachar [2], and H. G. Drexler [3]

A. Introduction

The analysis of various enzymes has been found to distinguish immunologic subsets of human leukemias. This is especially true for terminal deoxynucleotidyl transferase (TdT). This enzyme is present in 90% of all cases with common ALL, pre B-ALL, T-ALL, and it is negative in B-ALL. Some 5%–15% of AML are also positive for TdT. Interestingly, acute undifferentiated leukemias (HLA-DR positive, cALL-A negative) have been found to be TdT positive in 40%–60% of cases. This nuclear enzyme thus seems to be a very early marker of lymphohematopoietic development. The lysosomal enzyme β-hexosaminidase (*N*-acetyl-β-D-glucosaminidase) can be separated into two major forms: an isoenzyme A, which is constituted by two α and two β subunits, and in isoenzyme B, which consists of four β subunits. In cALL cells, a third isoenzyme was first observed by Ellis et al., eluted from an ion exchange chromatographic resin in an intermediate position between the A and B forms [1]. This intermediate isoenzyme I seems to consist of β subunits. Hexosaminidase C is a fourth isoenzyme with a more acidic isoelectric point than hexosaminidase A. In the study presented here, hexosaminidase isoenzymes were investigated as part of multiple marker analysis in various leukemia subtypes.

1 University of Ulm, Department of Pediatrics II,
2 Department of Transfusion Medicine, 7900 Ulm/Donau, FRG
3 Veterans Administration Edward Hines, Jr. Hospital, Hines, ILL 60141, 151 C USA
* Supported by the Deutsche Forschungsgesellschaft SFB 112, B 10

B. Methods

Leukemia cells were isolated from fresh bone marrow aspirates of leukemic patients, and separated by Ficoll and Percoll step gradients or by counterflow elutriation. Between 10^7 and 10^8 cells were used for the enzymatic tests. A crude extract was prepared by sonic disruption of the cells, isolation of the lysosomal fraction, and solubilization with a nonionic detergent. Activity was measured with the α-phenyl method, and protein concentration according to the Lowry procedure [2].

The enzyme was enriched either by phenyl–sepharose chromatography or by a Con-A–sepharose column prior to DEAE ion exchange chromatography. This was done with a LKB high performance system, using a linear NaCl gradient from 0 to 0.5 *M* NaCl. Crude extracts were used for separating the enzymatic activity into its isoenzymes by analytic isoelectric focusing or disk electrophoresis [2].

C. Results

1. In leukemic specimens, isoelectric focusing clearly demonstrates an anodic shift of hexosaminidase A. The same phenomenon is seen in DEAE ion exchange chromatography.

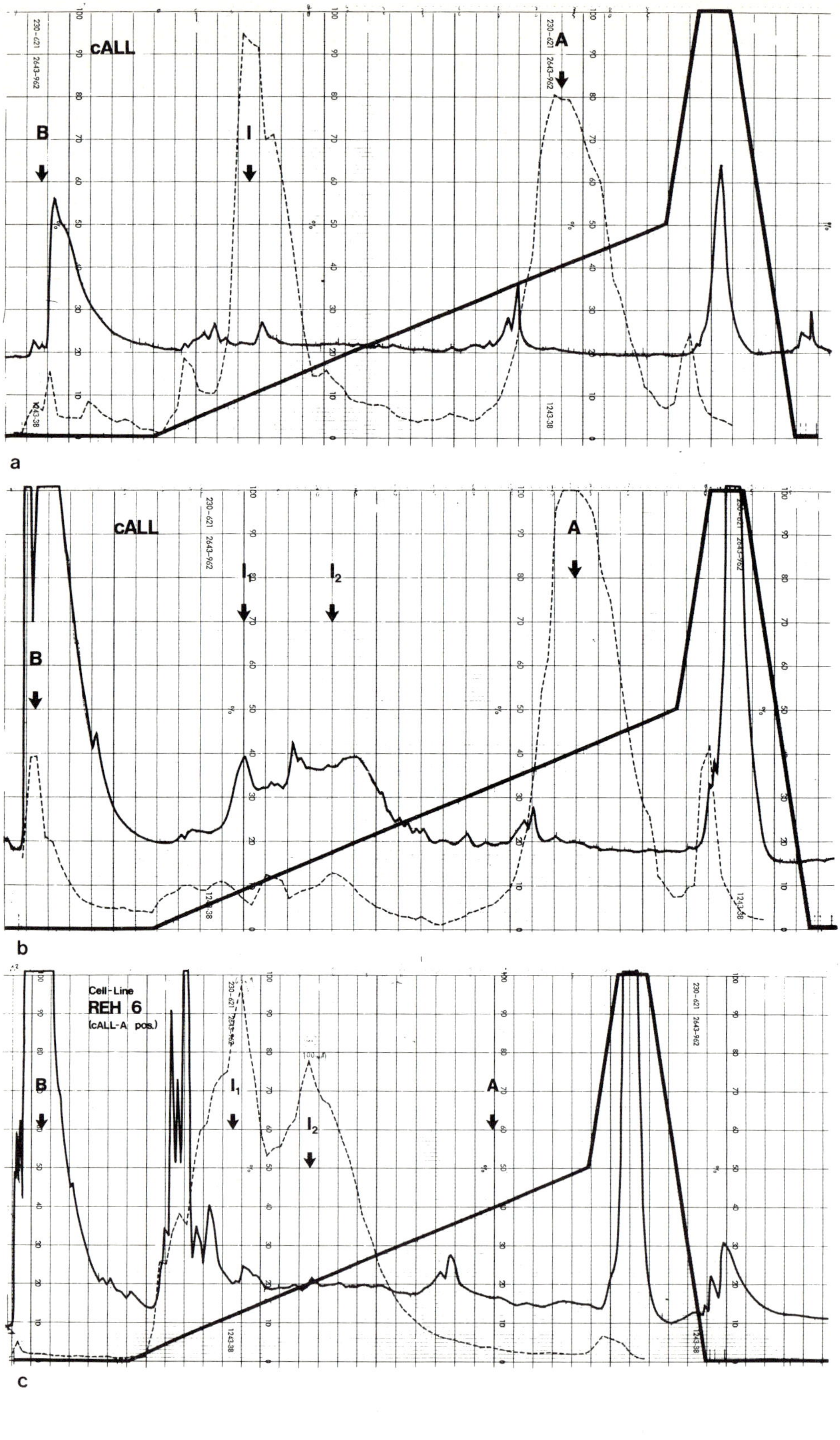
cALL
B
I
A
a
cALL
B
I1
I2
A
b
Cell-Line
REH 6
(cALL-A pos.)
B
I1
I2
A
c
230-621
2643-962
1243.38
%

Fig. 1 a–c. Ion exchange chromatographic patterns of hexosaminidase isoenzymes. *Thick full line* NaCl gradient; *thin full line* OD tracing; *broken line* hexosaminidase activity. *Arrows* indicate the position of isoenzymes A, B, and I. In the cell line REH 6, tow peaks with intermediate position are eluted from the DEAE column, indicating that isoenzyme I occurs in at least two variant forms

2. The investigation of 15 cases of acute childhood leukemias using a comparative analysis of multiple surface markers with hexosaminidase isoenzymes, showed that cALL could be further subdivided. Of 15 cases, 3 had no hexosaminidase activity; 10 cases demonstrated isoenzyme A, B, and I (Fig. 1 a), 2 cases isoenzymes A and B only (Fig. 1 b). Acute lymphocytic leukemias had imbalanced synthesis of A and B forms with a decrease of the hexosaminidase isoenzyme B. The cALL-positive celle line REH subclone 6 had two enzymatic activities in the intermediate region, and no A or B isoenzyme (Fig. 1 c). T cell leukemias (13 cases) had no isoenzyme I. Acute myeloblastic leukemias (8 cases) either had isoenzymes A and B only, or A, B and I. However, the ratio of A:B isoenzyme activity was balanced as is usually seen in normal granulocytes. Only one myeloblastic leukemia (M_1) had hexosaminidase A activity only.

All eight cases of AUL (HLA-DR positive, cALL-A negative, TdT±) had very low or absent enzymatic activity in the isoenzmye B region. To date, half of the cases investigated have had high levels of isoenzyme I and low levels of hexosaminidase A.

D. Discussion

Most of the surface and enzyme markers clearly demonstrate that leukemia cells correspond to a certain developmental stage of lymphohematopoiesis. This is called cell lineage fidelity [3]. As far as hexosaminidase isoenzyme I is concerned, it remains unknown if this isoenzyme occurs in normal hematopoietic precursor cells. It is well recognized that glycosphingolipids are the natural substrates for the hexosaminidases [4]. For hexosaminidase I this remains unknown. If it is assumed that hexosaminidase I activity represents elements of hexosaminidase B, it is possible to postulate that in leukemia cells there is lack of a factor necessary for the transformation of isoenzyme I to the B form. This suggestion is further supported by the observation of a shift from hexosaminidase I to hexosaminidase B when differentiation is induced in human leukemia cell lines by conditioned media or TPA (Drexler et al., this volume).

Hexosaminidase isoenzymes have been under investigation for a number of years in human leukemias and it has been observed that a shift to the anode occurs in hexosaminidase A, if the isoenzymes are separated by electrophoretic techniques [2, 5, 6]. This suggests that a posttranslational modification of this isoenzyme does not take place in leukemia cells. From our observations, one may conclude that hexosaminidase isoenzymes offer the opportunity of investigating the regulation of normal gene products in human leukemia cells.

References

1. Ellis RB, Rapson NT, Patrick AD, Greaves MF (1978) Expression of hexosaminidase isoenzymes in childhood leukemia. N Engl J Med 298:476
2. Drexler HG, Gaedicke G (1983) Isoenzyme studies in human leukemia – III. β-hexosaminidase (E.C. 3.2.1.30). Leuk Res 7:611–619
3. Greaves MF (1982) Target cells, cellular phenotypes and lineage fidelity in human leukemia. In: Mak TW, McCulloch EA (eds) Cellular and molecular biology of hematopoietic stemm cell differentiation. Liss, New York, p 113
4. Sandhoff K, Christomanou H (1979) Biochemistry and genetics of gangliosidoses. Hum Genet 50:107
5. Broadhead DM, Besley GTN, Moss SE, Bain ED, Eden OB, Sainsbury CPQ (1981) Recognition of abnormal lysosomal enzyme patterns in childhood leukemia by isoelectric focusing with special reference to some properties of abnormality expressed components. Leuk Res 5:29
6. Besley GTN, Moss SE, Bain AD, Dewar AE (1983) Correlation of lysosomal enzyme abnormalities in various forms of adults leukemia. J Clin Pathol 36:1000

Haematology and Blood Transfusion Vol. 29
Modern Trends in Human Leukemia VI
Edited by Neth, Gallo, Greaves, Janka

Analysis of Leukemic Cells with Monoclonal Antibodies in Acute Myelomonocytic Leukemia Suggests Abnormality at an Early Differentiation Stage in Certain Cases *

M. Gramatzki, A. Schaaff, G. R. Burmester, B. Koch, A. H. Tulusan, and J. R. Kalden

A. Introduction

Monoclonal antibodies (MoAb) are valuable tools in better defining hematologic malignancies, both for diagnostic purposes and for understanding normal and malignant differentiation [1–5]. In the present study, we characterized the bone marrow cells of a young child with acute myelomonocytic leukemia (AMML). The unusual immunologic phenotype in this case not only allows more insight into myelomonocytic differentiation, but also sheds some light on the origin of the malignant process in certain cases of AMML.

B. Clinical Information

A girl aged 2 years 2 months was admitted to the hospital with a history of low grade fever for several weeks, arthralgias, purpura, tonsillitis, mild generalized lymphadenopathy, and hepatosplenomegaly. Laboratory data showed elevated lactate dehydrogenase, HbF of 4%, and increased urine and serum lysozyme. Her Hb was 5.8 g/dl, thrombocytes $128 \times 10^9/l$, and the white blood cell count $57 \times 10^9/l$ with a differential count of 7% lymphocytes, 6% neutrophils and band forms, 4% metamyelocytes, 1% myelocytes, and 82% myelomonocytic blasts. Bone marrow analysis revealed a high percentage of polymorphic leukemic blasts, predominantly monocytoid with only a small number of cells with promyelocyte appearance. Almost all leukemic cells showed positive myeloperoxidase and nonspecific esterase reaction. Diagnosis of AMML, M4 according to FAB classification [6] was made.

C. Material and Methods

Heparinized bone marrow was layered over a Ficoll–Diatrozoate density gradient and interface cells were obtained after centrifugation as previously described [7]. These bone marrow mononuclear cells were evaluated for staining with MoAb in indirect immunofluorescence staining, using a goat anti-mouse immunoglobulin (Ig) as developing reagent, as described in detail [2, 8]. The following MoAb were used: 3A1 and 4F2 (kindly provided by Dr. A. Fauci) [3]; 9.6 and 20.2 (gift from Dr. J. Hansen) [5]; FMC7 (provided by Dr. H. Zola) [9]; Mo-P9, Mo-P15, Mo-S1, and Mo-S39 [8]; U-28 (gift from Dr. R. Winchester) [10]; the OKT/OKM/OKI series [1, 4]; B1 [11]; BA-1, BA-2, and TA-1 [12–15]; and My-1 [16]. Cytoplasmic Ig was detected on cytocentrifuge preparations stained with heteroantisera. Transmission electron microscopy was performed as previously described [2]. Analysis for lectin binding was done according to a recent paper by Koch et al. [17].

* Institute for Clinical Immunology and Rheumatology, and Department of Obstetrics and Gynecology, University of Erlangen, Erlangen; and Cnopf's Children's Hospital, Nürnberg, FRG

Table 1. Reactivity of the patient's bone marrow cells with different antibodies

Antibody	Characteristic specificity	Reactive cells (%)
9.6	Pan T cell	22
3A1	Major T cell subset	15
OKT4	Helper T cells	7
OKT8	Suppressor/cytotoxic T cells	10
B1	B cells	9
BA-1	B cells, granulocytes	40
BA-2	Lymphoid precursors	33
FMC7	B cell subset	2
Anti-IgA,G,M,D	Plasma cells	0[a]
Anti-κ/λ	Plasma cells	0[a]
Mo-S39	Monocytes	60
OKI1	HLA-DR-positive cells	60
OKT10	Activation antigen on different lineages, plasma cells	65

[a] Intracytoplasmic staining

Table 2. Reactivity with additional monoclonal antibodies detecting cells of myeloid/monocytoid lineage

Antibody	Characteristic specificity	Reactive cells (%)
Mo-P9	Monocytes	40
Mo-P15	Monocytes	40
Mo-S1	Monocytes	40
20.2	Monocytes, granulocytes	55
OKM1	Monocytes, granulocytes	54
TA-1	T cells, monocytes	45
4F2	Monocytes, activated/proliferating cells (not lineage specific)	80
My-1	Certain stages of myeloid differentiation, including promyelocytes and granulocytes	16
U-28	FAB M1 and some M5 cells	0

D. Results and Discussion

Immunologic characterization of the bone marrow cells of this patient revealed more than 70% leukemic cells, while the remaining population consisted of mature B and T lymphocytes as determined by positive staining with reagents 9.6, OKT4, OKT8, 3A1, and B1 (Table 1). The population of malignant cells reacted with six MoAb which have particular specificity for the monocyte lineage, namely Mo-P9, Mo-P15, Mo-S1, Mo-S39, 20.2, and OKM1, although some have additional reactivity with granulocytes and myeloid precursors (Tables 1 and 2). These cells were also stained by reagent 4F2, detecting monocytes and activated or proliferating cells of different origin. Furthermore, reactivity with MoAb OKT10 was found, an antibody which, besides reacting with plasma cells and certain thymocytes, serves as an activation marker in several lineages. Confirming the AMML differentiation stage, the leukemic cells reacted with TA-1, a MoAb detecting an antigen expressed on mature T cells, monocytes, and AMML cells, but not on cells of acute myelocytic leukemias (AML) [13]. A certain percentage of more immature myeloid cells was detected by antibody My-1, reactive mainly with FAB M2/M3 cells [16], a finding consistent with the morphological picture of a minor population of promyelocytes. Surprisingly, significant additional reactivity was found with two MoAb, namely BA-1 and BA-2. Antibody BA-1 primarily stains normal and malignant cells of B cell lineage, and, although also binding to granulocytes, is usually distinct unreactive with monocytes and AMML cells [10, 11]. Antibody BA-2 has been found primarily on lymphoid precursor cells and lymphoid malignancies of different differentiation stages, although additional reactivity with some nonlymphoid cells was found, particulary neuroblastoma and certain carcinomas [14, 15]. Finally, lectin binding studies showed 44% of the cells reactive with *Lotus tetragonolobus* agglutinin (LTA), consistent with the presence of myelomonocytic cells [17].

To evaluate whether MoAb BA-1, BA-2, and anti-monocyte MoAb did stain the same cell population, double-staining experiments were performed. Various combinations of two or more of these antibodies added to the same cell preparation did not result in additional positive cells, demonstrating that the corresponding antigens were expressed in the same cell population.

In this case, a rather homogeneous reactivity pattern with MoAb was seen, despite some degree of morphological variation. This has implications for models of myeloid differentiation and would be in favor of an uncommitted promyelocyte, still able to differentiate into the monocyte lineage as has recently been suggested [18]. Furthermore, the pattern of MoAb reactivity would classify this case of AMML as already differentiated primarily into the monocyte lineage.

Finally, the unusual occurrence of antigens normally detected on B lymphocytes and B lymphocyte precursors in these AMML cells suggests that in this case an abnormality may have developed at a very early differentiation stage with subsequent differentiation along the myeloid pathway. This idea would be consistent with genetic analysis of granulocyte/macrophage colonies in a case of AMML, where by karyotyping the malignant cells could be defined as arising shortly after stem cell differentiation. Thus, analysis with monoclonal reagents provides an additional tool in better defining the origin of malignant cells in addition to enzyme markers and chromosomal analysis.

Acknowledgment. This work was supported by SFB 118/B2 and DFG Bu 445/2–3.

References

1. Foon KA, Schroff RW, Gale RP (1982) Surface markers on leukemia and lymphoma cells: recent advances. Blood 60:1
2. Gramatzki M, Dolan MF, Fauci AS, Maples JA, Bonnard GD, Strong DM (1982) Immunologic characterization of a helper T-cell lymphoma. Blood 59:702
3. Haynes BF, Metzgar RS, Minna JD, Bunn PA (1981) Phenotypic characterization of cutaneous T-cell lymphoma. Use of monoclonal antibodies to compare with other malignant T-cells. N Engl J Med 304:1319
4. Kung PC, Goldstein G (1980) Functional and developmental compartments of human T lymphocytes. Vox Sang 39:121
5. Kadin ME, Kamoun M, Lamberg J (1981) Erythrophagocytic Tγ-lymphoma. A clinicopathological entity resembling malignant histiocytosis. N Engl J Med 304:648
6. Bennet JM, Catovsky D, Daniel MT, Flandrin G (1976) Proposals for the classification of the acute leukemias. Br J Haematol 33:451
7. Böyum A (1974) Separation of blood leukocytes, granulocytes, and lymphocytes. Tissue Antigens 4:269
8. Dimitriu-Bona A, Burmester GR, Waters SJ, Winchester RJ (1983) Human mononuclear phagocyte differentiation antigens I. Patterns of antigenic expression on the surface of human monocytes and macrophages defined by monoclonal antibodies. J Immunol 130:145
9. Brooks DA, Beckman IGR, Bradley J, McNamara PJ, Thomas ME, Zola H (1981) Human lymphocyte markers defined by antibodies derived from somatic cell hybrids. IV. A monoclonal antibody reacting specifically with a subpopulation of human B lymphocytes. J Immunol 126:1373
10. Dimitriu-Bona A, Winchester RJ, Szer I, Reilly M, Najfeld V, Cuttner J (1983) Expression of early or mature monocyte-related antigens on certain acute myeloid leukemias (AML) before and after culture. Clin Res 31:512A

11. Stashenko P, Nadler LM, Hardy R, Schlossman SF (1980) Characterization of a human B lymphocyte specific antigen. J Immunol 125:1506
12. Abramson C, Kersey J, Le Bien T (1981) A monoclonal antibody (BA-I) reactive with cells of human B lymphocyte lineage. J Immunol 126:83
13. Le Bien TW, McKennce RW, Abramson CS, Gajl-Peczalska KJ, Nesbit ME, Coccia PF, Bloomfield CD, Brunning RD, Kersey JH (1981) Use of monoclonal antibodies, morphology, and cytochemistry to probe cellular heterogeneity of acute leukemia and lymphoma. Cancer Res 41:4776
14. Kersey JH, Le Bien TW, Abramson CS, Newmann R, Sutherland R, Greaves M (1981) p24: a human leukemia-associated and lymphohemopoietic progenitor cell surface structure identified with monoclonal antibody. J Exp Med 153:726
15. Ash RC, Jansen J, Kersey JH, Le Bien TW, Zanjani ED (1982) Normal human pluripotential and committed hematopoietic progenitors do not express the p24 antigen detected by monoclonal antibody BA-2: Implications for immunotherapy of lymphocytic leukemia. Blood 60:1310
16. Civin CI, Mirro J, Benguerigo ML (1981) A new myeloid-specific antigen identified by a mouse monoclonal antibody. Blood 57:842
17. Koch B, Regnat W, Schedel I, Hermanek H, Leibold W, Kalden JR (1983) The binding of different lectins on peripheral blood mononuclear cells from patients with chronic inflammatory and malignant diseases. Immunobiology 164:99
18. Ball ED, Fanger MW (1983) The expression of myeloid-specific antigens on myeloid leukemia cells: correlations with leukemia subclasses and implications for normal myeloid differentiation. Blood 61:456
19. Reid MM, Tantravahi R, Grier HE, O'Toole S, Miller BA, Lipton JM, Weinstein HJ, Nathan DG (1983) Detection of leukemia-related karyotypes in granulocyte/macrophage colonies from a patient with acute myelomonocytic leukemia. N Engl J Med 308:1324

Haematology and Blood Transfusion Vol. 29
Modern Trends in Human Leukemia VI
Edited by Neth, Gallo, Greaves, Janka

Nonspecific Cross-Reacting Antigen as a Marker of Myelocytic Leukemias in Individual Stages of Myelocytic Cell Differentiation *

A. Harłozińska, A. Noworolska, and R. Richter

The aim of the study was to establish:

1. The distribution of nonspecific cross-reacting antigen (NCA) and carcinoembryonic antigen (CEA) in cells of different types of myelocytic leukemias
2. The presence of NCA in individual stages of granulocyte differentiation
3. NCA and CEA serum levels

A total of 17 acute myelocytic leukemia (AML) cases were studied, classified according to the proposals of the FAB cooperative group, and 14 cases of chronic granulocytic leukemia (CGL) – 5 of these were in myeloblastic crisis (CGL-BC) and formed a separate group. The control studies were performed on cells of 6 ALL patients and on granulocytes of 6 normal donors.

To separate the myelocyte cells into fractions containing granulocytes in individual stages of maturation, discontinuous density gradient centrifugation (Ficoll–Hypaque 1.05–1.105 g/ml) was applied. Dextran isolates were prepared in only some AML cases. The cells of each density layer were checked for NCA and CEA by immunofluorescence (IF) and were also stained with Wright–Giemsa to determine differential morphology.

The anti-CEA and anti-NCA sera used in IF were additionally absorbed on columns prepared by coupling purified CEA or NCA to CNBr-activated sepharose 4B to remove anti-CEA or anti-NCA activity, respectively. The results of NCA content in different types of AML are summarized in Table 1. The number of NCA-positive cells increased from individual blasts of AML with features of maturation (Fig. 1). Monoblastic leukemias were usually NCA negative and, in one erythroleukemia case, the percentage of fluorescent cells was similar to the amount of mature granulocytes. The analysis for NCA in patients with CGL-BC and CGL isolated by density gradient centrifugation showed that expression of this antigen increased as more mature cells in denser layers were obtained (Table 2). The comparison of fluorescence with phase-contrast pictures showed that some blasts from CGL-BC and individual blasts detectable in the chronic phase of CGL showed distinct cytoplasmic NCA-dependent staining. Many pathologic myelocytes and metamyelocytes were NCA positive (40%–70%), but their amount and fluorescence intensity varied from one case to another (Fig. 2). The fluorescence of mature neutrophils, focused mainly in fractions 1.09–1.105 g/ml, was observed in 80%–90% of cells. Lymphoblasts of ALL patients and healthy donors' lymphocytes were always negative. Anti-CEA serum stained neither AML, ALL, nor any fraction of CGL-BC and CGL cells.

Serum NCA levels in patients with AML and ALL were very low or undetectable (Table 1). In CGL-BC and CGL patients, circulating NCA was always elevated to a mean value of 100 and 140 ng/ml, respectively. Serum CEA was within the normal range (0–7 ng/ml) in all patients studied.

---

* Dept. Pathol. Anat. Sch. Med., 50-368 Wrocław, Poland

Table 1. NCA content in peripheral blood cells and serum of AML patients

Leukemias	Number of cases	Wright-Giemsa morphology (%)[b]				IF NCA-positive cells (%)	NAC serum level (ng/ml)
		Blasts	PMN	Mon	Lym		
AML classification[a]							
M0 (without maturation)	2	81	2		17	0.5	5.0
M1 (weak maturation)	2	88	4		8	6.0	3.0
M2 (distinct maturation)	4	81	9		10	13.0	0.0
M4 (myelomonocytic)	3	87	9		4	5.0	0.0
M5 (monoblastic)	5	77	6	6	11	4.0	7.0
M6 (erythroleukemia)	1	19	81			70.0	30.0
ALL	6	74	6		20	0.0	7.5

[a] According to FAB cooperative group

[b] Blasts = myeloblasts; PMN = polymorphonuclear neutrophils; Mon = monocytes; Lym = lymphocytes

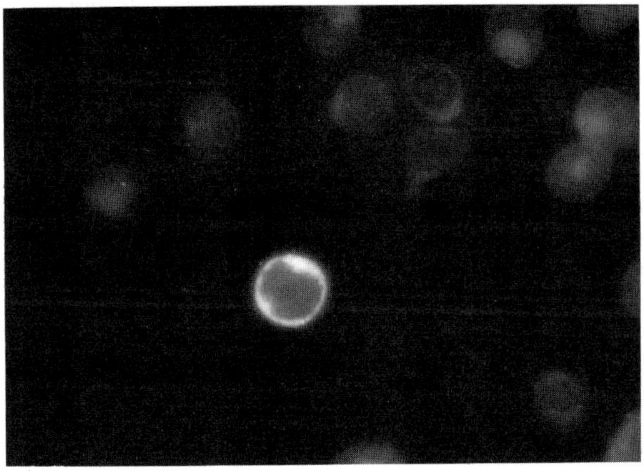

Fig. 1. AML (M2) cells treated with anti-NCA serum. Cytoplasmic fluorescence of an individual blast

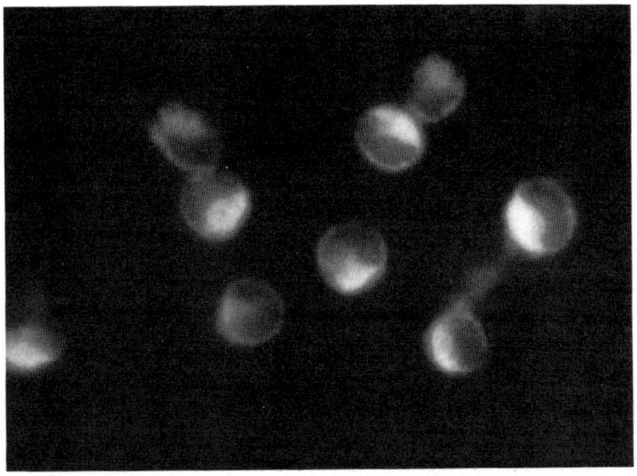

Fig. 2. CGL cells isolated in 1.07 g/ml fraction treated with anti-NCA serum. Cytoplasmic fluorescence of majority myelocytes and metamyelocytes

Table 2. NCA content in peripheral blood cells separated by density gradient centrifugation in CGL, CGL-BC patients, and normal donors

Material	Number of cases	Density layer (g/ml)	Wright-Giemsa morphology (mean %)					IF test NCA-positive cells (%)	NCA serum level (ng/ml)
			Blasts Pro	Myel[a] Mta	Band PMN	Eos Bas	Lym		
CGL	9	Dextran	6.7	36.5	50.0	2.6	4.2	79.8	142.0
		1.06–1.07	3.6	49.8	37.4	4.8	4.4	57.4	(20.0–410.0)
		1.08–1.09	1.2	25.0	67.9	5.2	0.7	92.5	
		1.105		21.5	70.3	8.2		92.8	
CGL-BC	5	Dextran	22.3	36.7	41.0			64.8	100.0
		1.05	62.0	30.0	8.0			18.3	
		1.06–1.07	21.0	38.3	37.0	3.0	0.7	53.6	
		1.08–1.09	9.0	21.7	65.3	3.5	0.5	86.1	
		1.105	0.7	14.6	82.0	2.7		83.7	
Normal granulocytes	6	1.105			92.0	3.0	5.0	90.0	30.0

[a] Myel = myelocytes; Band = band forms; Eos = eosinophils; Pro = promyelocytes; Mta = metamyelocytes; Bas = basophils. For other abbreviations see the legend to Table 1

Parallel studies by IF and immunodiffusion (ID) showed the immunologic relationship of the NCA extracted from CGL cells and purified from normal lung tissue.

Our results may be summarized as follows:

1. AML blasts without the ability to mature (M0) and monoblasts did not synthesize NCA.
2. Individual AML blasts with features of maturation (M1, M2) and some myeloblasts of CGL-BC showed limited ability to express cytoplasmic NCA.
3. The number of NCA-containing cells increased as the more mature granulocyte fractions were isolated on Ficoll–Hypaque density gradients.
4. Myelocytic NCA is immunologically related to NCA isolated from normal lung tissue.
5. CEA is undetectable in myelocytic cell series.

Haematology and Blood Transfusion Vol. 29
Modern Trends in Human Leukemia VI
Edited by Neth, Gallo, Greaves, Janka

Plasminogen Activator as a Prognostic Factor in Hematological Malignancies

E. L. Wilson [1, 3], P. Jacobs [2], and L. Oliver [1]

A. Introduction

The plasminogen–plasmin system is involved in many physiological processes such as fibrinolysis, tissue remodelling, destruction of intercellular matrix and cell migration [1]. Human cells release plasminogen activators of two distinct immunochemical types – urokinase and tissue plasminogen activator [2–4]. The activity of these enzymes in biological systems is regulated by a variety of agents such as hormones, retinoids and tumour promoters [5–11]. It is also regulated by protease inhibitors such as protease nexins [12] and by receptors for the enzyme on the surface of human fibroblasts [13]. Leukaemic cells secrete both species of plasminogen activator and patients with acute myeloid leukaemia whose cells release only tissue plasminogen do not respond to combination chemotherapy [14].

B. Methods

Heparinized blood samples were obtained from 117 patients with acute myeloid leukaemia (AML), from 31 patients with chronic myeloid leukaemia (CML), and from 89 patients with other myeloproliferative disorders. Cells were isolated by centrifugation on Ficoll–Hypaque and resuspended in RPMI containing 3% foetal calf serum to give 4×10^6 cells/ml [14]. The medium was harvested by centrifugation 24 h later and stored at – 80 °C for analysis of enzyme activity. Plasminogen activators were assayed by measuring the plasminogen-dependent release of soluble radioactive fibrin degradation peptides from insoluble ^{125}I-labelled fibrin-coated multiwell dishes as previously described [15]. Molecular species of plasminogen activators were identified by electrophoretic and immunochemical procedures as previously described [2].

C. Results and Discussion

Immunochemical analysis showed that granulocytes from 23 normal individuals released urokinase exclusively. Cells from 24/117 patients with AML secreted tissue plasminogen activator, cells from 67/117 patients secreted urokinase, cells from 14/117 patients secreted a mixture of both enzymes and cells from 12/117 patients secreted too little enzyme for identification (Table 1). The molecular species of enzyme appeared to have prognostic significance since none of the patients whose cells secreted tissue plasminogen activator entered remission with chemotherapy whereas remission was induced in 80% of patients whose cells secreted urokinase. There was a significant difference in median survival between those patients whose cells secreted tissue plasminogen activator (5 weeks) and those individuals whose cells secreted

1 Department of Clinical Science and Immunology
2 Department of Haematology, University of Cape Town Medical School, Observatory 7925, South Africa
3 Henry Kaplan Award for the best poster Clinical Session

Table 1. Correlation between clinical outcome and molecular species of plasminogen activator released by cultured cells from 117 patients with AML

Therapy	Group	Response	Nature of plasminogen activator				Totals
			TA[a]	UK[b]	TA and UK	Unknown	
Combination chemotherapy	A	Assessment completed					
		Complete remission	0	32	7	5	44
		No remission	14	10	2	1	27
		(Subtotals)	(14)	(42)	(9)	(6)	(71)
	B	Died before assessment	5	14	4	3	26
No/palliative therapy	C		5	11	1	3	20
Totals			24	67	14	12	117

[a] TA tissue activator
[b] UK urokinase

urokinase (32 weeks). No significant differences in age or white blood cell count at the time of presentation were found between those patients whose cells secreted tissue plasminogen activator and urokinase. Cells from approximately 20% of patients with AML secreted tissue plasminogen activator.

Cells from 31 patients with CML were examined for species of plasminogen activator produced. Cells from 15/31 patients secreted tissue plasminogen activator, cells from only 7/31 secreted urokinase and cells from 9/31 secreted both species of enzyme. Thus, the proportion of patients with CML whose cells secreted tissue plasminogen activator was much higher than in the AML group and cells from only 23% of these individuals secreted urokinase.

Cells isolated from 89 patients with other myeloproliferative and preleukaemic disorders have also been investigated. Cells from 47/89 patients secreted tissue plasminogen activator, cells from 16/89 patients secreted urokinase and cells from the remainder secreted both enzyme species. Thus, the myeloproliferative disorders contain a far higher percentage of individuals whose cells secrete tissue plasminogen activator – the enzyme which is associated with a failure to respond to chemotherapy in patients with AML. This is of interest as it is well known that when patients with CML or myelodysplastic states transform, they have a poor prognosis and do not respond to chemotherapy. We are investigating the plasminogen activator status of our patients with myeloproliferative disorders at regular intervals in order to ascertain whether those patients with tissue plasminogen activator have a worse prognosis than those patients whose cells secrete urokinase. It appears as if the type of plasminogen activator secreted by leukaemic cells cultured in vitro will serve as a useful aid to prognosis for patients with AML and possibly also for patients with other myeloproliferative disorders.

References

1. Reich E (1978) Activation of plasminogen: a general mechanism for producing localized extracellular proteolysis. In: Molecular basis of biological degradative processes. Berlin RD, Herman H, Lefow IH, Tanzer JM (eds). Academic, New York, pp 155–169
2. Wilson EL, Becker MLB, Hoal EG, Dowdle EB (1980) Molecular species of plasminogen activators secreted by normal and neoplastic human cells. Cancer Res 40:933
3. Vetterlein D, Bell TE, Young PL, Roblin R (1980) Immunological quantitation and immunoadsorption of urokinase-like plasmin-

ogen activators secreted by human cells. J Biol Chem 255:2665
4. Astedt B, Wallen P, Aasted B (1979) Occurrence of both urokinase and tissue plasminogen activator in human seminal plasma. Throm Res 16:463
5. Wigler M, Ford JP, Weinstein IB (1975) Glucocorticoid inhibition of the fibrinolytic activity of tumour cells. In: Rifkin D, Reich E, Shaw E (eds) Proteases in biological control. Cold Spring Harbor, Cold Spring Harbor, N.Y. p 849
6. Vassalli JD, Hamilton J, Reich E (1977) Macrophage plasminogen activator; induction of concanavalin A and phorbol myristate acetate. Cell 11:695
7. Ossowski L, Biegel D, Reich E (1979) Mammary plasminogen activator: correlation with involution, hormonal modulation and comparison between normal and neoplastic tissue. Cell 16:929
8. Wilson EL, Dowdle EB (1980) Effects of retinoids on normal and neoplastic human cells cultured in vitro. Cancer Res 40:4817
9. Wilson EL, Reich E (1978) Plasminogen activator in chick fibroblasts: induction of synthesis by retinoic acid; synergism with viral transformation and phorbol ester. Cell 15:385
10. Wigler M, Weinstein IB (1976) Tumour promoter induces plasminogen activator. Nature 259:232
11. Rifkin D (1978) Plasminogen activator synthesis by cultured human embryonic lung cells: characterization of the suppressive effect of corticosteroids. J Cell Physiol 97:421
12. Baker JB, Low DA, Simmer RL and Cunningham DD (1980) Protease-nexin: a cellular component that links thrombin and plasminogen activator and mediates their binding to cells. Cell 21:37
13. Hoal EG, Wilson EL, Dowdle EB (1983) The regulation of tissue plasminogen activator activity by human fibroblasts. Cell 34:273
14. Wilson EL, Jacobs P, Dowdle EB (1983) The secretion of plasminogen activators by human myeloid leukemic cells in vitro. Blood 61:568
15. Wilson EL, Dowdle E (1978) Secretion of plasminogen activator by normal reactive and neoplastic human tissues cultured in vitro. Int J Cancer 22:390

Haematology and Blood Transfusion Vol. 29
Modern Trends in Human Leukemia VI
Edited by Neth, Gallo, Greaves, Janka

Immune Status of Leukemia Patients

Y. Kaneko[1], H. Miyakoshi[2], Y. Aoyagi[3], and T. Aoki[2]

A. Introduction

The immune status of patients with hematologic disorders, especially various leukemias, may fluctuate according to the clinical course, e.g., acute phase, chronic phase, remission, and smoldering stage. In particular, since leukemia involves a variety of white blood cells, including subsets of lymphocytes, immunologic function as well as general function should be greatly modified, influencing the host defense mechanisms [1]. In this study, nonspecific and specific immune activities of patients with various hematologic disorders were investigated in the different phases of disease.

B. Nonspecific Immune Activity

NK activity of peripheral mononuclear cells (PM-NC) against human myeloid K562 cells generally fell in patients with almost all kinds of hematologic disorders and even with solid tumors or chronic infections diseases (Fig. 1). On the contrary, spontaneous DNA synthesis of PM-NC tends to be elevated in patients with various leukemias, including acute myelogenous leukemia (AML), acute lymphocytic leukemia (ALL), and chronic myelogenous leukemia (CML), and with polycythemia vera, primary myelofibrosis, and primary thrombocythemia (Fig. 1). However, PM-NC from patients with aplastic anemia, paroxysmal nocturnal hemoglobinuria, and solid tumors showed a decrease in spontaneous DNA synthesis. In detail, PM-NC from patients with AML or ALL showed relatively high NK activity, even below the normal range in complete remission, but relatively low levels of spontaneous DNA synthesis in complete remission (Fig. 2).

When PM-NC from patients with leukemias were stimulated with three different mitogens, PHA, SPL (staphage lysate), and Con-A, mitogen-induced DNA synthesis generally fell, except for slight elevation in the complete remission of AML and ALL (Fig. 3). Particularly, when stimulated with PHA, these PM-NC showed clear elevation in PHA-induced DNA synthesis.

C. Specific Immune Activity

As summarized in Table 1, one leukemia patient, four lymphoma patients, and two patients with solid tumors were investigated for autochthonous cell-mediated cytotoxicity in comparison with NK activity of their PM-NC against K562 cells. PM-NC from patients with ATL or Burkitt's malignant lymphomas (patients 1 and 2) did not lyse their own tumor cells by either direct killer T cell-mediated cytotoxicity or antibody-dependent cellular cytotoxicity

1 Pharmaceutical Department, Ajinomoto Company, 1-5-8 Kyobashi, Chuoku, Tokyo 104, Japan
2 Research Division, Shinrakuen Hospital, 1-27 Nishiariakecho, Niigata 950-21, Japan
3 1st Department of Internal Medicine, Gunma University School of Medicine, 3-39-22 Shohwacho, Maebashi 371, Japan

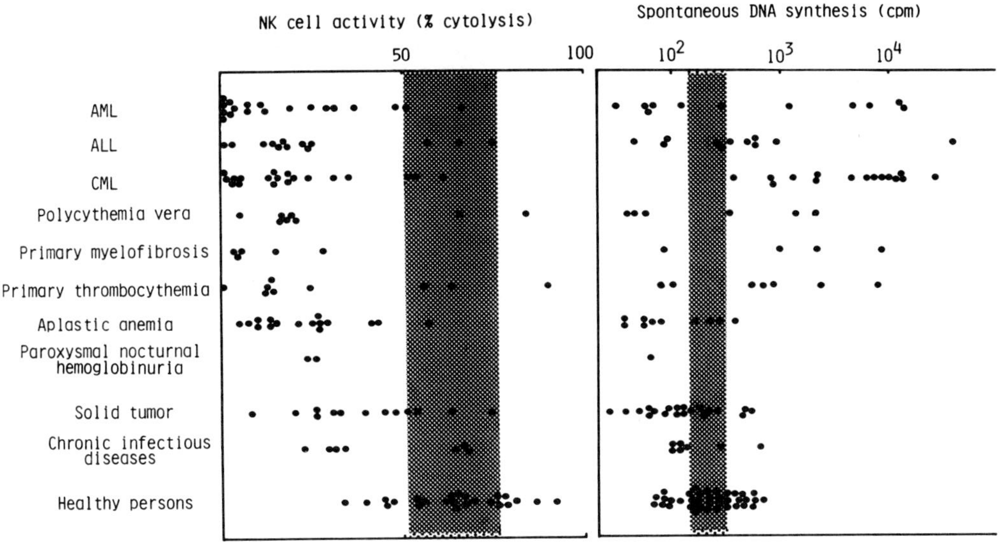

Fig. 1. NK activity and ^{3}H-TdR incorporation of peripheral mononuclear cells from leukemia patients

(ADCC) (Table 2), but showed significant NK activity. PM-NC from patients 3 and 4 with malignant lymphoma were positive for both ADCC and NK activity. Interestingly, PM-NC from patient 5 with T cell malignant lymphoma were negative for cell-mediated cytotoxicity (CMC) against malignant cells from the patient's own inguinal lymph nodes and positive for CMC against malignant cells from the patient's own neck lymph node, but positive for NK activity, suggesting a difference in the antigen specificity of malignant cells located in the different lymph nodes of a given patient. Another interesting fact is that PM-NC from patient 7 with paraganglioma were positive for both CMC and NK activity, but mononuclear cells from the malignant tissue were positive for CMC against the patient's own malignant cells, but negative for NK activity. These results

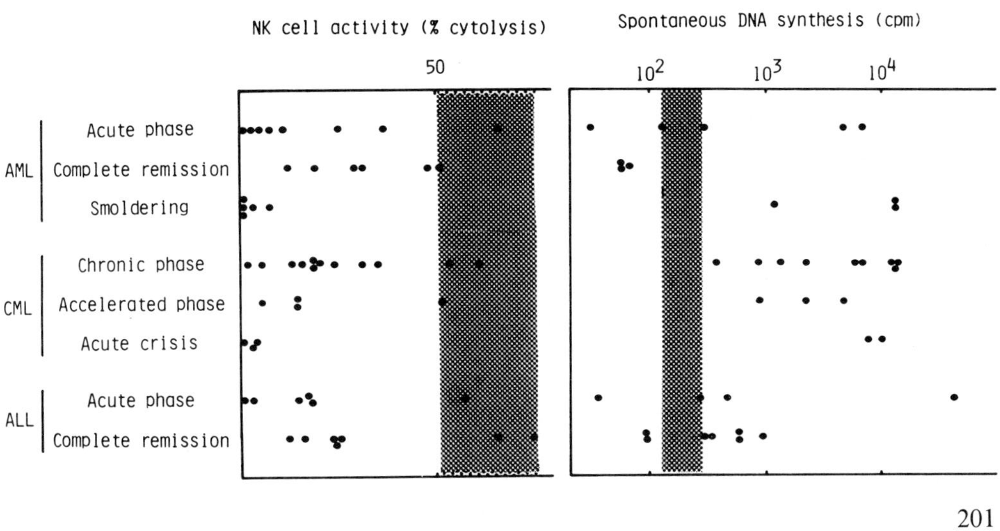

Fig. 2. NK activity and ^{3}H-TdR incorporation of peripheral mononuclear cells from leukemia patients in various phases

suggest that specific, cytotoxic effector cells selectively penetrated into the malignant tissue, or that, since morphologically these cells are large granular lymphocytes, there may be at least two different NK cell subsets one of which possesses such a specific CMC, but no NK activity and another which possesses NK activity, but no specific CMC [2].

In the light of this specific CMC, the following important observations seem appropriate: (a) tumor cells in different regional foci of one patient possess individual tumor-specific cell surface antigens; and (b) at least two different subgroups of cytotoxic mononuclear cells, even in the same subset, separately recognize individual cell surface antigens. In future, therefore, the immunotherapy of cancer might be achieved by combination of various specific antibodies, various effector cells of the subset, or several subsets of effector cells.

D. Remarks

The spontaneous DNA synthesis of PM-NC from most patients with hematologic disorders was higher than the normal level.

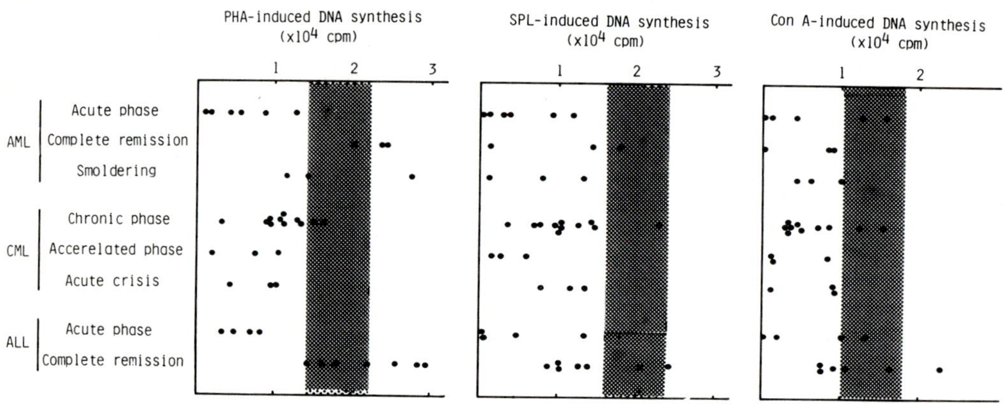

Fig. 3. Mitogen-induced DNA synthesis of peripheral mononuclear cells from leukemia patients in various phases

Table 1. Cell-mediated immunity in the autochthonous system of patients with malignant diseases

Patient No.	Diagnosis	Source of target malignant cells	Cell-mediated cytotoxicity to tumor cells	NK activity to K562 cells
1	Adult T-cell leukemia	Subcutaneous tumor of leg	(−)	(+)
2	Malignant lymphoma (Burkitt's)	Neck lymph node	(−)	(+)
3	Malignant lymphoma		(+) (ADCC)	(+)
4	Malignant lymphoma		(+) (ADCC)	(+)
5	Malignant lymphoma (T cell type)	Neck lymph node	(+) (Killer T?)	(+)
		Inguinal lymph nodes	(−)	
6	Metastatic squamous cell carcinoma	Neck lymph node	(±) (Killer T?)	(+)
7	Paraganglioma	Subcutaneous tumor of arm	(+) (Effector cell in tumor cells)	(−)
			(+) (PM-NC)	(+)

Table 2. Killer activity of peripheral mononuclear cells (PM-NC) from patients with malignant diseases

Target cells	Plasma	PM-NC donors: Adult T-cell leukemia (in remission) Patient 1	Malignant lymphoma: Patient 2	Patient 3	Patient 4	Patient 5: Neck tumor	Patient 5: Inguinal tumor	Metastatic squamous cell carcinoma Patient-6
Patient's own tumor cells	Patient's own	0.9[a]	3.7	*12.1*	*16.7*	*43.3*	7.0	9.1
	Healthy donor	0	9.1	–2.5	–13.4	*25.5*	0	*21.4*
	Pooled AB	N.D.[b]	10.3	5.4	–15.4	*35.1*	5.6	*19.8*
	Fetal calf serum	0.9	N.D.	N.D.	–22.9	1.4	15.5	N.D.
K562 cells	Patients own	*51.9*	*25.6*	*70.3*	*79.6*	*77.5*		*79.6*
	Healthy donor	*59.3*	*30.1*	*72.8*	*91.3*	*91.9*		N.D.
	Pooled AB	N.D.	*28.7*	*53.9*	*67.2*	*80.2*		*77.5*
	Fetal calf serum	N.D.	N.D.	N.D.	N.D.	*80.0*		N.D.

[a] Percentage cytolysis (target : PMNC = 1 : 40)
[b] Not done

This suggests that PM-NC with normal morphology from these patients may be functionally abnormal like those in the preleukemic stage, since PM-NC from most carriers of human T cell leukemia/lymphoma virus type I (HTLV-I) showed increased spontaneous DNA synthesis without malignant transformation [3]. HTLV-I infection may also change the function of PM-NC in HTLV-I carriers [4]. Even though no morphological changes occurred in the PM-NC, DNA synthesis became maximal so that a further increase in DNA synthesis was not induced by mitogen stimulation.

In terms of spontaneous DNA synthesis and NK activity of PM-NC, smoldering AML and CML are quite similar to each other, as described. Accordingly, these two diseases might be considered as one, especially from a nonspecific immunologic point of view [2]. The specificity of cell surface antigens, humoral antibodies, and CMC is very complicated indeed. Thus, diagnosis and treatment of leukemias by immunologic methods are extremely hard to establish. In particular, the immunotherapy of malignancies is not simple, but should be investigated from sophisticated and multiple standpoints.

References

1. Aoki T, Miyakoshi H, Horikawa Y, Shibata A, Aoyagi Y, Mizukoshi M (1982) Interaction between interferon and natural killer cells in humans after administration of immunomodulating agents. In: Herberman RB (ed) NK cells and other natural effector cells. Academic, New York, pp 1291–1302
2. Aoki T, Shibata A, Aoyagi Y, Miyakoshi H (1982) Immune status in leukemia patients. In: Yohn DS, Blakeslee JR (eds) Advances in comparative leukemia research 1981. Elsevier North Holland, Amsterdam, pp 547–549
3. Miyakoshi H, Aoki T (1984) Immunological study of HTLV-I-infected hosts. In: Aoki T, Tsubura E, Urushizaki I (eds) Manipulation of host defence mechanisms. Excerpta Medica, Amsterdam, pp 152–161
4. Miyakoshi H, Koide H, Aoki T (1984) *In vitro* antibody-dependent cellular cytotoxicity against human T-cell leukemia/lymphoma virus (HTLV)-producing cells. Int J Cancer 33:287–291

Haematology and Blood Transfusion Vol. 29
Modern Trends in Human Leukemia VI
Edited by Neth, Gallo, Greaves, Janka

Differential Expression of a Glycoprotein (p15E-RT) of Retroviral Origin in Patients Suffering from Various Hematological Disorders

P. C. Jacquemin [1]

A. Introduction

Sequences coding for human endogenous reverse transcriptases (RT) were recently identified in normal human DNA with the use of cDNA clones shown to be homologous to MuLV enzyme [1–3]. The expression of some of these endogenous retrovirus genes was also shown at the RNA level [4]. Earlier molecules with enzymatic properties of RT had been identified in the tissues of some leukemic patients [5–7]. We previously reported the presence of antibodies recognizing specific type C virus RT associated with the membrane of some hematopoetic cells, principally in leukemic patients, but also in some normal individuals [8, 9]. More recently, we purified a protein of 74 kilodaltons containing retroviral RT and p15E determinants [10]. This protein was purified to homogeneity and a specific radioimmunoassay was developed, allowing us to quantitate the level of this protein in the plasma of patients in various hematologic situations [11]. The level of the protein appeared elevated in hematologic situations where a stimulation of hematopoietic tissues was happening or was needed.

B. Results

A glycoprotein of 74 kilodaltons was purified to homogeneity from the plasma of a CML patient with the use of newly developed monoclonal antibodies. A similar protein was also partially purified from the plasma of a normal individual. This protein was analyzed immunologically with a battery of antibodies (hyperimmune and monoclonals) and was shown to contain RT and p15E antigenic determinants of retroviruses (Table 1).

By specific radioimmunoassay, the level of this protein was measured in normal individuals (25.5 μg/ml) and in various hematologic situations (Table 2). We could not correlate the level of the protein with the white blood cell count (WBC). Some leukemic patients with high WBC had a high level of antigen (patients with CML-BC, myeloproliferative syndromes, and acute leukemias) while others in bone marrow depletion harbored a high level of antigen (patients with aplastic anemia and congenital neutropenia). On the contrary, some patients who had undergone an intensive course of chemotherapy had a low level of antigen in their plasma. Follow-up studies of patients receiving chemotherapy are under way.

C. Discussion

The level of the 74 kilodaltons glycoprotein that we purified which contained RT and p15E of retroviruses, was measured in various patients. A high level (> 50 μg per milliliter plasma) appeared to correlate with a necessity of enhancement of hematopoietic cell proliferation or with an actual stimulation of cell proliferation. High levels of

1 Institut Pasteur du Brabant, Department of Virology, rue Engeland, 642, 1180 Brussels, Belgium

Table 1. Summary of the antibody results against the 74 kilodaltons glycoprotein

Source of antibodies	74 kilodaltons glycoprotein	
	Poly-G purified	Poly-G + Immuno-affinity purified
Normal sera: Rabbit, goat, mouse, cat, gibbon, human	– / – / – / – / – / –	– / – / – / – / – / –
Goat anti-SiSVp30, SiSVgp70	+ / –	– / –
Goat anti-HTLVp24	–	–
Rabbit anti-MuLVp30, MuLVgp70	– / –	– / –
Rabbit anti-FeLVp15E, anti-FeLVp15	+ / –	+ / –
Rabbit anti-RT of MuLV, BaEV, RD114, SiSV	+ / – / – / –	+ / – / – / –
Cat anti-FeLV RT	–	–
Gibbon anti-GaLV RT	–	–
Human anti-HLA (BW17, BW4,A2)	– / – / –	– / – / –
Rabbit anti-human α_1-glycoprotein	–	–
Rabbit anti-human albumin	–	–
Monoclonal antibodies:		
Mouse anti-MuLVp 15E	+	+
Mouse anti-MuLVgp70	–	–
Rat anti-MuLVp15	–	–
Rat anti-MuLVp30	–	–
Mouse anti-BaEVgp70	–	–
Mouse anti-BaEVp15	–	–
Mouse anti-HTLVp19	–	–
Newly developed mouse anti-74 kilodalton glycoprotein	+	+

Table 2. Plasma level of 74 kilodaltons glycoprotein in different hematologic situations

Clinical diagnosis	Cases	Age (years)	WBC/µl	Glycoprotein (µg/ml) (extreme values)
Normal individuals	10	22–52	5 000– 13 000	10– 37
Cord blood	10			8– 30
CML-BC	5	37–77	25 000–150 000	51–350
Myeloproliferative syndromes	3	55–61	11 000– 78 000	96–234
Myelofibrose	1	66	50 000	20
Acute leukemia	3	20–75	17 000–250 000	50–100
Aplastic anemia	3	11–60	~2 000	90–100
Congenital neutropenia	1	16	Low	125
Myeloma	1	60	3 400	90
ALL (post allogeneic bone marrow transplantation)	1	16	2 500	350
Post chemotherapy				
CML-BC	2	25–59	4 000– 8 000	2–3
AML	1	44	3 600	4
ALL	1	6	5 600	4

antigen were also recorded in patients with bone marrow aplasia as well as in patients in leukemia with high leukocyte counts. We tentatively explained the presence of this 74 kilodaltons glycoprotein as being a growth factor, maybe in an unprocessed form. This protein will be tested in vitro for different growth stimulation properties.

Acknowledgments. We thank Dr. R. C. Gallo, Dr. M. Essex, Dr. W. Hardy, and Dr. J. Portis for providing the various antiviral protein antisera, and Dr. P. Strijckmans for providing clinical samples.

References

1. Martin MA, Bryan T, Rasheed S, Khan AF (1981) Proc Natl Acad Sci USA 78:4892
2. Bonner TI, O'Connell C, Cohen M (1982) Proc Natl Acad Sci USA 79:4709
3. Repaske R, O'Neill RR, Steele PE, Martin MA (1983) Proc Natl Acad Sci USA 80:678
4. Rabson AB, Steele PE, Garon CF, Martin MA (1983) Nature 306:604
5. Sarngadharan MG, Sarin PS, Reitz MS, Gallo RC (1972) Nature New Biol 240:67
6. Todaro GJ, Gallo RC (1973) Nature 244:206
7. Witkin SS, Ohno T, Spiegelman S (1975) Proc Natl Acad Sci USA 72:4133
8. Jacquemin PC, Saxinger C, Gallo RC (1978) Nature 176:230
9. Jacquemin PC (1981) Eur J Cancer Clin Oncol 17:1283
10. Jacquemin PC (1983) Haematology and Blood Transfusion, vol 28, Modern trends in human leukemia V. Springer, Heidelberg, p 282
11. Jacquemin PC, Strijckmans P, Thiry L (1984) Blood 64:832

Haematology and Blood Transfusion Vol. 29
Modern Trends in Human Leukemia VI
Edited by Neth, Gallo, Greaves, Janka

Discrimination of Leukemias, Lymphomas, and Non-Neoplastic Controls by Retroviral Serum Markers

R. Hehlmann[1], M. A. Schreiber[2], G. Kreeb[1], V. Erfle[3], W. Weber[4], and P. Obrecht[4]

A. Introduction

Diagnostic and prognostic markers are urgently needed for early diagnosis and therapy of malignant neoplasias. One solution of this problem is the search for etiologic factors in the hope that they might indicate the presence or degree of progression of the disease. One possible factor are the retroviruses which are known to cause certain malignancies in several animal species [1]. These malignancies include leukemias, lymphomas, and sarcomas. Footprints of retroviruses have also been repeatedly described in man, and retroviral isolates have been grown from human neoplastic and non-neoplastic cells. These viral isolates include not only the human T lymphotropic viruses (HTLV-I–III), but also viruses that are very similar to the primate retroviruses simian sarcoma virus (SiSV) and baboon endogenous virus (BaEV) [2, 3, 6].

We have shown over the past few years that antigens and antibodies that are related to structural proteins of these primate viruses are present in human sera [4] and possibly possess prognostic relevance. For instance, one can correlate the presence of antigens and immune complexes that are related to the envelope glycoprotein gp70 of SiSV with shorter survival and poorer response to therapy in acute leukemias and chronic myelogenous leukemias in blast crisis [5]. We have therefore examined whether such retroviral markers, possibly in combination, can be utilized for diagnostic purposes.

1 Medizinische Poliklinik der Universität München, FRG
2 ISB der Universität München, FRG
3 Abteilung für Pathologie der GSF, Neuherberg, FRG
4 Abteilung für Onkologie, Kantonsspital Basel, CH

B. Materials and Methods

I. Patients

Sera from patients with leukemias, lymphomas, and from control subjects without neoplastic disease were treated with 5% trasylol and stored at $-20\,°C$. If possible, sera obtained at diagnosis or prior to treatment were used.

II. Antigens and Antibodies

p30 core proteins and gp70 envelope glycoproteins were prepared from purified SiSV and BaEV as described [7, 8]. Polyvalent antisera were prepared by injecting the purified viral antigens into rabbits [7]. Monoclonal antibodies (MoAB) against BaEV gp70 were the gift of Dr. L. Thiry, Liège, Belgium.

III. ELISA

The examination of the sera for cross-reacting antigens, antibodies (IgG and IgM), and immune complexes (IgG and IgM) was done with the enzyme-linked immuno-

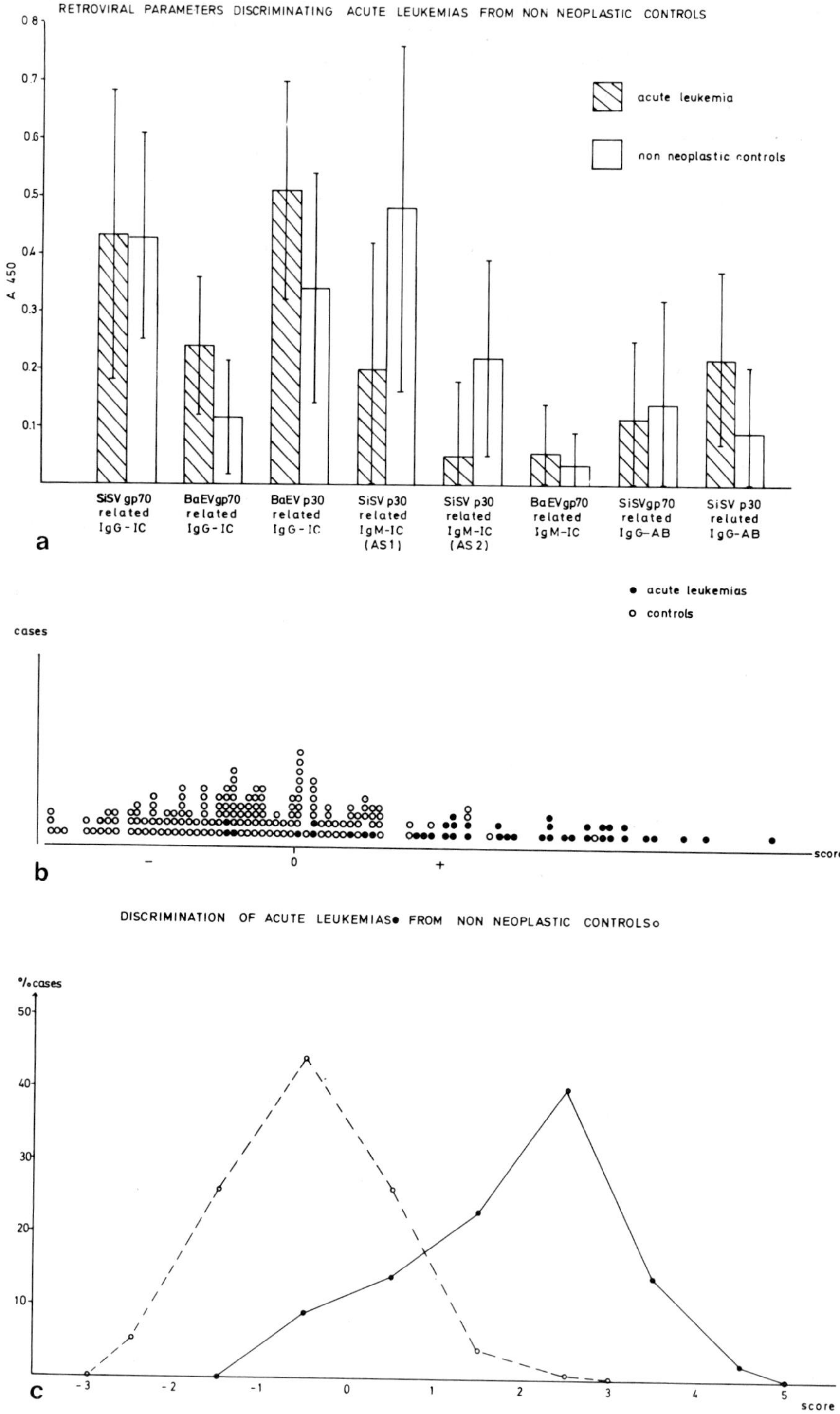

RETROVIRAL PARAMETERS DISCRIMINATING ACUTE LEUKEMIAS FROM NON NEOPLASTIC CONTROLS
A 450
acute leukemia
non neoplastic controls
SiSV gp70 related IgG-IC
BaEVgp70 related IgG-IC
BaEV p30 related IgG-IC
SiSV p30 related IgM-IC (AS1)
SiSV p30 related IgM-IC (AS2)
BaEVgp70 related IgM-IC
SiSVgp70 related IgG-AB
SiSV p30 related IgG-AB
a
acute leukemias
controls
cases
score
b
DISCRIMINATION OF ACUTE LEUKEMIAS FROM NON NEOPLASTIC CONTROLS
% cases
score
c

Table 1. Parameters for the discrimination of acute leukemias

a) Acute leukemias ($N=43$) vs controls ($N=154$)		
Parameters		
Immune complexes:	SiSV gp70 IgG	Sensitivity 82.4%
	BaEV gp70 IgG	Specificity 88.1%
	BaEV p30 IgG	
	SiSV p30 IgM (AS 1)	
	SiSV p30 IgM (AS 2)	
	BaEV gp70 IgM	
Antibodies	SiSV p30 IgG	
	SiSV gp70 IgG	
b) Acute leukemias ($N=43$) vs malignant lymphomas ($N=46$)		
Parameters		
Antigen	BaEV gp70 (MoAB)	Sensitivity 78.3%
Immune complexes	SiSV p30 IgG	Specificity 90.7%
	BaEV p30 IgG	
Antibodies	SiSV gp70 IgG	
	SiSV p30 IgG	
	BaEV gp70 IgG	
c) Acute leukemias ($N=43$) vs sarcomas ($N=17$)		
Parameters		
Antigen	BaEV gp70 (MoAB)	Sensitivity 100.0%
Antibodies	SiSV gp70 IgG	Specificity 97.7%
	SiSV p30 IgG	
	SiSV gp70 IgM	

sorbent assay (ELISA) technique [7, 8]; Kreeb et al., in preparation). For the detection of antigen-specific immune complexes, assays with immune and with preimmune sera were carried out in parallel. The extinction values obtained with the preimmune sera were subtracted from the values obtained with the immune sera (Kreeb et al., in preparation).

C. Results

We examined serum samples from 43 patients with acute leukemias, and from 46 patients with malignant lymphomas for antigens, antibodies (IgG and IgM), and immune complexes (IgG and IgM) that cross-react with the p30 core proteins and the gp70 envelope glycoproteins of SiSV and of BaEV and tried to distinguish the sera from each other and from three control groups (154 non-neoplastic controls, 10 benign lymphadenopathies, and 17 sarcomas). The enzyme-linked immunosorbent assay (ELISA) technique served as test system. The assay results were then subjected to stepwise discriminant analysis, and a score was determined. The results are shown in Tables 1 and 2.

Fig. 1a–c. Stepwise discriminant analysis of acute leukemias versus non-neoplastic controls. **a** means and standard deviations of the test results of each test parameter with acute leukemias and with controls; **b** scores calculated from the results with the test parameters for each individual leukemic and control sera; **c** distribution curves of leukemias and controls

I. Acute Leukemias

Acute leukemias can be distinguished from non-neoplastic controls with a sensitivity of 79.1% and a specificity of 90.9% (20.9% false negatives and 9.1% false positives) by eight parameters (Table 1a). The parameters are: IgG immune complexes related to SiSV gp70, BaEV gp70, and BaEV p30;

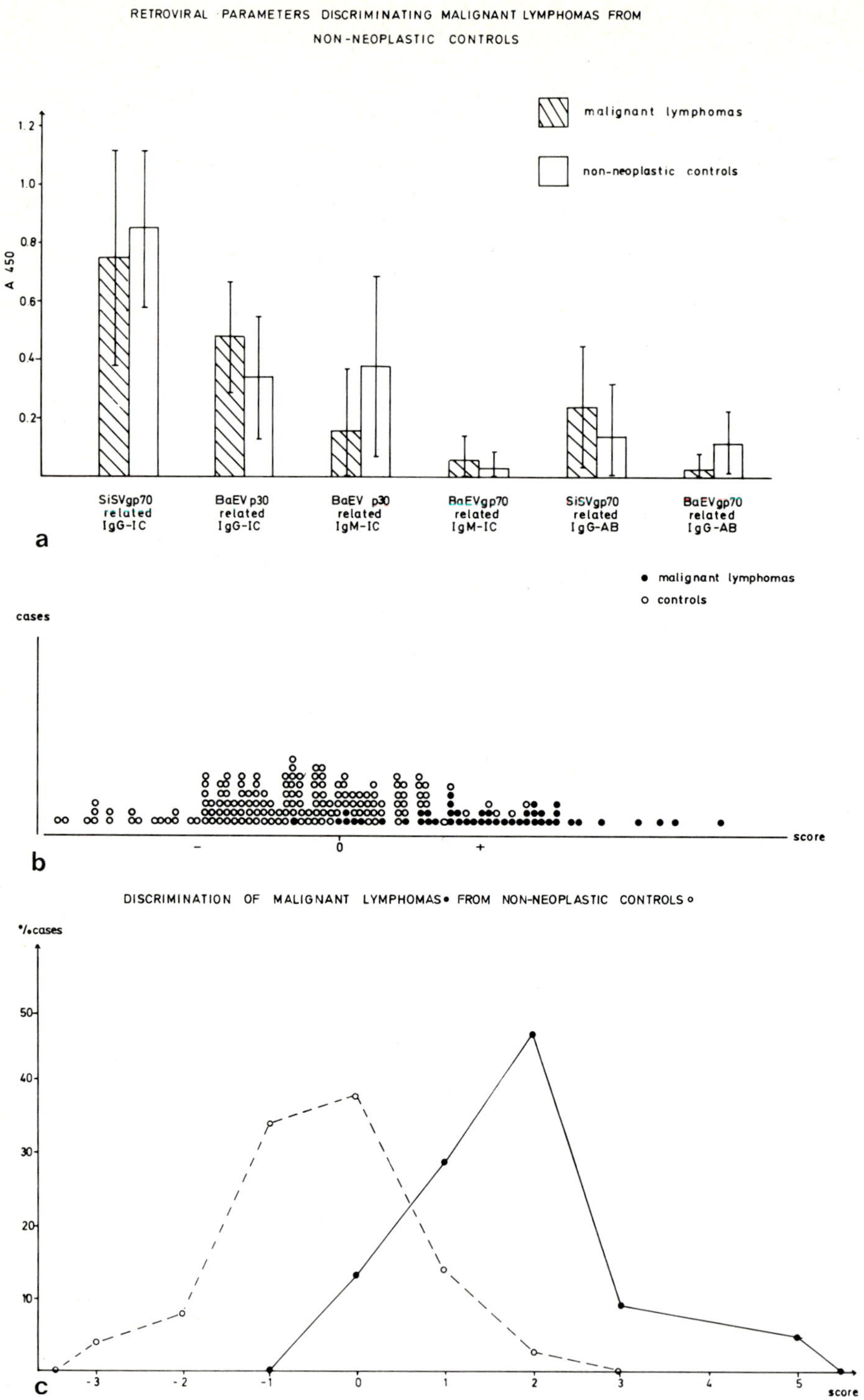

RETROVIRAL PARAMETERS DISCRIMINATING MALIGNANT LYMPHOMAS FROM NON-NEOPLASTIC CONTROLS
malignant lymphomas
non-neoplastic controls
A 450
1.2
1.0
0.8
0.6
0.4
0.2
SiSVgp70 related IgG-IC
BaEV p30 related IgG-IC
BaEV p30 related IgM-IC
BaEVgp70 related IgM-IC
SiSVgp70 related IgG-AB
BaEVgp70 related IgG-AB
a
• malignant lymphomas
o controls
cases
–
0
+
score
b
DISCRIMINATION OF MALIGNANT LYMPHOMAS • FROM NON-NEOPLASTIC CONTROLS o
%cases
50
40
30
20
10
-3
-2
-1
0
1
2
3
4
5
score
c

Table 2. Parameters for the discrimination of malignant lymphomas

a) Malignant lymphomas ($N=46$) vs controls ($N=154$)		
Parameters		
Immune complexes	SiSV gp70 IgG	Sensitivity 84.4%
	BaEV p30 IgG	Specificity 83.3%
	BAEV p30 IgM	
	BaEV gp70 IgM	
Antibodies	SiSV gp70 IgG	
	BaEV gp70 IgG	
b) Malignant lymphomas ($N=46$) vs benign lymphomas ($N=10$)		
Parameters		
Antigen	BaEV gp70 (MoAB)	Sensitivity 97.8%
Immune complexes	BaEV p30 IgG	Specificity 70.0%
	BaEV p30 IgM	
Antibodies	SiSV gp70 IgM	
c) Malignant lymphomas ($N=46$) vs sarcomas ($N=17$)		
Parameters		
Antibodies	SiSV gp70 IgM	Sensitivity 100.0%
	BaEV gp70 IgG	Specificity 94.1%
Antigen	BaEV gp70 (MoAB)	
	SiSV gp70 (rabbit AB)	
Antibodies	SiSV gp70 IgG	

IgM immune complexes related to SiSV p30 and BaEV gp70; and IgG antibodies cross-reacting with SiSV gp70 and SiSV p30. The means and standard deviations of the test results of each parameter with the acute leukemia group and with the control group are shown in Fig. 1a. The scores that are assigned to each leukemic and control serum were plotted and are shown in Fig. 1b. The good separation of the two groups is evident. In Fig. 1c, the numbers of patients per score unit are plotted, showing the relatively small overlap of the two groups. Similarly, acute leukemias were distinguished from malignant lymphomas with a sensitivity of 78.3% and a specificity of 90.7% by six parameters, and from sarcomas with a sensitivity of 100% and a specificity of 97.7% by the combination of four parameters (Table 1b and c).

Fig. 2a–c. Stepwise discriminant analysis of malignant lymphomas versus non-neoplastic controls. **a** means and standard deviations of the test results of each test parameter with malignant lymphomas and controls; **b** scores calculated from the results with the test parameters for individual lymphoma and control sera; **c** distribution curves of lymphomas and controls

II. Malignant Lymphomas

Malignant lymphomas are distinguished from non-neoplastic controls with a sensitivity of 84.4% and a specificity of 83.3% (15.6% false negatives and 16.7% false positives) by six parameters (Table 2a). The parameters are: IgG immune complexes related to SiSV gp70; IgG and IgM immune complexes related to BaEV p30; IgM immune complexes related to BaEV gp70; and IgG antibodies cross-reacting with SiSV gp70 and with BaEV gp70. The means and standard deviations of the test results of each of the six parameters with the malignant lymphoma group and with the control group are shown in Fig. 2a. Figure 2 also shows the scores of each serum as individual values (Fig. 2b) and as curves (Fig. 2c) as described. The distinction between malignant lymphomas and benign lymphadenopathies is depicted in Table 2b and Fig. 3. Malignant lymphomas are distinguished from benign lymphadenopathies with a sensitivity of 97.8% and a specificity of 70% by four parameters (Table 2b). The four parameters are: BaEV gp70-related antigen (as determined by monoclonal antibodies); IgG and IgM im-

RETROVIRAL PARAMETERS DISCRIMINATING MALIGNANT LYMPHOMAS FROM BENIGN LYMPHOMAS

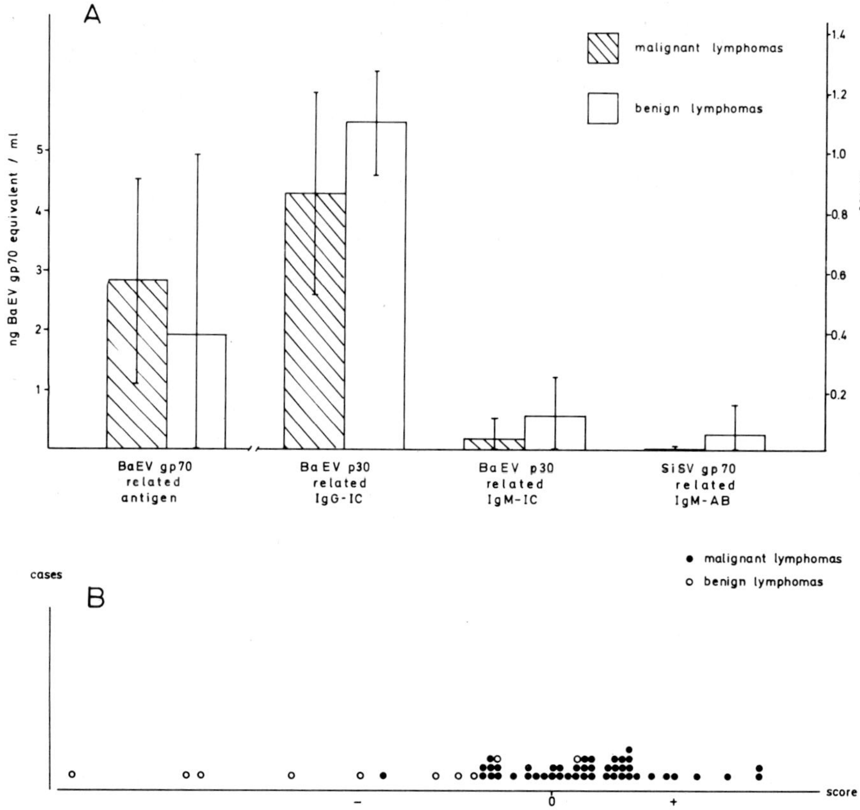

DISCRIMINATION OF MALIGNANT LYMPHOMAS ● FROM BENIGN LYMPHOMAS ○

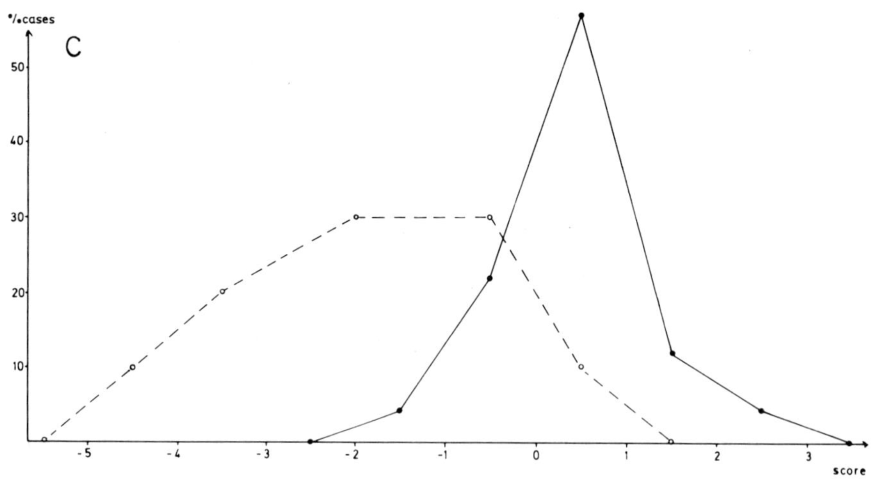

Fig. 3A–C. Stepwise discriminant analysis of malignant lymphomas versus benign lymphadenopathies. **A** means and standard deviations of the test results of each test parameter with malignant and benign lymphomas; **B** scores calculated from the results with the test parameters for individual lymphoma sera; **C** distribution curves of malignant and benign lymphomas

mune complexes related to BaEV p30; and IgM antibodies cross-reacting with SiSV gp70. Means and standard deviations of the test results with the individual test parameters (Fig. 3a), calculated scores as individual values (Fig. 3b), and as curves (Fig. 3c) are shown as already explained. Sarcomas are distinguished from malignant lymphomas with a sensitivity of 100% and a specificity of 94.1% by five test parameters (Table 2c): BaEV gp70-related antigen as determined by monoclonal antibodies; SiSV gp70-related antigen (by rabbit antiserum); IgG antibodies cross-reacting with BaEV gp70 and SiSV gp70; and IgM antibodies cross-reacting with SiSV gp70.

D. Discussion

On the basis of animal experiments, studies have been performed for several years to elucidate the etiologic role of retroviruses in human cancers, especially leukemias and lymphomas [1]. The first human candidate virus HTLV-I has been isolated and described by Gallo and co-workers [2], which can be regarded as the cause of T cell leukemias in humans in endemic areas. The detection of SiSV- and BaEV-related viruses or structural components of these primate viruses in human tissues or sera has been described independently by several groups [2, 3]. Their origin and their relevance for human malignancies has not been elucidated. Their ubiquitous appearance in humans makes it reasonable to regard them as of endogenous origin. This is supported by the description of homologous gene sequences to MuLV and BaEV [9, 10]. As with other endogenous retroviral entities, their etiologic role in tumors is likely, but far from being proven.

In human leukemias, we have detected a significant coincidence between the presence of cross-reacting envelope proteins of SiSV/SSAV and a poor prognosis and resistance to therapy [5]. We now describe the possibility of distinguishing certain human malignancies of mesenchymal origin on the basis of the presence of a number of primate retroviral markers. These include viral related antigens and antibodies and especially virus-specific immune complexes. The discrimination between the different patient groups or between patient groups and the control group could only be achieved with a certain number of parameters, but discrimination was unexpectedly high in comparison with other parameters used as special tumor markers. It is interesting to note the dominant role of virus-specific immune complexes of IgG and IgM classes in every discriminating pattern. This further supports the possible role of immune complex formation in the course of malignant diseases.

These results are a promising step in the direction of better diagnosis and more detailed classification of certain mesenchymal tumors. A prospective study is necessary to establish these parameters as diagnostic and prognostic factors. This may also be improved by the use of monoclonal antibodies, which is indicated by the fact that BaEV gp70 as detected by a monoclonal antibody has been included twice in discrimination patterns. Last, but not least, the prognostic and diagnostic relevance of the retroviral structures described here can be used as an argument for their possible etiologic significance in mesenchymal neoplasias.

Acknowledgments. This study was supported by the Bundesminister für Forschung und Technologie (BMFT-Projekt NT/A-MT 0299 01 ZO 0585). The authors thank Mrs. U. Böck for assistance with the tests and the documentation of the test results.

References

1. Gross L (1983) Oncogenic viruses, 3rd edn. Pergamon, Oxford
2. Gallo RC, Wong-Staal F, Ruscetti F (1982) Viruses and adult leukemia-lymphoma of

man and relevant animal models. In: Bloomfield CD (ed) Adult leukemias, pp 1–41

3. Hehlmann R, Schetters H, Kreeb G, Erfle V, Schmidt J, Luz A (1983a) RNA-tumorviruses, oncogenes, and their possible role in human carcinogenesis. Klin Wochenschr 61:1217–1231
4. Hehlmann R, Schetters H, Erfle V, Leib-Mösch C (1983b) Detection and biochemical characterization of antigens in human leukemic sera that cross-react with primate C-type viral proteins (M_r 30,000). Cancer Res 43:392–399
5. Hehlmann R, Erfle V, Schetters H, Luz A, Rohmer H, Schreiber MA, Essers U, Pralle H, Weber W (1984) Antigens and circulating immune complexes related to the primate retroviral-glycoprotein SiSV gp70: Indicators of early mortality in human acute leukemias and chronic myelogenous leukemia in blast crisis. Cancer 54:2927–2935
6. Popovic M, Sarngadharan MG, Read E, Gallo RC (1984) Detection, isolation, and continuous production of cytopathic retroviruses (HTLV-III) from patients with AIDS and pre-AIDS. Science 224:497–500
7. Schetters H, Hehlmann R, Erfle V, Ramanarayanan M (1980) Detection and quantification of type C viral proteins in tissues and sera with an enzyme immunoassay. Infect Immun 29:972–980
8. Schetters H, Hehlmann R, Erfle V (1981) ELISA for the detection and quantification of C-type viral glycoprotein (gp70) using antibodies that recognize the protein moieties of the glycoproteins. J Virol Methods 2:357–366
9. O'Brien SJ, Bonner TI, Cohen M, O'Connell C, Nash WG (1983) Mapping of an endogenous retroviral sequence to human chromosome 18. Nature 303:74–77
10. O'Connell C, O'Brien S, Nash WG, Cohen M (1984) ERV3, a full length human endogenous provirus: chromosomal localization and evolutionary relationships. Virology 138:225–235

Mechanism of Malignant Transformation

Cellular Human Oncogens, Chromosomes, and Viruses, Implication for Leukemia and Lymphoma

Haematology and Blood Transfusion Vol. 29
Modern Trends in Human Leukemia VI
Edited by Neth, Gallo, Greaves, Janka

Modulation of Gene Expression Through DNA-Binding Proteins: Is There a Regulatory Code?

M. Beato [1]

Introduction

The information stored in the DNA of a fertilized egg can be divided into two different classes: structural information, required for the synthesis of all macromolecules that build up the organism, and regulatory information, needed to modulate the expression of the structural information in time and space, that means during the development of the different tissues. The connection between the two types of information is provided by regulatory macromolecules, that are of course encoded in the structural information and regulate its expression through interaction with regulatory elements of the DNA, thus closing the information cycle (Fig. 1).

The structural information is stored in the DNA in the form of the genetic code that was unraveled in the 1960s. Part of the structural information are the signals for initiation and termination of transcription and translation, as well as the signals for RNA modification and splicing. On the other hand, little is known about the molecular mechanisms by which regulatory information is stored in the DNA. The general idea, however, is that recognition of specific features of the DNA molecule by regulatory DNA-binding macromolecules is essential for regulation. What exactly is recognized on the DNA and how the interaction modulates gene expression are the questions to be answered.

During the past decade, several DNA-binding regulatory proteins from prokaryotes have been purified to homogeneity, and their structure as well as their interaction with DNA have been studied in great detail. A comparison of the amino acid sequence of 13 DNA-binding regulatory proteins reveals two regions of homology overlapping the known DNA-binding domains (Fig. 2; [1, 2]). Interestingly, mutants that disturb the binding of the *lac*-repressor to the operator are clustered around these two regions [1].

The secondary, tertiary, and quaternary structure of several DNA-binding regulatory proteins from bacteria and bacteriophages exhibit striking similarities in their DNA-binding domains [2]. Not only are these proteins symmetric dimers or tetramers, but they contain a pair of twofold related α-helices connected by a β-turn that are responsible for most of the contacts with the B-form of the DNA double helix.

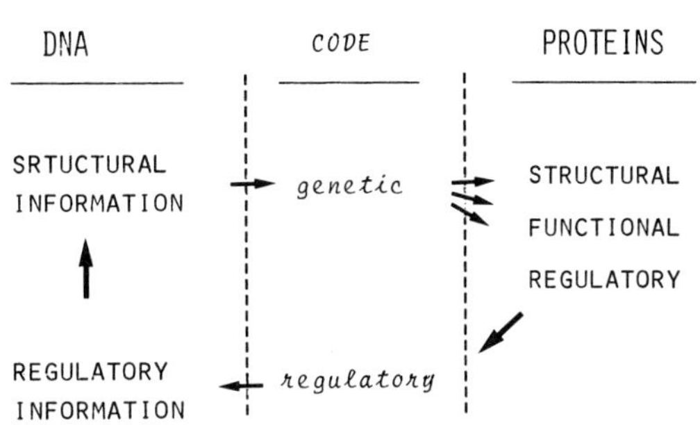

Fig. 1. The information cycle

1 Physiologisch-Chemisches Institut I der Philipps-Universität, Emil-Mannkopff-Str. 1–2, 3550 Marburg, FRG

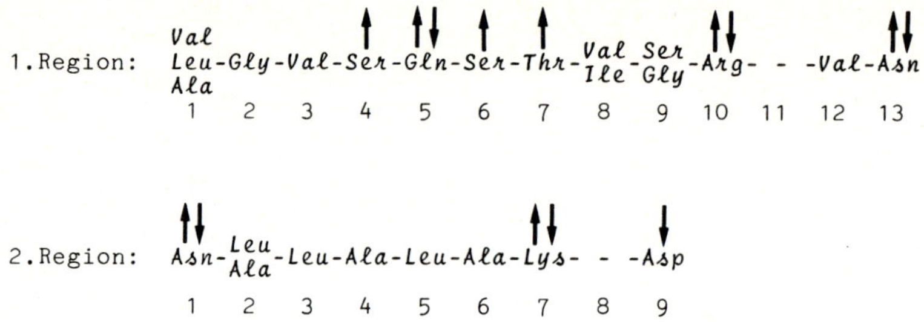

Fig. 2. Regions of homology among 13 prokaryotic DNA-binding regulatory proteins

One α-helix fits into the major groove of DNA while the other lies across it, holding it in position. If one looks at the relevant α-helices along their longitudinal axis, one observes that the orientation of the amino acid side chains exhibits a clear polarity. That means that the nonpolar amino acid side chains are oriented toward one side of the α-helix, whereas the polar and charged amino acid side chains are oriented toward the other side of the helix. This would be the site that contacts the DNA major groove.

This brief summary on the structure of prokaryotic regulatory proteins suggests that a basic protein structure has originated in evolution that can fulfill the requirements for DNA recognition. The actual function of a particular regulatory protein may depend on other domains of the protein that mediate the interaction with different modulator molecules.

As for the DNA sequences that are recognized by the regulatory proteins, they also show considerable homology. Two types of conserved sequences can be derived from a comparison of 23 sites recognized by 13 regulatory proteins [1].

I. TGTGT N_{6-10} ACACA
II. CAC N_{5-10} GTG

Both consensus sequences show a twofold rotational symmetry as expected from DNA sites recognized by dimeric or tetrameric proteins. Both conserved sequences are also similar in that they are composed of two short blocks (3–5 base pairs) of well-conserved nucleotides separated by a more variable region (7–8 base pairs on average). This structure of the binding sites is compatible with a model according to which the regulatory proteins contact the DNA only from one side and interact with two consecutive turns of the double helix (see later discussion). Most of the mutations that prevent binding of a particular regulatory protein to its binding site are located within the strictly conserved regions. It is striking that the homology between different binding sites for the same regulatory protein is not necessarily better than the homology between sites for different proteins, independent of whether they function as positive or negative modulators of transcription. In fact, the cyclic AMP receptor protein (CAP) of *Escherichia coli* can bind not only to its own sites in the regulated promoters, but also to the *lac* and *ara* operators [3, 4]. Thus, it appears that the mechanism by which regulatory proteins recognize their binding sites on DNA is similar regardless of the functional consequences of the interaction.

In higher organisms, several DNA-binding regulatory proteins have been described. The best characterized are probably the T antigens of DNA tumor viruses such as SV40 and polyoma. The behavior of these proteins is reminiscent of that found in the repressor systems of λ bacteriophages. By binding to three adjacent sites on the DNA, they can act as inhibitors of transcription from the early promoter or as activators of the late promoter [5].

I will concentrate on another group of regulatory proteins that have been extensively studied in our and other laboratories during the past 20 years, namely the receptors for steroid hormones. It is now well established that steroid hormones exert their effects on gene expres-

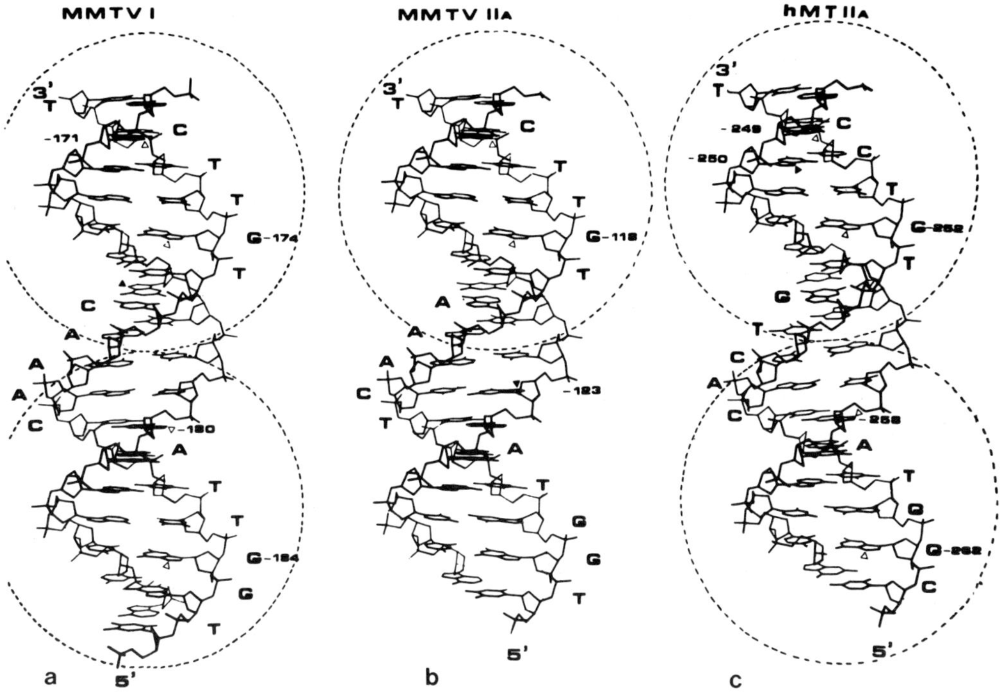

Fig. 3a–c. Structure of the glucocorticoid-binding sites of MMTV and hMTII$_A$. Computer graphic representation of the DNA double helix containing the nucleotide sequences of **a** MMTVI; **b** MMTVII$_A$; and **c** hMTII$_A$ (shown in Fig. 5). The sites of contact with the receptor are indicated by *open triangles.* Those positions hypermethylated in the presence of receptor are marked by *full triangles.* The receptor molecules are represented as *broken circles.* Numbers refer to the distance from the "cap" site

sion through interaction with intracellular receptors, that in their turn recognize regulatory elements in the neighborhood of the regulated promoters. Regulatory elements are defined as DNA sequences that in addition to being required for receptor binding, are needed for the hormonal regulation of transcription in gene transfer experiments. They were first reported in the long terminal repeat region (LTR) of mouse mammary tumor virus (MMTV), that contains the main promoter for proviral transcription [6–8]. Glucocorticoids were known to induce viral transcription in different cell lines [9], and gene transfer experiments with deletion mutants in the LTR region showed that the sequences relevant for hormonal regulation are located between 50 and 400 base pairs upstream of the initation of transcription [7, 10–12]. Within this region, several binding sites for the glucocorticoid receptor of rat liver have been described [8, 13]. Using a cloned proviral DNA from GR mice [8], we found four binding sites that share the hexanucleotide

5′-TGTTCT-3′
3′-ACAAGA-5′

Methylation protection studies have shown that both G residues in the hexanucleotides are in direct contact with the receptor [14]. In the binding site with the highest affinity for the receptor, further contacts are located in both strands 9–10 base pairs upstream of the hexanucleotide. These findings suggest an interaction of a dimer of the receptor with one side of the double-stranded DNA involving the major groove in two subsequent turns of the helix [14]. Such a model (Fig. 3a) is very similar to

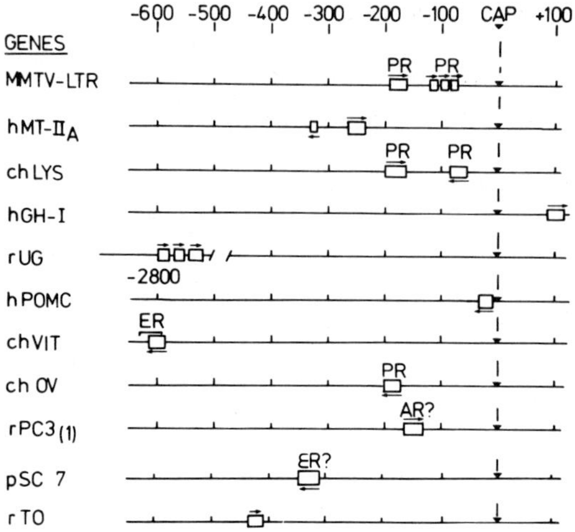

Fig. 4. Position and orientation of the binding sites for the glucocorticoid receptor in hormonally regulated genes. The binding sites are indicated by *open boxes*. The *horizontal arrows* show the orientation: to the right for the upper strand; to the left for the lower strand. The abbreviations are as follows: MMTV-LTD long terminal repeat region of mouse mammary tumor virus; hMT-II_A, human metallothioneine II_A; chLYS chicken lysozyme; hGH-I human growth hormone; rUG rabbit uteroglobin; hPOMC human proopiomelanocortin; chVIT chicken vitellogenin; chOV chicken ovalbumin; rPC3 [1] rat prostatic protein C3 [3]; pSC 7 *Drosophila* inducible gene at locus 74F; rTO rat tryptophanoxygenase; CAP initiation of transcription; PR progesterone receptor; ER estrogen receptor; AR androgen receptor; ER ecdysone receptor

that already mentioned for prokaryotic DNA-binding regulatory proteins.

An analysis of other glucocorticoid-regulated genes showed that the presence of a regulatory element is not an exclusive property of the retroviral genome. The human metallothioneine II_A gene (hMTII_A), that has been shown to be induced by glucocorticoids in many different cell lines, contains a glucocorticoid regulatory element about 250 base pairs upstream of the initiation of transcription [15]. This element is very similar to the strong binding site found in the LTR region of MMTV (compare a and c in Fig. 3). In addition, there is a weak binding site in the hMTII_A promoter located at around 320 base pairs upstream of the initiation of transcription [15]. Similarly to the weak binding site in the LTR region of MMTV (Fig. 3b), the shorter footprint and methylation protection pattern in the weak binding site of hMTII_A suggests binding of a receptor monomer. Interestingly, this weak site at – 320 can be deleted without influencing the hormonal inducibility of hMTII_A [15]. Thus, it could be that a functional interaction requires binding of a receptor dimer to a strong site on the DNA. In the meantime, we have identified binding sites for the glucocorticoid receptor in several hormonally regulated genes. A summary of these results along with data from the literature is shown in Fig. 4.

The promoter for the chicken lysozyme gene (chLYS), contains two binding sites for the glucocorticoid receptor, located at around 180 and 60 base pairs upstream of the initiation of transcription [16]. The upper binding site, that has a lower affinity for the glucocorticoid receptor, coincides with sequences required for hormone-dependent expression of the gene in oviduct cells [16]. In fact, these sequences mediate not only glucocorticoid regulation, but also induction by progesterone in microinjection experiments [16]. Interestingly, the partially purified progesterone receptor from rabbit uterus binds to the same sites as the glucocorticoid receptor, although with different affinity. Thus, it appears that the binding sites for the receptors of two different steroid hormones may be identical or at least share common sequences. That these similarities may not be limited to the progesterone and glucocorticoid receptors is suggested by studies with genes regulated by other steroid hormones (Fig. 4). The chicken vitellogenin II gene that is induced by estrogens in the liver, contains a binding site for the estrogen receptor around 600 nucleotides upstream of the transcription initiation site [17]. An analysis of the nucleotide sequences in this region reveals an element almost identical to the binding sites for the glucocorticoid receptor (Fig. 5).

A review of the literature showed that a rat gene for a prostatic protein, that is

		1	2	3	4	5	6	7	8	9	10	11	12	13	14	15	16	17
MMTV I	−186	T	G	G	T	T	A	C	A	A	A	C	T	G	T	T	C	T
MMTV IIa	−129	T	G	G	T	A	T	C	A	A	A	.	T	G	T	T	C	T
MrDNA	+2	C	T	G	A	C	A	C	A	C	G	C	T	G	T	C	C	T
rPC3(1)	−150	A	T	G	A	A	A	C	.	C	A	G	T	G	T	T	C	T
hMTIIA	−263	C	G	G	T	.	A	C	A	C	T	G	T	G	T	C	C	T
hGH-1	+92	G	G	G	C	.	A	C	A	A	T	G	T	G	T	C	C	T
hPOMC	−6	C	G	C	G	C	T	C	.	C	T	C	T	G	T	C	C	T
chLYS1	−50	T	T	G	A	T	T	C	.	C	T	C	T	G	T	T	C	T
chLYS2	−191	A	A	A	A	T	T	C	.	C	T	C	T	G	T	G	G	C
chVIT	−587	C	G	G	C	A	T	C	A	A	T	G	T	G	T	T	C	T
chOV	−177	G	G	G	C	.	A	C	A	A	T	G	T	G	T	C	C	T
RUG1	−2800	C	T	G	T	.	T	C	A	C	T	C	T	G	T	T	C	T
RUG2	−2820	C	C	G	G	.	A	C	A	C	G	G	A	G	T	C	C	T
RUG3	−2840	G	T	G	T	.	C	A	G	T	C	T	T	G	T	T	C	T
dSC7(2)	−315	T	C	G	A	T	T	T	G	A	T	C	T	G	T	T	C	T
rTO	−435	A	T	G	C	.	A	C	A	G	C	G	A	G	T	T	C	T
CONSENSUS.		C	G	G	T	A	A	C	A	C	T	G	T	G	T	T	C	T
		t	t		A	T	T			A	a	c				c		
YEAST Aktin		A	A	G	A	.	A	C	A	C	C	C	T	G	T	T	C	T

Fig. 5. Consensus sequence for the glucocorticoid regulatory element. The nucleotide sequences of the main binding sites for the glucocorticoid receptor are aligned to yield maximal homology. Abbreviations are as in Fig. 4

known to be induced by androgens, rPC 3(1), also contains a sequence homologous to the binding site for the glucocorticoid receptor some 140 nucleotides upstream of the initiation of transcription ([18]; Figs. 4 and 5). Finally, an ecdysone-inducible gene of *Drosophila* (pSC7) also contains a binding site for the glucocorticoid receptor some 330 nucleotides upstream of the transcription initiation site ([19]; Figs. 4 and 5). These findings, taken together, suggest that the regulatory elements for different steroid hormone receptors may be similar or at least overlap.

The rabbit uteroglobin gene is induced by glucocorticoids in the lung and by estrogen and progesterone in the endometrium [20]. We have looked for binding sites for the glucocorticoid receptor and found none in the neighborhood of the promoter. The closest binding region detected is located 2700 nucleotides upstream of the cap site, and is composed of three binding sites showing sequence homology to other glucocorticoid regulatory elements (Figs. 4 and 5). That this site may be relevant for regulation in vivo is suggested by the finding of a DNase I hypersensitive site in this region only in chromatin of hormonally stimulated endometrium (unpublished results).

The human growth hormone gene (hGHI) is induced by glucocorticoids in several cell lines [21]. In fact, gene transfer experiments with a chimeric gene suggested that a fragment of DNA containing 500 base pairs upstream of the initiation of transcription is sufficient for hormonal regulation [22]. In binding experiments with the glucocorticoid receptor, however, we found a main binding site located around position + 100, within the first intron (Figs. 4 and 5). If this site is involved in transcriptional regulation in vivo, it would mean that the regulatory element can act even when located downstream of the regulated promoter.

Taken together, the data shown in Fig. 4 show that the regulatory elements for steroid hormones share some of the properties of the so-called enhancer elements [23]. They can act at variable distance from the regulated promoters, both upstream and downstream, and in both orientations. There is in fact direct experimental evidence for an enhancer function of the glucocorticoid regulatory element in the LTR region of MMTV [7].

A comparison of the nucleotide sequences of ten different binding sites for the glucocorticoid receptor yields the consensus sequence shown in Fig. 5. Therefore, the glucocorticoid regulatory elements have been conserved in evolution between chicken, rodents, and humans. The best-conserved regions include all those sites that are involved in direct contacts with the receptor [14]. The symmetry in the element

	4	5	6	7		12	13	14	15	
5′	A	A	C	A	N_{8-11}	T	G	T	T	3′

is reminiscent of the binding sites for prokaryotic regulatory proteins, suggesting that molecular mechanisms similar to those operating in bacteria may be responsible for DNA recognition in higher organisms.

What could this mechanism be? And, how can a regulatory protein accommodate so much sequence variation in the central part of the recognition site? Of course, a model like the one shown in Fig. 3 will only require the binding sequence to be preserved in the two nucleotide blocks that are the sites of contact between the relevant α-helices and the major groove of double helix. This would explain the tolerance in the central part of the element, but what kind of interactions take place in the conserved regions? Certainly most of the overall energy of binding is sequence independence, and originates from ionic interactions with the phosphate backbone of the helix [2, 24]. This explains why all DNA-binding regulatory proteins also interact nonspecifically with DNA. In addition, specific base recognition is based on a complementary network of hydrogen bonds between amino acid side chains in the relevant α-helices and DNA base pair atoms exposed in the major groove of the double helix [24]. In fact several amino acid side chains such as Arg, Lys, Gln, and Asn, can form multiple hydrogen bonds with paired

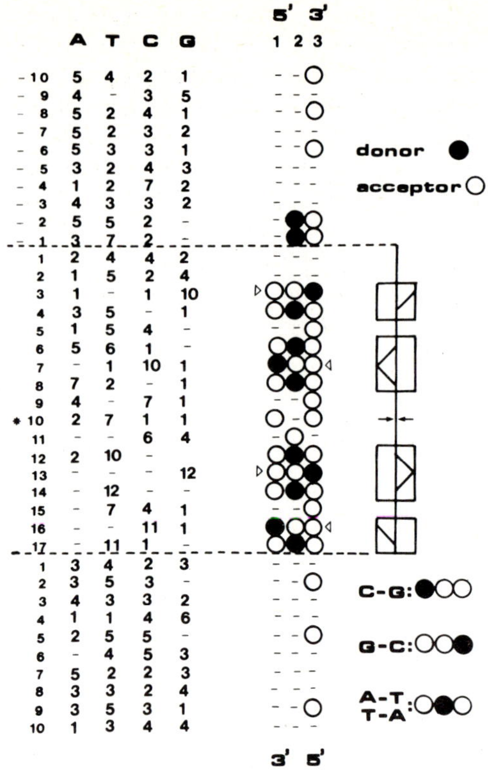

Fig. 6. Pattern of hydrogen bond donor–acceptor sites in the major groove of the DNA double helix in and around the receptor-binding sites. The conserved nucleotide sequences of twelve binding sites for the glucocorticoid receptor with the flanking base pairs on each side, have been analyzed for the pattern of hydrogen bond donor–acceptor sites in the major groove. Only those positions showing more than 90% conservation are shown (*open circles* acceptor sites; *full circles* donor sites). *Arrows* point to the conserved N-7 positions of guanines that represent sites of contact with the receptor [14]

bases on the DNA [25]. It has been proposed that if the regulatory protein moves a few Ångstroms away from the DNA, most of these hydrogen bonds would be broken or would not be formed, but many of the ionic interactions will be preserved. This mechanism may be utilized by the proteins for sliding along the DNA in search of their target sites [26].

If we consider the base pairs in the major groove in terms of their ability to form hydrogen bonds, we realize that an AT base pair has the structure acceptor–donor–acceptor and is therefore symmetric, whereas a GC base pair has the structure acceptor–acceptor–donor (Fig. 6). If one now compares the ten glucocorticoid receptor binding sites with their flanking sequences in terms of this hydrogen bond pattern, one observes a very good preservation of the donor–acceptor structure around the contact sites, with very little agreement outside the binding region (Fig. 6). A certain symmetry can be detected centered at position 10: two well-preserved blocks, 3 to 8 and 12 to 17, separated by less-preserved positions, and interrupted in symmetric positions at 5 and 15. Of course, other interactions are probably implicated in recognition, but the network of hydrogen bonds seems to be an essential part of the code in which regulatory information is stored in DNA. A precise understanding of the molecular mechanisms by which the regulatory code is read could derive from the fine structural analysis of cocrystals containing the DNA-binding domains of regulatory proteins bound to the corresponding nucleotide sequences [27, 28]. Only then will it be possible to decide whether there is a general rule underlying the mechanism of sequence-specific recognition by regulatory proteins.

Acknowledgments. The experimental work reviewed here has been supported by grants from the Deutsche Forschungsgemeinschaft and the Fond der Chemischen Industrie.

References

1. Gicquel-Sanzey B, Cossart P (1982) EMBO J 1:591–595
2. Takeda Y, Ohlendorf DH, Anderson WF, Matthews BW (1983) Science 221:1020–1026
3. Ogden S, Haggerty D, Stoner CM, Kolodrubetz D, Schleif R (1980) Proc Natl Acad Sci USA 77:3346–3350
4. Schmitz A (1981) Nucleic Acid Res 9:277–291
5. Tjian R (1978) Cell 13:165–179
6. Geisse S, Scheidereit C, Westphal HM, Hynes NE, Groner B, Beato M (1982) EMBO J 1:1613–1619
7. Chandler VL, Maler BA, Yamamoto KR (1983) Cell 33:489–499
8. Scheidereit C, Geisse S, Westphal HM, Beato M (1983) Nature 304:749–752
9. Ringold GM (1979) Biochim Biophys Acta 560:487–508
10. Hynes NH, van Ooyen AJJ, Kennedy N, Herrlich P, Ponta H, Groner B (1983) Proc Natl Acad Sci USA 80:3637–3641
11. Majors J, Varmus HE (1983) Proc Natl Acad Sci USA 80:5866–5870
12. Buetti E, Diggelmann H (1983) EMBO J 2:1423–1429
13. Payvar F, deFranco DF, Firestone GL, Edgar B, Wrange Ö, Okret S, Gustafsson JA, Yamamoto KR (1983) Cell 35:381–392
14. Scheidereit C, Beato M (1984) Proc Natl Acad Sci USA 81:3029–3033
15. Karin M, Haslinger A, Holtgreve H, Richards RI, Krauter P, Westphal HM, Beato M (1984) Nature 308:513–519
16. Renkawitz R, Schütz G, von der Ahe D, Beato M (1984) Cell 37:503–510
17. Jost JP, Seldran M, Geiser M (1984) Proc Natl Acad Sci USA 8:429–433
18. Parker M, Hurst H, Page M (1984) J Steroid Biochem 20:67–71
19. Moritz T, Edström JE, Pongs O (1984) EMBO J 3:289–295
20. Beato M, Arnemann J, Menne C, Müller H, Suske G, Wenz M (1983) In: McKerns KW (ed) Regulation of gene expression by hormones. Plenum, New York, pp 151–175
21. Martial JA, Baxter JD, Goodman HM, Seeburg PH (1977) Proc Natl Acad Sci USA 74:1816–1820
22. Robins DM, Paek I, Seeburg P, Axel R (1982) Cell 29:623–631
23. Banerji J, Rusconi S, Schaffner W (1981) Cell 27:299–308
24. Seeman NC, Rosenburg JM, Rich A (1979) Proc Natl Acad Sci USA 72:804–808
25. Rein R, Kieber-Emmons T, Haydock K, Garduno-Juarez R, Shibata M (1983) J Biomol Struct Dyn 1:1051–1079
26. Berg OG, Winter RB, von Hippel PH (1981) Biochemistry 20:6929–6948
27. Anderson J, Ptashne M, Harrison SC (1984) Proc Natl Acad Sci USA 81:1307–1311
28. Frederick CA, Grable J, Melia M, Samudzi C, Jen-Jacobson L, Wang BC, Greene P, Boyer HW, Rosenberg JM (1984) Nature 309:327–331

Haematology and Blood Transfusion Vol. 29
Modern Trends in Human Leukemia VI
Edited by Neth, Gallo, Greaves, Janka

Cellular Oncogenes as the Ancestors of Endocrine and Paracrine Growth Factors and Their Evolutionary Relic Status in Vertebrates

S. Ohno [1]

A. Introduction

The generally held belief that any gene whose expression is precisely regulated in development ought to perform an indispensable function to the host organism is not quite correct and, in fact, has no solid foundation. It should be recalled that the DNA replication mechanism of modern organisms has developed a high degree of precision (the error rate is 10^{-10} per base pair per replication or thereabout) and that whatever damage sustained by DNA is effectively rectified by multitudes of DNA repair mechanisms. Accordingly, even dispensable peptide chains such as fibrinopeptides A and B do not change their amino acid sequences very rapidly, a 1% change in their amino acid sequences taking roughly 1.0–1.6 million years [1]. Under these circumstances, a gene which has lost its usefulness to the host organism does not disappear quite so readily. The half-life of an enzyme gene that has become redundant has been estimated as 50 million years [2].

B. Redundant and Useless Genes May Persist for 50 Million Years or More

By becoming tetraploid, an organism initially gains four alleles at every gene locus. Subsequently, each set of four homologous chromosomes differentiates into two pairs, thus completing the process of diploidization. At this stage, freshly diploidized tetraploid species are endowed with twice the number of gene loci when compared with their diploid counterparts. This is the stage, at which trout and salmon of the teleost family Salmonidae, whitefish of the family Coregonidae, and grayling of the family Thymallidae find themselves [3]. A few of those duplicated, and therefore redundant, genes manage to acquire a new role; e.g., of all the vertebrates, only diploidized tetraploid teleost fish are endowed with liver-specific lactate dehydrogenase (LDH), in addition to the customary skeletal muscle and heart LDH. The mechanism of gene duplication as the means to acquire new genes with previously nonexistent functions, however, is very inefficient, having a very low success ratio: the phrase Salvandrum paucitas, dammnundrum multitudo gives ample testimony to its high failure ratio. Accordingly, older diploidized tetraploids of the teleost family Cyprinidae as well as Catostomidae have lost progressively larger numbers of these redundant, duplicated loci by silencing mutations. Since the fossil record gives the origin of these diploidized tetraploids, Ferris and Whitt [2] were able to calculate the average half-life of enzyme loci that became redundant as 50 million years. It should be noted here that this half-life refers to the average time needed for half of the redundant enzyme loci to lose their assigned functions. After losing their assigned functions, these redundant enzyme loci may continue to code for functionless polypeptide chains. The case in

1 Beckman Research Institute of The City of Hope, Duarte, California 91010, USA

point is the murine Slp locus, situated in the middle of the major histocompatibility (MHC) antigen gene complex region of the mouse genome. While the neighboring Ss locus specifies C4 (complement 4 of antibody-mediated lysis), a protein specified by the Slp locus has already lost its assigned function as C4 owing to accumulated mutations. Yet, this Slp locus was androgen dependent in most mouse strains, and operator constitutive mutation of this locus was found in wild mice [4]. It would thus appear that a substantial portion of the redundant gene loci may continue to specify functionless proteins even after 100 million years of independence from natural selection.

Although mammal-like reptiles were already an independent lineage at the time of the dinosaurs, mammals as we know them came into being only 70 million years ago. This should make us realize the unreality of the statement that any gene loci with precisely regulated expression must be indispensable to the host organism. The fact is that genes that have outlived their usefulness may linger on for 50–100 million years.

C. Most Oncogenes are Evolutionary Relics of the Cell Autonomous Stage of Development

Although multitudes of cellular oncogenes perform divergent functions (some of their products are found in the nucleus, while others are found inside the plasma membrane), it is clear that all of them function as intracellular cell growth factors. In unicellular eukaryotes such as baker's yeast as well as in many of the multicellular eukaryotes with underdeveloped circulatory systems such as insects, these intracellular growth factors have apparently played a vital role, for it should be recalled that embryonic development of insects is still largely a cell autonomous process as discussed in detail elsewhere [5]. With the advent of the cardiovascular system, development of vertebrates became a centrally controlled affair via multitudes of peptide and steroid hormones and cellular autonomy was suppressed. While intracellular growth factors of earlier times served as ancestors of these peptide hormones as well as of their plasma membrane receptors, they themselves largely became evolutionary relics whose functions have become redundant [5].

D. Near Immortality of Certain Oncogenes Conferred on Them by Their Original Construction

If cellular oncogenes became redundant at the onset of vertebrate evolution, most of them should have become silent by now, in spite of their long estimated half-life of 50 million years, for primitive vertebrates were already in evidence more than 300 million years ago. However, the continued performance of essential functions need not be invoked to explain this persistence for more than 300 million years.

The view first expressed in 1981 [6] that all the coding sequences originally were repeats of base oligomers has found increasing support from independent sources [7–9]. Provided that the number of bases in the oligomeric unit is not a multiple of three, coding sequences made of oligomeric repeats are inherently impervious to normally very damaging base substitutions, deletions, and insertions, thus possessing a near immortality. In this kind of oligomeric repeat, three consecutive copies of the oligomeric unit translated in three different reading frames gives the unit periodicity to their polypeptide chains: while nonameric repeats, the unit sequence being a multiple of three, can give only tripeptide periodicity to their peptide chains, three consecutive copies of decameric repeats encode the decapeptidic periodicity to its polypeptide chain. Thus, if one reading frame of this kind of oligomeric repeat is open, the other two are automatically open as well. It follows then that the potentially most damaging base substitution that changes an amino acid-specifying codon to the chain terminator (e.g., Trp codon TGG to chain-terminating TAG or TGA) merely silences one of the three open reading frames. Deletions or insertions of bases that are not multiples of three are usually as damaging, for resulting frame shifts alter downstream amino acid sequences and most often result in premature chain terminations. In this type of oligomeric repeat, such insertions and deletions are of no consequence either, for downstream amino acid sequences are not at all affected by frame shifts.

In a previous paper [10], we have analyzed the published coding sequence of human c-*myc* gene [11] in detail. Within the 5′ half of c-*myc* coding sequence, we identified one each of recurring base tetradecamer, duodecamer, and two monodecamers. The significance of this becomes clear once it is realized that if c-*myc* is a unique sequence *sensu stricto*, even a given base decamer is expected to recur only once every 1 048 576 bases. Yet, here we found a recurring base tetradecamer within a mere 687-base 5′ half c-*myc* coding sequence. Furthermore, recurring duodecamer and monodecamers were found to represent slightly modified parts of the tetradecameric sequence GGCCGCCGCCTCCT. Thus, it was concluded that the entire 5′ half of the c-*myc* coding sequence originated from repeats of the previously noted base tetradecamer. Since 14 is not a multiple of 3, three consecutive copies of it translated in three different reading frames would have given the following tetradecapeptidic periodicity to the original c-*myc* polypeptide chain, at least the amino terminal half of it

Gly	Arg	Arg	Leu	Leu
GGC	CGC	CGC	CTC	CT/G
Ala	Ala	Ala	Ser	Trp
GCC	GCC	GCC	TCC	T/GG
Pro	Pro	Pro	Pro	
CCG	CCG	CCT	CCT	

Indeed, the human c-*myc* coding sequence, at least the 5′ half of it, apparently inherited a measure of immortality from its original construction, for we found two long, alternative open reading frames, one covering the first 301 bases and the other from the 599th to 952nd bases. When this region of human c-*myc* coding sequence [11] was compared with the corresponding region of v-*myc* coding sequence of avian retrovirus MC29 [12], we found that the two differed from each other not so much by amino acid substitutions as by five stretches of insertions and two stretches of deletions. Thus, c-*myc*'s inherent imperviousness to deletions and insertions was shown [10].

E. Resurrection of a Silenced v-*src* Gene by Utilization of its Alternative Open Reading Frame

A measure of immortality inherited by some of the oncogenes from their original construction was indeed shown by the following experiment of Mardon and Varmus [13]. First, they established the rat cell line that was transformed by the integration into the genome of a single copy of strain B77 Rous sarcoma virus v-*src* coding sequence. One of the defective mutations sustained by the integrated v-*src* that deprived from the rat cell line of the transformed phenotype was identified as an insertion of a single base A between 146th Glu codon GAA and 147th Glu codon GAG. A resulting frame shift created a new chain terminator 51 bases further downstream, thus, silencing a mutated v-*src* [13]. The surprise was the second mutation that resurrected a silenced v-*src* as a transforming gene. This second event was an insertion of a duplicated 242-base segment into the position between T and GG of the 148th Trp codon in the original reading frame. This 242-base segment started from GAT representing the 68th Asp codon in the original reading frame and ended in T of 148th Trp also in the original reading frame, thus including a previously inserted A. Since the inserted segment is now translated in an alternative reading frame, the resulting double frame shifts restored the original reading frame, starting from GAG of the 147th Glu of the wild-type v-*src* and downward which in the resurrected v-*src* became the 228th Glu.

Such restoration of function by an insertion in the midst of the polypeptide chain of an 81-residue new amino acid sequence is hardly believable, unless a new sequence specified by a repeated coding segment translated in an alternative open reading frame resembles parts of the preexisting amino acid sequence. Such a resemblance, in turn, is expected only if the coding sequence itself still maintains a sufficient vestige of the ancestral construction;

i.e., the coding sequence originating from repeats of a base oligomer in which the number of bases in the oligomeric unit was not a multiple of three. Indeed, the existence of so long an alternative open reading frame itself is a reflection of the v-*src* coding sequence's ultimate derivation from oligomeric repeats, the number of bases in the oligomeric unit not being a multiple of three. As might be expected, when translated in an alternative open reading frame, amino acid residues 1–8 encoded by a duplicated 242-base segment were Thr-Pro-Se-Arg-Arg-Arg-Ser-Val. In the standard amino acid sequence of Rous sarcoma v-*src*, the very similar nonapeptide, Thr-Pro-Ser-(Gln)-Arg-Arg-Arg-Ser-Leu customarily occupies positions 10–18 [5].

F. Summary

Contrary to the popularly held view, genes that have lost their usefulness to the host organism may continue to encode proteins for 50 million years or longer. Accordingly, precisely regulated expression of genes can not be taken as proof of their indispensability. My view is that multitudes of oncogenes of vertebrates are evolutionary relics harking back to the days of invertebrate ancestors in which embryogenesis was still a cell autonomous process. Parts of certain oncogene coding sequences originated from repeats of base oligomers whose numbers of bases were not multiples of three. Thus, these segments are still endowed with a measure of immortality in that they are impervious to normally very deleterious base substitutions, insertions, and deletions.

References

1. Dayhoff MO (ed) (1972) Atlas of protein sequences and structure. National biomedical research foundation, Silver Springs, Maryland
2. Ferris SD, Whitt GS (1977) Loss of duplicated gene expression after polyploidization. Nature 265:258–260
3. Ohno S (1970) Evolution by gene duplication. Springer, Heidelberg Berlin New York
4. Hansen TH, Shreffler DC (1976) Characterization of a constitutive variant of the murine serum protein allotype, *Slp*. J Immunol 117:1507–1513
5. Ohno S (1984) Repeats of base oligomers as the primordial coding sequence of the primeval earth and their vestiges in modern genes. J Mol Evol 20:313–321 (1984)
6. Ohno S (1981) Original domain for the serum albumin family arose from repeated sequences. Proc Natl Acad Sci USA 79:1999–2002
7. Blake C (1983) Exon – present from the beginning? Nature 306:535–537
8. Gō M (1983) Modular structural units, exons and functions in chicken lysozyme. Proc Natl Acad Sci USA 80:1964–1968
9. Alexander F, Young PR, Tilghman SM (1984) Evolution of the albumin: α-fetoprotein ancestral gene from the amplification of a 27 nucleotide sequence. J Mol Biol 173:159–174
10. Ohno S, Yazaki A (1983) Simple construction of human c-*myc* gene implicated in B-cell neoplasms and its relationship with avian v-*myc* and human lymphokines. Scand J Immunol 18:373–388
11. Watt R, Stanton LW, Marcu KB, Gallo RC, Croce CN, Tovera G (1983) Nucleotide sequence of cloned cDNA of human c-*myc* oncogene. Nature 303:725–727
12. Alitalo K, Bishop MJ, Smith DH, Chen E, Colby WW, Levinson AD (1983) Nucleotide sequence of the v-*myc* oncogene of avian retrovirus MC29. Proc Natl Acad Sci USA 80: 100–105
13. Mardon G, Vermus HE (1983) Frameshift and intragenic suppressor mutations in a Rous sarcoma provirus suggest *SRC* encodes two proteins. Cell 32:871–879

Haematology and Blood Transfusion Vol. 29
Modern Trends in Human Leukemia VI
Edited by Neth, Gallo, Greaves, Janka

The Genes That Carcinogens Act Upon *

F. Anders, M. Schartl, A. Barnekow, C. R. Schmidt, W. Lüke, G. Jaenel-Dess and A. Anders

A. Introduction

Currently in cancer research much emphasis is being placed on mutation [2–4], rearrangement [5], amplification [6–8], and demethylation [9] of oncogenes that are supposed to represent the primary events leading to oncogene activation when carcinogens trigger neoplasia in animals or humans (the reader is referred to ref. [10] for more extensive details on this topic). The data underlying this supposition were mainly derived from experiments performed with tumor cells in vitro. In vivo studies on this issue are rare.

A model which has proven to be suitable for such in vivo studies is *Xiphophorus,* i.e., a fish genus from Central America known as the platyfish and swordtails [11]. All individuals of this genus carry an oncogene, designated *Tu,* which was analyzed by formal genetics long before the viral and cellular oncogenes were identified by methods of modern molecular biology [12–16]. Our phenogenetic, cytogenetic, and developmental genetic studies on *Xiphophorus,* however, have failed so far to detect any structural alterations of the *Tu* oncogene which were expected to occur when the gene switches over from the silent to the tumorigenic state. In contrast, it appears that impairment of the *Tu* oncogene might reduce rather than promote its tumorigenic potential and, therefore, it is difficult to detect.

By means of seven experiments the present study aims to show that the common primary events in the causation of neoplasia in *Xiphophorus* are changes in the regulatory gene systems controlling the oncogenes rather than changes in the oncogenes themselves.

B. The Oncogene and the Neoplasm Used in This Study

I. The Oncogene

It appears that the genetically identified oncogene *Tu* may mediate neoplastic transformation in poorly differentiated cells of all tissues. The type of tissue in which transformation occurs (for instance in the pigment-cell system) depends on regulatory genes of *Tu.* Oncogenes other than *Tu* which were expected to exist in *Xiphophorus* were not detected by genetic methods (for discussion of this problem see [16]).

From the eleven cellular oncogenes (*c-oncs*) that were identified molecularly in *Xiphophorus* (*c-erb, c-src, c-myc, c-fgr, c-abl, c-fes, c-myb,* c-ras^H, c-ras^K, *c-sis, c-yes*) [16] only *c-src* will be taken into con-

* This work was generously supported by the Deutsche Forschungsgemeinschaft (SFB 47 "Virologie", 103 "Zellenergetik und Zelldifferenzierung", 118 "Früherkennung des Krebses"), by the Bundesminister für Forschung und Technologie, by the President of the University of Giessen, 6300 Giessen, FRG, and by the President of the University of Erlangen, 8520 Erlangen, FRG
The present paper supplements that of "The Biology of an Oncogene" published in vol. 28 of this series [1]

sideration because most of our knowledge comes from this gene. Its inheritance was identified by molecular hybridization of viral *src* probes with genomic *Xiphophorus* DNA, and its activity was monitored by the transcript and by the $pp60^{c\text{-}src}$ kinase activity assayed according to Collet and Erikson [17]. The results parallel completely the inheritance and phenotypic expression of the *Tu* oncogene, specified by tumor development [1, 18–20].

II. The Neoplasm

Out of the 25 different types of neurogenic (neuroblastoma, melanoma, etc.), mesenchymal (fibrosarcoma, reticulosarcoma, etc.), and epithelial (adenocarcinoma, hepatoma, etc.) neoplasms that have been induced and identified in *Xiphophorus* only melanoma is taken into consideration in this study. This tumor has the advantage over the tumors of other histogenesis in that its development can easily be traced from a single transformed pigment cell detectable by its typical heavy black pigmentation, up to the extreme malignant melanoma that is lethal (Fig. 1).

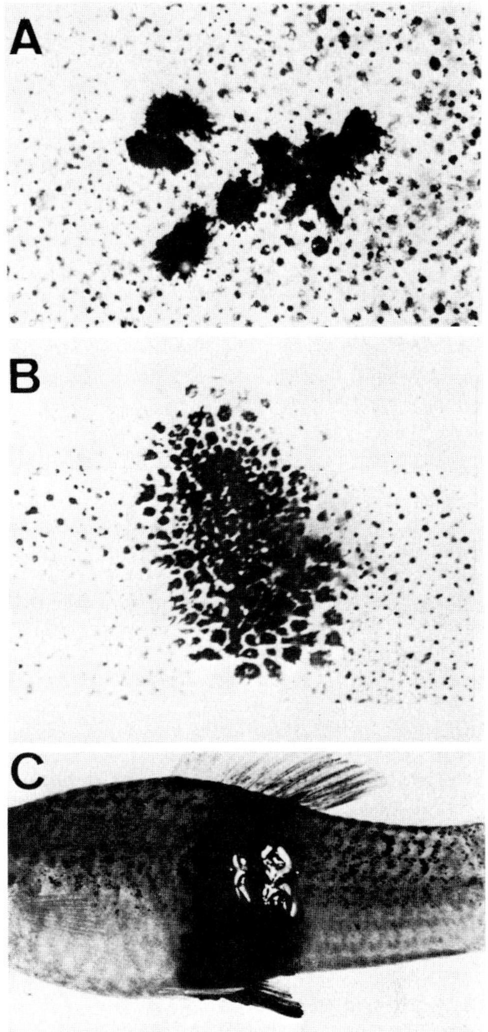

Fig. 1 A–C. Development of a somatic mutation-conditioned melanoma. **A** Cell clone consisting of eight transformed melanocytes; **B** Clone consisting of some hundreds of transformed melanoblasts and melanocytes; **C** Lethal malignant melanoma

C. Results and Discussion

I. First Experiment: Tumors Induced by Dislocation of Regulatory Genes for the Oncogene in a Germ Line Cell

Information about the crucial event in the causation of this type of hereditary melanoma comes from an X-ray-induced structural chromosome change involving a translocation of the *Tu* oncogene from the X chromosome of *Xiphophorus maculatus* (platyfish) to an autosome of *Xiphophorus helleri* (swordtail) and the corresponding *Tu* deletion that took place in meiosis of an F_1-hybrid female [13] (see Fig. 2 a–d). In its new position (Fig. 2 c) *Tu* is no longer controlled by its formerly linked regulatory genes that act only in the *cis* position [13]. A powerful regulatory gene nonlinked to *Tu* that acts in the *trans* position persisted in the system. Fertilization of the egg with sperm of the swordtail and breeding the mutant using the swordtail as the recurrent parent resulted in offspring in which all animals containing the *Tu* translocation segregated into a 1 : 1 ratio of animals lacking or containing the nonlinked regulatory gene for *Tu*.

In both segregants, as a consequence of the lack of the linked regulatory genes,

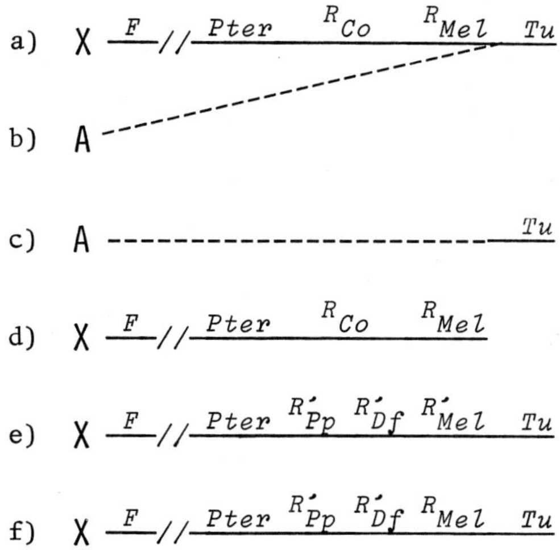

Fig. 2a–f. a–c Translocation of the *Tu* oncogene from the X chromosome (*X*) of *X. maculatus* to an autosome (*A*) of *X. helleri* and **d** the respective *Tu* deletion. Note separation of *Tu* from its linked regulatory genes R_{Mel} and R_{Co} (see first experiment of this study); **e** X chromosome of *X. maculatus* that is used in the second experiment (see Figs. 5, 9); **f** The X chromosome used in the third experiment (see Fig. 10). Note that **e** and **f** differ only in the R_{Mel} locus. *F,* female-sex-determining region; *Pter,* pterinophore locus. R_{Co} region containing at least 13 compartment-specific regulatory genes such as R_{Pp} (posterior part-specific) and R_{Df} (dorsal fin-specific); R_{Mel}, melanophore-specific regulatory gene; *Tu,* oncogene

neoplastic transformation takes place in the pigment-cell precursors of the early embryo. In the segregants lacking both the linked and the nonlinked regulatory genes, neoplastic transformation continues in pigment-cell precursors in all areas of the body, thus forming a "whole body melanoma" (Fig. 3B) which kills the fish before or shortly after birth. If, however, the nonlinked regulatory gene is present in the system, melanoma development is retarded at the time of birth (Fig. 3C). The fish develop melanoma but may reach sexual maturity, thus providing the possibility to breed by further backcrosses with *X. helleri,* a stock that continuously produces lethal-melanoma-developing and nonlethal-melanoma-developing embryos. If, furthermore, the regulatory gene is introduced into the system in the homozygous state, no *Tu*-mediated melanoma develops (Fig. 3A). Fish carrying the *Tu* deletion chromosome (see Fig. 2d) have a highly diminished potential for the formation of all kinds of neoplasms.

The development of the whole body melanoma in the early embryo reflects the genuine oncogenic effect of the completely deregulated *Tu* on the pigment-cell system. These observations suggest to us that in the early embryo *Tu* normally exerts important functions in cytodifferentiation, which, if *Tu* is completely deregulated, cannot be stopped (see below).

So far we have not tested pp60$^{c\text{-}src}$ kinase activity in the embryos that develop melanoma. However, pp60$^{c\text{-}src}$ kinase activity was measured in the normal developing embryos (Fig. 4) [21]. The activity is detectable from the very outset of cleavage and strongly increases during early organogenesis. While organogenesis morphologically culminates, kinase activity apparently becomes choked, decreases during the growth phase before and after birth to a lower level, and thereafter (not shown in Fig. 4) remains constant at a basic level throughout the whole life of the fish [19]. In adults it was found that pp60$^{c\text{-}src}$ kinase activity is organ specific, with the brain always showing the highest values [18, 19]. The results suggest that *c-src* activity is related to differentiation and specificity of organs rather than to cell growth. Similar sequences of pp60$^{c\text{-}src}$ kinase activity during life were found in frogs and chickens (see Fig. 4), indicating that our results are more general rather than fish specific [21].

These genetic, embryological, and molecular biological observations suggest to us that the melanoma-mediating oncogene, irrespective of its appearance as *Tu* or *c-src,* exerts important normal functions as a developmental gene in the early embryo. Moreover, we assume that in normal embryogenesis these functions become switched off or choked by regulatory genes after cell differentiation progresses to organogenesis. If, however, the regulatory genes (i.e. the entire choke in the lethal *Tu* translocation) are lacking, the oncogene continues to exert its early embryo-specific functions which, as an extension of the cellular development in the early embryo,

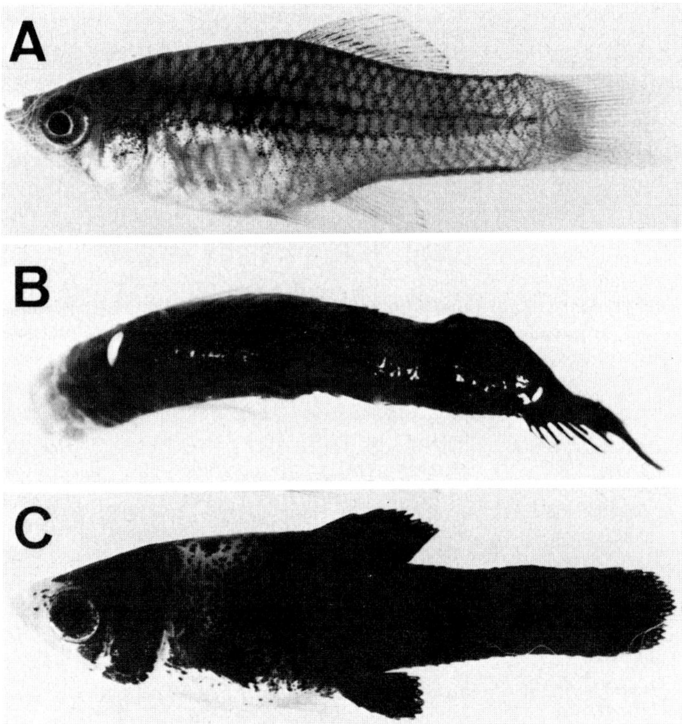

Fig. 3 A–C. Backcross hybrids (*X. maculatus* × *X. helleri* × *X. helleri*) carrying the *Tu* translocation according to Fig. 2c. **A** A nonlinked regulatory gene is present in the homozygous state. There is no tumor; **B** The nonlinked regulatory gene is lacking. Lethal "whole body melanoma" develops; **C** One copy of the nonlinked regulatory gene is present. Melanoma develops but the animals reach sexual maturity. **A** Adult fish, 5 cm long; **B, C** neonates, 6 mm long

appear as neoplastic transformation. Support for this idea comes from the high pp60$^{c\text{-}src}$ kinase activity that is found in the melanoma of young and adult fish (see second and third experiments). In any case, the crucial event leading to neoplasia in this experiment is the X-ray-induced translocation-conditioned loss of oncogene-specific regulatory genes.

II. Second Experiment: Tumors Induced by Crossing-Conditioned Elimination of Regulatory Genes for the Oncogene from the Germ Line

The basic crossing procedure for the production of melanoma-developing *Xiphophorus* is shown in Fig. 5: Crosses of a wild platyfish female from Rio Jamapa (Fig. 5 A) with a wild swordtail male from Rio Lancetilla (Fig. 5 B) result in F_1 hybrids (Fig. 5 C) that develop uniformly in all individuals, with melanomas consisting mainly of well-differentiated transformed pigment cells that are morphologically similar to those of certain spots of the parental platyfish. They occur only in those compartments of the body where the platyfish parent infrequently exhibits the spots, e.g., in the skin of the dorsal fin and the posterior part of the body. In older F_1 animals, the compartment-specific melanomas combine to form a large benign melanoma. Backcrosses of the F_1 hybrids with the swordtail as the recurrent parent (Fig. 5 D) result in offspring (BC_1) exhibiting three types of segregants: 25% of the BC_1 (Fig. 5 E) develop benign melanoma like that of the F_1, 25% (Fig. 5 F) develop malignant melanoma consisting mainly of incompletely differentiated transformed cells which invade other tissues (except for brain, gonads, intestine) and eventually kill the fish, whereas 50% (Fig. G, H) develop neither spots nor melanomas. Further backcrosses (not shown in Fig. 5) of the fish carrying benign melanoma with the swordtail result in a BC_2 that exhibits the same segregation pattern as the BC_1. The same applies for further backcrosses of this kind.

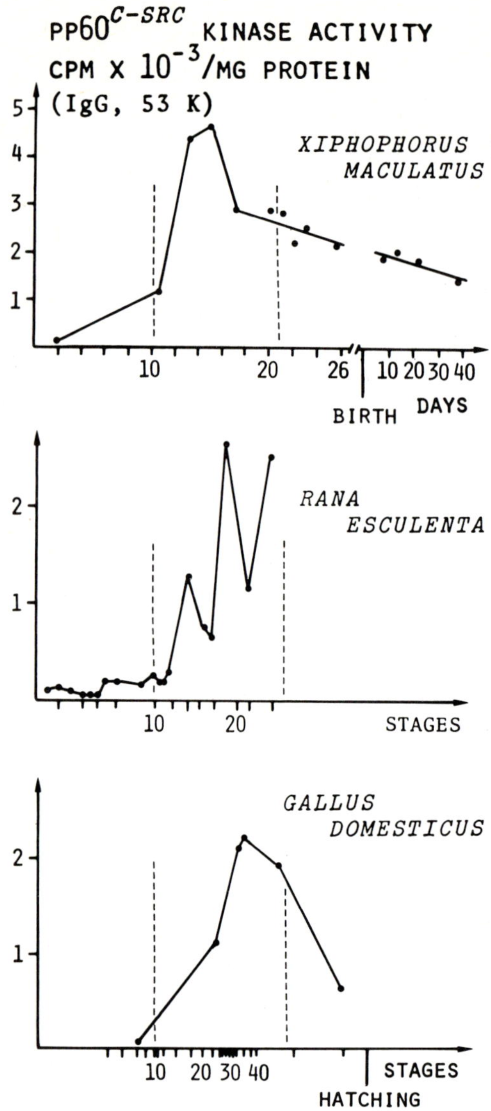

Fig. 4. pp60$^{c\text{-}src}$ Kinase activity during cleavage, organogenesis, and growth. Data from [21]

Backcrosses of the fish carrying the malignant melanoma with the swordtail show a different result: 50% of the BC segregants develop malignant melanoma, whereas the remaining 50% are melanoma free; benign melanomas do not occur. Whenever melanomas occur in these crossing experiments, they develop in both the compartment of the dorsal fin and the compartment of the posterior part of the body.

The results obtained in this crossing experiment (and a large variety of similar experiments) may be explained by the assumption of four prominent genetic components that are involved in melanoma formation or protection from melanoma, respectively. They are contributed by *X. maculatus* (for those contributed by *X. helleri* but not involved in melanoma formation in this crossing experiment, see below) and are normal homozygous constituents of the natural gene pool of the wild platyfish population from Rio Jamapa. Three of the genetic components (see the following points 1, 2, 3), as was confirmed by about 70 structural changes, are closely linked together at the end of the X chromosome (see Fig. 2). The fourth (point 4) is autosomally located.

1. The *Tu* oncogene. This gene is apparently responsible for neoplastic transformation. The restriction of neoplastic transformation to pigment cells and to the development of melanoma in the dorsal fin and in the skin of the posterior part of the body comes from other genes.

2. The regulatory gene R_{Mel}. Impairment of this gene (R'_{Mel}) specifies the tumorigenic effect of *Tu* to the melanophore system. R_{Mel} is a member of a series of tissue-specific regulatory genes which, in the impaired state, determine the histogenesis of the tumors (mesenchymal, epithelial, and neurogenic neoplasms). The mutations of these genes indicate that tissue specificity of neoplasia depends on regulatory genes rather than on oncogenes.

3. The regulatory genes R_{Pp} and R_{Df}. Impairment of these genes (R'_{Pp}, R'_{Df}) permits the development of melanoma in the skin of the posterior part of the body (*Pp*) and in the dorsal fin (*Df*) provided that R_{Mel} is also impaired. Thirteen compartments of the body (anal fin, tail fin, mouth, eye, peritoneum, meninx, etc.) that have been identified correspond to a series of different regulatory genes (R_{Co} in total) which in turn correspond to sites of the body where melanomas may occur (see Fig. 13).

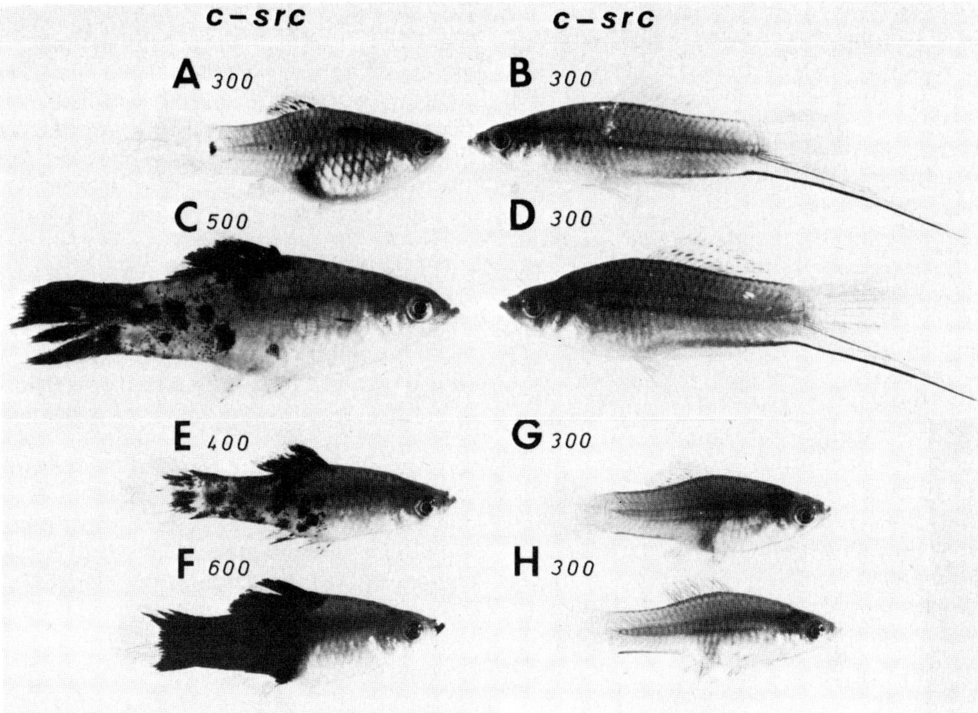

Fig. 5A–H. Crossing procedure for the production of melanoma-developing hybrids of *Xiphophorus*. **A** *X. maculatus* from Rio Jamapa (Mexico); some small spots in the skin of the dorsal fin and the side of the body are visible. The spots consist of terminally differentiated, neoplastically transformed pigment cells. **B** *X. helleri* from Rio Lancetilla (Mexico), always lacking the spots. **C** F_1, developing benign melanoma instead of spots (100% of the F_1). **D** *X. helleri* from **B** used in the backcross as the recurrent parent. **E** Backcross hybrid with benign melanoma (25% of the BC generation). **F** Backcross hybrid with malignant melanoma (25% of the BC generation). **G, H** Backcross hybrids that do not develop melanoma (50% of the BC generation). Spots and melanomas (in the posterior part of the body and the dorsal fin) depend on the deregulated *Tu* of the X chromosome shown in Fig. 2e. Depending on the pterinophore locus (*Pter* of this chromosome), spotted and tumorous fish (**A, C, E** and **F**) exhibit a reddish coloration. $pp60^{c\text{-}src}$ Kinase activity expressed as counts/min per milligram protein; *note* basic and excessive activity and correlation between *c-src* expression and *Tu* expression. Data from [15, 19] were combined. See Figs. 9 and 10

4. The differentiation gene *Diff*. This gene is indicated by the 1:1 segregation of benign- and malignant-melanoma-bearing fish. If it is present, the majority of the melanoma cells are well differentiated (benign melanoma). If, however, *Diff* is lacking, the majority of the melanoma cells are poorly differentiated (malignant melanoma).

Additional regulatory genes contributed by the platyfish to the hybrid genome have been identified but are considered only in general in this experiment.

Xiphophorus helleri also contains the *Tu* oncogene and presumably the linked regulatory genes, which, however, are not mutated and thus are fully active. *Tu* and its linked regulatory genes, therefore, are not detectable with the methods used in this experiment. Furthermore, since the linked regulatory genes act only in the *cis* position, this "oncogene-regulatory-gene complex," contributed by the swordtail, does not significantly influence the expression of the platyfish-derived melanoma-mediating *Tu* copy. No *Diff* and nor any other nonlinked regulatory gene was found in the swordtail that might correspond to those of the platyfish.

The outcome of this crossing experiment suggests the following interpretation: Following crossings and backcrossings according to Fig. 5, the regulatory-gene-carrying chromosomes of the platyfish are replaced stepwise by the homologous chromosomes of the swordtail, resulting in the gradual disintegration of the regulatory gene system for the platyfish-derived *Tu*. Thus the *Tu* hybrids spontaneously develop benign melanoma if some regulatory genes such as *Diff* are still present in the genome and malignant melanoma if the regulatory genes are lacking. If the platyfish-derived *Tu* is lacking, no melanomas occur.

Based on the assumption that the activity of the $pp60^{c\text{-}src}$-associated phosphokinase monitors the activity of the *c-src* oncogene, we carried out comparisons between kinase activity, i.e., *c-src* expression, and tumor development, i.e., *Tu* expression. The preparatory work to this study showed that $pp60^{c\text{-}src}$ kinase activity in normal tissues of nontumorous and tumorous fish is tissue specific, with the brain always showing the highest values [18]. It furthermore showed that this activity is elevated in the brain of benign-melanoma-bearing fish, and even higher in the brain of malignant-melanoma-bearing fish. In any case, $pp60^{c\text{-}src}$ kinase activity varies in both melanoma and the brain in the same direction. Hence, we were able to determine $pp60^{c\text{-}src}$-associated protein kinase activity mainly in brain extracts and relate the activity observed to the expression of *Tu* ascertained by the development of melanoma. The possibility that the differences in kinase activity measured in the fish of different *Tu* genotypes are due to secondary processes in the melanoma appears unlikely. Therefore, the results reflect the actual genetic activity of the *c-src* oncogene in the nontumorous brain tissue of the tumorous and nontumorous fish. For critical evaluation of the methods see refs. [18, 19].

As indicated in Fig. 5, the purebred platyfish female (Fig. 5 A) carrying the population-specific "*Tu*-regulatory-gene complex" in both of its X chromosomes, as well as the purebred swordtail and the BC hybrids lacking this special complex, display the same activity of *c-src* kinase. We interpret this activity to be the basic expression of *c-src*. In contrast, the melanoma-bearing hybrids which contain the derepressed *Tu* show an increase in *c-src* activity, with the malignant-melanoma-bearing BC hybrids displaying the highest activities.

To accomplish the crossing experiment (not shown in Fig. 5) we crossed two melanoma-bearing BC hybrids (F×F) that exceptionally reached sexual maturity. The resulting *Tu*/*Tu* hybrids (25% of the offspring) are of special interest. They show an oncogene dosage effect in both melanoma formation and $pp60^{c\text{-}src}$ kinase activity as compared with the parental BC hybrids [1, 20].

In summary, all experiments of this kind showed a clear-cut correlation between *c-src* expression (measured by $pp60^{c\text{-}src}$ kinase activity) and *Tu* expression (measured by melanoma formation).

Many features that are assumed to be involved in the causation of neoplasia have been found in melanoma of *Xiphophorus*. About 70% of the melanomatous cells in cell cultures derived from embryos exhibit at least two pairs of double minute chromosomes (Fig. 6) [22] that might be interpret-

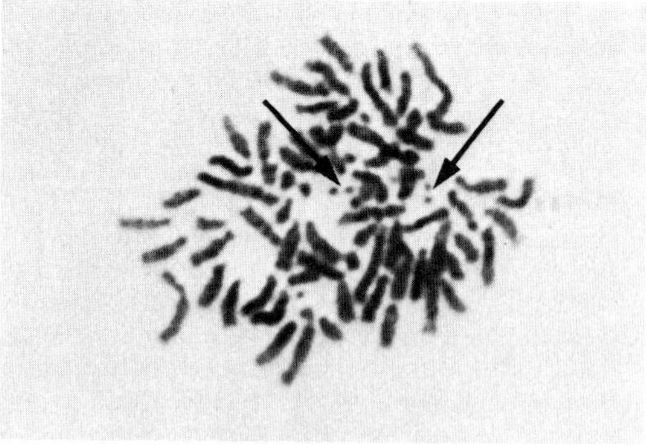

Fig. 6. Metaphase showing double minute chromosomes (DM). DMs were always found in cell cultures derived from melanomatous embryos [22]

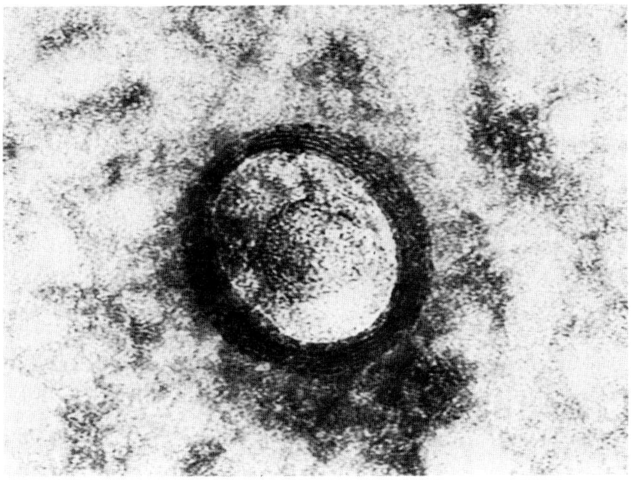

Fig. 7. Virus particle (iridovirus-like [24]). These particles were always found in the supernatant of cell cultures mentioned in the legend of Fig. 6

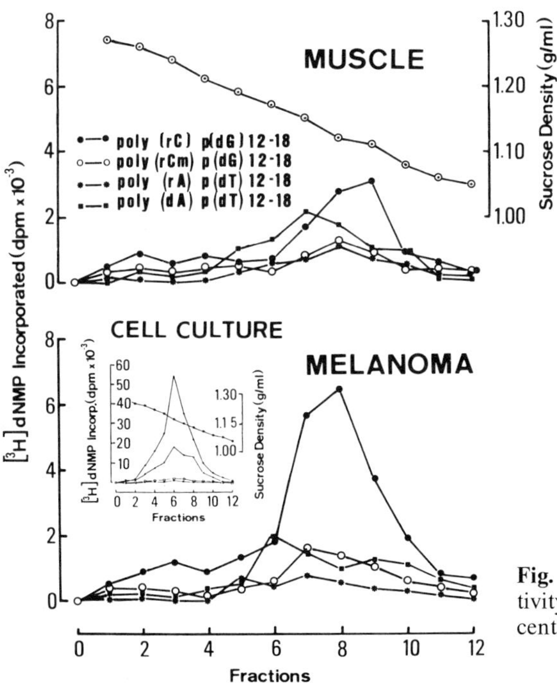

Fig. 8. RNA-dependent DNA polymerase activity in *Xiphophorus.* Sucrose density gradient centrifugation of the microsomal pellet

ed as carriers of amplified oncogenes [7, 8]. Virus particles have been found in the melanoma following treatment with bromodesoxyuridine [23]. Following sucrose density centrifugation, in the supernatant of nontreated melanomatous cells of cultures mentioned above, RNA-dependent DNA polymerase associated with particles similar to fish iridovirus [24] (Fig. 7) was found in the density range of 1.15–1.17 g/ml. Three to five particles have been counted per grid, which is equivalent to 10^5 particles/ml. RNA-dependent DNA polymerase activity has also been detected in the melanoma tissue and, although three to five times lower, in the muscle (Fig. 8). Activity of many other enzymes, such as tyrosinase [25], lactate dehydrogenase [26, 27], malate dehydrogenase, and pyruvate kinase [27], is changed in the melanoma.

Table 1. SCE frequency in intestinal cells of *Xiphophorus* [29]

Xiphophorus	Metaphases scored	Cells with SCE (%)	Range (SCE/cell)	Mean SCE/metaphase (SE)
X. maculatus				
Tu/Tu;Diff/Diff	131	31.9	0–3	0.41±0.05
X. helleri				
–/–;–/–	166	32.0	0–3	0.40±0.03
Hybrids carrying *melanoma*				
F_1: benign				
Tu/–;Diff/–	153	56.8	0–4	0.82±0.05
BC: benign				
Tu/–;Diff/–	113	61.9	0–4	0.97±0.09
BC: malignant				
Tu/–;–/–	137	66.5	0–4	0.92±0.10
BC hybrids carrying *no melanoma*				
–/–;Diff/–	188	33.6	0–3	0.38±0.03
–/–;–/–	145	38.7	0–4	0.47±0.04

Sister chromatid exchange (SCE) is elevated in melanoma cells [28]. Interestingly, its high frequency is in parallel with that of nontumorous intestinal cells of melanomatous fish, and is low in intestine of the nonmelanomatous fish (Table 1) [29]. This is a striking similarity to the parallels of pp60$^{c\text{-}src}$ kinase activity measured in the melanoma and in the healthy brain.

These factors and many others not mentioned in this study are certainly important in melanoma formation, but probably none of them is involved in the primary event of tumorigenesis in this experiment. The primary event of tumor initiation in this experiment, without any doubt, happens when the egg and sperm contribute a normal set of oncogenes to the zygote but fail to contribute the adequate regulatory gene systems for control of the oncogenes. The confirmation of this view comes from the final crossing series of this experiment outlined in Fig. 9: Backcrosses of malignant-melanoma-bearing hybrids (Fig. 9A) (i.e., Fig. 5F) with the platyfish (Fig. 9B) (like those of Fig. 5A, but containing the *Tu* deletion according to Fig. 2d) result in a quasi F_1 that segregates in 50% of animals displaying benign melanoma (Fig. 9C) and 50% exhibiting neither melanomas nor spots (not shown in Fig. 9). Further backcrosses of the benign melanoma bearing quasi-F_1 hybrids with the platyfish (Fig. 9D) result in spotted and nonspotted fish that are similar to the purebred platyfish (Fig. 9E–H). Genetically they segregate into those that inherit the capability to develop melanoma after crossings with swordtails and those that do not inherit the capability to develop melanoma (not shown in Fig. 9). The outcome of this final series of backcrosses indicates the stepwise reintroduction of the platyfish chromosomes carrying the regulatory genes for the oncogene into the descendants, and the reconstruction of the original regulatory gene system that suppresses the activity of the oncogene in the platyfish genome.

Fig. 9A–H. Crossing procedure for the suppression of melanoma in *Xiphophorus.* **A** Malignant melanoma-bearing backcross hybrid according to Fig. 5F. **B** *X. maculatus* according to Fig. 5A as the recurrent parent. **C** Quasi F_1-exhibiting benign melanoma. **D** *X. maculatus* as the recurrent parent. **E–H** Backcross hybrids (quasi *X. maculatus*) exhibiting spots only. Melanomas and spots depend on *Tu* of the X chromosome shown in Fig. 2e. See Fig. 5

Fig. 10A–H. Crossing procedure for the production of *Xiphophorus* hybrids that are sensitive to carcinogens. The procedure is basically the same as that outlined in Fig. 5 (**A** *X. maculatus;* **B** *X. helleri;* **C** F_1; **D** *X. helleri*). **A**, **C**, **E**, and **F** exhibit a reddish coloration. *c-src*, pp60$^{c\text{-}src}$ kinase activity. See text

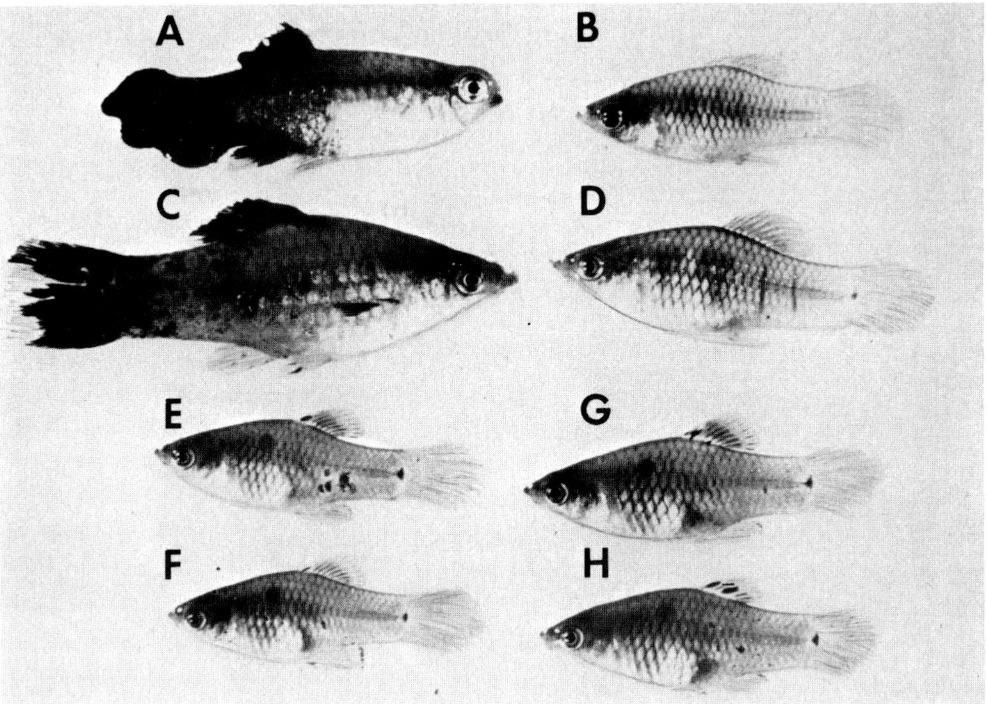
A
B
C
D
E
G
F
H

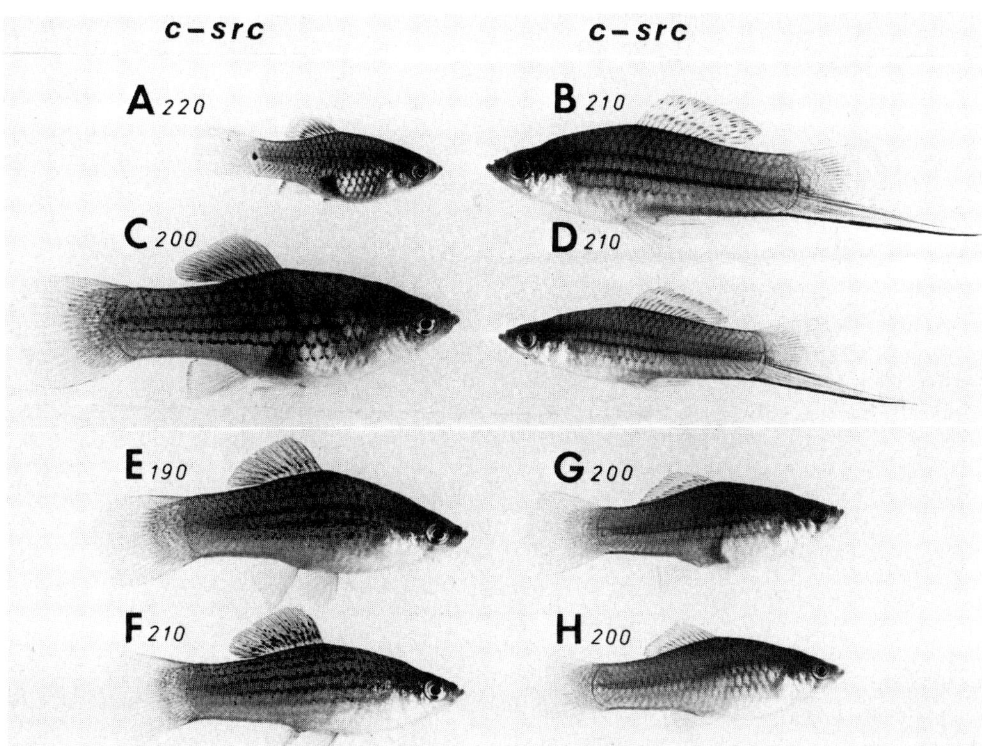
c-src
c-src
A 220
B 210
C 200
D 210
E 190
G 200
F 210
H 200

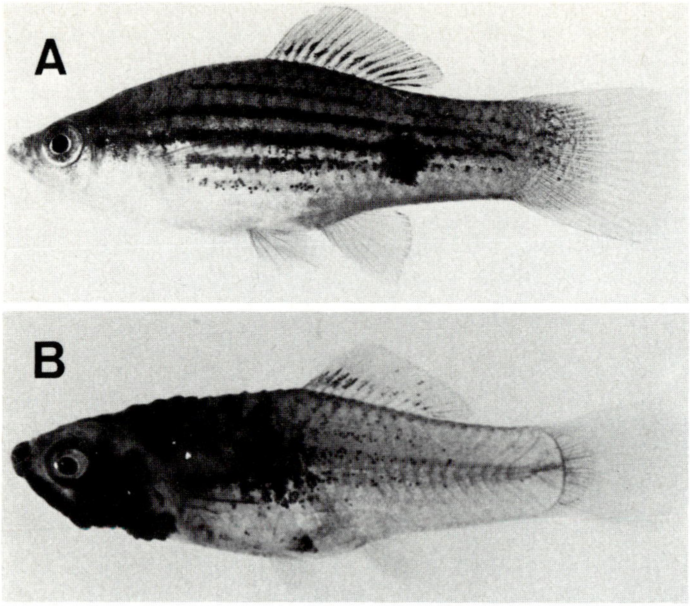

Fig. 11 A, B. Backcross hybrids according to Fig. 10 E and F after treatment with MNU. **A** *Diff*-carrying segregant (identified by an esterase) developing benign melanoma; **B** *Diff*-lacking segregant (identified by lack of the esterase) developing malignant melanoma

Presumably the oncogene itself remained unchanged during the crossing procedure (Figs. 5, 9) that first induced and thereafter suppressed melanoma formation. Carcinogens or tumor-suppressing agents were not required in this experiment. The outcome of the experiment, however, indicates that the experimenter must interfere in the regulatory gene system of the oncogene to be able to induce or suppress melanoma (or any other neoplasm). To examine this idea, we carried out the following experiment.

III. Third Experiment: Tumors Induced by Impairment of Cell-Type-Specific Regulatory Genes for the Oncogene in Somatic Cells

This experiment is based on the two assumptions that (a) the total number of pigment-cell precursors competent for neoplastic transformation is 10^6 (this is the average number in the pigment-cell system of a young fish) and (b) the mutation rate for a given gene in these cells is 10^{-6}. Then tumor incidence is one (on average 100% of the treated animals develop one tumor) provided the oncogene is under control of only one regulatory gene. If, however, the oncogene is regulated by two genes, the rate of simultaneous mutations of both regulatory genes in one cell is 10^{-12} and the tumor incidence is 10^{-6}. This calculation shows that if the oncogene is controlled by more than one regulatory gene, it is difficult to succeed in inducing somatic mutation-conditioned neoplasms at a frequency suitable for mutagenesis experiments.

To establish a *Xiphophorus* strain suitable for mutagenesis studies on a single regulatory gene of the *Tu* oncogene, we replaced the R'_{Pp} R'_{Df} R'_{Mel} platyfish X chromosome used so far (Fig. 2e) by the R'_{Pp} R'_{Df} R_{Mel} *Tu* X chromosome (Fig. 2f), which, instead of the impaired R'_{Mel}, contains the normal R_{Mel}. Crossings were performed according to Fig. 10, which are essentially the same as those described in the first part of the previous experiment (Fig. 5).

Due to the active R_{Mel} that controls the oncogene in the pigment cell system, no melanomas develop in the hybrids. The BC hybrids E and F that correspond to the melanoma-developing BC hybrids in the former experiment (they can be recognized by a reddish coloration encoded in the pteridine marker gene *Pter* also linked to the *Tu* oncogene; see Fig. 2) are, however, sensitive to carcinogens and may develop

Table 2. Tumor initiation (somatic mutation) and promotion (promotion of cell differentiation) distinguished by tester strains of *Xiphophorus* constructed according to the third and sixth experiments

Agents	Dose	Period	Initiation		Promotion	
			Survivors	Tumors (%)	Survivors	Tumors (%)
MNU	10^5 μg/liter	5×14 days 45 min	457	88 (19)	36	18 (50)
ENU	10^5 μg/liter	5×7 days 1 h	235	21 (9)	21	2 (10)
Diethylnitrosamine	45×10^3 μg/liter	2×/week for 8 weeks	23	2 (9)	24	0
TPA (in DMSO)	1 μg/liter/day	10 weeks	121	0	23	11 (48)
4-*O*-Methyl TPA	1 μg/liter/day	10 weeks	20	0	15	0
DMSO	2×10^6 μg/liter/8 days	10 weeks	98	0	12	1 (8)
Diazepam	500 μg/liter/day	48 weeks	27	0	24	0
Phenobarbital	7.5×10^3 μg/liter/day	10 weeks	25	0	11	7 (64)
Cyclamate	10^6 μg/liter	8 weeks	28	0	22	12 (55)
	2×10^6 μg/liter	8 weeks	NT	NT	10	6 (60)
Saccharin	5×10^6 μg/liter	10 weeks	21	0	23	3 (13)
5-Azacytidine	1.25×10^3 μg/liter/day	8 weeks	47	0	12	7 (58)
L-Ethionin	500 μg/liter/day	8 weeks	18	0	16	0
Actinomycin D	20 μg/liter/day	8 weeks	15	0	10	0
Testosterone	2–20 μg/liter/day	24 weeks	NT	NT	22	22 (100)
Methyltestosterone	2–20 μg/liter/day	24 weeks	113	0	30	30 (100)
5-Dihydrotestosterone	2–20 μg/liter/day	24 weeks	NT	NT	11	11 (100)
Methylandrostenolone	2–20 μg/liter/day	24 weeks	NT	NT	21	21 (100)
Estrogen	2–20 μg/liter/day	48 weeks	NT	NT	5	0
Diethylstilbestrol	2–20 μg/liter/day	48 weeks	NT	NT	16	0
17-Hydroprogesterone	2–20 μg/liter/day	48 weeks	NT	NT	9	0
Progesterone	2–20 μg/liter/day	48 weeks	NT	NT	8	0
X-rays	1000 R	3×45 min/6 week interval	805	163 (20)	45	45 (100)

DMSO, dimethylsulfoxide; NT, not tested. Data were compiled from theses of C.-R. Schmidt, A. Schartl, A. Herbert (Univ. of Giessen)

melanoma after carcinogen treatment. Those BC hybrids carrying the *Diff* gene (autosomal; identified by a *Diff*-linked esterase marker gene [30, 31]) may develop benign melanomas and those lacking *Diff* may develop malignant ones (see Figs. 1, 11). Crosses between two BC hybrids of the latter genotype were the basis for the establishment of a strain homozygous for the R'_{Pp} R'_{Df} R_{Mel} *Tu* chromosome [32, 33]. Because each of the two copies of the *Tu* oncogene is repressed by its own linked R_{Mel}, which acts in the *cis* position only, the incidence of animals developing melanoma following treatment with carcinogens potentially doubles. These fish are highly suitable as test animals for mutagenic carcinogens in the water (Table 2, see column "Initiation").

In contrast to the crossing-conditioned hereditary melanomas that, due to their multicellular origin [15], cover large areas in the compartments of the body from their very beginning, the carcinogen-induced melanomas appear first as small foci of cells in these compartments (Fig. 1), indicating that they originate from the expected single mutational event in a particular regulatory gene of the oncogene in a particular somatic cell in a particular compartment of the body.

All purebred and hybrid animals of this experiment display uniform $pp60^{c\text{-}src}$ kinase activity in the brain [19]. This activity seems to represent the basic *c-src* expression like that of the nontumorous fish in the previous experiment (cf. Figs. 5, 10). Following the induction of melanomas and of any other kind of neoplasia, $pp60^{c\text{-}src}$ kinase activity in the brain remains unchanged. Kinase activity in the melanomas, however, is heterogeneous, with the malig-

Table 3. Elevated pp60$^{c\text{-}src}$ kinase activity in *Xiphophorus* bearing tumors as compared with nontumorous controls

Tumor	Elevation of kinase activity	
	In tumors	In brain
Hereditary		
Melanoma, benign ($n=15$)	+	+
Melanoma, malignant ($n=13$)	+ +	+ +
Induced		
Melanoma, malignant ($n=2$)	+ +	0
Melanoma, malignant	+ + +	0
Melanoma, amelanotic	+ + + +	0
Retinoblastoma ($n=2$)	+ + +	0
Fibrosarcoma	+ +	NT
Fibrosarcoma	+ + +	0
Fibrosarcoma	+ + + + +	0
Rhabdomyosarcoma	+	NT
Rhabdomyosarcoma	+ + + +	0
Epithelioma	+ +	0
Squamous-cell carcinoma	+ +	0

NT, not tested

nant melanoma showing values that are at least as high as those of the corresponding melanomas of crossing-conditioned hereditary origin. In an induced malignant amelanotic melanoma pp60$^{c\text{-}src}$ kinase activity was even six times higher than that of the brain. As in melanomas, elevated levels of kinase activity were also found in other carcinogen-induced neoplasms such as fibrosarcoma, retinoblastoma, and epithelioma (see Table 3). However, changes in the pp60$^{c\text{-}src}$ kinase activity in the brain that are typical in the hereditary tumor-bearing animals were not observed. More studies are necessary to find out whether the elevation of pp60$^{c\text{-}src}$ activity found in the neoplasms is due to the same impaired regulatory gene that permits the *Tu* oncogene to mediate carcinogenesis.

IV. Fourth Experiment: Transfer of the Regulatory Gene-Dependent Tumorigenic Potential by Genomic DNA

To perform this transfection experiment we used different laboratory stocks of *X. maculatus* as donors. These stocks were uniform with respect to *Tu* and the impairment of the compartment-specific regulatory genes R_{Ap} and R_{Pp} (see fifth experiment). They were, however, different in the condition of the melanophore-specific regulatory gene R_{Mel}, which was normal, impaired, strongly impaired, or deleted (Fig. 12). Total genomic DNA of the donors was injected into the neural crest region of early embryos (where the pigment-cell precursors originate) of *X. helleri*. This species has excellent potential for expressing a deregulated oncogene (see previous experiments). If a donor containing the normal R_{Mel}-*Tu* complex (Fig. 12A) was used, no recipient exhibited transformed pigment cells. If a donor strain was used that carried a *Tu* slightly derepressed in the pigment-cell system by a "weak" mutation of its linked R_{Mel}, i.e., R'_{Mel} *Tu* (Fig. 12B), then 0.4% of the recipients developed colonies of neoplastically transformed cells. If the DNA originated from a strain that carries the *Tu* derepressed to a greater degree, due to a "stronger" mutation of R_{Mel}, i.e., R''_{Mel} (Fig. 12C), the incidence of recipients exhibiting transformed pigment cells increased to 2.6%. If, finally, a donor was used in which the *Tu* lacks the R_{Mel} (due to a chromosomal translocation) (Fig. 12D), this incidence increased to 6.3%. DNA from animals carrying additional but rigidly repressed accessory *Tu* copies (not shown in Fig. 12) did not influence the incidence of transformants [34].

Besides the fact that the information for neoplastic transformation, presumably the

Donors		No. of Recipients	
Phenotype	Chromosomes	Survived	Showing Tr cells
A 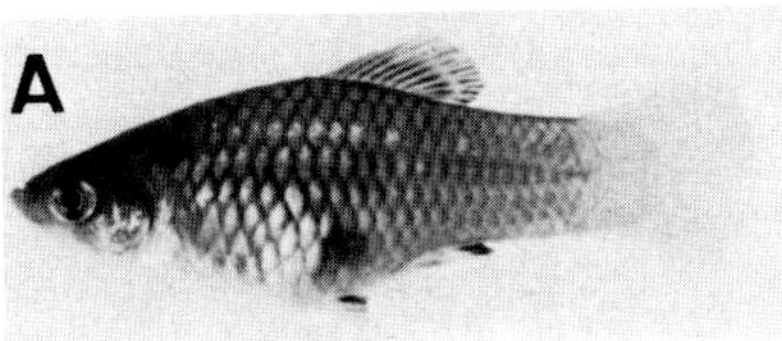	$X\frac{R\,Mel\,Tu}{}$ $Y\frac{R\,Mel\,Tu}{}$	2 010	0
B 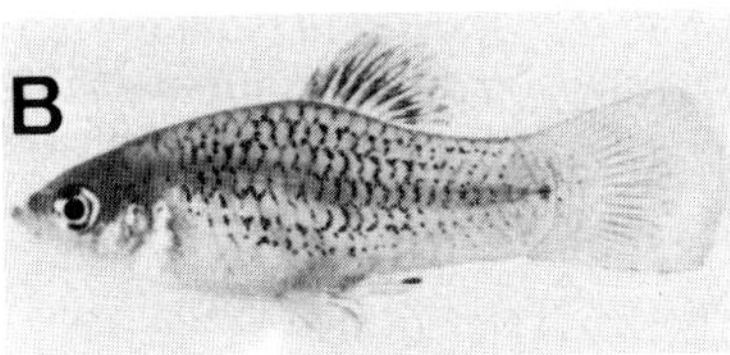	$X\frac{R'\,Mel\,Tu}{}$ $Y\frac{R'\,Mel\,Tu}{}$	535	2 (0.4%)
C 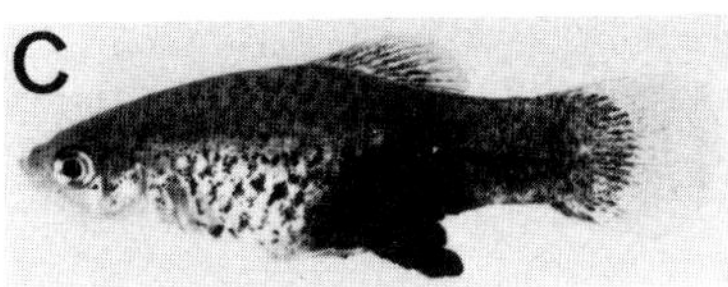	$X\frac{R''\,Mel\,Tu}{}$ $Y\frac{R''\,Mel\,Tu}{}$	1 052	27 (2.6%)
D 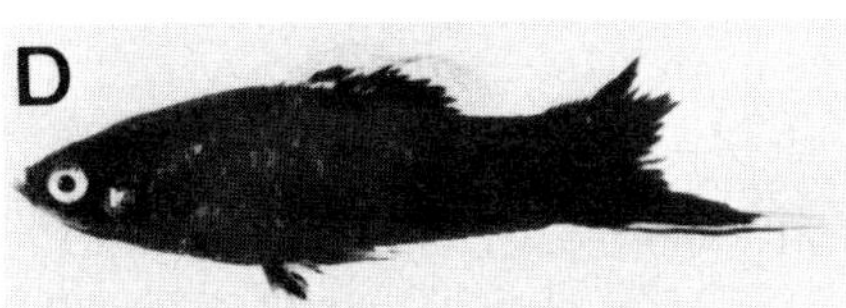	A - - - $\frac{Tu}{}$ A - - - $\frac{Tu}{}$	1 032	65 (6.3%)
DNase degraded DNA of C and D		710	0

Fig. 12 A–D. Transfection activity of donor DNA extracted from male gonads of fish differing in *Tu* control by the pigment-cell-specific regulatory gene R_{Mel}. Data from [34]. See text

oncogene itself, was transferred via total genomic DNA, it is important to note that the transforming donor DNA did not originate from tumor cells but from the nonneoplastic testes, indicating that oncogenes must not necessarily be changed or amplified in order to acquire the transforming potential. The many oncogene transfection experiments accomplished during the past years by several authors with other systems in which DNA extracts from tumors were used [2, 3, 35–37], with the expectation that tumor DNA differs from DNA from normal tissues, should be, in our opinion, reconsidered from the viewpoint of repression and derepression of oncogenes exerted by intact and defective regulatory genes. The main factors responsible for neoplasia are, in view of our results on *Xiphophorus*, not the *onc* genes, but their regulatory genes.

This view is supported by the fact that the incidence of transformants, i.e., the incidence of transformation events mediated by *Tu*, was independent of the number of *Tu* copies in the donor DNA (we tested DNA containing up to eight copies), but was exclusively dependent on the degree of impairment of R_{Mel}. In this light it also appears reasonable to assume that R_{Mel}, if present, is so closely linked to *Tu* that both *Tu* and R_{Mel} are always cotransferred [34].

Although the donor DNA originated from fish exhibiting different degrees of *Tu* expression, the transformed cells of the recipients all looked alike, and the cell colonies were all about the same size. This indicates that growth of the tumor is influenced neither by *Tu* nor by the intact or impaired R_{Mel}.

V. Fifth Experiment: Tumors Induced by Impairment of Compartment-Specific Regulatory Genes for the Oncogene in Germ Line Cells and/or in Somatic Cells

The compartment-specific regulatory genes for the oncogene, designated R_{Co} in total (see Fig. 2), have been studied mainly by means of X-ray-induced germ line mutations that affect one or several sites of the crossing-conditioned melanomas (Fig. 13). These melanomas develop in BC hybrids, for instance (a) in the dorsal fin; (b) in the tail fin; (c) in both the dorsal fin and tail fin; (d) in the anal fin; (e) in the tail fin, dorsal fin, anal fin, mouth tip, and posterior part of the side of the body (mutations of five compartment-specific regulatory genes are involved); (f) in the anterior and posterior parts of the side of the body; (g) in all compartments except for the mouth, belly, eye, dorsal fin, and tail fin; or (h) even in all compartments of the body. The phenotypes of additional combinations of impaired R_{Co} genes have been described previously [13, 15, 16].

The compartment-specific distribution of these melanomas is inherited according to the segregation of the parental *Tu*-carrying chromosome, indicating that the respective R_{Co} genes are linked to *Tu,* and structural changes of the chromosome have verified that this linkage is very close. At least 14 genes corresponding to 14 different compartments have been identified. They represent regulatory genes that were designated R_{Ap} (anterior part), R_{Pp} (posterior part), R_{Df} (dorsal fin), R_{Tf} (tail fin), etc. in reference to each specific body compartment. Intact R_{Co} genes repress *Tu,* and impaired R_{Co} genes permit *Tu* activity. They act in the *cis* position only, indicating that the compartment-specific regulation of *Tu* exerted by the R_{Co} genes acts at the DNA level.

In the active state the R_{Co} genes appear to delay the differentiation of pigment cells in the stem-cell stage (S-melanoblasts; see R_{Co} in Fig. 14). Additional mechanisms that are not understood provide the fish with differentiating pigment cells that mostly escape neoplastic transformation, but very exceptionally may be transformed. If, however, one or several R_{Co} genes are impaired by mutation, compartment-specific melanomas develop in the hybrids and are inherited according to Mendelian prediction.

To study whether melanoma can also be induced by impairment of a compartment-specific regulatory gene in a somatic cell we carried out the following experiment: BC hybrids, which, due to the impairment of the pigment-cell-specific regulatory gene (R'_{Mel}) and of the dorsal-fin-specific regulatory gene (R'_{Df}), develop hereditary melanoma in the dorsal fin only, were irradiated with X-rays. These animals frequently developed additional melanomas in other compartments of the body (Fig. 15) which, in contrast to the hereditary melanoma of the dorsal fin, are nonhereditary and develop from small foci of transformed cells in the skin. This indicates a mutational event in a particular compartment-specific regulatory gene in a particular competent pigment-cell precursor in a particular compartment of the body. The oncogene itself that mediates neoplastic transformation probably remained unchanged.

VI. Sixth Experiment: Tumors Induced by Promotion of Cell Differentiation

The *neutral crest cells* of *Xiphophorus* which are, like those of all vertebrates, the precursors of different cell types, start migrating and differentiating at the outset of organogenesis in the embryo (Fig. 14) [38, 39]. Those entering their final locations in the skin and extracutaneous tissues become determined to differentiate to *chromatoblasts.* These chromatoblasts are the common precursors of all types of pigment cells (chromatophores), including pterinophores, purinophores, and melanophores. Those chromatoblasts committed to differentiate to melanophores give rise to *stem melanoblasts* (S-melanoblasts). These may reproduce throughout the life of the fish,

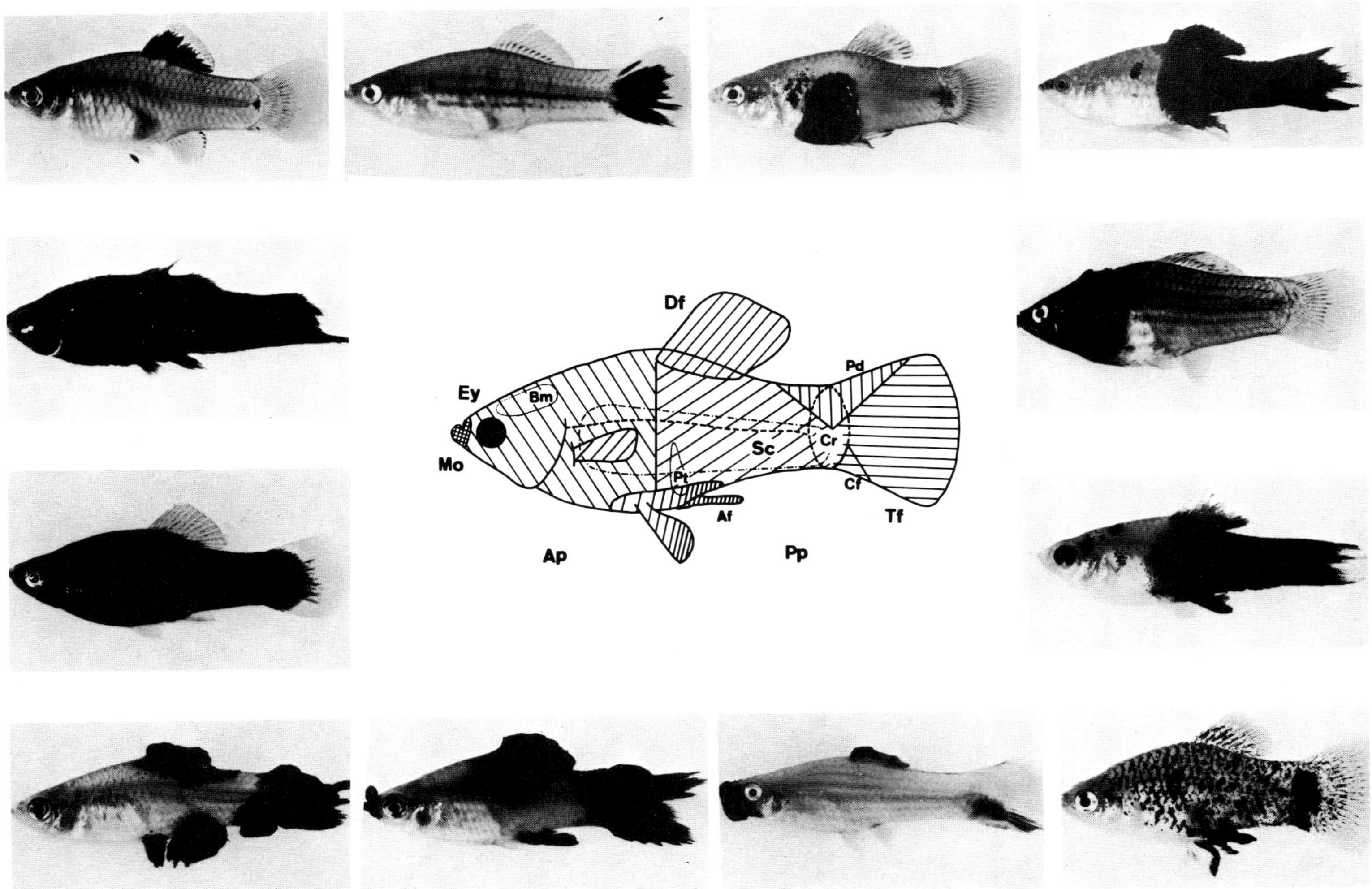

Fig. 13. Compartments for the development of melanomas in the fish. *Mo*, mouth; *Ey*, eye; *Bm*, brain membrane; *Ap*, anterior part; *Df*, dorsal fin; *Pt*, peritoneum; *Af*, anal fin; *Sc*, spinal cord; *Pp*, posterior part; *Cr*, crescent region; *Pd*, peduncle of the tail fin; *Cf*, caudal fin stripe; *Tf*, tail fin (see text)

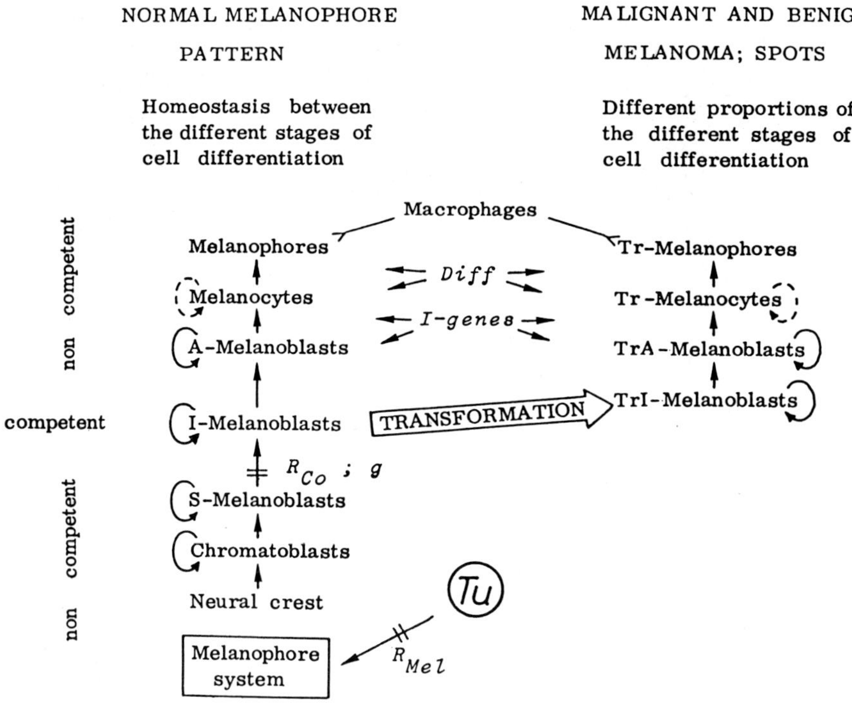

Fig. 14. Schematic presentation of the differentiation of normal and neoplastically transformed pigment cells. *S-, I-, and A-melanoblasts* are stem, intermediate, and advanced melanoblasts, respectively. The Tr cells represent the transformed cells. Only I-melanoblasts are competent for neoplastic transformation. *Tu,* tumor gene (oncogene); R_{Mel}, regulatory gene for control of *Tu* in the melanophore system; R_{Co}, compartment-specific regulatory genes; *g,* "golden" gene that blocks pigment-cell differentiation; *Diff,* differentiation gene; *I-genes,* intensifier genes, which support proliferation of poorly differentiated transformed pigment cells. Macrophages attack melanophores and Tr-melanophores. Modified from [16]

but may also differentiate to *intermediate-stage melanoblasts* (I-melanoblasts) that continue differentiation to the *advanced-stage melanoblasts* (A-melanoblasts) that can be distinguished from their precursors by their reaction to dopa. These cells differentiate to *melanocytes,* and these, finally, to *melanophores.* Genetic, cytological, and ultrastructural studies of the differentiation of the pigment cells have shown that the I-melanoblasts are the only cells of the system that are competent to undergo neoplastic transformation, i.e., competent to undergo the transforming activity of the *Tu* oncogene [38, 39].

The I-melanoblasts, after being transformed to *TrI-melanoblasts* (all transformed cells are called *Tr* cells) differentiate to the easily recognizable, proliferating *TrA melanoblasts.* These *Tr* cells differentiate to the heavily pigmented *Tr melanocytes,* which proceed to the terminal stage of differentiation of the transformed pigment cells, represented by the *Tr melanophores* [15].

We have analyzed several genes that are involved in pigment-cell differentiation. One of these genes is the "golden" gene (g^+), which, if present as a mutation in the homozygous state (g/g), creates an almost complete stop of melanophore differentiation at the stage of S-melanoblasts (see *g* in Fig. 14). The always present drosopterines become more visible in the skin, thus giving the fish the "golden" coloration.

This *g* mutation was introduced into the hereditary melanoma-bearing hybrids by

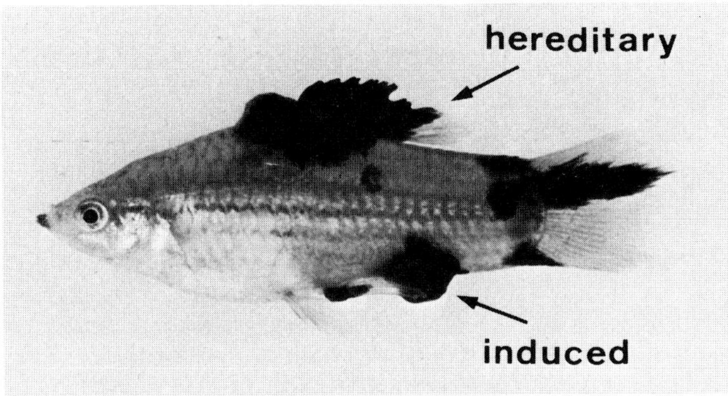

Fig. 15. Fish exhibiting crossing-conditioned hereditary melanoma in the compartment of the dorsal fin and X-ray-induced somatic mutation-conditioned melanoma in the compartment of the posterior part of the body (see *Df* and *Pp* in Fig. 13)

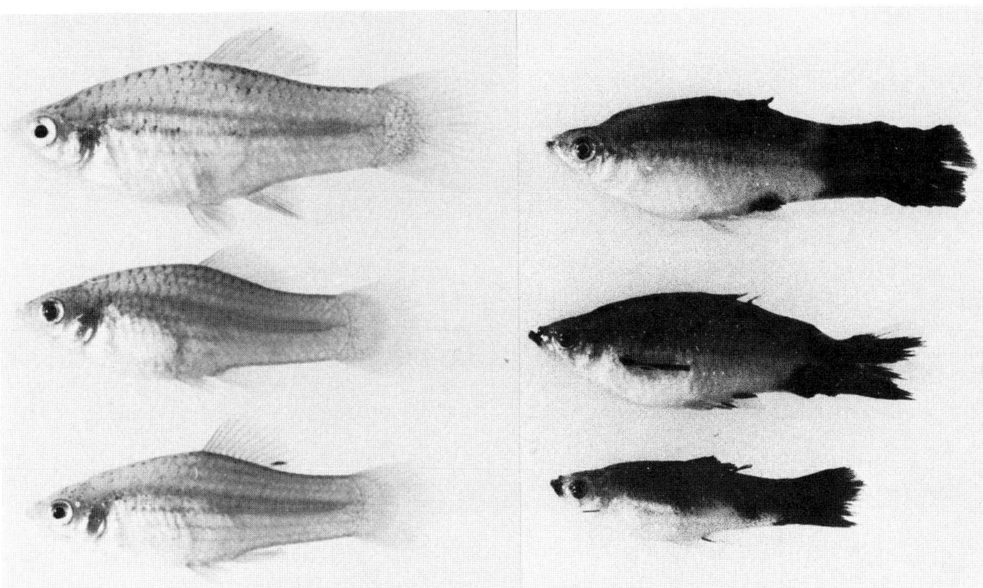

Fig. 16. Littermates that segregate into "golden" (g/g) animals (*left*) and tumor (g^+/g) animals (*right*). The g/g animals are protected from melanoma by a block of pigment-cell differentiation in the stage of the stem melanoblasts (see Fig. 14). Following treatment with promoters of cell differentiation (see Table 2) they develop melanoma similar to their heterozygous littermates

introgressive breeding, i.e., by the replacement of the g^+-bearing chromosome by the g-bearing homolog. In animals heterozygous for g (g/g^+) the derepressed *Tu* oncogene still mediates melanoma formation (Fig. 16, right). In the littermates that are homozygous for g (g/g), however, no melanomas develop (Fig. 16, left): The block of differentiation at the stage of the stem melanoblasts exerted by the homozygous g-mutation protects the fish from melanoma formation or from the activity of its own derepressed oncogene.

To break this protection mechanism we tested a large variety of mutagenic and nonmutagenic agents. Most of these agents (see Table 2, column "Promotion") promote almost simultaneously the differentiation of large amounts of the noncompetent cells to the competent stage, which subsequently become neoplastically transformed and give rise to melanomas.

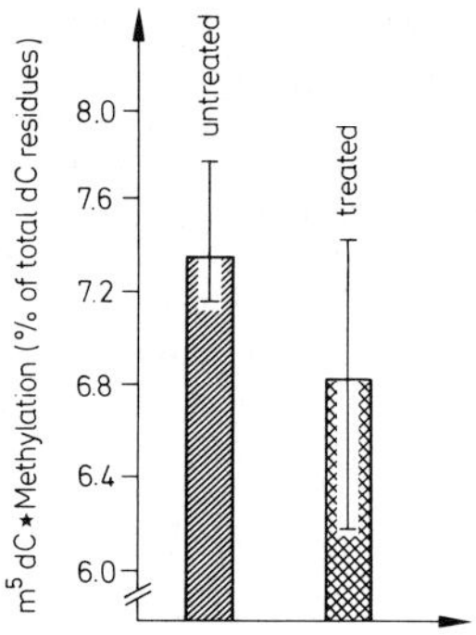

Fig. 17. Decrease of m^5dC methylation of DNA in *Xiphophorus* hybrids after treatment with 2.5 mg/liter per day 5-azacytidine. Fish were treated for 3 months, beginning at birth. HPLC analysis (filling, Supelco 4C-18-DB). Untreated, six animals; treated, five animals [63]

speculate that the *g* mutation undergoes a general modification that brings the function of *g* close to the normal function of the original g^+. The promoting effect of 5-azacytidine could be interpreted in this direction. This agent creates undermethylation in the DNA and, as a consequence, presumably gene activation [9, 40, 41]. As shown in Fig. 17, 5-azacytidine, which promotes differentiation, also demethylates DNA of *Xiphophorus*. More data are required to correlate the removal of the tumor-protecting effect of the *g*-mutation by 5-azacytidine with DNA methylation.

The crucial event leading to neoplasia in this experiment is the promotion of cell differentiation and possibly a more general modification of a gene that is involved in cell differentiation. The oncogene itself probably remained unchanged.

These tumors are morphologically similar to the spontaneously developing melanomas of the g/g^+ littermates, develop in the same compartments of the body, and are, similar to all hereditary melanomas, of multicellular origin. X-rays, *N*-methyl-*N*-nitrosourea (MNU), and *N*-ethyl-*N*-nitrosourea (ENU), which are powerful mutagens or tumor initiators, respectively, may also trigger melanoma by promotion of cell differentiation. It appears, however, that in this case neither of these agents acts as a mutagen, but as a differentiation-promoting agent such as testosterone, TPA, and cyclamate, which are certainly not mutagens.

The assumption that any somatic mutation, including that of a possible back mutation or suppressor mutation for the *g* mutation, is not involved in the promoting effect is compatible with the multicellular origin of the melanoma and with the high frequency of the respondents, which, in the case of 17-methyltestosterone, even reaches 100%. Optimization of the treatment in future experiments will show whether the promoting effect of a certain agent is an all-or-nothing effect, as is conceivable on the basis of the concept of this experiment.

Since somatic mutations are probably not involved in the trigger for melanoma development in this experiment, one could

VII. Seventh Experiment: Tumors Induced by Elimination of a Differentiation Gene from the Germ Line and Impairment of That Gene in Somatic Cells

To study the effect of the differentiation gene (*Diff*), thousands of melanoma-bearing BC segregants were produced according to the crossing procedure shown in Fig. 5, and all showed a clear-cut 1 : 1 segregation into animals developing spontaneously benign (Fig. 5E) or malignant melanomas (Fig. 5F). BC hybrids that require the carcinogenic trigger for the development of melanoma also show a clear-cut *Diff* effect (Fig. 11, see third experiment).

Morphological, histological, cytological, fine structural, biochemical, and molecular studies showed that the majority of the cells of the benign melanoma are well differentiated whereas those of the malignant melanoma are poorly differentiated, and that differentiation of the transformed cells is controlled by *Diff* [42, 43]. The most convincing data supporting *Diff*-dependent control of pigment-cell differentiation in melanoma come from transplantation experiments which have shown that pigment-cell precursors present in the transplants taken from fish carrying the deregulated *Tu* and lacking *Diff* (material of still tumor-free early embryos of the malignant-mela-

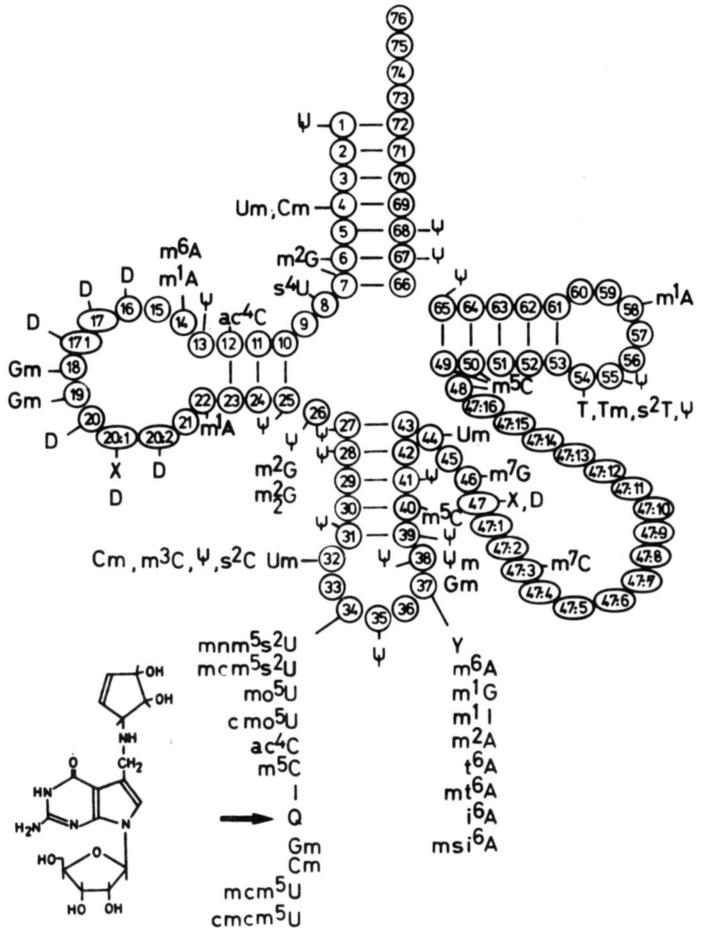

Fig. 18. General cloverleaf structure of the tRNA and positions of modified nucleosides. *Bottom left,* structure of queuosine (*Q*). Modified from [49]

noma-developing genotype according to the fish shown in Fig. 5 F) become transformed and remain incompletely differentiated if transplanted into embryos lacking *Tu* and *Diff:* The resulting animals develop malignant melanoma. If, however, the pigment-cell precursors of the same genotype are transplanted into *Tu*-lacking embryos that contain the *Diff* gene, the cells of the developing melanoma become terminally differentiated and regain their distance regulation: These resulting animals develop extreme benign melanomas which regress and eventually may become removed by macrophages (see [1]).

Further studies on the *Diff* effect on melanoma in *Xiphophorus* were stimulated by the experimental results of other laboratories that have focused on the involvement of nucleotide modifications of a certain tRNA family in cell differentiation in eubacteria, slime molds, and cell cultures from different vertebrates [43–48]. These tRNAs include $tRNA^{Asn}$, $tRNA^{Asp}$, $tRNA^{His}$, and $tRNA^{Tyr}$, which usually contain queuosine (Q) instead of guanosine (G) in the first position of the anticodon (position 34; see arrow in Fig. 18). The Q nucleoside (7-(((4,5-*cis*-dihydroxy-2-cyclopenten-1-yl)-amino)-methyl-7-deazaguanosine) is unique in that its purine skeleton is modified to a 7-deazastructure. Eubacteria synthesize the base queuine de novo whereas vertebrates are supplied with queuine by nutrition or the intestinal flora. Queuine itself is inserted into the nucleotide chain of tRNA by an exchange with guanine. This process is catalyzed by

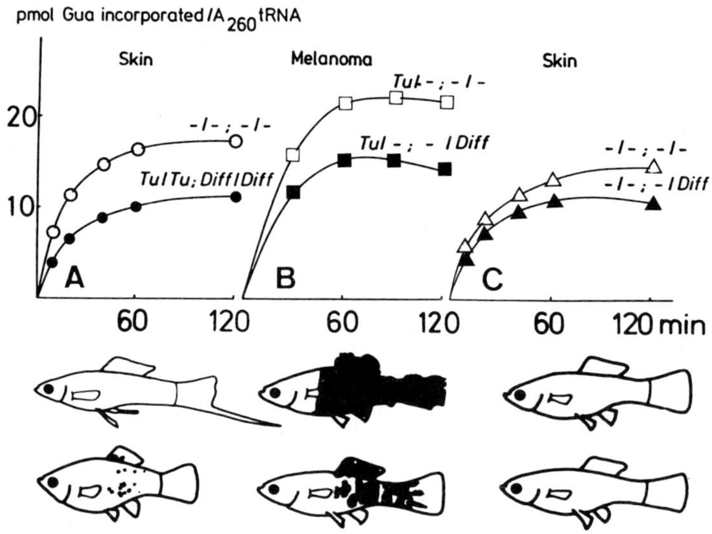

Fig. 19 A–C. Incorporation of [^{3}H]guanine in position 34 of tRNA for Asp, Asn, His, and Tyr of *Xiphophorus* catalyzed by tRNA-guanine-transglycosylase (insertase) of *E. coli.* The graphs show the kinetics of the exchange of G34 of tRNA by [^{3}H]guanine, a reaction used to evaluate the amount of (Q^-)tRNA [50]. **A–C** according to the fish shown below the curves. These fish correspond to those shown in Fig. 5. High incorporation of [^{3}H]guanine in *Diff*-lacking animals corresponds to a low content of Q, whereas low incorporation of [^{3}H]guanine in *Diff*-containing animals corresponds to a high content of Q. **A** Skin of purebred *Xiphophorus:* ○, X. helleri; ●, *X. maculatus.* **B** Melanoma of BC segregants: □, malignant; ■, benign. **C** Skin of nonmelanomatous BC segregants: △, lacking *Diff;* ▲, containing *Diff. Note* that comparable *Diff*-containing animals always have a lower G content and a higher Q content than *Diff*-lacking ones. Data from [43, 44, 51]

tRNA-guanine-transglycosylases. The more the cells are differentiated, the more replacement of G by Q is observed in position 34.

The method for estimating the G : Q ratio in a given population of the tRNA family consisted of following the replacement of guanine in position 34 by a ^{3}H-labeled guanine exerted by a guanine-transglycosylase (insertase) of *Escherichia coli* [50, 51].

The results obtained in *Xiphophorus* by measurement of [^{3}H]guanine incorporation into the tRNAs of the Q family, differing in the ratio of G : Q in position 34, are summarized in Fig. 19. The graphs show the kinetics of the exchange of G 34 of the tRNA family by [^{3}H]guanine, which is the reaction used to evaluate the amount of (Q^-)-tRNA. The fish genotypes and phenotypes are identical to those shown in Fig. 5.

In accordance with the findings of many investigators working with other differentiation systems [52], [^{3}H]guanine incorporation is high in tRNAs from malignant melanomas that consist predominantly of poorly differentiated cells. In contrast, the incorporation is lower if the tRNAs are derived from benign melanomas that consist predominantly of well-differentiated cells. Therefore, tRNAs of malignant melanomas have a higher amount of G in place of Q than those of the benign melanomas (Fig. 19 B).

To decide whether the distinct difference in G : Q ratios between benign and malignant melanoma is *Diff* dependent or represents an epiphenomenon of benignancy and malignancy, the skin of nontumorous littermates that segregate into animals carrying *Diff* and lacking *Diff* like the tumorous fish in a 1 : 1 ratio was used for analysis (Fig. 19 C). The *Diff*-lacking segregants always had higher amounts of Q-lacking tRNA than the *Diff*-carrying animals. The skin of the parent animals used

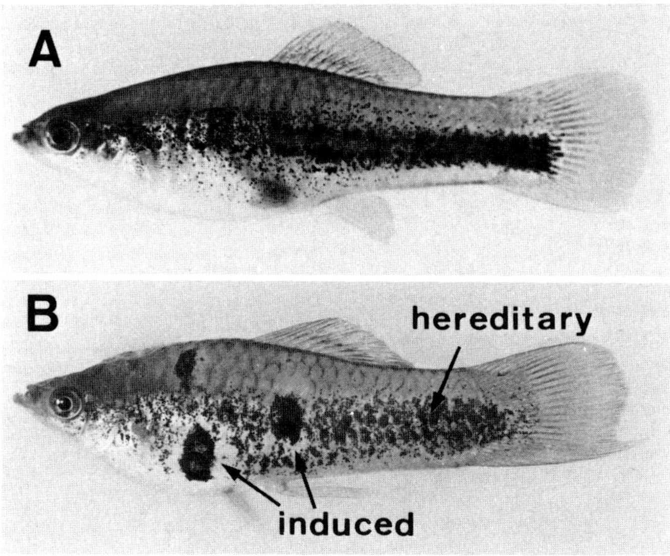

Fig. 20 A, B. Development of induced somatic mutation-conditioned malignant melanomas on a crossing-conditioned superficial hereditary melanoma. **A** Untreated fish; **B** Fish treated with X-rays. It is assumed that the induced melanomas are due to an impairment of the differentiation gene *Diff* in a pigment-cell precursor each

for the initial crosses showed the same differences (Fig. 19A): *X. helleri,* which lacks the *Diff* gene, has a high [^{3}H]guanine incorporation (i.e., is G-rich) whereas *X. maculatus,* which contains the *Diff* gene, has a lower [^{3}H]guanine incorporation. From these results we suggest that the difference of G : Q ratios between benign and malignant melanoma are not epiphenomena of benignancy and malignancy, but are closely related to the primary effect of the *Diff* gene.

The differences in the functional properties of Q-containing and Q-lacking tRNAs require further elucidation. The (Q)tRNAs have been suggested to prefer codons NAU to NAC, whereas the Q-lacking tRNAs read NAC and NAU equally well [46]. This may be an important mechanism in the regulation of translation. For eukaryotic $tRNA^{Tyr}$ it has been shown that the Q-lacking species reads a terminator codon, probably UAG. Therefore the Q-lacking and Q-containing tRNAs of vertebrates might select mRNAs for translation by a regulatory mechanism similar to that of termination transcription control (see discussions in ref. [51]).

If benignancy depends on the presence of a single copy of *Diff* and malignancy on the lack of this copy then it should be possible to induce easily somatic mutation-conditioned malignant melanoma in the area of germinal-conditioned benign melanoma. For this purpose we treated superficial benign melanoma with MNU or X-rays and observed the development of focal malignant melanoma in the area of the benign melanoma (Fig. 20). This is not to say that the benign melanoma changes to the malignant state. In contrast, the somatic mutation-conditioned malignant melanoma develops independently from the already present germ-line-conditioned benign melanoma. The induced malignant melanoma, however, competes with the hereditary benign melanoma for pigment-cell precursors. As a consequence of this competition the focal malignant melanomas are surrounded by a halo-like zone that is sparsely polulated by the cells of the benign melanoma.

This experiment shows once more that the genes that carcinogens act upon if they trigger neoplasia are not necessarily the oncogenes themselves, but their regulatory genes in the broadest sense.

D. Conclusions

In our *Xiphophorus* model we have not found any genetic change of the Mendelian inherited oncogene *Tu* that might lead to neoplasia, although one would expect this

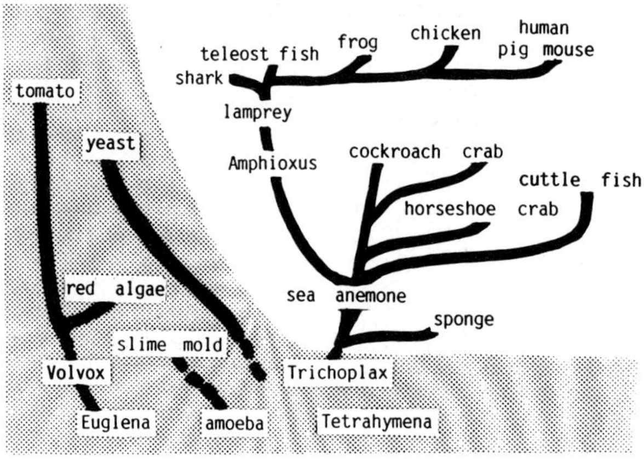

Fig. 21. Distribution of the *c-src* oncogene in living organisms. All organisms listed have been tested. *c-src* was found in all multicellular animals

to be possible based on the molecular findings of other laboratories that mutation, rearrangement, amplification, and demethylation can convert a silent oncogene to the transforming state. In contrast, our carcinogenesis studies show that the most important process involved in neoplasia in these animals is loss, impairment, or any other dysfunction of the regulatory gene system of the *Tu* oncogene. About 20 regulatory genes controlling the oncogene *Tu* at the gene level have been identified genetically and phenotypically. These genes comprise tissue-specific and compartment-specific (eye, mouth, etc.) regulatory genes (first to fifth experiments). Once the system of these regulatory genes controlling *Tu* is impaired, a chain of events is begun that can lead straight to neoplasia, but can also be interrupted by a genetic block of cell differentiation which protects the animal from the transforming activity of the oncogene. This protection mechanism can, however, easily be broken by promotion of cell differentiation (sixth experiment). If, finally, the cells are transformed, tumor growth can be stopped by terminal differentiation of the tumor cells exerted by the differentiation gene. Loss or impairment of the differentiation gene, then, leads definitely to neoplasia (seventh experiment). Our carcinogenesis experiments indicate that it is the regulatory genes (in the broadest sense) and not the oncogene itself that the carcinogens commonly act on, when they trigger neoplasia in *Xiphophorus.*

The inheritance and phenotypic expression of the genetically defined *Tu* oncogene parallels completely the expression of the molecularly defined *c-src* oncogene. Regardless of any future findings that might bring *Tu* substantially in relation to *c-src* and/or any other *c-onc,* both *Tu* and *c-src* act, are regulated, and are inherited as if they were the same chromosomal gene of the natural gene pool of the *Xiphophorus* fish.

c-src has been found functioning in all taxonomic groups of multicellular animals ranging from mammals down to the sponges (Fig. 21) [16, 53], and intensive efforts are being made in many laboratories to determine whether a cellular oncogene, such as *c-src,* is capable of mediating neoplastic transformation like its viral counterpart [3, 54–59]. If this should be proven we suggest that all individuals of all metazoa are endowed with the capacity to develop neoplasia. Support for this idea comes from the fact that neoplasia is distributed – although sporadically – in all groups of multicellular animals [60–62]. Ubiquity of the oncogene in metazoa including humans on the one hand and the infrequent occurrence of neoplasia in all these organisms on the other hand raises the question of the mechanisms that protect the majority of the individuals of all metazoans from the action of their own oncogenes. The *Xiphophorus* model provides an opportunity to contribute to the study of this problem.

Acknowledgment. Thanks are due to Kristine Krüger for valuable help in the preparation of this paper.

References

1. Anders F (1983) In: Neth R, Gallo RC, Greaves MF, Moore MAS, Winkler K (eds) Modern trends in human leukemia V. Springer, Berlin New York, pp 186–206 (Haematology and Blood Transfusion, vol 28)
2. Reddy EP, Reynolds RK, Santos E, Barbacid M (1982) Nature 300: 149–152
3. Tabin CJ, Bradley SM, Bargmann CI, Weinberg RA, Papageorge AG, Scolnick EM, Dhar R, Lowy DR, Chang EH (1982) Nature 300: 143–149
4. Taparowsky E, Suard Y, Fasano O, Shimizu K, Goldfarb M, Wigler M (1982) Nature 300: 762–764
5. Payne GS, Bishop JM, Varmus HE (1982) Nature 295:209–213
6. Dalla Favera R, Wong-Staal F, Gallo R (1982) Nature 299:61–63
7. Schwab M, Alitalo K, Varmus HE, Bishop JM, George D (1983) Nature 303:497–501
8. Schimke RT (1984) Cancer Res 44:1735–1742
9. Riggs AD, Jones PA (1983) Adv Cancer Res 40:1–30
10. Pimentel E (1985) Cancer Genet Cytogenet 14:347–368
11. Kallman KD (1975) Handb Genet 4:81–132
12. Anders F (1967) Experientia 23:1–10
13. Anders A, Anders F, Klinke K (1973) In: Schröder JH (ed) Genetics and mutagenesis of fish. Springer, Berlin New York, pp 33–63
14. Anders F, Anders A, Vielkind U (1974) Int Cancer Congr 11th Florence 3:305 (Abstr)
15. Anders A, Anders F (1978) Biochim Biophys Acta 516:61–95
16. Anders F, Schartl M, Barnekow A, Anders A (1984) Adv Cancer Res 42: 191–275
17. Collet MS, Erikson RL (1978) Proc Natl Acad Sci USA 75:2021–2024
18. Barnekow A, Schartl M, Anders F, Bauer H (1982) Cancer Res 42:2429–2433
19. Schartl M, Barnekow A, Bauer H, Anders F (1982) Cancer Res 42:4222–4227
20. Anders F, Schartl M, Barnekow A (1984) Natl Cancer Inst Monogr 65:97–109
21. Schartl M, Barnekow A (1984) Developmental Biology 105:415–422
22. Heil M (1984) Thesis, University of Giessen
23. Kollinger G, Schwab M, Anders F (1979) J Cancer Res Clin Oncol 95:239–246
24. Berthiaume L (1984) Virology 135:10–19
25. Vielkind U, Schlage W, Anders F (1977) Z Krebsforsch 90:285–299
26. Ahuja MR, Schwab M, Anders F (1975) Experientia 31:296–297
27. Mäueler W (1984) Thesis, University of Giessen
28. El-Zawahri MM, Hamdoon NT, Anders F (to be published) Cancer Genet Cytogenet
29. Hamdoon NT (1984) Thesis, University of Giessen
30. Ahuja MR, Schwab M, Anders F (1980) J Hered 71:403–407
31. Morizot DC, Sicliano MJ (1982) Genetics 102:539–566
32. Anders F, Schwab M, Scholl E (1981) In: Stich HF, San RHC (eds) Short-term tests for chemical carcinogens. Springer, Berlin New York, pp 399–407
33. Anders F, Schmidt CR, Herbert A, Anders A (1983) In: Prüfung von Chemikalien auf Kanzerogenität, Mutagenität und Teratogenität. Ges. f. Strahlen- und Umweltforschung, München, pp 253–274
34. Vielkind J, Haas-Andela H, Vielkind U, Anders F (1982) Mol Gen Genet 185:379–389
35. Krontiris TG, Cooper GM (1981) Proc Natl Acad Sci USA 78:1181–1184
36. Perucho M, Goldfarb M, Shimizu K, Lama C, Fogh J, Wigler M (1981) Cell 27:467–476
37. Der CJ, Krontiris TG, Cooper GM (1982) Proc Natl Acad Sci USA 79:3637–3640
38. Anders F, Diehl H, Schwab M, Anders A (1979) In: Klaus SN (ed) Pigment cell; vol 4, Karger, Basel, pp 142–149
39. Anders F, Diehl H, Scholl E (1980) Linnean Soc Symp Ser 9:211–224
40. Constantinides PG, Taylor SM, Jones PA (1978) Dev Biology 66:57–71
41. Jones PA, Taylor SM (1981) Nucleic Acid Res 3:2933–2947
42. Vielkind U (1976) J Exp Zool 196:197–204
43. Anders A, Dess G, Nishimura S, Kersten H (to be published) In: Bagnara JT, Klaus S, Paul E, Schartl M (eds) Pigment Cell 1985
44. Kersten H (1982) In: Jaenicke L (ed) Biochemistry of differentiation and morphogenesis. Springer, Berlin New York, pp 116–119
45. Kersten H (1983) in: Nass G (ed) Recent results in cancer research: modified nucleosides and cancer. Springer, Berlin New York, pp 255–263
46. Nishimura S (1983) Prog Nucleic Acid Res Mol Biol 28:49–74
47. Katze JR, Beck WT, Cheng CS, McCloskey JA (1983) In: Nass G (ed) Recent results in cancer research: modified nucleosides and cancer. Springer, Berlin New York, pp 146 –159
48. Katze JR, Gündüz U, Smith DL, Cheng CS, McCloskey JA (1984) Biochemistry 23:1171 –1176
49. Sprinzl M, Gauss DH (1982) Nucleic Acids Res 10:r1–r55
50. Okada N, Nishimura S (1979) J Biol Chem 254:3062–3066
51. Kersten H, Schachner E, Dess G, Anders A, Nishimura S, Shindo-Okada N (1983) In: Curtis HC, Pfleiderer W, Wachter H (eds)

Biochemical and clinical aspects of pteridines. Walter de Gruyter, Berlin, pp 367–382
52. Nass G (1983) Recent results in cancer research. Modified nucleosides and cancer. Springer, Berlin New York
53. Barnekow A, Schartl M (1984) Mol Cell Biol 4:1179–1181
54. Takeya T, Hanafusa H (1982) J Virol 44: 12–18
55. de Klein A, van Kessel AG, Grosveld G, Bartram CR, Hagemeijer A, Bootsma D, Spurr NK, Heisterkamp N, Groffen J, Stephenson JR (1982) Nature 300:765–767
56. Duesberg P (1983) Nature 304:219–225
57. Bishop JM (1982) Sci Am 246:68–78
58. Weinberg RA (1983) Sci Am 249:102–116
59. Hunter T (1984) Sci Am 251:60–69
60. Kraybill HF, Dawe CJ, Harshbarger JC, Tardiff RG (1977) Ann NY Acad Sci 298
61. Kaiser HE (1981) Neoplasms – comparative pathology of growth in animals, plants and man. Williams and Wilkins, Baltimore
62. Dawe CJ, Harshbarger JC, Kondo S, Sugimura T, Takayama S (1981) Phyletic approaches to cancer. Japan Scientific Societies Press, Tokyo
63. Schmiedel A (1984) Thesis. University of Giessen

Haematology and Blood Transfusion Vol. 29
Modern Trends in Human Leukemia VI
Edited by Neth, Gallo, Greaves, Janka

Chromosome Alterations in Oncogenesis

P. C. Nowell[1], B. S. Emanuel[2], J. B. Finan[1], J. Erikson[3], and C. M. Croce[3]

A. Introduction

Recently there has been increased interest in the study of chromosomal alterations in neoplastic cells. Such investigations have already begun to contribute significantly to our understanding of fundamental tumor biology, particularly with respect to the role of specific genes in carcinogenesis. This brief review will focus on this aspect of tumor cytogenetics, and particularly our own recent studies, but some generalizations will be offered first to help provide an appropriate perspective.

Based on the work from many laboratories, four general statements can be made about karyotypic alteration in neoplasia:

1. Most tumors have chromosome abnormalities. These usually are not present in other cells of the body.
2. In a given tumor, all the neoplastic cells often have the same cytogenetic change, or related changes.
3. Chromosome abnormalities are more extensive in advanced tumors.
4. Chromosome alterations are frequently different between tumors, but there are nonrandom patterns.

The cytogenetic findings that support the first two statements represent a significant portion of the increasing evidence that somatic genetic changes are important in tumorigenesis. In addition, the second generalization, along with related biochemical and immunoglobulin data, has been the basis for the now generally accepted view that most neoplasms are unicellular in origin [1, 2]. The fact that in a given tumor all of the cells show the same chromosome abnormality (or related abnormalities) suggests the origin of the tumor from a single altered cell. Presumably, the particular karyotypic change confers on the progenitor cell a selective growth advantage, allowing its progeny to expand as a neoplastic clone [1].

The third generalization listed has also contributed to our understanding of the natural history of tumor development. The observation that more advanced neoplasms typically show more extensive karyotypic alterations has led to the suggestion that clinical and biologic tumor progression may reflect the appearance in a neoplastic clone, over time, of subpopulations of cells with increasingly altered genetic makeup [1, 3]. Experimental evidence indicates that neoplastic cells show increased genetic instability, and so are more likely than normal cells to generate genetic variants [3]. Occasionally, such a variant cell may have more aggressive biologic characteristics, and so its progeny may grow out as the predominant malignant population, providing the basis for clinical tumor progression.

This concept has been well documented in chronic granulocytic leukemia, where

1 Department of Pathology and Laboratory Medicine, University of Pennsylvania School of Medicine, Philadelphia, Pennsylvania, USA
2 The Children's Hospital of Philadelphia, Philadelphia, Pennsylvania, USA
3 The Wistar Institute of Anatomy and Biology, Philadelphia, Pennsylvania, USA

the cells in the early indolent stage of the disorder typically show only the Philadelphia chromosome, but the terminal accelerated phase of the disease apparently results from overgrowth of this initial population by one or more subclones having additional karyotypic changes [4]. A similar sequence of events has been documented in other human and experimental tumors [3]. It has also been possible, through cytogenetic studies, to demonstrate the coexistence of multiple variant subpopulations within many advanced malignancies, thus providing at least one explanation for the biologically and clinically important phenomenon of tumor cell heterogeneity [3, 4].

B. Nonrandom Chromosome Abnormalities in Neoplasia

It is the final generalization listed that has engendered most of the very recent interest in tumor cytogenetics. With improved staining methods, it has become increasingly apparent that specific alterations in particular chromosomes are associated, with varying degrees of consistency, with specific types of tumors or with neoplasia in general [4, 5]. It has been hypothesized that these nonrandom karyotypic changes are indicating sites in the genome where particular genes, important in carcinogenesis, may be located, and also how the function of these "oncogenes" might be significantly altered [4–6]. In some instances, the consistent abnormality has been the gain or loss of a whole chromosome, or parts of a chromosome, suggesting a critical role for gene dosage in oncogenesis [4–6]. This has also been suggested by the observation in tumor cells of unusual chromosome structures that include elongated homogeneously staining regions (HSR), small extrachromosomal paired chromatin bodies – double minutes (DM), and abnormal banded regions (ABR), that all apparently represent alternative forms of gene amplification [7, 8].

Specific reciprocal chromosome translocations, without apparent addition or loss of genetic material, have also been identified as occurring nonrandomly in a variety of neoplasms, particularly leukemias and lymphomas [1, 4, 5]. Because such translocations, as well as a few of the HSR-type aberrations, are the only karyotypic abnormalities in tumor cells which thus far have been clearly related to altered function of known oncogenes, the remainder of this discussion will be restricted to these phenomena. Also, since most of the relevant data have been derived from hematopoietic neoplasms, only limited reference will be made to findings in other types of tumor.

C. Chromosome Translocations and Oncogenesis

Cytogenetic details of a number of the translocations recognized in various human leukemias and lymphomas have been the subject of several recent reviews [4, 5]. It has been suggested that their importance in carcinogenesis results from position effects, with the translocation bringing an inactive "proto-"oncogene into juxtaposition with "activating" sequences elsewhere in the genome [4, 6]. This hypothesis has now been investigated in cells of Burkitt's lymphoma, with very recent extension of such concepts to other leukemias and lymphomas. Current findings will be summarized in the subsequent sections.

I. Burkitt's Lymphoma

In most cases of Burkitt's tumor [9, 10], there is a reciprocal translocation between chromosomes 8 and 14. Variant translocations have been described in a small minority of these neoplasms [11, 12], one involving chromosomes 8 and 22, the other involving chromosomes 2 and 8. In all instances, the breakpoint in chromosome 8 is the same, at band q24 in the terminal portion of the long arm of the chromosome.

It has also been shown [13–16] that the genes for human immunoglobulin heavy chains map to chromosome 14, for λ light chain genes to chromosome 22, and for the $\varkappa$ light chain genes to chromosome 2. At the same time, one of the human homologs of known retroviral oncogenes, the so-called c-*myc* gene that is homologous to the

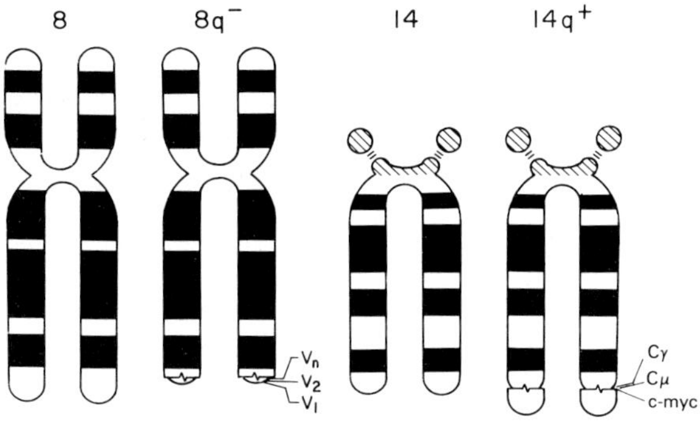

Fig. 1. Diagram of the t(8; 14) chromosome translocation in a Burkitt's lymphoma cell line. The V_H genes translocate from chromosome 14 to the involved chromosome 8 (8q–), while the c-*myc* oncogene translocates to the heavy chain locus, and shows greatly increased transcriptional activity in its new location. Reproduced from [21]

avian virus oncogene v-*myc*, was found [17, 18] to be located on the terminal portion of the long arm of chromosome 8. These observations suggested that the immunoglobulin genes and the c-*myc* oncogene might have important roles in the development of Burkitt's tumor, and this has subsequently been demonstrated, in our laboratory and by others, to be the case.

It was first shown, in a Burkitt's tumor cell line [19], that the immunoglobulin heavy chain locus in these cells was split, with a portion translocated to the involved chromosome 8, and a portion retained on chromosome 14. Subsequently, similar methods were used to show that the segment of chromosome 8 translocated to the long arm of chromosome 14 contained the c-*myc* oncogene [17, 18, 20], as shown in Fig. 1. It was also demonstrated [21] that in its new location, adjacent to a transcriptionally active immunoglobulin gene, the c-*myc* oncogene showed markedly increased transcription.

These studies have since been extended to Burkitt's lymphomas with the variant 8;22 and 2;8 chromosome translocations, using both somatic cell genetic and in situ hybridization methods [22–25]. In these circumstances, the results again indicate involvement of both the c-*myc* gene and an immunoglobulin gene, but with interesting differences in the apparent mechanism of activation of the oncogene. In a study of a Burkitt's lymphoma cell line with the 8;22 translocation, we found [23] that the c-*myc* gene remains on the number 8 chromosome, and the constant region portion of the λ light chain gene is translocated from chromosome 22 to this chromosome 8. The c-*myc* oncogene on the rearranged chromosome 8 (8q+) shows enhanced transcriptional activity as a result of the translocation, whereas the c-*myc* oncogene on the normal chromosome 8 is transcriptionally silent [23]. Similar results have been obtained with a Burkitt's cell line containing the variant 2;8 chromosome translocation that involves the $\varkappa$ light chain locus [24, 25], and here again it was possible to demonstrate that high levels of transcripts of the c-*myc* gene were found when it resided on the 8q+ chromosome, but not on the normal chromosome 8.

Taken together, these various findings with Burkitt's lymphomas clearly suggest that a chromosomal rearrangement in a B lymphocyte that places the c-*myc* oncogene adjacent to a transcriptionally active immunoglobulin gene can lead to markedly increased transcription of the oncogene in circumstances where it is not normally active. Additional support for this conclusion comes from concurrent observations with mouse plasmacytomas, in which it recently has been shown that a characteristic nonrandom chromosomal translocation involves the same immunoglobulin and *myc* genes as in Burkitt's tumor [26], with the same effect of increased transcription of c-*myc* [27]. The same circumstance may also obtain in the rat [28]. It is not yet clear to what extent such findings may be applicable to other hemic tumors, but the results have stimulated initial investigations in a number of directions. Several of these will be summarized briefly in the next section.

II. Other Human Leukemias and Lymphomas

A number of lymphomas have translocations that involve the terminal portion of 14q (band q32) and either the long arm of chromosome 11 (q13) or the long arm of chromosome 18 (q21) [29, 30]. It appeared very likely that these rearrangements might involve the immunoglobulin heavy chain locus, as in the 8; 14 translocation of Burkitt's tumor. At present, however, there is no candidate oncogene that has been mapped to the relevant regions of 11q and 18q that might be activated in the same fashion as the c-*myc* gene in Burkitt's tumor.

We have recently begun to study a number of these translocations, and have cloned the chromosomal breakpoint of a human B cell tumor with the characteristic 11; 14 translocation already mentioned [31]. We have found [32] that the breakpoint is indeed within the immunoglobulin heavy chain locus on chromosome 14. Furthermore, it was possible to demonstrate that DNA sequences from chromosome 11 had been translocated immediately adjacent to the breakpoint on the involved chromosome 14 and that these chromosome 11 sequences were rearranged. This rearranged DNA segment was also present in the cells of another B cell lymphoma with the same 11; 14 translocation, but not in Burkitt's lymphoma cells with the 8; 14 translocation or in non-neoplastic human lymphoblastoid cells [31]. Thus, it may be possible to identify and characterize a gene, for which we have suggested the name bcl-1, located at band q13 of chromosome 11, which appears to be involved in the malignant transformation of human B cells carrying the 11; 14 translocation. Similar studies are now under way with neoplastic B cells having the 14; 18 translocation that also occurs nonrandomly in a significant number of non-Hodgkin's lymphomas.

A different situation is found in several types of human myeloid leukemia. In these disorders, characteristic chromosomal translocations have been identified that appear to involve the human homolog of a known retroviral oncogene, but a mechanism for activation, analogous to the role of the immunoglobulin genes in the B cell tumors, has not been readily apparent.

For example, in chronic myelogenous leukemia (CML), several laboratories [33, 34] have now demonstrated that the typical t(9 ; 22)(q34; q11) translocation, which produces the Philadelphia chromosome, uniformly involves translocation of the c-*abl* oncogene from its normal site on chromosome 9 to a position adjacent to the breakpoint on chromosome 22. In this new location, the c-*abl* oncogene is close to the immunoglobulin λ light chain locus, which remains on chromosome 22 (unlike the circumstance in the 8; 22 translocation of the variant Burkitt's tumors) [35]. There is, however, evidence that in most CML cells the λ light chain gene is not rearranged or transcriptionally active, and so it does not appear to be a likely candidate for "activating" the newly juxtaposed c-*abl* [36]. Nor is there yet strong evidence that there is an alteration in the structure or function of the translocated c-*abl* oncogene, except for one report of an abnormal RNA transcript [37]. At present, the role of c-*abl* in the pathogenesis of CML remains under active investigation.

Similar circumstances may obtain with respect to the 15; 17 chromosome translocation commonly seen in acute promyelocytic leukemia (APL) and the 8; 21 translocation that characterizes a subgroup of patients with acute myelogenous leukemia (AML) [4]. Several laboratories have been investigating the possibility that a human homolog of the retroviral oncogene erbA might be involved in the typical translocation of APL [38, 39]. We have recently obtained evidence [39] that supports the localization of this gene to the q21-22 region of human chromosome 17, closely proximal to the breakpoint in the t(15; 17)(q22; q21-22) translocation in APL [4]. Perhaps unidentified "activating" sequences are translocated from chromosome 15 and are influencing the erbA oncogene on chromosome 17, but there are as yet no specific data to support this hypothesis.

A similar phenomenon might also be occurring in those cases of AML with a characteristic t(8; 21)(q22; q22) translocation [4]. In this instance, the candidate proto-oncogene for activation is c-*mos*, which has been mapped to the q22 region of chromosome 8, with the suggestion that sequences from 21q might be serving in the activating role [4, 5, 18]. Again, no direct data are currently available to support this concept, but our study of the c-*erbA* oncogene may have provided some relevant information. In that investigation [39], we were also able to study leukemic cells with an unusual t(17;21)(q21-22;q22) translocation involving the breakpoints on chromosomes 17 and 21 typically observed in the 15;17 translocation of APL and the 8;21 translocation of AML [40]. Here again, the erbA oncogene appeared to be located closely proximal to the breakpoint on chromosome 17, suggesting the possibility that activating sequences, in this case from chromosome 21, were being brought adjacent to it. These would be the same activating sequences presumably brought adjacent to c-*mos* in the 8;21 translocation of AML.

At present, these studies of translocations in hematopoietic tumors other than Burkitt's lymphoma are still in their early stages. It does already appear, however, that they will provide important information on other oncogenes and other activating mechanisms that could have wide applicability in tumor biology.

D. Chromosome Alterations and Oncogene Amplification Units

As already indicated, the types of visible chromosomal changes in malignant tumors, other than translocations, that have been most definitely associated with known oncogenes to date are certain of the HSR, DM, and ABR that appear to represent gene amplification units. In earlier studies of tissue culture cell lines, it was demonstrated that these unusual cytogenetic structures represented, in some cases, multiple copies of genes necessary for cell growth under specific culture conditions [8, 41]; and also that they might be alternative forms of gene amplification, with HSR breaking down to form DM, and DM integrating into various chromosomal sites to generate HSR and ABR [7, 8]. Although these structures do not show the same consistent localization within the genome as do the nonrandom chromosome translocations, it has been shown that they can involve human homologs of retroviral oncogenes.

Perhaps most interesting is the recent report [42] that the HSR observed in a significant proportion of cases of freshly isolated neuroblastoma cells involved DNA sequences related, but not identical, to the c-*myc* oncogene. This new gene, which they designated N-*myc*, maps to the short arm of chromosome 2 in normal cells, but in the neuroblastoma cells studied, the amplified N-*myc* was found to be located at a variety of sites within the genome [42].

Related observations have been made in our laboratory and elsewhere on several cell lines derived from human carcinomas and leukemias [43–45]. For example, it has recently been demonstrated that in cells of the HL-60 cell line, originally established from a patient with APL, there are 20–40 copies of the c-*myc* gene [46, 47], and that these are associated with an ABR on chromosome 8 in the normal location of c-*myc* [45] (Fig. 2). Alitalo et al. [43] have shown similar amplification of c-*myc* in a human intestinal carcinoma cell line, related either to an HSR at an abnormal location in the genome or to DM chromosomes. In a study involving another oncogene, we have been able to demonstrate that multiple copies of the c-*abl* oncogene in the K562 cell line (from a case of CML), as well as similarly amplified copies of the C-λ immunoglobulin gene, are associated in an ABR located on what appears to be a modified Philadelphia chromosome [44].

These various data, although still limited, certainly suggest that gene amplification units, recognizable cytogenetically as HSR, DM, and ABR, can represent another mechanism by which oncogene function may be so altered as to play a singificant role in tumorigenesis. This appears already well documented with respect to chromosomal translocations. As additional studies of oncogene structure and function are linked in the near future to various other types of nonrandom chromosomal alterations in neoplasia, it may be expected that similar associations will be made with respect to specific additions and losses of

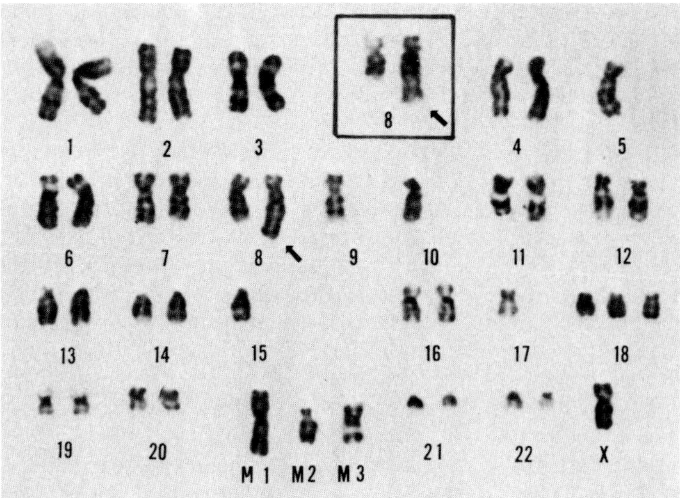

Fig. 2. Karyotype of human leukemic cell line HL-60, in which amplification of the c-*myc* oncogene was shown to be associated with the abnormally banded region of chromosome 8 (*arrows*). Reproduced from [45]

chromosomal material as well. It is equally clear that not all specific genetic changes important in carcinogenesis will be demonstrable through karyotypic studies, and that many will be submicroscopic, but meanwhile a wealth of visible changes are available for exploitation by combining modern cytogenetic and molecular genetic techniques.

References

1. Nowell P (1976) The clonal evolution of tumor cell populations. Science 194:23
2. Fialkow P (1979) Clonal origin of human tumors. Annu Rev Med 30:135
3. Nowell P (1983) Tumor progression and clonal evolution: the role of genetic instability. In: German J (ed) Chromosome mutation and neoplasia. Liss, New York, p 413
4. Rowley JD, Testa JR (1983) Chromosome abnormalities in malignant hematologic diseases. In: Advances in cancer research. Academic, New York, p 103
5. Yunis JJ (1983) The chromosomal basis of human neoplasia. Science 221:227
6. Klein G (1981) The role of gene dosage and genetic transpositions in carcinogenesis. Nature 294:313
7. Balaban-Malenbaum G, Gilbert F (1977) Double minute chromosomes and the homogeneously staining regions in chromosomes of a human neuroblastoma cells line. Science 198:739
8. Biedler JL, Melera PW, Spengler BA (1983) Chromosome abnormalities and gene amplification: comparison of antifolate-resistant and human neuroblastoma cell systems. In: Rowley JD, Ultmann JE (eds) Chromosomes and cancer: from molecules to man. Academic Press, New York, p 117
9. Manolov G, Manolova Y (1972) Marker band in one chromosome 14 from Burkitt lymphoma. Nature 237:33
10. Zech L, Haglund V, Nilsson N, Klein G (1976) Characteristic chromosomal abnormalities in biopsied and lymphoid cell lines from patients with Burkitt and non-Burkitt lymphoma. Int J Cancer 17:47
11. Van den Berghe H, Paloir C, Gosseye S, Englebienne V, Cornu G, Sokal G (1979) Variant translocation in Burkitt lymphoma. Cancer Genet Cytogenet 1:9
12. Lenoir GM, Preud'homme JL, Bernheim A, Berger R (1982) Correlation between immunoglobulin light chain expression and variant translocation in Burkitt's lymphoma. Nature 298:474
13. Croce CM, Shander M, Martinis J, Cicurel L, D'Ancona GG, Dolby TW, Koprowski H (1979) Chromosomal location of the human immunoglobulin heavy chain genes. Proc Natl Acad Sci USA 76:3416
14. Erikson J, Martinis J, Croce CM (1981) Assignment of the human genes for immunoglobulin chains to chromosome 22. Nature 294:173
15. McBride OW, Heiter PA, Hollis GF, Swan D, Otey MC, Leder P (1982) Chromosomal location of human kappa and lambda im-

munoglobulin light chain constant region genes. J Exp Med 155:1480
16. Malcolm S, Barton P, Murphy C, Ferguson-Smith MA, Bentley DL, Rabbitts TH (1982) Localization of the human immunoglobulin light chain variable region genes to the short arm of chromosome 2 by in situ hybridization. Proc Natl Acad Sci USA 79:4957
17. Dalla Favera R, Bregni M, Erikson J, Patterson D, Gallo RC, Croce CM (1982) Assignment of the human c-myc onc-gene to the region of chromosome 8 which is translocated in Burkitt lymphoma cells. Proc Natl Acad Sci USA 79:7824
18. Neel B, Jhanwar S, Chaganti R, Hayward W (1982) Two human c-onc genes are located on the long arm of chromosome 8. Natl Acad Sci USA 79:7842
19. Erikson J, Finan J, Nowell PC, Croce CM (1982) Translocation of immunoglobulin V_H genes in Burkitt lymphoma. Proc Natl Acad Sci USA 79:5611
20. Taub R, Kirsch I, Morton C, Lenoir G, Swan D, Tronick S, Aaronson S, Leder P (1982) Translocation of the c-myc gene into the immunoglobulin heavy chain locus in human Burkitt lymphoma and murine plasmacytoma cells. Proc Natl Acad Sci USA 79:7837
21. Erikson J, ar-Rushdi A, Drwinga H, Nowell P, Croce C (1983) Transcriptional activation of the translocated c-myc oncogene in Burkitt lymphoma. Proc Natl Acad Sci USA 80:820
22. De la Chapelle A, Lenoir G, Boue J, Boue A, Gallano P, Huerre C, Szajnert M-F, Jeanpierre M, Lalouel JM, Kaplan JC (1983) Lambda Ig constant region genes are translocated to chromosome 8 in Burkitt's lymphoma with t(8;22). Nucleic Acids Res 11:1133
23. Croce C, Thierfelder W, Erikson J, Nishikura K, Finan J, Lenoir G, Rabbitts T, Nowell P (1983) Transcriptional activation of an unrearranged and untranslocated c-myc oncogene by translocation of a C-lambda locus in Burkitt lymphoma cells. Proc Natl Acad Sci USA 80:6922
24. Erikson J, Nishikura K, ar-Rushdi A, Finan J, Emanuel B, Lenoir G, Nowell PC, Croce CM (1983) Translocation of an immunoglobulin kappa locus to a region 3′ of an unrearranged c-myc oncogene enhances c-myc transcription. Proc Natl Acad Sci USA 80:7581
25. Emanuel B, Selden J, Chaganti RSK, Jhanwar S, Nowell PC, Croce CM (1984) The 2p breakpoint of a 2;8 translocation in Burkitt's lymphoma interrupts the V_k locus. Proc Natl Acad Sci USA 81:2444
26. Shen-Ong GLC, Keath EJ, Piccoli SP, Cole MD (1982) Novel myc oncogene RNA from abortive immunoglobulin-gene recombination in mouse plasmacytomas. Cell 31:443
27. Marcu K, Harris L, Stanton L, Erikson J, Watt R, Croce CM (1983) Transcriptionally active c-*myc* oncogene is contained within NIARD, a DNA sequence associated with chromosomal translocations in B-cell neoplasia. Proc Natl Acad Sci USA 80:523
28. Sumegi J, Spira J, Bazin H, Szpirer J, Levan G, Klein G (1983) Rat c-myc oncogene is located on chromosome 7 and rearranges in immunocytomas with t(6;7) chromosomal translocation. Nature 306:497
29. Fukuhara S, Rowley JD, Variakojis D, Golomb HM (1979) Chromosome abnormalities in poorly differentiated lymphocytic lymphoma. Cancer Res 39:3119
30. Yunis JJ, Oken MM, Kaplan ME, Ensrud KM, Howe RR, Theologides A (1982) Distinctive chromosomal abnormalities in histologic subtypes of non-Hodgkin's lymphoma. N Engl J Med 307:1231
31. Tsujimoto Y, Yunis J, Onorato-Showe L, Nowell P, Croce C (1984) Science 224:1403
32. Erikson J, Finan J, Tsujimoto Y, Nowell P, Croce C (1984) The chromosome 14 breakpoint in neoplastic B cells with the t(11;14) translocation involves the immunoglobulin heavy chain locus. Proc Natl Acad Sci USA 81:2444
33. De Klein A, van Kessel AG, Grosveld G, Bartram CR, Hagemeijer A, Boatsma D, Spurr NK, Heisterkamp N, Groffen J, Stephenson JR (1982) A cellular oncogene is translocated to the Philadelphia chromosome in chronic myelocytic leukemia. Nature 300:765
34. Heisterkamp N, Stephenson JR, Groffen J, Hansen PF, de Klein A, Bartram CR, Grosveld G (1983) Localization of the c-abl oncogene adjacent to a translocation break point in chronic myelocytic leukaemia. Nature 306:239
35. Emanuel B, Wang E, Nowell P, Selden J, Croce C (1984) Non-identical 22q11 breakpoint for the t(9;22) of CML and the 6(8;22) of Burkitt's lymphoma. Cytogenet Cell Genet 38:127
36. Bakhshi A, Minowada J, Arnold A, Cossman J, Jensen JP, Whang-Peng J, Waldman TA, Korsmeyer SJ (1983) Lymphoid blast crises of chronic myelogenous leukemia represent stages in the development of B-cell precursors. N Engl J Med 309:826
37. Canaani E, Steiner-Saltz D, Aghai A, Gale RP, Berrebi A, Januszewicz E (1984) Altered transcription of an oncogene in chronic myeloid leukemia. Lancet 1:593

38. Spurr NK, Solomon E, Jannson M, Sheer D, Goodfellow PN, Bodmer WF, Vennstrom B (1984) Mapping of cellular oncogenes: ErbAl is on chromosome 17. EMBO J 3:159
39. Dayton AI, Selden JR, Laws G, Dorney DJ, Finan J, Tripputi P, Emanuel BS, Rovera G, Nowell PC, Croce CM (1984) A human c-*erbA* oncogene homologue is closely proximal to the chromosome 17 breakpoint in acute promyelocytic leukemia. Proc Natl Acad Sci USA 81:4495
40. Nowell P, Wilmoth D, Hoxie J, Lyss A (1984) Ph-positive acute leukemia with a 17q;21q translocation. Cancer Genet Cytogenet 12:51
41. Kaufman RJ, Brown PC, Schimke RT (1979) Amplified dihydrofolate reductase genes in unstably methotrexate-resistant cells are associated with double minute chromosomes. Proc Natl Acad Sci USA 76:5669
42. Schwab M, Alitalo K, Klempnauer K-H, Varmus HE, Bishop JM, Gilbert F, Brodeur G, Goldstein M, Trent J (1983) Amplified DNA with limited homology to myc cellular oncogene is shared by human neuroblastoma cell lines and a neuroblastoma tumor. Nature 305:245
43. Alitalo K, Schwab M, Lin CC, Varmus HE, Bishop JM (1983) Homogeneously staining chromosomal regions contain amplified copies of an abundantly expressed cellular oncogene (c-myc) in malignant neuroendocrine cells from a human colon carcinoma. Proc Natl Acad Sci USA 80:1707
44. Selden J, Emanuel B, Wang E, Cannizzaro L, Palumbo A, Erikson J, Nowell P, Rovera G, Croce C (1983) Amplified C-lambda and c-*abl* genes on the same marker chromosome in K562 leukemic cells. Proc Natl Acad Sci USA 80:7289
45. Nowell P, Finan J, Dalla Favera R, Gallo R, ar-Rushdi A, Ramanczuk P, Selden J, Emanuel B, Rovera G, Croce C (1983) Association of amplified oncogene c-*myc* with an abnormally banded chromosomes 8 in a human leukemia cell line. Nature 306:494
46. Collins S, Groudine M (1982) Amplification of endogenous *myc*-related DNA sequences in a human myeloid leukaemia cell line. Nature 298:679
47. Dalla Favera R, Wong-Staal F, Gallo RC (1982) Onc-gene amplification in promyelocytic leukaemia cell line HL-60 and primary leukaemic cells of the same patient. Nature 299:61

Haematology and Blood Transfusion Vol. 29
Modern Trends in Human Leukemia VI
Edited by Neth, Gallo, Greaves, Janka

Chromatin Structure of the Human c-*myc* Oncogene: Definition of Regulatory Regions and Changes in Burkitt's Lymphomas

U. Siebenlist[1], L. Hennighausen[2], J. Battey[3], and P. Leder[2]

A. Introduction

Chromosomal translocations of the *myc* oncogene are a consistent feature of all Burkitt's lymphomas and are also observed in many murine plasmacytomas. These translocations of *myc* occur into the immunoglobulin loci and they result in a general increase in *myc* transcription, but this increase in *myc* is variable [2, 6, 7, 10, 11, 21, 22]. Since *myc* may be regulated during the cell cycle (see [9]), deregulation may mean expression at the inappropriate time, which in turn may result in only a modest overall increase in transcription of *myc* in Burkitt's lymphomas. On the other hand, the true (and unidentified) precursor cell of Burkitt's lymphomas may have a very low level of *myc* transcription and we are as yet unable to assess properly the true increase in transcription as a consequence of translocations.

In any case, another observation points to a loss of the normal control mechanism governing *myc* in Burkitt's lymphomas. The nontranslocated *myc* allele is transcriptionally silent in Burkitt's lymphomas as well as in plasmacytomas [2, 19, 21] and this has led to the prediction that the *myc* gene is under negative control [10, 13]. Thus, to understand how translocations affect *myc* expression it is critical to understand how *myc* is regulated. We therefore identified the presumed regulatory sequences near *myc* by DNAase I hypersensitivity studies [17].

DNAase I hypersensitivity is due to a discrete region on chromatin that is very sensitive to DNAase I [18, 23]. Hypersensitive sites appear near many different DNA sequences which are known to be functionally important for gene expression, as is the case of the immunoglobulin kappa light chain and heavy chain enhancers [14]. In fact, hypersensitive regions may bind regulatory proteins [5].

We will discuss here the location of DNAase I hypersensitivity sites immediately 5′ of *myc* near sequences that we suspect on the basis of other data to be functionally important. We will also dicuss the dramatic difference in chromatin structure between the translocated and the nontranslocated alleles in two Burkitt's lymphomas, BL 31 and BL 22. The nontranslocated allele features one strong hypersensitive site, a probable site for mediating negative transcriptional control of *myc*. The deregulation of the translocated *myc* allele in BL 31 is likely to be the result of the immunoglobulin heavy chain enhancer, juxtaposed with the *myc* gene in that lymphoma.

B. Results and Discussion

In order to study the effect of a translocation on the chromatin structure of *myc*,

1 Laboratory of Immunoregulation, Niaid, Nih, Bethesda, MD
2 Department of Genetics, Harvard Medical School, Boston, MA
3 Nci Navy Oncology-Hematology Department, National Naval Medical Center, Bethesda, MD

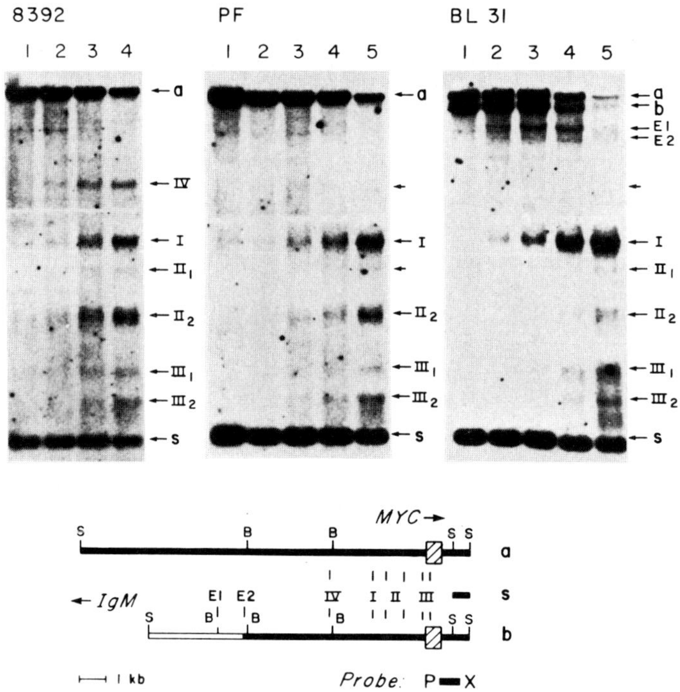

Fig. 1. DNAase-I-hypersensitive sites near *myc* in PF, 8392, and BL 31 cells. Nuclei were digested with increasing amounts of DNAase I (*from left to right*) (for details see [17]) and the isolated genomic DNA was restricted with *Sst*I, electrophoresed, blotted onto nitrocellulose, and hybridized with the PX probe. The hypersensitive sites are labeled I, II_1, II_2, III_1, III_2, IV, E1, and E2. E1 is the location of the immunoglobulin enhancer. *a* represents the germline *myc* fragment and *b* is the translocated *myc* allele, both of which are detected by the probe. *S* is an internal size marker genomic *Sst*I fragment which the probe overlaps. *Solid bar* indicates *myc*-derived sequences, while *open bar* indicates Ig- derived sequences. *The box* represents the untranslated first *myc* exon. *S, Sst*I; *B, Bgl*II; *P, Pvu*II; *X, Xba*I

we initially chose a Burkitt's lymphoma in which the translocation point occurs at a considerable distance from the *myc* oncogene. This less common situation occurs in BL 31. Here the *myc* gene is translocated into the IgM locus, with the crossover point occurring about 6 kb upstream of the first and untranslated *myc* exon. Also unusual, though not unique, is that *myc* is now juxtaposed with the immunoglobulin heavy chain enhancer.

DNAase-I-hypersensitive sites in this Burkitt's cell and in the nonmalignant B-cell lines PF and 8392 (EBV-transformed lymphoblastoid lines) were determined essentially as described by Wu [23] (for details see [17]). In this method, nuclei are digested with increasing amounts of DNAase I. Upon isolating and restricting the DNA, the DNAase-I-cutting sites (hypersensitive sites) can be visualized as subbands on genomic Southern blots, in addition to the original genomic restriction fragment. As is shown in Fig. 1 for the lymphoblastoid lines PF and 8392 and the Burkitt's line BL 31, these subbands appear with increasing amounts of DNAase I, from left to right. PF and 8392 cells contain two germline *myc* alleles (fragment a in Fig. 1), whereas BL 31 cells have one translocated (b) and one germline (a) *myc* band. Clearly several DNAase-I-hypersensitive sites emerge and their positions are indicated on the map in Fig. 1 and summarized in Fig. 2.

The DNAase-I-hypersensitive sites I through III are consistently observed,

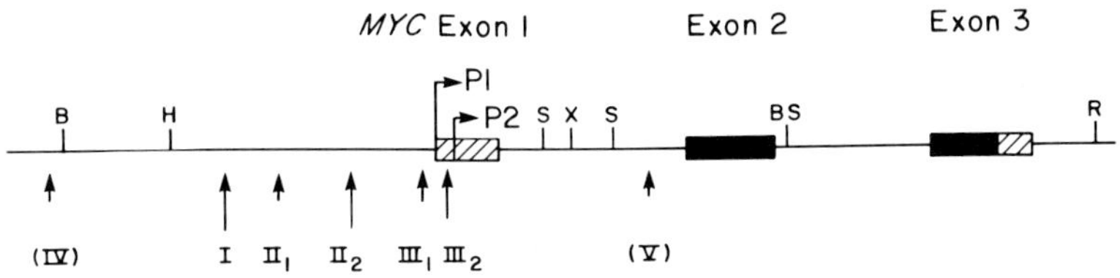

Fig. 2. Location of DNAase-I-hypersensitive sites. The sizes of the *arrows* reflect the approximate relative intensities of the hypersensitive sites in the lymphoblastoid lines. *H, Hind*III; *R, Eco*RI; *P1* and *P2* are the two *myc* promoters; for further description see Fig. 1 and text

whereas sites IV and V are not (site IV is only seen in 8392 cells and site V is very weak in these cells, but much more intense in peripheral T cells; U. Siebenlist, unpublished observation). E1 is located at the immunoglobulin enhancer and E2 lies close to or at the crossover point.

Hypersensitive sites I through III lie within a 2-kb region immediately 5′ of the *myc* gene, a region we thus presume to contain regulatory sequences. Indeed all of these hypersensitive sites coincide with positions that we suspect on the basis of other data to be functionally important. This strengthens our notion that the DNAase-I-hypersensitive sites reflect regions critical to *myc* regulation.

To begin with, the very strong hypersensitive site I is located about 2 kb upstream of the P2 promoter start site, within a sequence region that is well conserved between mouse and man, as seen in a cross-species heteroduplex [1]. Such conservation is usually indicative of functional importance, and, as we will discuss below, this region possibly mediates negative control of *myc*.

The hypersensitive sites III-1 and III-2 are located directly upstream of the two *myc* promoters P1 and P2, respectively. III-1 maps about 100 basepairs 5′ of the P1 'TATA' box in a cystosine-rich stretch of DNA that is very homologous to the – 100 region described by Dierks [4], a region of functional significance for several genes. This sequence may therefore bind a more general transcription factor.

The relatively weak hypersensitive site II-1 lies just 5′ of a sequence which is recognized by a protein from nuclear extracts in vitro (see [17]). Interestingly, site II-2 lies next to a similar sequence. We speculate that the in vitro binding also occurs in vivo, resulting in a hypersensitive site II-1 and possibly also II-2. By comparing these sequences with other competing binding sites next to the human immunoglobulin *mu* gene (L. Henninghausen, unpublished observation) or in the long terminal repeat of adenovirus [17], a conserved sequence emerges (TGGCN$_5$ GCCAA). The binding site on adenovirus is in fact also recognized by nuclear factor 1, a nuclear protein which has been shown to be necessary for adenovirus replication in vitro [12]. Since purified nuclear factor 1 also binds to the immunoglobulin and *myc* sites (L. Henninghausen, unpublished observation), it is likely to be the protein detected in our nuclear extracts. Although this protein has an identified role in replication of adenovirus, its function at the *myc* locus is yet to be defined.

Is the fact that only the translocated allele in Burkitt's lymphomas is transcribed reflected in the chromatin structures of the two *myc* alleles within the same cell? In BL 31 the two *myc* alleles can be differentiated by employing a probe which hybridizes only to the nontranslocated (germline) *myc* (a), but not to the translocated *myc*, as seen in Fig. 3. The germline *myc* allele in BL 31 has only one hypersensitive site, I, and it is very intense when compared with the contribution from both chromosomes in PF; sites II and III are undetectable. A similar situation exists in BL 22, where the breakpoint on the translocated allele occurs between hypersensitive sites II$_1$ and II$_2$ (U. Siebenlist, unpublished observation and [1]). We therefore hypothesize that site I mediates the nega-

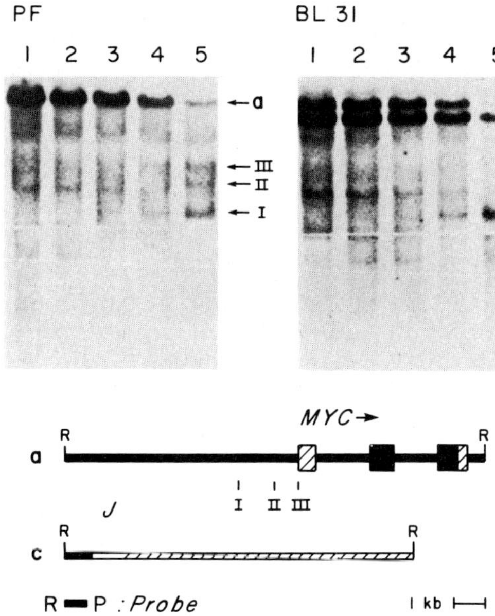

Fig. 3. The nontranslocated *myc* allele in BL 31 has only one very intense DNAase-I-hypersensitive site. The analysis was similar to the one described in Fig. 1, except that a different probe was used (*R-P*), which hybridizes to the germline *myc* allele (*Eco*RI: fragment *a*) and the reciprocal product of the translocation process (*Eco*RI: fragment *c*). *J*, immunoglobulin J region; *hatched bar* indicates an immunoglobulin rearrangement; *R*, *Eco*RI; *P*, *Pst*I; for further description see Fig. 1

tive transcriptional control that appears to operate on the germline *myc* gene in all Burkitt's cells and plasmacytomas where this could be analyzed (see "Introduction"). In one of several possible scenarios then, we imagine that the abnormally high production of *myc* from the translocated allele precipitates increased activity in a *trans*-acting repressor which functions through site I on the germline *myc* allele. This, in turn, represses transcription of *myc*, possibly by preventing transcriptional factors from binding at site III.

Elimination of site I by the translocation process may explain deregulation of *myc* in BL 22, but how does the translocated *myc* allele escape repression in BL 31, where the chromosomal breakpoint does not cut the regulatory region apart? Sites III_1 and III_2 are very intense on the translocated allele, suggesting that the translocation interferes with the function of the hypothetical *trans*-acting repressor proposed above. In BL 31, this may be due to the immunoglobulin heavy chain enhancer, which is presumably functional, since it is itself associated with a hypersensitive site (see Fig. 1). Interestingly, insertion of an ALV LTR 5′ of the chicken *myc* gene changes the chromatin structure of that gene as well [16]. Here, the enhancer may directly activate the promoters, possibly by allowing transcriptional factors to bind near sites III-1 and III-2. Of course other not yet identified elements either removed or introduced by the translocation could also contribute the chromatin changes observed and thus lead to the deregulation of *myc*.

The presented data lead to a new interpretation of how translocations in general may deregulate the *myc* gene. We would like to suggest that the structural alteration or elimination of site I (like in BL 22) might account for the observed loss of the normal control mechanisms governing this gene. Many translocations interrupt or eliminate this site and the untranslated first exon [2, 3, 8, 15, 20, 21]. In addition, it is possible that this region is mutated as a consequence of a translocation [15, 21]. Of course, other mutational changes of elements may further affect the deregulation of the *myc* gene. In BL 31, site I is retained and most likely not mutated and here the strong dominant effect of the immunoglobulin enhancer may cause deregulation. Experiments testing these hypotheses are in progress.

References

1. Battey J, Moulding C, Taub R, Murphy W, Stewart T, Potter H, Lenoir G, Leder P (1983) The human *c-myc* oncogene: structural consequences of translocation into the IgH in Burkitt lymphoma. Cell 34:779–789
2. Bernard O, Cory S, Gerondakis S, Webb E, Adams JM (1983) Sequence of the murine and human cellular *myc* oncogenes and two modes of *myc* transcription resulting from chromosome translocation in B lymphoid tumors. EMBO J 2:2375–2383
3. Dalla-Favera R, Martinotti S, Gallo R, Erikson J, Croce C (1983) Translocation and rearrangements of the *c-myc* oncogene locus in human and undifferentiated B-cell lymphomas. Science 219:963–967
4. Dierks P, van Ooyen A, Cochran M, Dobkin C, Riser J, Weissmann C (1983) Three regions upstream from the CAP site are required for efficient and accurate transcription of the rabbit beta-globin gene in mouse 3T6 cells. Cell 32:695–706
5. Emerson BM, Felsenfeld G (1984) Specific factor conferring nuclease hypersensitivity at the 5′ end of the chicken adult beta-globin gene. Proc Natl Acad Sci USA 81:95–99
6. Erikson J, ar-Rushdi A, Drwinga HL, Nowell PC, Croce C (1983) Transcriptional activation of the translocated *c-myc* oncogene in Burkitt lymphoma. Proc Natl Acad Sci USA 80:820–824
7. Hamlyn PH, Rabbitts TH (1983) Translocation joins *c-myc* and immunoglobulin gamma-1 genes in Burkitt lymphoma revealing a third exon in the *c-myc* oncogene. Nature 304:135–139
8. Hayday A, Gillies S, Saito H, Wood C, Wiman K, Hayward W, Tonegawa S (1984) Activation of a translocated human *c-myc* gene by an enhancer in the immunoglobulin heavy chain locus. Nature 307:334–340
9. Kelly K, Cochran B, Stiles C, Leder P (1983) Cell-specific regulation of the *c-myc* gene by lymphocyte mitogens and platelet derived growth factor. Cell 35:603–610
10. Leder P, Battey J, Lenoir G, Moulding C, Murphy W, Potter H, Stewart T, Taub R (1983) Translocations among antibody genes in human cancer. Science 222:765–771
11. Maguire RT, Robins TS, Thorgeirsson S, Heilman CA (1983) Expression of cellular *myc* and *mos* genes in undifferentiated B cell lymphomas of Burkitt and non-Burkitt types. Proc Natl Acad Sci USA 80:1947–1950
12. Nagata K, Guggenheimer RA, Hurwitz J (1983) Specific binding of a cellular DNA replication protein to the origin of replication of adenovirus DNA. Proc Natl Acad Sci USA 80:6177–6181
13. Nishikura K, ar-Rushdi A, Erikson J, Watt R, Rovera G, Croce CM (1983) Differential expression of the normal and of the translocated human *c-myc* oncogenes in B cells. Proc Natl Acad Sci USA 80:4822–4826
14. Parslow T, Granner D (1983) Structure of a nuclease-sensitive region inside the immunoglobulin kappa gene: evidence for a role in gene regulation. Nucleic Acids Res 11:4775–4792
15. Rabbitts TH, Hamlyn PH, Baer R (1983) Altered nucleotide sequence of a translocated *c-myc* gene in Burkitt lymphoma. Nature 306:760–765
16. Schubach W, Groudine M (1984) Alteration of *c-myc* chromatin structure by avian leukosis virus integration. Nature 307:702–708
17. Siebenlist U, Hennighausen L, Battey J, Leder P (1984) Chromatin structure and protein binding in the putative regulatory region of the *c-myc* gene in Burkitt lymphoma. Cell 37:381–391
18. Stalder J, Larsen A, Engel J, Dolan M, Groudine M, Weintraub H (1980) Tissue-specific DNA cleavages in the globin chromatin domain introduced by DNAase I. Cell 20:451–460
19. Stanton LW, Watt R, Marcu KB (1983) Translocation, breakage and truncated transcripts of *c-myc* oncogene in murine plasmacytomas. Nature 303:401–406
20. Taub R, Kirsch I, Morton C, Lenoir G, Swan D, Tronick S, Aaronson S, Leder P (1982) Translocation of the *c-myc* gene into the immunoglobulin heavy chain locus in human Burkitt lymphoma and murine plasmacytoma cells. Proc Natl Acad Sci USA 79:7837–7841
21. Taub R, Moulding C, Battey J, Murphy W, Vasicek T, Lenoir G, Leder P (1984) Activation and somatic mutation of the translocated *c-myc* gene in Burkitt lymphoma cells. Cell 36:339–348
22. Westin EH, Wong-Staal F, Gelman EP, Dalla-Favera R, Papas T, Lautenberger JA, Eva A, Reddy EP, Tronick SR, Aaronson SA, Gallo RC (1982) Expression of cellular homologs of retroviral *onc* genes in human hematopoietic cells. Proc Natl Acad Sci USA 79:2490–2494
23. Wu C (1980) The 5′ ends of *Drosophila* heat shock genes in chromatin are hypersensitive to DNAase I. Nature 286:854–860

Haematology and Blood Transfusion Vol. 29
Modern Trends in Human Leukemia VI
Edited by Neth, Gallo, Greaves, Janka

Identification of the Human Cellular *myc* Gene Product by Antibody Against the Bacterially Expressed Protein

T. Benter[1], P. Beimling[1], E. Pfaff[2], T. Sander[1], B. Heimann[1], and K. Moelling[1]

Retroviruses code for oncogenes which are related to normal cellular genes. The oncogenes code for products which, according to their properties, can be classified into two groups, one group comprising those gene products which reside in the nucleus, like *myb* and *myc*, and the other, larger group represented by the *src* gene family, which codes for membrane-associated proteins, some of which exhibit protein kinase activities (for review see [4]).

The *myc* gene is the transforming gene of MC29 viruses. Its normal cellular homologous gene may play a role in certain types of tumor such as Burkitt's lymphoma and small cell cancer of the lung (SCCL) [3]; and for review see [6]. To identify the human cellular *myc* (*hu-c-myc*) gene product, the production of antibodies was required. For that purpose a portion of the *hu-c-myc* gene has been cloned into an expression vector for protein expression in bacteria. The expression vector pPLc24 codes for the replicase gene of the bacteriophage MS2 [5] and has been used previously for the expression of a MS2–viral *myc* fusion protein [1] (see Fig. 1, clone *p-myc* 5/30 Sal). The viral *myc* gene was replaced by the ClaI-BclI fragment of the human cellular *myc* gene (clone *p-myc* 6/4, Fig. 1). Expression of the MS2-*hu-c-myc* fusion protein is controlled by a thermolabile repressor. Cells grown overnight at 28 °C are shifted to 42 °C for 2 h which results in expression of the fusion protein. About 10% of the total bacterial protein content is represented by the fusion protein abbreviated as MS2-*myc* in Fig. 2a, which has a molecular weight of about 30 000, 20 000 of which are *myc* specific.

This protein was eluted from gels or purified by differential centrifugation and solubilization in 6 *M* urea. Antibodies were raised in rabbits and the serum applied to immobilized MS2-containing bacterial lysate to remove MS2-specific IgG from the serum and subsequently *hu-c-myc*-specific IgG was recovered from MS2-*hu-c-myc*-containing bacterial protein lysates. Details of a similar IgG isolation procedure have been described [1]. The *hu-c-myc*-specific IgG was used for immunoblotting of HeLa and MC29-Q8-NP cellular lysates which were lysed in RIPA buffer as described [2]. The result is shown in Fig. 2b. The *hu-c-myc*-specific IgG cross-reacts with the $p110^{gag\text{-}myc}$ protein from MC29-Q8 fibroblasts and recognizes a protein of molecular weight 64 000, designated $p64^{hu\text{-}c\text{-}myc}$. A faint larger band of molecular weight 67 000 is also detectable. Figure 3 shows that the *hu-c-myc* gene product in HeLa cells gives rise to nuclear fluorescence. The experiment was performed as described [2]. Whether the *hu-c-myc* gene product is also a DNA-binding protein similar to $p110^{gag\text{-}myc}$ [2], needs to be demonstrated. The *myc*- gene product is expected to be a transcriptional control element. Experiments are in progress to demonstrate this effect.

1 Max-Planck-Institut für Molekulare Genetik, Ihnestrasse 63, 1000 Berlin 33, FRG
2 Zentrum für Molekulare Biologie, Universität Heidelberg, Im Neuenheimer Feld 230, 6900 Heidelberg, FRG

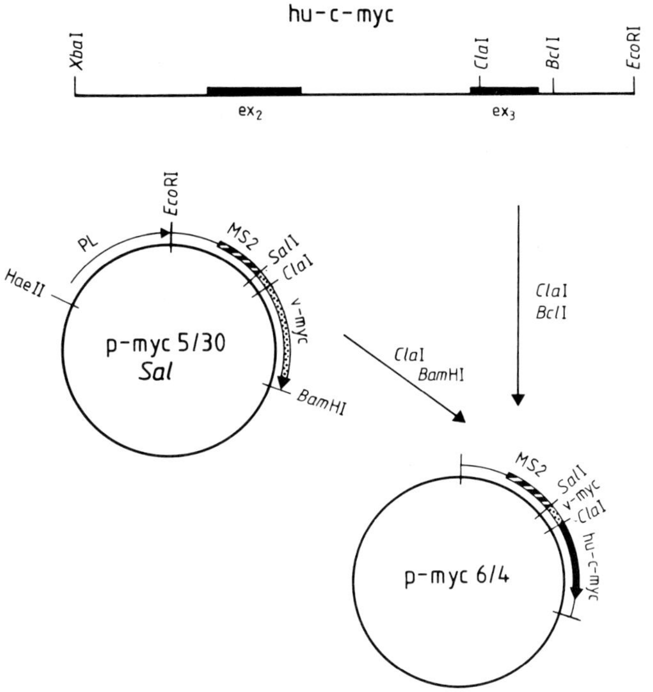

Fig. 1. The *hu-c-myc* clone was constructed from pPLc24 containing a portion of the *v-myc* gene previously designated *p-myc* 5/30 Sal [1]. The *v-myc* gene was replaced by the ClaI/Bcl fragment of the *hu-c-myc* clone and the clone designated *p-myc* 6/4

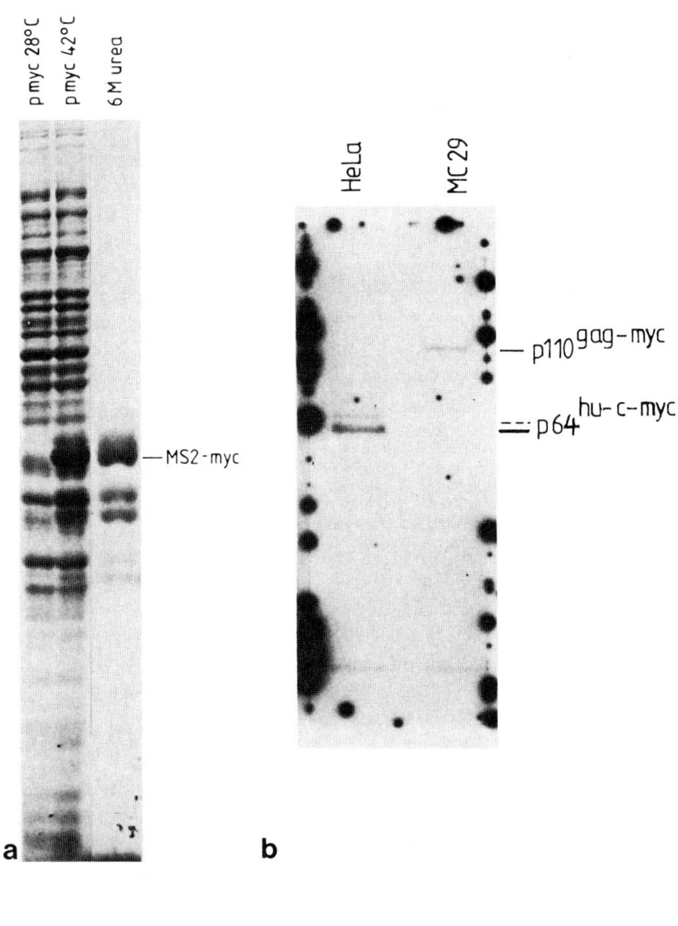

Fig. 2 a, b. **a** The *p-myc* 6/4 clone described in Fig. 1 was expressed in bacteria. At 42 °C, the MS2-*hu-c-myc* protein (abbreviated MS2-*myc*) is expressed. The protein was purified and solubilized in 6 *M* urea; **b** *hu-c-myc*-specific IgG was isolated from antibodies against the MS2-*hu-c-myc* protein and used in an immunoblot with HeLa and MC29-Q8-NP cell lysates

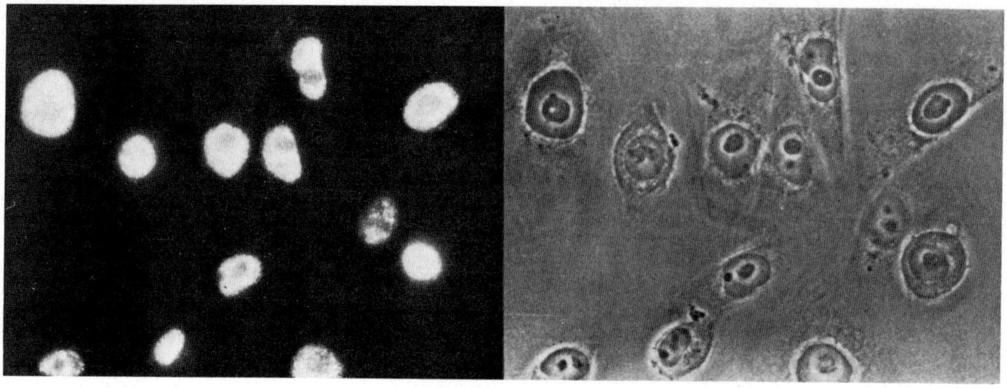

Fig. 3. Indirect immunofluorescence with HeLa cells using *hu-c-myc*-specific antiserum (1:40 dilution)

References

1. Bunte T, Donner P, Pfaff E, Reis B, Greiser-Wilke I, Schaller H, Moelling K (1984) Inhibition of DNA-binding of purified $p55^{v\text{-}myc}$ in vitro by antibodies against bacterially expressed *myc* protein and a synthetic peptide. EMBO J 3 (in press)
2. Donner P, Grieser-Wilke I, Moelling K (1982) Nuclear localization and DNA-binding of the transforming gene product of avian myelocytomatosis virus. Nature 296:262–266
3. Little CD, Nau MM, Carney DN, Gazdar AF, Minna JD (1983) Amplification and expression of the *c-myc* oncogene in human lung cancer cell lines. Nature 306:194–196
4. Moelling K (1985) Fusion proteins in retroviral transformation. In: Weinhouse S, Klein G (eds) Advances in cancer research, vol 43. Academic, New York, pp 205–239
5. Remaut E, Stanssen P, Fiers W (1981) Plasmid vectors for high-efficiency expression controlled by the PL promoter of coliphage lambda. Gene 15:81–93
6. Robertson M (1984) Message of myc in context. Nature 309:585–587

Haematology and Blood Transfusion Vol. 29
Modern Trends in Human Leukemia VI
Edited by Neth, Gallo, Greaves, Janka

Oncogenes of Avian Acute Leukemia Viruses are Subsets of Normal Cellular Genes

T. S. Papas [1], N. C. Kan [1], D. K. Watson [1], J. A. Lautenberger [1], C. Flordellis [1], K. P. Samuel [1], U. G. Rovigatti [1], M. Psallidopoulos [1], R. Ascione [1], and P. H. Duesberg [2]

A. Introduction

Avian acute leukemia viruses are a group of defective retroviruses which cause neoplasia in animals after short periods of latency. Transformation induced by the acute leukemia viruses usually manifest the direct expression of one or two viral *onc* genes that include characteristic elements transduced from cellular genes termed proto-oncogenes. Table 1 demonstrates the oncogenic properties of these viruses. Of particular interest to our laboratory is the MC29 subgroup of acute transforming viruses with *onc*-specific sequence termed *myc* as well as the avian myeloblastosis virus (AMV) subgroup with an *onc*-specific sequence termed *myb*. There are dramatic biologic differences between these two subgroups of viruses. As illustrated in Table 1, the MC29 subgroup possesses a broad spectrum of oncogenicity in vivo, causing leukemia and solid tumors in animals, and the ability to transform a variety of cells such as fibroblasts and hematopoietic cells in vitro. By contrast, the AMV subgroup has a much narrower spectrum of oncogenicity in vivo, causing leukemia, but not solid tumors, and possesses the ability to transform only hematopoietic cells in vitro.

Significant biologic differences exist among the viruses of the MC29 subgroup. To understand these biologic differences, we have cloned the integrated proviral genomes of the MC29 and MH2 viruses and analyzed their genetic structures. The *onc* gene of MC29 is a genetic hybrid (*Δgag-myc*), that consists of an element derived from the retroviral *gag* gene linked to the two 3′ exons of the cellular proto-*myc* gene. Thus in MC29-infected cells, the transforming *onc* gene product is expressed as a hybrid protein that includes both *gag* and *myc* sequences. A unique characteristic of the MH2 virus that has been described in our laboratory is that this virus contains two different *onc* genes, each of which is different from the *Δgag-myc* gene of MC29. One MH2 *onc*-gene has the genetic structure *Δgag-mht,* the other exists in two exons, a small 5′ exon of 6 *gag* codons and a major 3′ *myc* exon that is almost colinear with the *myc* sequence of MC29 [1, 2], Finally, our studies on the proto-*myc* and proto-*mht* genes have enabled us to reconstruct how the *myc* and *mht* sequences of MC29 and MH2 were transduced from proto-*myc* and proto-*mht* by the retroviruses that must have generated MC29 and MH2.

B. Results and Discussion

I. Sequence Analysis of MC29 and Chicken and Human Proto-*myc* Oncogenes

We have cloned [3] and sequenced the *Δgag-myc* gene of MC29 as well as the chicken proto-*myc* gene, and the cor-

1 National Cancer Institute-FCRF, National Institutes of Health, Frederick, MD 21701
2 Department of Molecular Biology, University of California, Berkeley, California 94740, USA

Table 1. Oncogenic properties of acute leukemia virus

Virus Strain	Neoplastic growth induced in vivo			Cell Types Transformed in vitro	Viral *onc* sequences
	Sarcoma (Fibrosarcoma = F) (Hepatocytoma = H)	*Carcinoma* (Renal adenocarcinoma = RC) (Carcinoma = C)	*Acute leukemia* (Myelocytomatosis = M) (Erythroblastosis = E) (Myeloblastosis = My)	(Fibroblastic = f) (Epitheloid = ep) (Myeloid = m) (Erythroid = e)	
MC29 subgroup					
MC29	F, H	C, RC	M, E	f, ep, m, e	*myc*
MH2	F, H	C, RC	M, E	f, ep, m, e	*myc, mht*
OK10	F, H	C, RC	M, E	f, ep, m, e	*myc*
CMII	F, H	C, RC	M, E	f, ep, m, e	*myc*
AMV subgroup					
AMV			My	m	*myb*
E26			My, E	m, e	*myb, ets*
AEV subgroup					
AEV	F	C	E, M	f, e	*erb* A, *erb* B

responding human proto-*myc* gene [4–6]. We have then aligned the sequences of the viral and cellular *myc*-related genes on the basis of their nucleotide homology, to identify similarities and dissimilarities, and have reached the conclusions presented elsewhere [7].

II. Molecular Structure of MH2

We have molecularly cloned the MH2 provirus, and determined its exact genetic structure by sequence analysis shown in Fig. 1 [2]. As expected, the virus contained a *gag*-derived sequence as the 5′ end of the viral genome and a *myc*-sequence as its 3′ end. Unexpectedly, this analysis revealed an MH2-specific sequence of 1.2 kilobases, termed *mht*, which is unrelated to the *myc* sequence and which maps between *Δgag* and *myc* [4, 5]. The nucleotide sequence of the MH2 viral genome indicates that the *gag* region and the *mht* gene form an open reading frame starting at the known AUG codon of the *gag* gene and terminating at a TAG stop codon near the 3′ end of *mht*. This open reading frame contains 894 amino acids capable of encoding a protein of about 100 kilodaltons. This prediction is in accord with the size of the p100 *gag-mht* protein observed in MH2-transformed cells [8].

III. Sequence Homology Between *mht* and *raf*

When the *mht* sequence of MH2 was compared with the *onc*-specific *raf* sequence of mouse sarcoma virus (MSV) 3611, a striking homology extending from the 5′ end of *mht* sequence for over 969 nucleotides was observed (Fig. 1) [9–10]. At the nucleotide level, the homology is 80%. Most nucleotide changes are third-base substitutions that result in no amino acid changes. The *raf* sequence differs from the *mht* sequence by having one inserted codon (proline) at position 1170 and by 19 amino acid substitutions. The absence of proline at position 1170 in the *mht* sequence is confirmed by MH2-specific oligonucleotide 6a [1]. Thus, the homology is 94% at the deduced amino acid level. This region of homology is flanked in both viruses by MH2- and

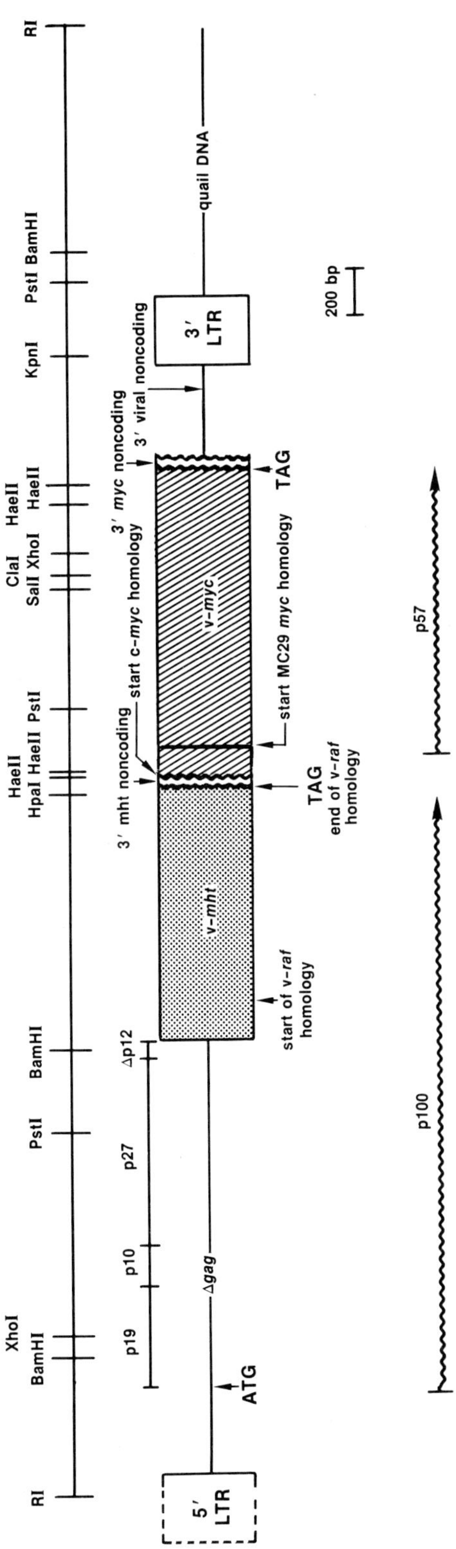

MSV-specific sequences with essentially no homology between the two viruses. At the 5′ end, the homology begins 174 base pairs 3′ to the *gag-mht* junction in MH2. Thus, the first 57 amino acids of *mht* preceding the start of homology with *raf* are MH2 specific, whereas *raf* is a completely colinear subset of *mht* [10]. At the 3′ end, the two sequences share a common termination codon at position 1186 and diverge beyond this position. Following the termination codon, there are 12 and 175 presumably cell-derived noncoding nucleotides in *mht* and *raf*, respectively.

IV. Relation of *mht* to Cellular proto-*mht* Genes

We have recently shown that the *mht* sequence, like the specific sequences of other retroviral *onc* genes, has a cellular counterpart in the chicken chromosome [7] as well as in the chromosomes of mice and humans (data not shown). Because a 3.8 kilobases cellular *mht*-related mRNA was detected by RNA blot hybridization in normal chicken cells [7], the chicken proto-*mht* gene may contain a coding sequence of about 3.8 kilobases. Therefore, the 1.3 kilobases *mht* sequence of MH2 probably represents only a subset of the proto-*mht* gene. The fact that the *mht* sequence terminates with several translation stop codons, suggests that it represents the 3′ end of the proto-*mht* gene. The same is true for the relation between the viral *myc* and proto-*myc* genes [7, 11]. Thus, the *Δgag-mht* gene and the cellular proto-*mht* gene are coterminal, but not isogenic. This is consistent with the

Fig. 1. Genetic structure of MH2 proviral genome. A restriction enzyme map of the 6.5 kilobases *Eco*RI-resistant quail DNA fragment that includes the MH2 provirus [1] is shown above the genetic map of MH2 proviral genome. *Broken lines* represent sequences not present in the 6.5 kilobases *Eco*RI fragment; *boxes* between the 5′ and 3′ LTR represent cell-derived sequences; *full lines* between the two LTR represent viral sequences; p100 and p57 represent the *Δgag-mht* hybrid protein and the *myc*-containing protein in MH2-transformed cells, respectively

Table 2. Cellular genes transduced by avian acute leukemia viruses

Cellular gene	Transcript (kilobases)	Virus	Segment transduced (kilobases)
myc	2.5	MC29	1.4
		MH2	1.5
mht	3.8	MH2	1.2
myb	4.0	AMV	1.2
		E26	0.8
ets	7.4	E26	1.5

notion that the *onc* genes of most retroviruses are subsets of their cellular prototypes. By the same analogy, our parallel observation with AMV and MV29 viruses compared with their proto-*onc* transcripts seem to support this overall scheme (Table 2). The most dramatic example is the segment of the *ets* gene transduced by E26 virus which is four times smaller than the proto-*ets* transcript identified in normal chicken embryo fibroblasts (Table 2) [12, 13].

References

1. Kan N, Flordellis C, Garon C, Duesberg P, Papas T (1983) Proc Natl Acad Sci USA 80:6566
2. Kan N, Flordellis C, Mark G, Duesberg P, Papas T (1984) Proc Natl Acad Sci USA 81:3000
3. Lautenberger J, Schultz R, Garon C, Tsichlis P, Papas T (1981) Proc Natl Acad Sci USA 78:1518
4. Reddy E, Reynolds K, Watson D, Schulz R, Lautenberger J, Papas T (1983) Proc Natl Acad Sci USA 80:2500
5. Watson D, Reddy E, Duesberg P, Papas T (1983) Proc Natl Acad Sci USA 80:2146
6. Watson D, Psallidopoulos M, Samuel D, Dalla Favera R, Papas T (1983) Proc Natl Acad Sci USA 80:3642
7. Papas T, Kan N, Watson D, Flordellis C, Psallidopoulos M, Lautenberger J, Samuel K, Duesberg P (1984) In: Levin A, Topp W, Vande Woude GF, Watson JD (eds) Cancer cells. Cold Spring Harbor, New York, pp 153–160
8. Hu S, Moscovici C, Vogt P (1978) Virology 89:162
9. Rapp U, Godsborough M, Mark G, Bonner T, Groffen J, Reynolds F, Stephenson J (1983) Proc Natl Acad Sci USA 80:4218
10. Kan N, Flordellis C, Mark G, Duesberg P, Papas T (1984) Science 233:813
11. Watson D, Reddy E, Duesberg P, Papas T (1983) Proc Natl Acad Sci USA 80:2146
12. Leprince D, Genonne A, Coll J, de Taisne C, Schneeberger A, Lagrou C, Stehelin D (1983) Nature 306:395
13. Nunn M, Seeburg P, Moscovici C, Duesberg P (1983) Nature 306:391

Haematology and Blood Transfusion Vol. 29
Modern Trends in Human Leukemia VI
Edited by Neth, Gallo, Greaves, Janka

Structure and Function of *ras* and *Blym* Oncogenes

G. M. Cooper [1]

A. Introduction

The biologic activity of tumor DNA, detected by transfection of NIH 3T3 mouse cells, has led to the identification of transforming genes which are activated in a variety of human, rodent, and avian neoplasms (see [5] for recent review). The transforming genes of some neoplasms are cellular homologs of the *ras* genes of Harvey and Kirsten sarcoma viruses. Other neoplasm transforming genes, such as *Blym-1,* are unrelated to *ras* or to other retroviral transforming genes. In this article, I will discuss recent work related to functional analysis of the *ras* and *Blym-1* gene products.

B. *ras* Genes

Three different members of the *ras* gene family have been identified as biologically active transforming genes in neoplasm DNA: ras^H, ras^K, and ras^N [8, 15, 16, 18, 22]. These genes have been detected in many different types of neoplasms, including carcinomas, sarcomas, melanomas, neuroblastomas, lymphomas, and leukemias of myeloid and lymphoid origin. Thus, it appears that *ras* genes can contribute to the development of neoplasms arising from multiple types of differentiated cells. This is consistent with the fact that *ras* genes are expressed in all normal vertebrate cells which have been examined. In addition, yeast contains functional *ras* genes, suggesting that these genes play a fundamental role in cell proliferation which is highly conserved in evolution. However, *ras* genes are found as active transforming genes in only a small fraction (approximately 10%–20%) of individual neoplasms. Thus, although *ras* activation can occur in many different types of tumors, it is apparently not a necessary event for development of any particular type of neoplasm. In addition, recent data suggest that *ras* activation may be a late event in tumor progression. For example, Albino et al. [1] have reported detection of an activated ras^N gene in only one in five metastases of an individual melanoma patient. This finding suggests the possibility that *ras* activation may, when it occurs, impart a selective advantage to a clone of neoplastic cells, but is not essential for formation of a primary neoplasm or even its metastatic derivatives.

The *ras* genes all encode proteins of approximately 21 000 daltons which are designated p21. Experimental manipulations of the normal human ras^H gene have shown that overexpression of the normal gene product is sufficient to induce cell transformation [4]. However, activation of *ras* genes in human tumors is commonly a consequence of structural, rather than regulatory, mutations [2, 3, 7, 17, 21, 23–25, 27]. The mutations in tumors which have been analyzed to date alter either codon 12 or codon 61. At either of these positions, substitution of multiple different amino acids is sufficient to endow p21 with transforming activity. In addition, most activat-

1 Dana Farber Cancer Institute and Department of Pathology, Harvard Medical School Boston, MA 02115, USA

ing mutations appear to induce conformational alterations in p21 which are detectable by abnormal electophoretic mobilities [7, 23, 27]. Taken together, these observations suggest that substitution of a variety of abnormal amino acids at these critical loci may inactivate a regulatory domain of p21, thus resulting in abnormal p21 function in vivo.

Studies of viral *ras* proteins have indicated that they are localized at the inner face of the plasma membrane [12, 26] and modified by acylation [20]. The only established biochemical activity common to all viral *ras* transforming proteins is guanine nucleotide binding [12, 19].

To attempt to elucidate the biochemical basis for the transforming activity of mutant p21 in human tumors, we have compared the biochemical properties of p21 encoded by normal and activated human *ras* genes. These experiments indicated that both normal and transforming human p21 were localized at the plasma membrane and were modified to similar extents by posttranslational acylation [11]. Neither normal nor activated p21 were glycosylated or phosphorylated [7, 11]. Thus, the subcellular localization and posttranslational processing of human p21 were not altered by *ras* gene activation.

Since guanine nucleotide binding represented the only known biochemical activity of p21, we investigated the possibility that the affinity or specificity of p21 for nucleotides was altered as a consequence of mutational activation. However, the GTP binding affinities of both normal and activated human p21 were indistinguishable ($K_D = 1{-}2 \times 10^{-8}$ M) and both the normal and activated proteins were specific for GTP and GDP binding [11]. Thus, mutational activation of p21 does not directly affect its intrinsic nucleotide binding properties.

In order to investigate the physiologic function of *ras* proteins, we have attempted to identify other cellular proteins with which p21 might interact [10]. Immunoprecipitation of extracts of human carcinoma cell lines with anti-p21 monoclonal antibodies revealed the coprecipitation of a second protein of approximately 90 000 daltons. This coprecipitated protein was identified as the transferrin receptor by three criteria: (a) comigration in both reducing and nonreducing gels; (b) immunologic reactivity with monoclonal antibody raised against transferrin receptor; and (c) identity of partial proteolysis maps of the 90 000 daltons coprecipitated protein and transferrin receptor. Coprecipitation of transferrin receptor was detected with three different *ras* monoclonal antibodies and was dependent on the presence of *ras* proteins in cell extracts, indicating that p21 and transferrin receptor form a molecular complex. This complex was dissociated by addition of transferrin to cell extracts, suggesting that transferrin binding induced a conformational change in the receptor which led to the dissociation of *ras* proteins.

Transferrin is an iron binding protein which is required for the growth of most cells in culture. Expression of transferrin receptor is closely correlated with cell proliferation. Furthermore, monoclonal antibodies against transferrin receptor inhibit cell growth, in some cases even if iron is supplied in an alternate form. Transferrin and its receptor thus appear to play a fundamental role in the growth of many differentiated cell types. The findings of interaction between *ras* proteins and transferrin receptor therefore suggest that p21 may function in conjunction with this cell surface receptor in regulation of cell growth, perhaps by transducing growth signals mediated by transferrin binding. It is possible that the role of p21 in this respect is analogous to other membrane guanine nucleotide binding proteins, such as the adenyl cyclase G proteins and transducin [13].

C. *Blym* Genes

In contrast to *ras*, the *Blym*-1 gene is representative of several transforming genes which are activated highly reproducibly in neoplasms of specific cell types. Thus, *Blym*-1 has been detected as an active transforming sequence in all chicken B cell lymphomas [6] and all human Burkitt's lymphomas [9] which have been examined. It thus appears to play a highly reproducible role in the development of similar B cell neoplasms in both chickens and humans.

The *Blym*-1 transforming gene activated in chicken B cell lymphomas was isolated as a molecular clone by sib-selection [14]. The cloned chicken *Blym*-1 gene was unusually small (only about 600 nucleotides) and its nucleotide sequence indicated that it encoded a small protein of 65 amino acids [14]. Comparison of the predicted chicken *Blym*-1 amino acid sequence with sequences of known cellular proteins revealed partial homology (36%) between the chicken *Blym*-1 protein and the NH, terminal region of transferrin family proteins [14]. This homology was concentrated in regions which were conserved between different members of the transferrin family, suggesting a common ancestry for chicken *Blym*-1 and a region of the transferrins, as well as stimulating the speculation that this homology might also suggest a functional relationship.

Blot hybridization analysis indicated that the chicken *Blym*-1 gene was a member of a small family of related genes which were present in human as well as chicken DNA. We therefore investigated the possibility that the transforming gene detected by transfection of Burkitt's lymphoma DNA might be a member of the human gene family defined by homology to chicken *Blym*-1. A genomic library of DNA from a Burkitt's lymphoma was screened using chicken *Blym*-1 probe and a biologically active human transforming gene, designated human *Blym*-1, was isolated [9]. This human homolog of chicken *Blym*-1 was found to represent the transforming gene detected by transfection of all six Burkitt's lymphoma DNA samples studied.

Restriction mapping and nucleotide sequencing indicate that human *Blym*-1, like chicken *Blym*-1, is quite small (approximately 700 nucleotides) (Diamond et al., manuscript submitted [9]). Also like chicken *Blym*-1, the sequence of human *Blym*-1 predicts a small protein (58 amino acids) which consists of two exons and is rich in lysine and arginine. Alignment of the human and chicken *Blym*-1 amino acid sequences indicates 33% amino acid identities. The human and chicken *Blym*-1 proteins are therefore clearly related ($P < 0.005$), but significant divergence between the two sequences has occurred. This divergence suggests the possibility that the chicken and human genes may represent relatively distant members of the *Blym* family.

In spite of the divergence between the chicken and human *Blym*-1 genes, the human *Blym*-1 sequence also displays significant homology (20%) to the NH_2 terminal region of transferrins. Significantly, amino acids which are conserved between the chicken and human *Blym*-1 genes also tend to be conserved between different members of the transferrin family. It is unlikely that such divergent sequences as chicken and human *Blym*-1 have maintained homology to transferrin by chance. Rather, the conservation of transferrin homology in these *Blym* transforming genes suggests that this homology reflects some functional property of the *Blym* transforming proteins. In view of the molecular interaction between *ras* proteins and transferrin receptor, these findings suggest the hypothesis that the *Blym* transforming genes may also affect cell proliferation via a pathway related to transferrin and its surface receptor. Further understanding of the function of the *Blym* gene products will require direct biochemical analysis of these proteins.

References

1. Albino AP, LeStrange R, Oliff AI, Furth ME, Old LJ (1984) Nature 308:69–72
2. Capon DJ, Chen EY, Levinson AD, Seeburg PH, Goeddel DV (1983a) Nature 302:33–37
3. Capon DJ, Seeburg PH, McGrath JP, Hayflick JS, Edman U, Levinson AD, Goeddel DV (1983b) Nature 304:507–513
4. Chang EH, Furth ME, Scolnick EM, Lowy DR (1982) Nature 297:497–483
5. Cooper GM, Lane M-A (1984) Biochim Biophys Acta Rev Cancer (in press)
6. Cooper GM, Neiman PE (1980) Nature 287:656–658
7. Der CJ, Cooper GM (1983) Cell 32:201–208
8. Der CJ, Krontiris TG, Cooper GM (1982) Proc Natl Acad Sci, USA 79:3637–3640
9. Diamond AD, Cooper GM, Ritz J, Lane, MA (1983) Nature 305:112–116
10. Finkel T, Cooper GM (1984) Cell 36:1115–1121

11. Finkel T, Der CJ, Cooper GM (1984) Cell 37:151–158
12. Furth ME, Davis LJ, Fleurdelys B, Scolnick EM (1982) J Virol 43:294–304
13. Gilman AG (1984) Cell 36:577–579
14. Goubin G, Goldman DS, Luce J, Neiman PE, Cooper GM (1983) Nature 302:114–119
15. Hall A, Marshall CJ, Spurr NK, Weiss RA (1983) Nature 303:396–400
16. Parada LF, Tabin CJ, Shih C, Weinberg RA (1982) Nature 297:474–478
17. Reddy EP, Reynolds RK, Santos E, Barbacid M (1982) Nature 300:149–152
18. Santos E, Tronick SR, Aaronson SA, Pulciani S, Barbacid M (1982) Nature 298:343–347
19. Scolnick EM, Papageorge AG, Shih TY (1979) Proc Natl Acad Sci USA 76:5355–5359
20. Sefton BM, Trowbridge IS, Cooper JA, Scolnick EM (1982) Cell 31:465–474
21. Shimizu K, Birnbaum D, Ruley MA, Fasano O, Suard Y, Edlund L, Taparowsky E, Goldfarb M, Wigler M (1983a) Nature 304:497–500
22. Shimizu K, Goldfarb M, Perucho M, Wigler M (1983b) Proc Natl Acad Sci USA 80:383–387
23. Tabin CJ, Bradley SM, Bargmann CI, Weinberg RA, Papageorge AG, Scolnick EM, Dhar R, Lowy DR, Chang EH (1982) Nature 300:143–149
24. Taparowsky E, Suard Y, Fasano O, Shimizu K, Goldfarb M, Wigler M (1982) Nature 300:762–765
25. Taparowsky E, Shimizu K, Goldfarb M, Wigler M (1983) Cell 34:581–586
26. Willingham MC, Pastan I, Shih TY, Scolnick (1980) Cell 19:1005–1014
27. Yuasa Y, Srivastava SK, Dunn CY, Rhim JS, Reddy EP, Aaronson SA (1983) Nature 303:775–779

Haematology and Blood Transfusion Vol. 29
Modern Trends in Human Leukemia VI
Edited by Neth, Gallo, Greaves, Janka

TLym 1, a Stage-Specific Transforming Gene Which Shares Homology to MHCI Genes and Encodes a Secreted Protein

M. A. Lane[1,2], H. A. F. Stephens[1,2], K. M. Doherty[1], and M. Tobin[1]

We previously reported the identification of five different genes activated in human and mouse leukemias and lymphomas [1]. Three of these genes were found to be activated in a stage-specific manner in B cell lineage neoplasms. The gene activated in multiple human intermediate B stage tumors, BLym 1 which shares substantial homology with chicken BLym 1 [2] was isolated from human Burkitt's lymphomas. This gene encodes a small protein of about 8 kilodaltons, the bulk of which is present in the nucleus of transformed cells (Nieman and Cooper, personal communication).

We recently isolated a second stage-specific transforming gene from mouse T lymphomas, representative of an intermediate stage of T lymphocyte differentiation. This gene differs by restriction endonuclease sensitivity from the transforming gene activated in multiple mature T neoplasms. TLym 1 has been found to be activated in four human and 12 mouse T cell neoplasms, but has not been found to be activated in cells from other lineages or cells at other stages of differentiation. TLym 1 shares no homology with Blym 1 nor does it share homology with any of the identified retrovirally transduced oncogenes. Thus, it represents a new cellular transforming gene highly specific for T lymphocytes at an intermediate stage of differentiation [3].

1 Laboratory of Molecular Immunobiology, Dana-Farber Cancer Institute, USA
2 Dept. of Pathology, Harvard Medical School, USA

TLym 1 was isolated from the S49 BALB/c T lymphoma by sib-selection and transfection of a transforming gene-enriched recombinant library prepared in the bacteriophage Charon 30. The isolated bacteriophage clone had a transforming efficiency of 10^4 foci per microgram cell DNA insert as assayed on NIH 3T3 cells. From Southern blot analysis using a flanking sequence probe, we determined that the gene did not become activated as a result of gross inversions, deletions, or rearrangements. TLym 1 is a small gene, approximately 3 kilobases in length and was originally thought to be a member of a small gene family, consisting of only two genes as defined by sequences hybridizing to the flanking region probe. Recent findings described in the following paragraphs, however, may alter this conclusion [3].

Hybridization of TLym 1 to T cell RNA indicated that three major messages could be identified in helper T cells which were 0.6, 0.7, and 1.6 kilobases in length. An additional message of 1.8 kilobases was identified in a suppressor T cell clone. As the size classes of meassages identified by TLym 1 were quite similar to those reported by Peter Rigby for his Set 1 genes, thought to encode a major histocompatibility class I gene [4], it was of interest to us to determine whether our gene shared homology to MHCI genes as well.

Southern blot hybridization was carried out using the following probes: pAG64C, a cDNA clone obtained from P. Rigby containing half of exon 4, and exons 5 and 6 of his Set 1 gene; pAG64E, which contained the Set 1 transposon-like direct repeat sequence; and pMHCI, and MHCI cross-reactive probe containing exons 2, 3, 4, and 5 which was obtained from John Seidman [5]. Additional hybridizations carried out by Steven Hunt in the laboratory of Lee Hood included hybridization utilizing MHC cross-reactive 5′ and 3′ probes. These studies indicated that our TLym 1 gene shared homology to genes mapped to the MHCI region and that the direct repeat sequence described by Rigby and co-workers was present in our gene. This sequence has also been detected by Hood and co-workers and was found in the third intron of their QA pseudogene 27.1 [6]. We were also able to determine from these hybridizations the orientation of our gene in the pBR322 plasmid to which it was subcloned.

As TLym 1 contained a ClaI site, some further analysis was possible based upon the report by Steinmetz et al. [7] defining 13 clusters containing 36 genes within the BALB/c MHCI region. From their reported analysis of ClaI sites within the gene clusters. Clusters 1 and 6 map to QA regions, while clusters 3 and 5 map to TL regions as determined by these authors. If the genes contained in the 13 clusters constitute all of the genes encoding MHCI sequences, then this retrospective analysis further localizes TLym 1 to the QA/TL region of the MHCI complex.

We have determined that our gene differs from that identified by Rigby and co-workers based upon hybridization of our flanking sequence probe to mouse DNA digested with the enzyme BAMH1 which identified two bands of 8.6 and 18.0 kilobases while hybridization of Rigby and co-workers' pAG64C probe to the same filter identified bands of 6.0, 3.5, 3.2, and 2.2 kilobases, as the 8.6 kilobases genomic BamH1 fragment is analogous to the cell DNA insert which contains the TLym 1 transforming gene isolated in Charon 30. We concluded that although these genes share some homology, they are in fact different genes. Genes within the MHCI region may share as much as 80% homology. Thus, analysis of these genes at the level of Southern blot hybridization is sometimes complicated, however, utilization in this case of low or single-copy probes has facilitated this analysis.

To analyze the protein encoded by TLym 1 we utilized a series of monoclonal or heteroantibodies prepared against H-2, TL, or QA region determinants. Immunoprecipitations carried out utilizing these reagents have failed to detect the TLym 1-encoded protein. Utilization of an antiserum cross-reactive with all MHCI-encoded proteins, however, detected a 44 kilodaltons protein in the supernatants of NIH 3T3 cells transformed by TLym 1 which was not present in supernatants from normal NIH 3T3 cells, spontaneously transformed 3T3 cells, NIH 3T3 cells transformed by *ras*^{H}, or NIH 3T3 cells transformed by the Blym 1 gene. These findings further substantiate the relatedness of the TLym 1 product to MHCI-encoded proteins and indicate that TLym 1 is the first transforming gene found to encode a secreted protein product. While most MHCI products have been localized to the cell surface, Jay and co-workers have reported a liver-specific MHCI protein which appears to be secreted, but which is not involved in transformation [8].

As TLym 1 appears to encode a secreted protein, we have begun preliminary experiments to determine whether this protein can behave as a growth factor. We therefore utilized supernatants from untransformed NIH 3T3 cells and supernatants from NIH 3T3 cells transformed by TLym 1 in a soft agar colony growth factor assay [9] with NIH 3T3 cells as the target cells.

After 14 days in culture, plates were scored for numbers of colonies having 20 or more cells. A total of 77 colonies were detected on seven plates treated with supernatants from NIH 3T3 cells whereas 960 colonies were detected on seven plates treated with supernatant from NIH 3T3 cells transformed by TLym 1. It will be of great interest to determine whether supernatants from TLym 1-transformed NIH 3T3 cells will have similiar effects upon T lymphocytes.

To summarize these findings, TLym 1 is an intermediate T-specific transforming gene which transforms NIH 3T3 cells with high efficiencies. This gene appears to share homology with genes encoded in the MHCI region and may be the transforming analog of a TL/QA region gene. TLym 1 encodes a secreted protein of 44 kilodaltons which preliminary evidence indicates behaves as a transforming growth factor.

Acknowledgments. The authors wish to thank Dr. John Seidman, Dr. Peter Rigby, Dr. Leroy Hood, Dr. Stephen Hunt, F. W. Shen, E. A. Boyse and Gordon Freeman for reagents and useful discussions. This work was supported by CA 33108. M. A. Lane is a scholar of the Leukemia Society of America.

References

1. Lane MA, Sainten A, Cooper GM (1982) Cell 28:873
2. Goubin G, Goldman DS, Luce J, Nieman P, Cooper GM (1983) Nature 302:114
3. Lane MA, Sainten A, Doherty K, Cooper GM (1984) Proc Natl Acad Sci USA 81:2227
4. Brickell PM, Latchman DS, Murphy D, Willison K, Rigby PWJ (1983) Nature 306:756
5. Evans GA, Marguiles DH, Camerini-Otero RD, Ozato K, Seidman JG (1982) Proc Natl Acad Sci USA 79:1994
6. Winoto A, Steinmets M, Hood L (1983) Proc Natl Acad Sci 80:3425
7. Steinmetz M, Winoto A, Minard K, Hood L (1982) Cell 28:489
8. Maloy WL, Coligan JE, Barra Y, Jay G (1984) Proc Natl Acad Sci USA 81:1216
9. Ozanne B (1982) Nature 299:744

Haematology and Blood Transfusion Vol. 29
Modern Trends in Human Leukemia VI
Edited by Neth, Gallo, Greaves, Janka

The *mil/raf* and *myc* Oncogenes: Molecular Cloning and In Vitro Mutagenesis *

H. W. Jansen, C. Trachmann, T. Patschinsky, and K. Bister

A. Introduction

Avian retrovirus MH2 is a member of the MC29 subgroup of avian acute leukemia viruses which includes the four independently isolated viruses MC29, CMII, OK10, and MH2 [4]. The genetic hallmark of these viruses is the presence in their genomes of unique transformation-specific sequences, termed v-*myc* [4, 5], which are of cellular origin [3–5, 13]. In contrast to MC29, CMII, and OK10 which induce predominantly leukemic diseases, MH2 induces predominantly liver and kidney carcinomas [1, 2].

The genetic structure of MH2 was recently analyzed in detail. A molecularly cloned MH2 provirus was shown to contain a novel oncogene, termed v-*mil,* in addition

* Otto-Warburg-Laboratorium, Max-Planck-Institut für Molekulare Genetik, Ihnestr. 63–73, 1000 Berlin 33 (Dahlem), FRG

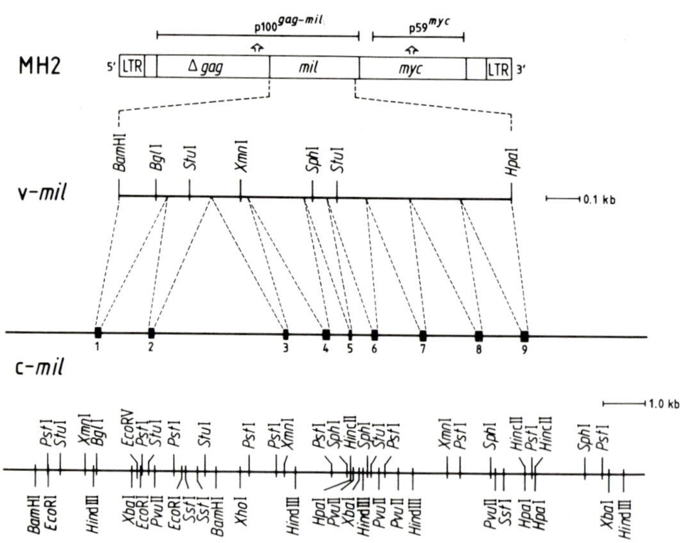

Fig. 1. Genome structure of MH2 and relationship between v-*mil* and c-*mil.* A schematic diagram of cloned proviral MH2 DNA and of its gene products is shown at the top. *Δgag* indicates the presence of partial complements of the *gag* gene. Below this diagram a restriction map of the v-*mil* oncogene is shown. At the bottom of the figure a detailed restriction map of the chicken c-*mil* locus is presented. The exon–intron arrangement as determined from Southern blots and from heteroduplex analysis is shown between the restriction maps of the viral and the cellular oncogene. *Numbered black boxes* represent the regions of c-*mil* homologous to v-*mil* sequences. These presumed exons are numbered in the 5′–3′ direction (see note added in proof)

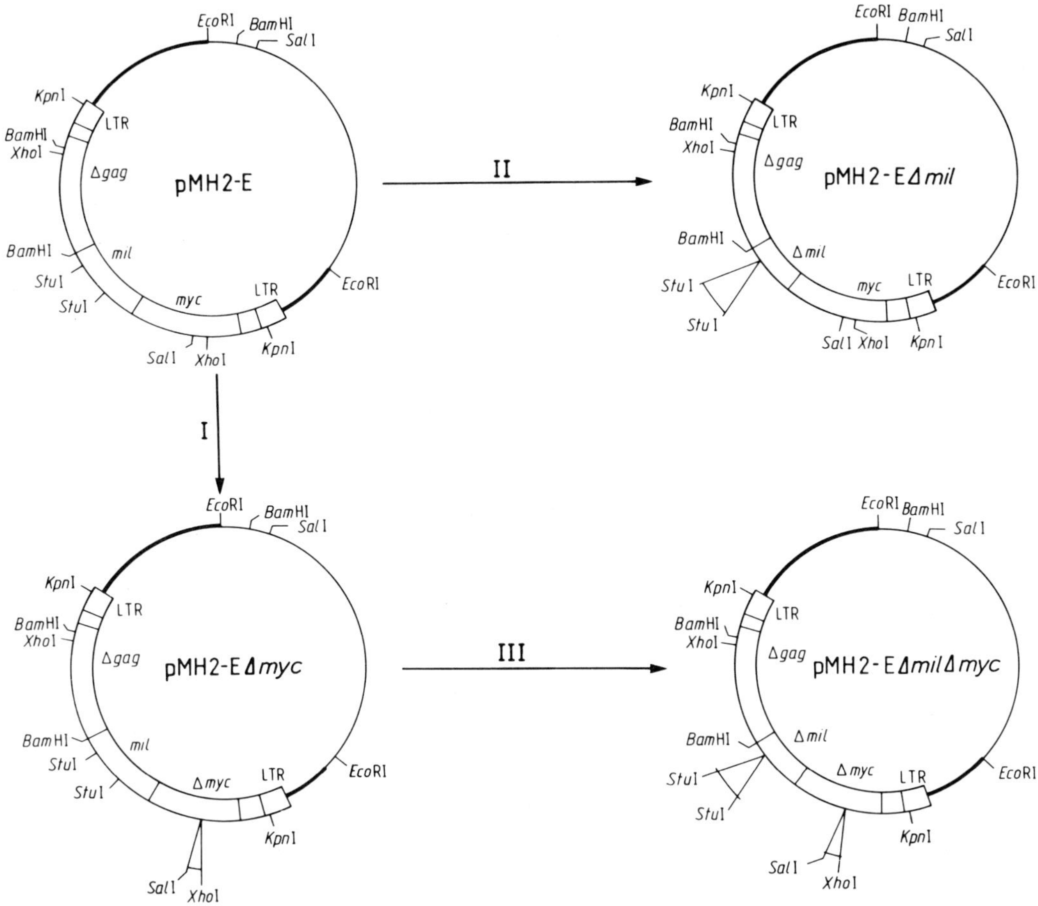

Fig. 2. In vitro mutagenesis of the cloned MH2 provirus. I: construction of an MH2 *Δmyc* provirus. The cloned MH2 provirus was digested with *Sal*I. The ~ 6.5 kilobases fragment containing 5′-LTR-*Δgag-mil*-5′-*myc* of the provirus was isolated. In parallel, the MH2 provirus was digested with *Sal*I and *Xho*I. The ~ 5.6 kilobases fragment containing all plasmid sequences essential for ampicillin resistance and all MH2 proviral sequences 3′ of the *Xho*I site in v-*myc* was isolated. After ligation of these two fragments and transformation of competent bacterial cells, the desired plasmids were selected by growth on tetracycline plates. The structure of four recombinant plasmids was verified and all four turned out to contain the desired MH2 *Δmyc* provirus. The *Δmyc* preserves the reading frame for the v-*myc* protein 3′ of the *Xho*I site. II: construction of an MH2 *Δmil* provirus. The cloned MH2 provirus was digested with *Stu*I. The ~ 11.9 kilobases fragment containing all of the provirus with the exception of a ~ 440 base pairs v-*mil* fragment was isolated and religated. III: construction of an MH2 *ΔmilΔmyc* provirus. To obtain the double deletion mutant the MH2 *Δmyc* provirus was cleaved with *Stu*I, the ~ 11.7 kilobases fragment was isolated and religated. *Boxes* proviral DNA; *thick lines* cellular DNA; *thin lines* plasmid DNA (pBR322)

to v-*myc* [8, 10]. This novel oncogene, like all other viral oncogenes, is of cellular origin [9, 10], and it was shown to be the avian counterpart of the murine *raf* gene [11, 14], the oncogene of the murine retrovirus 3611-MSV. In this communication, we report on two different strategies for the construction of proviral DNA species which will be useful to resolve the individual contributions of the *mil* and *myc* oncogenes in the induction of the specific tumors observed in chickens infected by MH2.

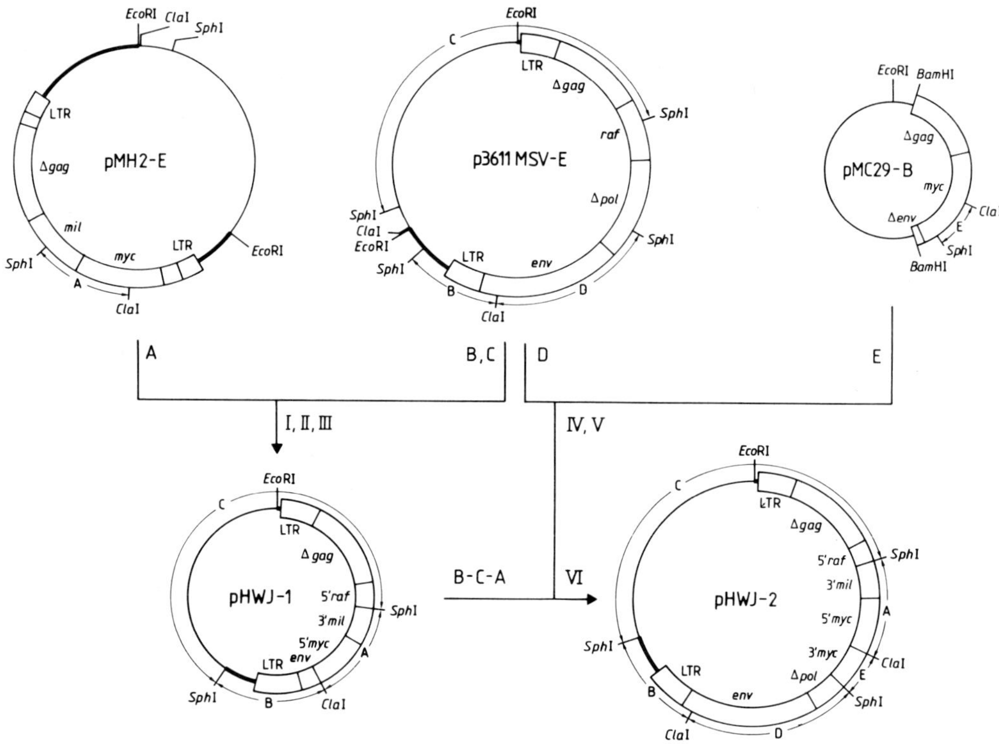

Fig. 3. Construction of a murine provirus containing the *raf/mil* and the *myc* oncogene. For the assembly of pHWJ-1 which contains a v-*raf/mil* hybrid oncogene and the 5′ half of MH2 v-*myc*, plasmids containing the cloned proviruses of MH2 or of 3611-MSV were cleaved with the restriction endonucleases *Cla*I and *Sph*I. The fragments denoted *A–C* were electroeluted from an agarose gel (I). Fragments *A* and *B* were ligated and subsequently cleaved with *Sph*I (II). The products of these reactions were ligated to fragment *C* which had been dephosphorylated with bacterial alkaline phosphatase in advance. The plasmids obtained after transformation of competent *Escherichia coli* cells with this reaction mixture were selected for size and orientation (III). For the construction of the plasmid pHWJ-2 which contains the v-*raf/mil* hybrid oncogene and a complete v-*myc* gene, plasmids containing the cloned provirus of 3611-MSV or the 3.0 kilobases *Bam*HI fragment of the MC29 provirus were cleaved with *Cla*I and *Sph*I. The fragments denoted *D* and *E* were isolated (IV), ligated, and subsequently cleaved with *Cla*I. The desired *D–E* fragment was gel-purified (V) and ligated with the *B–C–A* DNA of pHWJ-1 which had been dephosphorylated after cleavage with *Cla*I. The plasmids obtained after transformation were selected for size and orientation (VI)

B. Results and Discussion

The basic structures of the cloned MH2 provirus, of its oncogene v-*mil*, and of the chicken c-*mil* locus are shown in Fig. 1. In order to get information on the role of the *mil* and *myc* oncogenes in tumor induction by MH2 virus, mutants of MH2 were constructed which are deleted in their oncogenes (Fig. 2). A *Δmil* mutant was constructed by deletion of a 443 base pairs *Stu*I fragment of v-*mil* resulting in an out-of-frame deletion. A *Δmyc* mutant was constructed by deletion of an 171 base pairs *Sal*I-*Xho*I fragment of MH2 v-*myc* resulting in an in-frame deletion. This constructed *Δmyc* deletion is similar to deletions observed in natural mutants of MC29 [6] which are still able to transform fibroblasts, but not macrophages efficiently [12] and which are unable to induce tumors in chickens [7]. A mutant with deletions in both oncogenes (*ΔmilΔmyc*) was constructed by a combination of the strategies described. Biologic studies of the *Δmil* and *Δmyc* mutants are under way. First results suggest that *mil* enhances the induction of cell proliferation and transformation by the *myc* oncogene both in vivo and in vitro (T. Graf, H. W. Jansen, T. Patschinsky, K. Bister, in preparation).

The observation that the avian oncogene v-*mil* and the murine oncogene v-*raf* were derived from cognate cellular genes [11, 14] led to studies of the transforming capacities of the *mil* and *myc* oncogenes in mice. Upon transfection of NIH/3T3 cells with cloned MH2 proviral DNA, no focus formation was observed. Therefore, we decided to construct murine retroviruses containing the avian *mil* and *myc* oncogenes. The detailed strategy for the construction of pHWJ-1, a plasmid containing a complete *raf/mil* oncogene and the 5′ part of v-*myc*, and of pHWJ-2, a plasmid containing both a complete *raf/mil* and a complete *myc* oncogene, is shown in Fig. 3. Upon transfection, both plasmids gave rise to foci on NIH/3T3 cells with those induced by pHWJ-2 being much more prominent. A first striking result from in vivo experiments with these viruses is the observation that the oncogenicity of HWJ-2 virus is markedly higher than that of 3611-MSV (U. R. Rapp, H. W. Jansen, K. Bister, in preparation).

Note added in proof

A recent nucleotide sequence analysis [15] of the c-*mil* locus revealed that there are two additional small regions of homology to v-*mil* 5′ from exon 1 (Fig. 1).

References

1. Alexander RW, Moscovici C, Vogt PK (1979) Avian oncovirus Mill Hill No. 2: pathogenicity in chickens. J Natl Cancer Inst 62: 359–366
2. Beard JW (1980) Biology of avian oncornaviruses. In: Klein G (ed) Viral oncology. Raven, New York, pp 55–87
3. Bishop JM (1983) Cellular oncogenes and retroviruses. Ann Rev Biochem 52:301–354
4. Bister K (1984) Molecular biology of avian acute leukaemia viruses. In: Goldman JM, Jarrett JO (eds) Leukaemia and lymphoma research, vol 1. Mechanisms of viral leukaemogenesis. Churchill-Livingstone, Edinburgh, pp 38–63
5. Bister K, Duesberg PH (1982) Genetic structure and transforming genes of avian retroviruses. In: Klein G (ed) Advances in viral oncology, vol 1. Raven, New York, pp 3–42
6. Bister K, Ramsay GM, Hayman MJ (1982) Deletions within the transformation-specific RNA sequences of acute leukemia virus MC29 give rise to partially transformation-defective mutants. J Virol 41:754–766
7. Enrietto PJ, Hayman MJ, Ramsay GM, Wyke JA, Payne LN (1983) Altered pathogenicity of avian myelocytomatosis (MC29) viruses with mutations in the v-*myc* gene. Virology 124:164–172
8. Jansen HW, Patschinsky T, Bister K (1983) Avian oncovirus MH2: Molecular cloning of proviral DNA and structural analysis of viral RNA and protein. J Virol 48:61–73
9. Jansen HW, Trachmann C, Bister K (1984) Structural relationship between the chicken protooncogene c-*mil* and the retroviral oncogene v-*mil*. Virology 137:217–224
10. Jansen HW, Rückert B, Lurz R, Bister K (1983) Two unrelated cell-derived sequences in the genome of avian leukemia and carcinoma inducing retrovirus MH2. EMBO J 2:1969–1975
11. Jansen HW, Lurz R, Bister K, Bonner TI, Mark GE, Rapp UR (1984) Homologous cell-derived oncogenes in avian carcinoma virus MH2 and murine sarcoma virus 3611. Nature 307:281–284
12. Ramsay GM, Graf T, Hayman MJ (1980) Mutants of avian myelocytomatosis virus with smaller *gag* gene-related proteins have an altered transforming ability. Nature 288: 170–172
13. Robins TS, Bister K, Garon C, Papas TS, Duesberg PH (1982) Structural relationship between a normal chicken DNA locus and the transforming gene of the avian acute leukemia virus MC29. J Virol 41:635–642
14. Sutrave P, Bonner TI, Rapp UR, Jansen HW, Patschinsky T, Bister K (1984) Nucleotide sequence of avian retroviral oncogene v-*mil*: homologue of murine retroviral oncogene v-*raf*. Nature 309:85–88
15. Jansen HW, Bister K (1985) Nucleotide sequence analysis of the chicken gene c-*mil*, the progenitor of the retroviral oncogene v-*mil*. Virology 143 (in press)

Haematology and Blood Transfusion Vol. 29
Modern Trends in Human Leukemia VI
Edited by Neth, Gallo, Greaves, Janka

Characterization of the Number of Carbohydrate Chains on the Avian Erythroblastosis Virus *erb* B Gene Product and Their Role in Transformation

M. J. Hayman [1], J. A. Schmidt [1], G. Kitchener [1], J. Marshall [1], and H. Beug [2]

A. Introduction

Avian erythroblastosis virus, AEV, is a replication-defective avian acute leukemia virus that causes acute erythroid leukemia and sarcomas on injection into young chicks. Analysis of the genome of AEV revealed that it was 5.0 kilobases in length and that the gene order was 5′-*gag-erb-env-poly* A-3′ where *gag* and *env* represent partially deleted structural genes and *erb* is a 3.25 kilobases sequence of nonviral origin [2, 13]. Subsequently, sequences homologous to *erb* could be found in cellular DNA from all vertebrate species tested [16, 19]. This evidence suggested that the *erb* sequences represented the viral oncogene of AEV, and led to studies attempting to define the products of this gene.

Studies rapidly revealed that AEV contained an oncogene capable of coding for two gene products. Consequently, *erb* was divided into two regions known as *erb* A and *erb* B. The first gene product identified was the *erb* A protein, a 75 000 molecular weight protein, $p75^{erb\,A}$ that could be shown to be composed of NH_2 terminal *gag* sequences plus approximately 50 000 daltons of *erb* A sequences [10]. Recently, the *erb* B protein has also been identified in AEV-transformed cells and was shown to be a membrane glycoprotein [9, 14]. This protein has a molecular weight of 62 500 in the nonglycosylated state, but is modified by glycosylation first to a 66 000 molecular weight form, $gp66^{erb\,B}$ and then through a 68 000 molecular weight phosphorylated form, $gp68^{erb\,B}$ to a plasma membrane form, $gp74^{erb\,B}$ [8, 9].

Interest in the *erb* B protein was heightened by several recent observations. First, site-directed mutagenesis experiments on the AEV genome demonstrated that it was primarily the *erb* B gene that was responsible for the transformation of both erythroid cells and fibroblasts [6, 18]. The *erb* A gene did, however, play some role in the development of the fully transformed erythroblast phenotype. Second, characterization of a new isolate of AEV, termed AEV-H, which was capable of causing both erythroblastosis and fibrosarcoma, revealed that the only *erb*-related sequence it contained in its genome was *erb* B [11, 23]. Finally, it was demonstrated that avian leukosis virus-induced erythroblastosis was associated with insertion of the viral long terminal repeat, LTR, into the cellular *erb* B locus, c-*erb*, resulting in the elevation of c-*erb* B transcription [7]. Thus, the central role of *erb* B in erythroblasosis and fibrosarcoma induction has encouraged us to characterize the product of this gene in greater detail.

Digestion of the v-*erb* B protein with the enzyme endoglycosidase H, endo-H, had previously shown that both $gp66^{erb\,B}$ and $gp68^{erb\,B}$ were sensitive to digestion with this enzyme [9], whereas $gp74^{erb\,B}$ was resistant [8]. This enzyme specifically cleaves

1 Imperial Cancer Research Fund Laboratories, St. Bartholomew's Hospital, Dominion House, Bartholomew Close, London EC1A 7BE, England
2 EMB Laboratories, Postfach 10, 2209, Meyerhofstrasse 1, 6900 Heidelberg, FRG

off the high mannose core sugars which are associated with the immature forms of glycoproteins [20]. Therefore, these results were consistent with gp66 and gp68 being the immature forms and gp74 being the mature form of the *erb* B gene product. Recently, analysis of mutants of AEV which are temperature sensitive for cell transformation have shown that the mutation blocks the processing of gp68 into gp74 and hence there is no surface expression of *erb* B [1]. Consequently, we have examined the number of carbohydrate units and their role in the function of the *erb* B protein.

B. Results and Discussion

I. Endoglycosidase H Digestion of the *erb* B Protein

Previous analysis of the gp68 product by endo-H digestion had employed complete digestion in order to remove all the available high mannose glycan units. By using limited digestion with endo-H it is possible to remove these units sequentially and thus ascertain how many units there are on the protein. Figure 1 shows the results of such an experiment. The gp68 form of *erb* B is first converted into a gp66 form (lane 4) and then finally into the p62 form (lane 5), which is the same size as the in vitro translation product and the form synthesized in the presence of tunicamycin [9, 14]. As demonstrated previously, gp74 is resistant to digestion (lane 5). These data indicate that there are two *N*-linked carbohydrate chains present on the *erb* B protein which can be released with endo-H. Recent sequence analysis of the *erb* B gene of AEV-ES4 ([3] and our unpublished data), which is the strain used in our experiments, indicate that there are three consensus sequences for *N*-linked carbohydrate addition. Therefore, only two of the three possible sites for addition are being used. At the present time we are unable to say which these two sites are. However, one of the three sites is located only four amino acids from the presumptive membrane spanning region and therefore may not be available. Also, *erb* B has recently been reported to be highly homologous to the human epidermal growth factor receptor, EGF-R [4, 22] and comparison of the glycosylation sites between *erb* B and EGF-R shows that this site is not conserved whereas the other two are. In summary, it appears as if the v-*erb* B protein contains two *N*-linked carbohydrate chains.

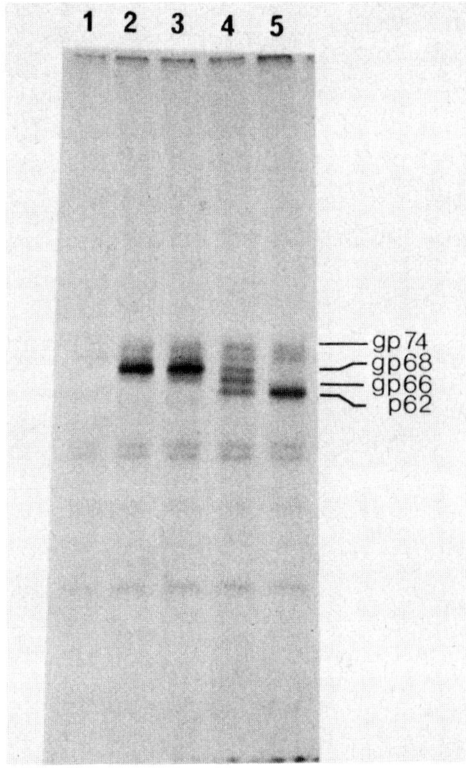

Fig. 1. Endoglycosidase H (endo-H) digestion of v-*erb* B. Erythroblasts transformed with *ts* 34 AEV were labelled with methionine ^{35}S under optimal conditions to label gp68$^{erb\,B}$ and gp74$^{erb\,B}$ [8]. Digestions of endo-H on immunoprecipitated v-*erb* B were performed as described [8]. Reactions contained either 0.01 mU (*lane* 3), 0.1 mU (*lane* 4) or 1 mU (*lane* 5) endo-H, in addition to a negative control (*lane* 2). *Lane* 1 is a normal rat serum immunoprecipitation of the same cell extract treated with 1 mU endo-H. Products were identified by fluorography after polyacrylamide gel electrophoresis

II. Effect of Inhibitors of Glycosylation on the Function of *erb* B

Recently, inhibitors of the processing of carbohydrate side chains have proved very

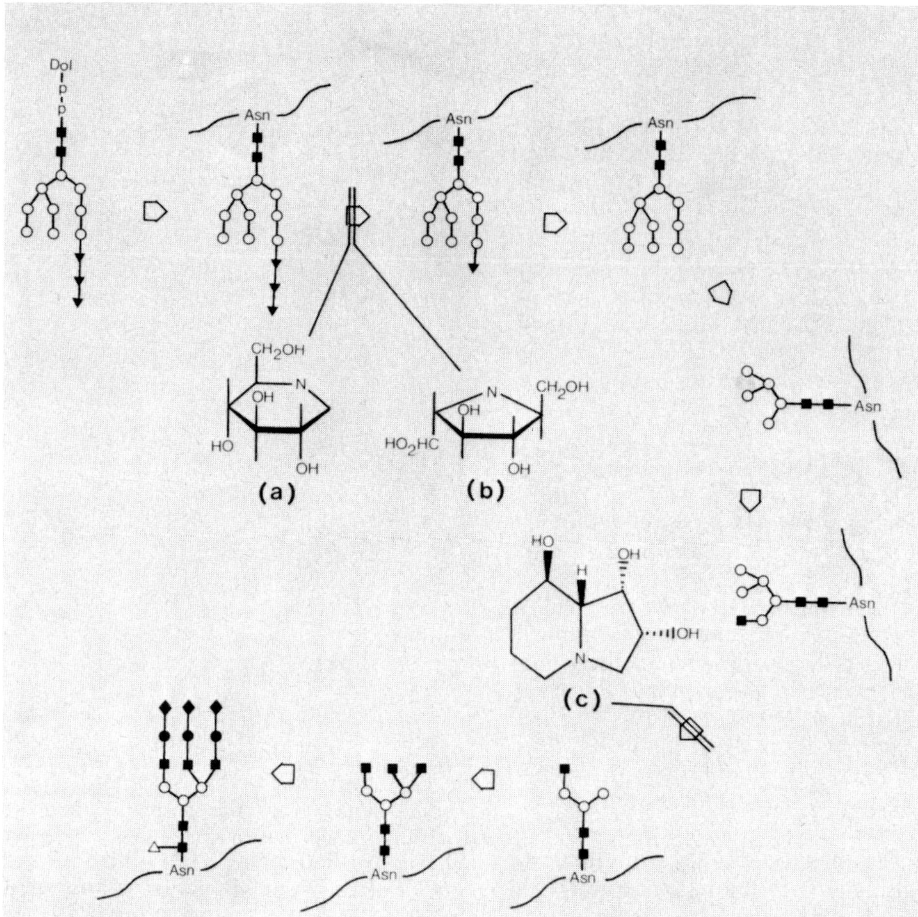

Fig. 2. Structures and the sites of action of the glycosylation inhibitors. ■ GlcNAc, ○ Man, ▲ Glc, ● Gal, ◆ NeuAc, △ Fuc; (a) 1-Deoxynojirimycin, (b) 2,5-Dihydroxymethyl-3,4-dihydroxypyrrolidine, (c) Swainsonine

useful in delineating the pathways of processing in addition to the functional role of carbohydrate side chains on a variety of proteins (see [17] for review). We have used three such inhibitors to study the processing of the *erb* B proteins. These are swainsonine, which inhibits the Golgi mannosidase II [21] leading to decreased expression of complex oligosaccharide chains on cell surface glycoproteins [5] and 1-deoxynojirimycin and 2,5-dihydroxymethyl-3,4-dihydroxypyrrolidine which are both inhibitors of glucosidase I and interfere with the release of the outermost glucose ([15]; Elbein and Fellows, in press). These sites of action are shown diagrammatically in Fig. 2. AEV-transformed cells were grown in the presence of predetermined amounts of the three inhibitors to give maximum inhibition of the processing enzymes [Schmidt et al., in press]. Interestingly, there was no effect of these inhibitors on the transformed phenotype of the AEV-transformed cells, either erythroblasts or fibroblasts, by any criteria tested. Since these inhibitors had no effect on transformation it was obviously necessary to show that they were having the expected effect in chicken cells. Accordingly AEV-transformed cells grown in the presence of three different inhibitors were labelled with

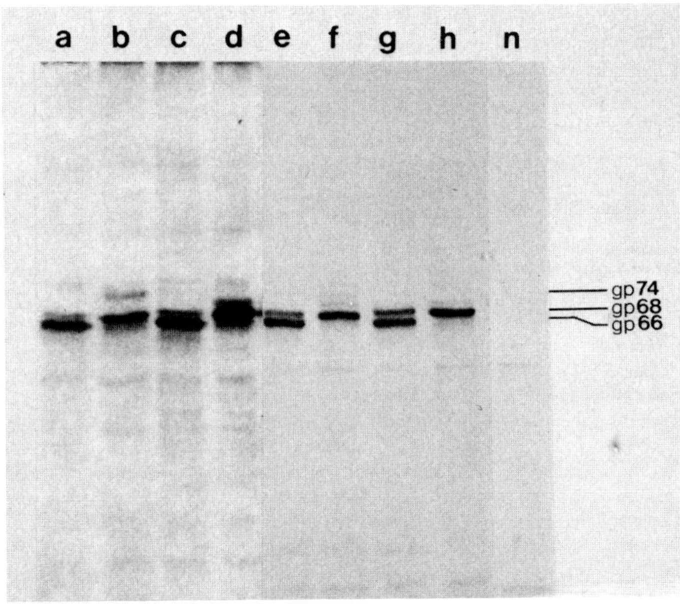

Fig. 3. Pulse-chase analysis of the synthesis of v-*erb* B in the presence or absence of glycoprotein processing inhibitors. Erythroblasts transformed with *ts* 34 AEV were pulse labelled with methionine ^{35}S for 1 h, samples taken (*lanes a, c, e, g*) and then chased in excess cold methionine for a further 4 h (*lanes b, d, f, h*). Glycoprotein processing inhibitors were added to a final concentration of either 10 μ*M* (swainsonine, *lanes c* and *d*) or 2 m*M* (1-deoxynojirimycin, *lanes g* and *h* and 2,5-dihydroxymethyl- 3,4- dihydroxypyrrolidine, *lanes e* and *f*) at least 2 h before addition of label and were present throughout the labelling period. Cell extracts were immunoprecipitated with *erb* B-specific serum and analysed by polyacrylamide gel electrophoresis. *Lanes a* and *b* are control AEV cells grown in the absence of any inhibitors, *lane n* is a control cell extract immunoprecipitated with normal rat serum

methionine ^{35}S and then chased to allow the processing to take place. Detergent extracts were prepared and immunoprecipitated with anti-*erb* B-specific serum [8]. Figure 3 shows the results of such an experiment. In control cells grown in the absence of inhibitors, methionine ^{35}S can be chased from gp66$^{erb\,B}$ through gp68 and into gp74 as shown previously (Fig. 3 lanes a and b). Similar pulse-chase analysis of v-*erb* B in cells grown in the presence of swainsonine contained a 70 000 molecular weight protein instead of gp74 (Fig. 3 lanes c and d) as would be predicted for a protein containing a "hybrid" oligosaccharide structure often formed on glycoproteins synthesized in the presence of swainsonine [12]. Cells grown in the presence of 2 m*M* 1-deoxynojirimycin or 2,5-dihydroxymethyl-3,4-dihydroxypyrrolidine had arrested the processing of *erb* B at the gp68 form (Fig. 3 lanes e–h); again this is the result predicted (see Fig. 2). Therefore the inhibitors are having their predicted effects on the processing of *erb* B, but this inhibition does not affect the ability of this protein to maintain the transformed phenotype.

Preliminary results indicate that these abnormally processed forms of *erb* B synthesized in the presence of the inhibitors are nevertheless transported to the plasma membrane (unpublished observations). These data, together with those on the *ts* mutants of AEV [1] would indicate that it is the expression of the *erb* B product in the plasma membrane that is crucial for it to exert its oncogenic effect. Given the recently described homology of this protein with EGF-R [4, 22] this result is perhaps not surprising since the plasma membrane is most likely the site of action of growth factor receptors. Having identified the compartment within the cell where *erb* B exerts its effect, further experiments will now be necessary to identify potential target molecules for this oncogenic protein.

Acknowledgments. We would like to thank Peter Dorling for providing purified swainsonine, Linda Fellows for 1-deoxynojirimycin and 2,5-dihydroxymethyl-3,4-dihydroxypyrrolidine, and Irene Esmond for typing the manuscript.

References

1. Beug H, Hayman MJ (1984) Temperature-sensitive mutants of avian erythroblastosis virus: surface expression of the *erb* B product correlates with transformation. Cell 36:963–972
2. Bister K, Duesberg PH (1979) Structure and specific sequences of avian erythroblastosis virus RNA; evidence for multiple classes of transforming genes among avian tumor virus. Proc Natl Acad Sci USA 76:5023–5027
3. Debuire B, Henry C, Benaissa M, Biserte G, Claverie JM, Saule S, Martin P, Stehelin D (1984) Sequencing the *erb* A gene of avian erythroblastosis virus reveals a new type of oncogene. Science 224:1456–1459
4. Downward J, Yarden Y, Mayes E, Scrace G, Totty N, Stockwell P, Ullrich A, Schlessinger J, Waterfield MD (1984) Close similarity of epidermal growth factor receptor and *v-erb* B oncogene protein sequences. Nature 307: 521–527
5. Elbein AD, Pan YT, Solf R, Vosbeck K (1983) Effect of swainsonine, an inhibitor of glycoprotein processing, on cultured mammalian cells. J Cell Physiol 115:265–275
6. Frykberg L, Palmieri S, Beug H, Graf T, Hayman MJ, Vennstrom B (1983) Transforming capacities of avian erythroblastosis virus mutants deleted in the *erb* A or *erb* B oncogenes. Cell 32:227–238
7. Fung YKT, Lewis WG, Kung HJ, Crittenden LB (1983) Activation of the cellular oncogene C-*erb* B by LTR insertion: molecular basis for induction of erythroblastosis by avian leukosis virus. Cell 33:357–368
8. Hayman MJ, Beug H (1984) Identification of a form of the avian erythroblastosis virus *erb*-B gene product at the cell surface. Nature 309:460–462
9. Hayman MJ, Ramsay G, Savin K, Kitchener G, Graf T, Beug H (1983) Identification and characterisation of the avian erythroblastosis virus *erb* B gene product as a membrane glycoprotein. Cell 32:579–588
10. Hayman MJ, Royer-Pokora B, Graf T (1979) Defectiveness of avian erythroblastosis virus: synthesis of a 75k *gag*-related protein. Virology 92:31–45
11. Hihara H, Yamamoto H, Shimohira H, Arai K, Shimizu T (1983) Avian erythroblastosis virus isolated from chicken erythroblastosis induced by lymphatic leukemia virus subgroup A. JNCI 70:891–898
12. Kang MS, Elbein AD (1983) Alterations in the structure of the oligosaccharide of vesicular stomatitis virus G protein by swainsonine. J Virol 46:60–69
13. Lai MMC, Hu SSF, Vogt PK (1979) Avian erythroblastosis virus: transformation-specific sequences form a contiguous segment of 3.25 kb located in the middle of the 6 kb genome. Virology 97:366–377
14. Privalsky ML, Sealy L, Bishop JM, McGrath JP, Levinson AD (1983) The product of the avian erythroblastosis virus *erb* B locus is a glycoprotein. Cell 32:1257–1267
15. Romero PA, Datema R, Schwartz RT (1983) N-methyl-1-deoxynojirimycin, a novel inhibitor of glycoprotein processing and its effect on fowl plague virus maturation. Virology 130:238–242
16. Roussel M, Saule S, Lagron C, Rommens C, Beug H, Graf T, Stehelin D (1979) Three new types of viral oncogene of cellular origin specific for haematopoietic cell transformation. Nature 281:452–455
17. Schwartz RT, Datema R (1984) Inhibitors of trimming: new tools in glycoprotein research. Trends Biol Sci 9:31–34
18. Sealy L, Privalsky ML, Moscovici G, Moscovici C, Bishop JM (1983) Site-specific mutagenesis of avian erythroblastosis virus: *erb* B is required for oncogenicity. Virology 130:155–178
19. Stehelin D, Saule S, Roussel M, Sergeant A, Lagrou C, Rommeno C, Raes MB (1980) Three new types of viral oncogenes in defective avian leukemia viruses. 1. specific nucleotide sequences of cellular origin correlate with specific transformation. Cold Spring Harbor Symp Quant Biol 44:1215–1223
20. Tarentino AL, Maley F (1974) Purification and properties of an endo-β-N-acetylglucosaminidase from Streptomyces griseus. J Biol Chem 249:811–817
21. Tulsiani DPR, Harris TM, Touster O (1982) Swainsonine inhibits the biosynthesis of complex glycoproteins by inhibition of golgi α-mannosidase II. J Biol Chem 257: 7936–7939

22. Ullrich A, Cousseno L, Hayflick JS, Dull TJ, Gray A, Tam AW, Lee J, Yarden Y, Libermann TA, Schlessinger J, Downward J, Mayes ELV, Whittle N, Waterfield MD, Seeburg PH (1984) Human epidermal growth factor receptor; cDNA sequence and aberrant expression of the amplified gene in A431 epidermoid carcinoma cells. Nature 309:418–425

23. Yamamoto T, Hihara H, Nishida T, Kawai S, Toyashima K (1983) A new avian erythroblastosis virus, AEV-H, carries *erb* B gene responsible for the induction of both erythroblastosis and sarcomas. Cell 34:225–232

Haematology and Blood Transfusion Vol. 29
Modern Trends in Human Leukemia VI
Edited by Neth, Gallo, Greaves, Janka

Characterization of Hematopoietic Cells Transformed In Vitro by AEV-H, a *v-erbB*-Containing Avian Erythroblastosis Virus

H. Beug[1], P. Kahn[1], G. Doederlein[1], M. J. Hayman[2], and T. Graf[1]

A. Introduction

Avian erythroblastosis virus ES4 (AEV-ES4) is a replication-defective avian leukemia virus that causes erythroleukemia and fibrosarcomas in chicks and transforms bone marrow cells and fibroblasts in vitro (for review, see [7]). The 5.5 kb genome of AEV-ES4 contains two oncogenes, *v-erbA* and *v-erbB* [1, 5, 21] which code for a *gag*-related cytoplasmic protein, $p75^{gag\text{-}erbA}$, and for an integral membrane glycoprotein, $gp74^{erbB}$, respectively [10–12, 18]. Studies using deletion mutants in either *v-erbA* or *v-erbB* indicate that *v-erbB* is sufficient to transform fibroblasts and erythroblasts, whereas *v-erbA* does not transform by itself but cooperates with *v-erbB* in erythroblasts to generate a more transformed phenotype [6, 7, 20].

Recently, another strain of avian erythroblastosis virus (AEV-H) was isolated [13] and shown to contain *v-erbB* as its only oncogene [23]. In vivo, this strain induced both erythroblastosis and sarcomas which were anatomically and histologically indistinguishable from the respective diseases induced by AEV-ES4 [13]; in vitro, it induced foci of transformed fibroblasts (Hihara et al., 1983). Here we show that AEV-H is also able to transform bone marrow cells in vitro using specific culture conditions. The transformed erythroblasts undergo self-renewal as well as spontaneous differentiation into erythrocytes and do not require exogenous erythropoietin for either process. They express an *erbB*-coded cell surface glycoprotein ($gp79^{erbB}$) which is 5 kilodaltons larger than $gp74^{erbB}$, the *erbB* gene product of AEV-ES4.

B. Materials and Methods

I. Viruses

Avian erythroblastosis virus strain H was obtained as a gift from Dr. Toyoshima, Tokyo. Its origin has been described elsewhere [13]. The origin of avian erythroblastosis virus strains AEV-ES4 and AEV193 has been described earlier [8, 12].

II. Cells and Cell Culture

Bone marrow cells from 3- to 14-day-old chicks were prepared, infected with virus, and seeded into Methocel under standard or CFU-E (Colony-Forming Unit Erythroid) conditions as described earlier [9, 19]. Colonies were isolated 6–8 days later with a drawn-out Pasteur pipette and expanded in either standard growth medium (AEV-ES4, 193 strains) or CFU-E medium (AEV-H strain). These media were prepared as described by Radke et al. [19].

III. Assays for Erythroid Differentiation Markers

The morphology and hemoglobin content of AEV-H-transformed erythroblasts were

1 European Molecular Biology Laboratory, Meyerhofstrasse 1, 6900 Heidelberg, FRG
2 Imperial Cancer Research Fund Laboratories, St. Bartholomews Hospital, Dominion House, London EC1A 7BE, UK

analyzed by staining cytospin preparations with neutral benzidine plus histological dyes as described earlier [4]. Alternatively, a more sensitive staining for hemoglobin content using acid benzidine was done according to Orkin et al. [17]. Detection of erythroid-specific cell surface antigens by indirect immunofluorescence using antisera to mature erythroid cells and to immature erythroblasts (anti-Ery and anti-Ebl; [3]) was carried out as described previously [4]. The possible presence of myeloid cells in the transformed cultures was assessed using the myeloid-specific monoclonal antibody MC51-2 [15].

IV. Percoll Fractionation of AEV-H Erythroblasts

Erythroblasts ($10-20 \times 10^6$) from a single clone (ID4) were loaded on a discontinous Percoll gradient (prepared as described by Beug and Hayman [2]; densities from top to bottom: 1.070, 1.072, 1.075 and 1.085 g/cm³) and centrifuged for 10 min at 2000 *g*. The least-dense cells (fraction I, 1.070) and the cells banding at 1.072 and 1.075 g/cm (fraction II) were retrieved, seeded in CFU-E medium containing either normal or anemic chicken serum, and analyzed by cytocentrifugation and staining as described above. Alternatively, cells from the least-dense fraction were seeded into plasma clot cultures, which were processed and stained 3–4 days later as described earlier [4].

V. Protein Analysis

Using methionine-free differentiation medium [2], $5-10 \times 10^6$ cells were labeled with 100–250 μCi ^{35}methionine for 2 h. They were then lysed and immunoprecipitated with anti-*erbB* serum according to published procedures and analyzed on sodium dodecyl sulfate polyacrylamide gels (SDS-PAGE) [10–12].

C. Results and Discussion

I. In Vitro Transformation of Bone Marrow Cells by AEV-H

Since AEV-H was negative in standard bone marrow transformation assays (T. Graf and H. Beug, unpublished observations) we tested whether bone marrow cells could be transformed under conditions (CFU-E-Methocel; Radke et al., 1982) which had been successfully employed to obtain erythroblasts transformed by AEV-ES4 mutants that carry a deletion in the *erbA* gene (AEV-A$^-$B$^+$; [6]). Bone marrow cells were infected with AEV-H and, in controls, with two other AEV strains (AEV-ES4 and AEV193, both containing *erbA* and *erbB* oncogenes). The infected cells were then seeded into Methocel under both standard [9] and CFU-E conditions. Numerous colonies were obtained from AEV-H-infected bone marrow in CFU-E Methocel, whereas no transformed colonies were seen with this virus under standard conditions. In contrast, the two other AEV strains tested yielded comparable numbers of colonies under standard and CFU-E conditions.

Several of the AEV-H-induced colonies were isolated and then cultivated in CFU-E medium. Most clones grew in this medium for 20–35 generations, exhibiting doubling times of 24 h or less. When transferred to standard growth medium, however, the AEV-H cells ceased proliferating, developed large vacuoles, and disintegrated within 4–7 days. In contrast, AEV-ES4- and AEV193-derived clones exhibited similar growth rates and life spans in standard and CFU-E media.

II. AEV-H-Transformed Cells Consist of Erythroid Precursors at Different Stages of Maturation

To determine the lineage and degree of maturation of bone marrow cells transformed in vitro by AEV-H, the AEV-H clones were analyzed for a set of erythroid differentiation markers [3, 4] as well as for the myeloid-cell-specific antigen 51-2 [15]. Table 1 and Fig. 1 show that all AEV-H clones tested consisted entirely of erythroid cells, representing a mixture of immature erythroblasts and more mature reticulocytes and erythrocytes. In contrast, AEV-ES4- and AEV193-transformed clones consisted exclusively of immature erythroblasts.

Table 1. Characterization of erythroblast clones transformed by AEV-H

AEV-H clone No.	Hemoglobin-positive cells (%)[a]	Cells classified as LR+E (%)[b]	Cells stained with		
			α Erb (%)[c]	α Erb (%)	α Mbl (%)
I B 4	78	11	40 (10)[d]	80	ND[f]
I B 6	27	0.9	10 (3)	>95	<0.1
I C 1	100	68	[e]	[e]	ND
I C 2	71	10	55 (30)	50	ND
I C 6	63	3.2	40 (10)	80	<0.1
I D 1	95	46	[e]	[e]	ND
I D 4	89	17	80 (60)	40	ND

[a] Determined by staining with acid benzidine (Beug et al. 1982)

[b] Cell types were defined by neutral benzine plus histological staining (Beug et al. 1982). LR, late reticulocytes; E, erythrocytes

[c] The characterization of these antisera has been described elsewhere (Beug et al. 1979; Kornfeld et al. 1983). α Erb, anti-erythroblast serum; α Ery, anti-erythrocyte; α Mbl, anti-myeloblast monoclone MC 51/2

[d] Figures in parenthesis; cells strongly stained in a ring-like fashion (Beug et al. 1979)

[e] These clones differentiated into erythrocytes before sufficient cell numbers for fluorescent staining were built up

[f] ND: not determined

The data in Table 1 also indicate that the AEV-H clones tested varied with respect to the proportion of mature cells. Furthermore, an inverse relationship was seen between the frequency of mature cells in a particular clone and its growth rate. A few clones could not be propagated more than 7–10 days after isolation because all cells differentiated into erythrocytes.

III. AEV-H Erythroblasts Proliferate and Differentiate in an Erythropoietin-Independent Fashion

To study how the heterogeneity of cells within single erythroblast clones was generated and maintained during culture, cells from a clone (ID4) containing about 20% mature cells were fractionated according to density using a discontinuous Percoll gradient [2]. The individual fractions were then seeded in CFU-E medium in the absence or presence of anemic chicken serum as a source of erythropoietin [4] and aliquots analyzed for their stage of differentiation during the following few days. As illustrated in Fig. 2A, four fractions were obtained from the Percoll gradient; the top fraction (I) and the pooled intermediate-density fractions (II) were analyzed further. Fraction I contained exclusively immature erythroblasts that grew rapidly and regenerated the initial proportion of mature cells within 3 days, regardless of whether or not erythropoietin was present (Fig. 2B and data not shown). In contrast, fraction II, which contained partially mature, hemoglobinized cells ceased proliferating after 2 days, at which time essentially all cells exhibited an erythrocyte-like phenotype. The most dense fraction consisted of erythrocyte-like cells with no in vitro proliferative capacity.

Similar results were obtained by seeding cells from the above Percoll-density fractions into plasma clot cultures [4]. Whereas the immature cells from fraction I frequently grew into large colonies consisting of either immature or a mixture of immature and mature erythroid cells, CFU-E-like erythrocyte colonies and single erythrocytes were formed exclusively by the cells from fraction II. Similar numbers

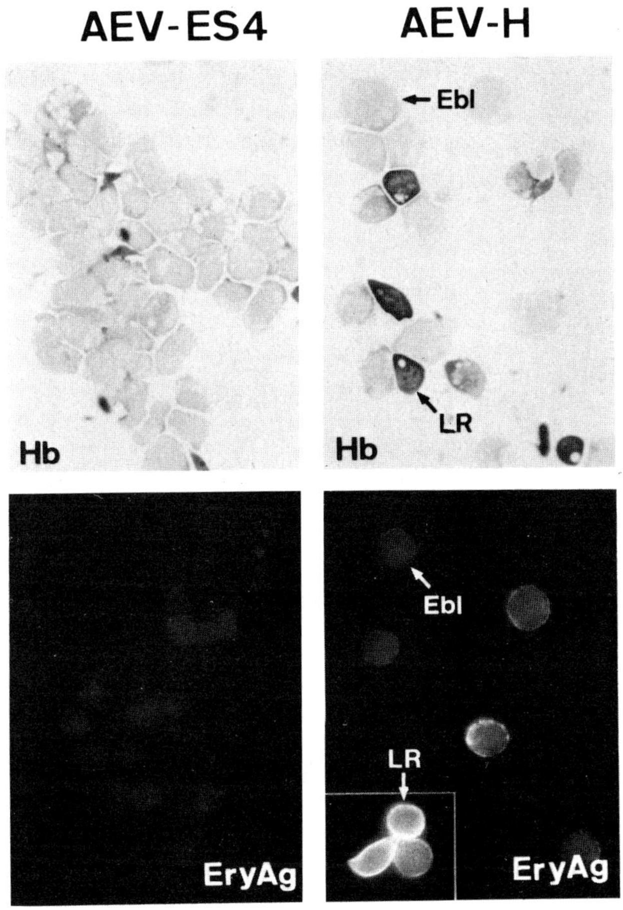

Fig. 1. Characterization of AEV-H-transformed erythroblasts. Cells from an AEV-H-transformed erythroblast clone (ID4) and from a culture of AEV-ES4-transformed erythroblasts were cytocentrifuged onto slides and stained with neutral benzidine (*Hb*). Live cells from the same preparations were also stained with anti-erythrocyte serum by indirect immunoflouorescence (*ErgAg*) (Beug et al., 1979). *Ebl,* cells classified as erythroblasts; *LR,* cells classified as late reticulocytes. (Beug et al., 1982)

and proportions of these colonies were obtained in the absence and presence of erythropoietin (data not shown). These results suggest that AEV-H-transformed erythroblasts can either self-renew or become committed to terminal differentiation with a frequency characteristic for the particular clone. In contrast to normal erythroid progenitors, AEV-H erythroblasts carry out both these functions in the absence of exogenous erythropoietin.

IV. In Vitro Transformed AEV-H Erythroblasts Express High Levels of an *erbB*-Coded Cell Surface Glycoprotein

To study expression of *erbB*-related proteins by AEV-H erythroblasts, cells were labeled with [^{35}S]methionine and immunoprecipitated with *erbB*-specific sera. Figure 3 shows that proteins of 72 and 74 kilodaltons were immunoprecipitated from AEV-H cell lysates. Thus, the AEV-H *erbB* gene products are approximately 5 kilodaltons larger than *erbB* gene products of AEV-ES4 but only slightly larger than the respective proteins expressed by AEV193 [12]. As expected, no *erbA*-related proteins could be immunoprecipitated from AEV-H cells [23].

The *erbB* protein produced by AEV-H erythroblasts is expressed at the cell surface, since live cells were strongly stained by *erbB*-specific sera by indirect immunofluorescence (Fig. 4; [12]). Interestingly, most if not all mature cells (as classified by staining with antierythrocyte

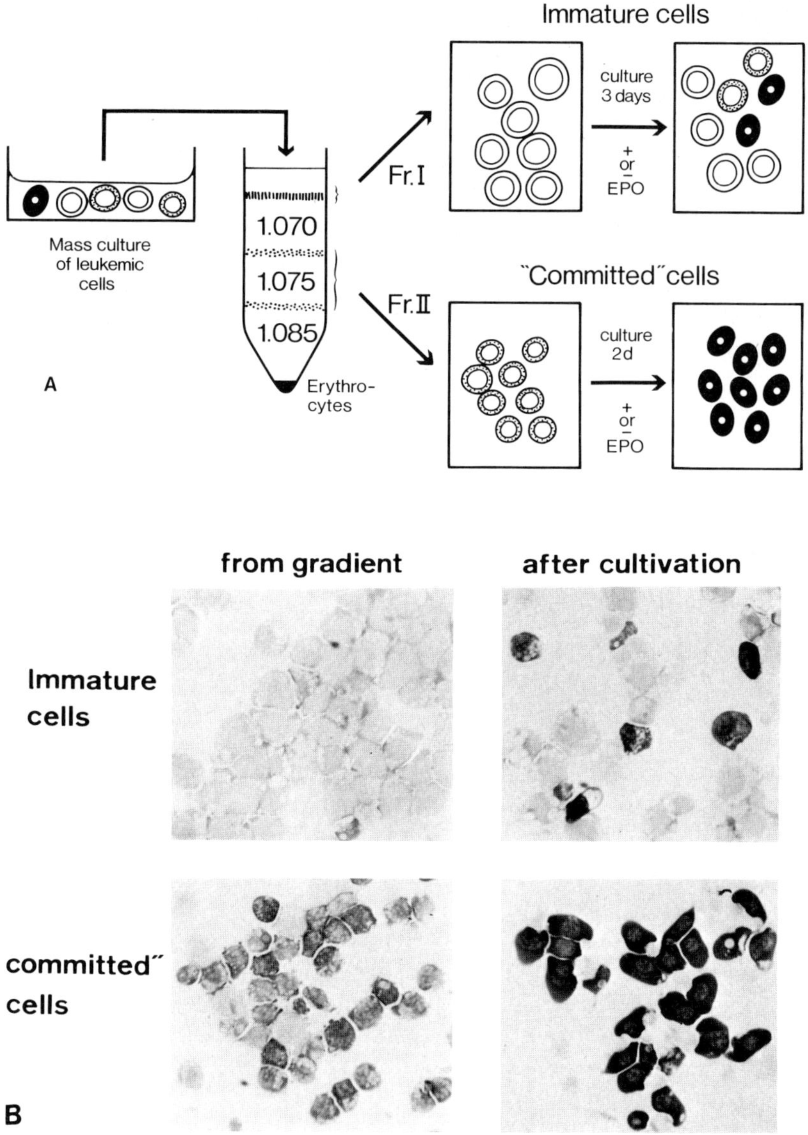

Fig. 2 A, B. Self-renewal and differentiation capacity of AEV-H erythroblasts fractionated according to density. **A** Schematic diagram showing Percoll fractionation of AEV-H-transformed erythroblasts and phenotypes of cells retrieved from the gradient before and after cultivation in the presence and absence of anemic chicken serum (*EPO*); **B** Cytospin preparations from the cell populations described in **A** were stained with neutral benzidine and then photographed

serum) were negative or only weakly positive with anti-*erbB* serum. This suggests a down-regulation of *erbB* protein expression during erythroid differentiation, as also seen in differentiating tsAEV erythroblasts [2].

V. What is the Role of *v-erbA* in Erythroid Transformation?

The results presented above clearly demonstrate that erythroblasts transformed by the *v-erbB* gene of AEV-H both self-renew and differentiate into erythrocytes, whereas erythroblasts transformed by two viruses that contain *v-erbA* in addition to *v-erbB* are restricted to the self-renewal pathway (Fig. 5). At the same time, *v-erbB*-transformed cells require specific growth conditions (including pH and ionic strength optima) similar to those required by normal erythroid progenitors, whereas erythroblasts transformed by both *v-erbB* and *v-erbA* grow in standard growth media. This suggests that *v-erbA* enhances the effect of *v-erbB* by abolishing two characteristics of normal erythroid precursors expressed by AEV-H erythroblasts, i.e., spontaneous differentiation into erythrocytes and specific growth requirements.

VI. The Phenotype of AEV-H Erythroblasts is Common Among Erythroid Cells Transformed by Other Avian Retroviruses

Recently, several avian retroviruses containing oncogenes other than *v-erbB* have been found to transform erythroid bone

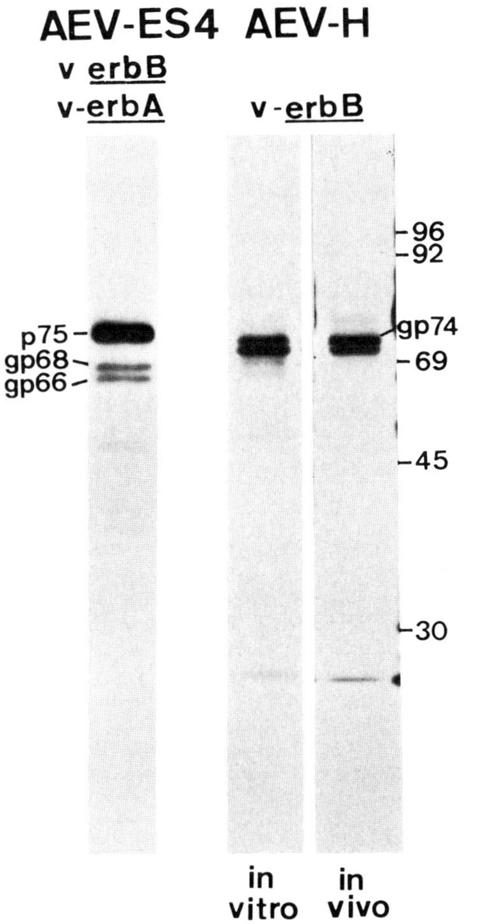

Fig. 3. Expression of *v-erbB*-encoded proteins in AEV-H-transformed erythroblasts; AEV-H erythroblasts (clone IB6, in vitro), erythroblasts grown from the blood of a leukemic chicken infected with AEV-H virus (Kahn et al., 1984; in vivo), and AEV-ES4 erythroblasts (as controls) were labeled with [^{35}S]methionine. Cell extracts were immunoprecipitated with anti-*erbA* + *B* serum followed by gel electrophoresis and autoradiography as described earlier (Hayman et al., 1979, 1983). *Gp66/68*, gp66/68^{erbB} from AEV-ES4; *p75*, p75$^{gag\text{-}erbA}$; *gp74*, gp72/74^{erbB} from AEV-H

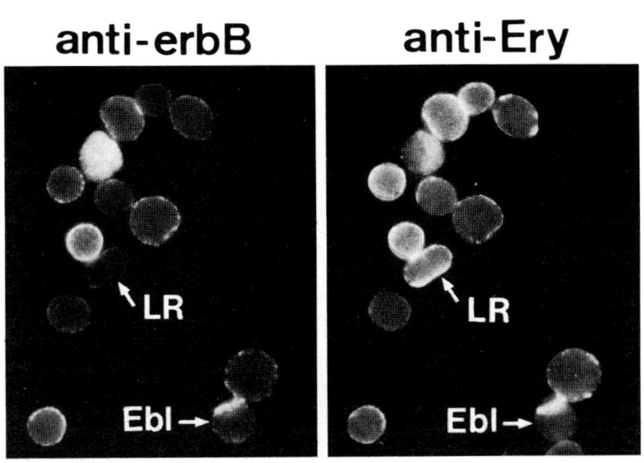

Fig. 4. AEV-H erythroblasts express *v-erbB* protein at the cell surface. AEV-H erythroblasts (clone ID4) were double stained by indirect immunofluorescence with anti-*erbB* serum (anti-*erbB*) and anti-erythroblast serum (anti-*Ery*) as described earlier (Beug and Hayman, 1984). Note absence of *erbB* fluorescence in some late reticulocytes (*LR*)

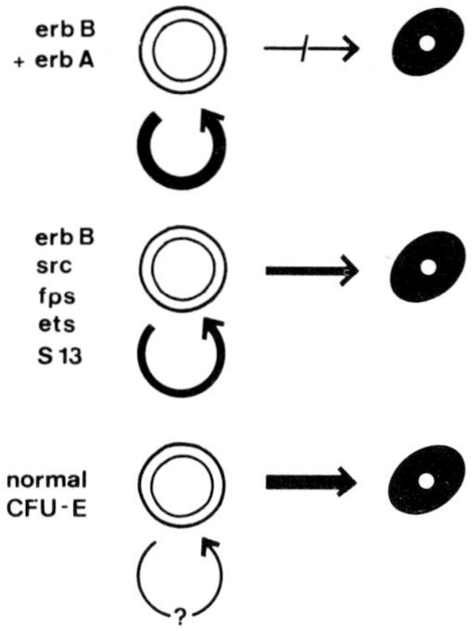

Fig. 5. Transformation phenotypes of erythroid cells containing various retroviral oncogenes. The diagram illustrates how different retroviral oncogenes modulate the self-renewal capacity (*circular arrows*) and the probability of undergoing terminal differentiation into erythrocytes (*straight arrows*). *Thick arrows* indicate high probability; *thin arrows* indicate low probability. *The bar across the straight arrow in the upper diagram* (*erbB + erbA*) indicates that these two oncogenes together completely arrest differentiation

marrow cells. Using growth conditions similar to those required by AEV-H erythroblasts, the *myb,ets*-oncogene-containing E26 virus [16, 19], the *src*-containing RSV (Rous sarcoma virus), the *fps*-containing FSV (Fujinami sarcoma virus) [14], and the S13 erythroblastosis virus (H. Beug et al., submitted for publication) were shown to induce transformed erythroblasts that closely resembled AEV-H erythroblasts (Table 1, Fig. 5). All these oncogenes cause two types of transformation-specific changes in the infected erythroid progenitors: they induce in them the ability to self-renew and render them independent of the erythroid differentiation hormone erythropoietin with respect to in vitro survival, self-renewal, and differentiation. It will be interesting to determine whether *v-erbA* can cooperate with these oncogenes in a similar manner as with *v-erb*B.

References

1. Anderson SM, Hayward WS, Neel BG, Hanafusa H (1980) Avian erythroblastosis virus produces two mRNAs. J Virol 36:676–683
2. Beug H, Hayman MJ (1984) Temperature-sensitive mutants of avian erythroblastosis virus: surface expression of the *erbB* product correlates with transformation. Cell 36:963–972
3. Beug H, von Kirchbach A, Doederlein G, Conscience J-F, Graf T (1979) Chicken hematopoietic cells transformed by seven strains of defective avian leukemia viruses display three distinct phenotypes of differentiation. Cell 18:375–390
4. Beug H, Palmieri S, Freudenstein C, Zentgraf H, Graf T (1982) Hormone-dependent terminal differentiation in vitro of chicken erythroleukemia cells transformed by *ts* mutants of avian erythroblastosis virus. Cell 28:907–919
5. Coffin JM, Varmus HE, Bishop JM, Essex M, Hardy WD Jr, Martin GS, Rosenberg NE, Scolnick EM, Weinberg RA, Vogt PK (1981) A proposal for naming host cell-derived inserts in retrovirus genome. J Virol 40:953–957
6. Frykberg L, Palmieri S, Beug H, Graf T, Hayman MJ, Vennström B (1983) Transforming capacities of avian erythroblastosis virus mutants deleted in the *erbA* or *erbB* oncogenes. Cell 32:227–238
7. Graf T, Beug H (1983) Role of the v-*erbA* and v-*erbB* oncogenes of avian erythroblastosis virus in erythroid cell transformation. Cell 34:7–9
8. Graf T, Royer-Pokora B, Schubert GE, Beug H (1976) Evidence for the multiple oncogenic potential of cloned leukemia virus: in vitro and in vivo studies with avian erythroblastosis virus. Virology 71:423–433
9. Graf T, von Kirchbach A, Beug H (1981) Characterization of the hematopoietic target cells of AEV, MC29 and AMV avian leukemia viruses. Exp Cell Res 131:331–343
10. Hayman MJ, Beug H (1984) Identification of a form of the avian erythroblastosis virus *erbB* gene product at the cell surface. Nature 309:460–462
11. Hayman MJ, Royer-Pokora B, Graf T (1979) Defectiveness of avian erythroblastosis virus: synthesis of a 75k *gag*-related protein. Virology 92:31–45
12. Hayman MJ, Ramsay GM, Savin K, Kitchener G, Graf T, Beug H (1983) Identification and characterization of the avian erythroblastosis virus *erbB* gene product as a membrane glycoprotein. Cell 32:579–588

13. Hihara H, Yamamoto H, Shimohira H, Arai K, Shimizu T (1983) Avian erythroblastosis virus isolated from chick erythroblastosis induced by lymphatic leukemia virus subgroup A. JNCI 70:891–897
14. Kahn P, Adkins B, Beug H, Graf T (1984) *Src*- and *fps*-containing avian sarcoma viruses transform chicken erythroid cells. Proc Natl Acad Sci USA 81:7122–7126
15. Kornfeld S, Beug H, Doederlein G, Graf T (1983) Detection of avian hematopoietic cell surface antigens with monoclonal antibodies to myeloid cells. Exp Cell Res 143:383–394
16. Leprince D, Gegonne A, Coll J, deTaisne C, Schneeberger A, Lagrou C, Stehelin D (1983) A putative second cell-derived oncogene of the avian leukaemia retrovirus E26. Nature 306:391–395
17. Orkin SH, Harosi FI, Leder P (1975) Differentiation in erythroleukemic cells and their somatic hybrids. Proc Natl Acad Sci USA 72: 98–102
18. Privalsky ML, Sealy L, Bishop JM, McGrath JP, Levinson AD (1983) The product of the avian erythroblastosis virus *erbB* locus is a glycoprotein. Cell 32:1257–1267
19. Radke K, Beug H, Kornfeld S, Graf T (1982) Transformation of both erythroid and myeloid cells by E26, an avian leukemia virus that contains the *myb* gene. Cell 31:643–653
20. Sealy L, Moscovici G, Moscovici C, Bishop JM (1983) Site-specific mutagenesis of avian erythroblastosis virus: v-erbA is not required for transformation of fibroblasts. Virology 130:179–194
21. Sheiness D, Vennström B, Bishop JM (1981) Virus-specific RNAs in cells infected by avian myelocytomatosis virus and avian erythroblastosis virus: modes of oncogene expression. Cell 23:291–300
22. Vennström B, Fanshier S, Moscovici C, Bishop JM (1980) Molecular cloning of the avian erythroblastosis virus genome and recovery of oncogenic virus by transfection of chicken cells. J Virol 36:575–585
23. Yamamoto T, Hihara T, Nishida T, Kawai S, Toyoshima K (1983) A new avian erythroblastosis virus, AEV-H, carries *erbB* gene responsible for the induction of both erythroblastosis and sarcomas. Cell 34:225–232

Haematology and Blood Transfusion Vol. 29
Modern Trends in Human Leukemia VI
Edited by Neth, Gallo, Greaves, Janka

Different Cellular Substrates of Abelson Leukemia Virus Transforming Protein Kinase in Murine Fibroblasts and Lymphocytes

D. Saggioro [1], M. F. Di Renzo [2], P. M. Comoglio [2], and L. Chieco-Bianchi [1, 3]

A. Introduction

Abelson murine leukemia virus (A-MuLV) is a replication-defective retrovirus capable of rapidly inducing leukemia in mice as well as of transforming in vitro mouse bone marrow cells and fibroblasts [1, 2, 14]; the A-MuLV was derived by passage in vivo of the replication-competent Moloney leukemia virus (M-MuLV) and its genome codes for a single polypeptide which is a hybrid molecule containing a portion of the parental M-MuLV genome (*gag* gene) and a portion of the cellular gene termed *abl* [18]. This protein, which varies in size from 160 to 90 kilodaltons, depending on the specific A-MuLV strain, is associated mainly with the detergent-insoluble cell fraction and possesses a tyrosine kinase activity [4, 15, 19]. In this regard, the A-MuLV protein resembles the pp60*src* encoded by the Rous sarcoma virus (RSV) [10] and the protein kinases encoded by other retroviruses such as the feline sarcoma virus (FeSV) [3, 17] and the Fujinami sarcoma virus (FuSV) [9]. The fact that the RSV pp60*src* is linked with specialized cellular areas such as cell–cell junctions and adhesion plaques has suggested that the alteration of these structures is involved in the origin of the transformed phenotype [12, 13] (Marchisio et al., Exp. Cell Res., in press). However, it has also been demonstrated that, in the same cell type, different cellular substrates are phosphorylated at tyrosine residues by diverse protein kinases (Di Renzo et al., submitted). Accordingly, we found it of interest to study the cellular substrates of the A-MuLV protein kinase in cells having different cytoskeletal architecture and adhesion properties such as fibroblasts and lymphocytes.

B. Materials and Methods

I. Cell Lines

TA-3 and TA-4, non-B lymphoma cell lines were established from two independent thymic lymphomas induced by inoculating intrathymically (i.t.) newborn BALB/c mice with the complex A-MuLV(M-MuLV). MZ-5, a pre-B lymphoma cell line, was established from a splenic lymphoma induced by inoculating the complex A-MuLV(M-MuLV) subcutaneously (s.c.) in newborn BALB/c mice. ABC-1, a A-MuLV-transformed line of pre-B cells, was kindly provided by Dr. Natalie Teich [16]. ANN-1 is an A-MuLV-transformed line of fibroblasts [14]. As control, a T cell lymphoma line (TB-5) induced by M-MuLV in BALB/c mice was also included in this study.

Lymphoma cell lines were cultured in complete medium consisting of Dulbecco-MEM (Gibco Europe, Glasgow, Scotland) supplemented with L-glutamine, HEPES, 2-mercaptoethanol, antibiotics, and 10%

1 Cattedra di Oncologia, Università di Padova, via Gattamelata 64, 35128 Padova, Italy
2 Istituto di Istologia ed Embriologia Generale, Università di Torino, Corso M. D'Azeglio, 10126 Torino, Italy
3 Henry Kaplan Award for the best poster Virological Session

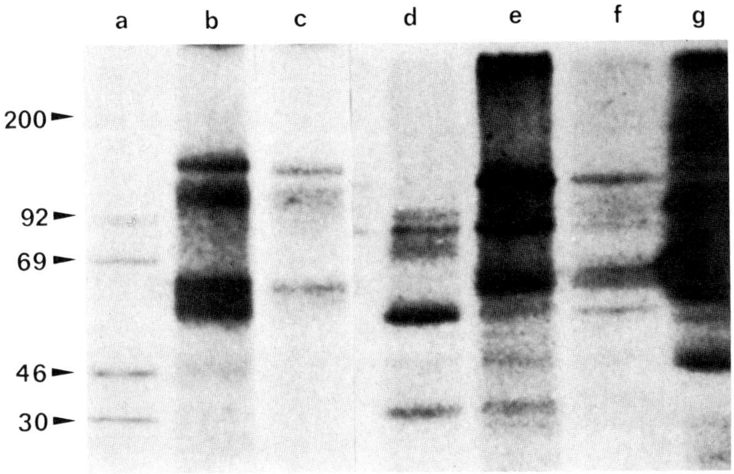

Fig. 1. Immunoprecipitation by anti-phosphotyrosine (anti-P-Tyr) antibodies of ^{32}P-labeled detergent-insoluble proteins from A-MuLV-transformed lymphocytes and fibroblasts. *Lane a* molecular weight markers; *lanes b* and *f* pre-B lymphoma cells MZ-5 and ABC-1; *lanes c* and *e* non-B lymphoma cells TA-4 and TA-3; *lane d* TB-5, M-MuLV-transformed T-cells; *lane g* ANN-1 fibroblasts

heat-inactivated fetal calf serum (FCS Gibco). ANN-1 fibroblasts were cultured in Dulbecco-MEM plus 10% FCS.

II. Specific Antisera

Antibodies against phosphotyrosine residues (anti-P-Tyr antibodies) were produced as previously described [6]. Anti-M-MuLV serum (Lot No. 71S/161) was obtained from the Office of Program Resources and Logistics, NCI, Bethesda, Maryland.

III. Immunoprecipitation Assay

Detergent-insoluble fractions were labeled according to Burr [5] by incubating detergent-insoluble proteins with ^{32}P-labeled γ-ATP (specific activity 5000 mCi/m*M*, Amersham) in conditions allowing phosphorylation catalyzed by the kinase coded by A-MuLV [4, 5]. After phosphorylation, the proteins were immunoprecipitated either by anti-P-Tyr antibodies or by anti-M-MuLV serum, as previously described [6]. After elution from protein A-Sepharose with Laemmli buffer [11], proteins were separated by SDS-PAGE. Dried gels were exposed to Kodak X-Omat film and processed for autoradiography.

C. Results and Discussion

The natural targets for in vivo transformation by A-MuLV are pre-B lymphocytes [1, 2]; however, the A-MuLV, if inoculated i.t., is also able to induce thymic lymphomas [7]. Thus, in addition to ABC-1 cells we also studied some lines derived from A-MuLV-induced thymic lymphomas; these cells do not express either T cell or B cell markers, even after stimulation with Con-A or LPS, respectively, and accordingly were putatively defined as non-B cells.

In order to investigate whether a specific substrate for A-MuLV kinase could be detected in different A-MuLV transformed cell types, the detergent-insoluble cellular fraction was studied with the aid of monospecific antibodies directed against the phosphorylated form of protein tyrosine residues (anti-P-Tyr antibodies).

As shown in Fig. 1, two main proteins of 70 and 120 kilodaltons were precipitated from ANN-1 fibroblasts (Fig. 1, lane *g*),

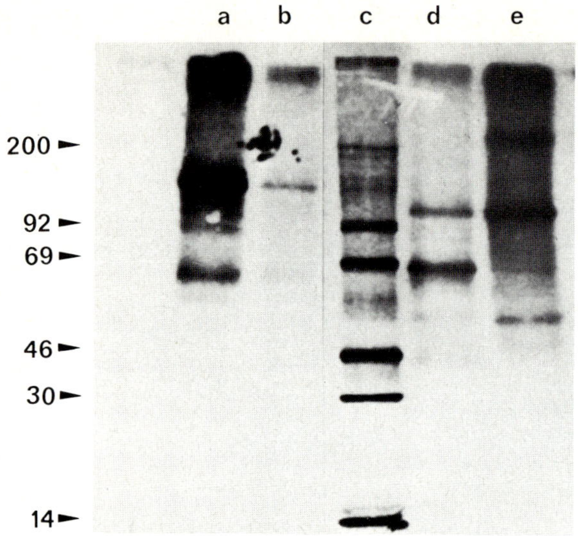

Fig. 2. Immunoprecipitation of phosphotyrosine proteins by anti M-MuLV serum and anti P-Tyr antibodies in TA-3 lymphoma cells and ANN-1 fibroblasts. *Lane c* molecular weight markers; *lanes a* and *b* detergent-insoluble fraction from TA-3 lymphoma cells immunoprecipitated by anti P-Tyr antibodies and anti M-MuLV serum, respectively; *lanes d* and *e* detergent-insoluble fraction from ANN-1 fibroblasts immunoprecipitated by anti-P-Tyr antibodies and anti-M-MuLV serum, respectively

whereas three different tyrosine phosphorylated proteins of 150, 100, and 65 kilodaltons were immunoprecipitated from pre-B and non-B lymphoma cells (Fig. 1, lanes *b, c, e, f*). No phosphorylated proteins were detected in nontransformed fibroblasts and normal thymus cells (data not shown in Fig. 1). On the contrary, in the TB-5 M-MuLV lymphoma cells, two proteins of 55 and 30 kilodaltons and an additional one of 100 kilodaltons, comigrating with the corresponding protein of A-MuLV lymphoma cells, were detected (Fig. 1, lane *d*). Moreover, in a preliminary experiment, using the anti-M-MuLV serum, which is able to recognize the *gag*-coded portion of the kinase protein, we observed only one immunoprecipitate band of 120 kilodaltons in ANN-1 fibroblasts (Fig. 2, lane *e*) and of 150 kilodaltons in lymphoma cells (Fig. 2, lane *b*). The anti-M-MuLV serum was not able to precipitate either the 70 kilodaltons phosphoprotein in fibroblasts (Fig. 2, lane *d*) or the 100 and 65 kilodaltons phosphoproteins in lymphoma cells (Fig. 2, lane *b*), suggesting that these latter are probably cellular substrates and not degradation products of the A-MuLV tyrosine itself.

These data seem to indicate that A-MuLV protein kinase, under identical experimental conditions, is able to phosphorylate at tyrosine residues different substrates in cells possessing diverse cytoskeletal architecture. It is known that A-MuLV-coded protein kinase, like other transforming protein kinases, does not discriminate for substrate phosphorylation [8, 18]; consequently, the different pattern of phosphorylation induced by A-MuLV protein kinase in fibroblasts and lymphocytes is probably imputable to a different association of the tyrosine kinase with the cytoskeletal macromolecules.

Acknowledgments. This work was supported by the Consiglio Nazionale delle Ricerche, Progetto Finalizzato Oncologia, and Associazione Italiana per la Ricerca sul Cancro. D.S. is a recipient of a Fondazione Assicurazioni Generali training grant.

References

1. Abelson HT, Rabstein LS (1970) Lymphosarcoma: virus-induced thymic-independent disease in mice. Cancer Res 30:2213–2222
2. Baltimore D, Rosemberg N, Witte ON (1979) Transformation of immature lymphoid cells by Abelson murine leukemia virus. Immunol Rev 48:1–22
3. Barbacid M, Beemon K, Devare SG (1980) Origin and functional properties of the major gene product of the Snyder-Theilen strain of feline sarcoma virus. Proc Natl Acad Sci USA 77:5158–5162

4. Boss MA, Dreyfuss G, Baltimore D (1981) Localization of the Abelson murine leukemia virus protein in a detergent-insoluble subcellular matrix: architecture of the protein. J Virol 40:472–481
5. Burr JG, Dreyfuss G, Penman S, Buchanan JM (1981) Association of the src gene product of Rous sarcoma virus with cytoskeletal structures of chicken embryo fibroblasts. Proc Natl Acad Sci USA 77:3484–3488
6. Comoglio PM, DiRenzo MF, Tarone G, Giancotti FG, Naldini L, Marchisio PC (1984) Detection of phosphotyrosine-containing proteins in the detergent-insoluble fraction of RSV-transformed fibroblasts by azobenzene phosphonate antibodies. EMBO J 3:483–489
7. Cook WD (1982) Rapid thymomas induced by Abelson murine leukemia virus. Proc Natl Acad Sci USA 79:2917–2921
8. Erikson RL, Collett MS, Erikson E, Purchio AF (1979) Evidence that the avian sarcoma virus transforming gene product is a cyclic AMP-independent protein kinase. Proc Natl Acad Sci USA 76:6260–6264
9. Feldman RA, Wang E, Hanafusa H (1983) Cytoplasmic localization of the transforming protein of Fujinami sarcoma virus: salt-sensitive association with subcellular components. J Virol 45:782–791
10. Hunter T, Sefton BM (1980) Transforming gene product of Rous sarcoma virus phosphorylates tyrosine. Proc Natl Acad Sci USA 77:1311–1315
11. Laemmli UK (1970) Cleavage of structural proteins during the assembly of the head of bacteriophage T_4. Nature 277:680–685
12. Rohrschneider LR (1979) Immunofluorescence on avian sarcoma virus transformed cells: localization of the src gene product. Cell 16:11–14
13. Rohrschneider LR (1980) Adhesion plaques of Rous sarcoma virus-transformed cells contain the src gene product. Proc Natl Acad Sci USA 77:3514–3518
14. Scher CD, Siegler R (1975) Direct transformation of 3T3 cells by Abelson murine leukaemia virus. Nature 253:729–731
15. Sefton BM, Hunter T, Raschke WC (1981) Evidence that the Abelson virus protein functions in vivo as a protein kinase that phosphorylates tyrosine. Proc Natl Acad Sci USA 78:1552–1556
16. Teich N, Boss M, Dexter TM (1979) Infection of mouse bone marrow cells with Abelson murine leukemia virus and establishment of producer cells. In: Neth R, Gallo RC, Hofscheider PM, Mannweiler K (eds) Modern trends in human leukemia III. Springer, Heidelberg, pp 487–490
17. Van de Ven WJM, Reynolds FH, Stephenson JR (1980) The nonstructural components of polyproteins encoded by replication-defective mammalian transforming retroviruses are phosphorylated and have associated protein kinase activity. Virology 101:185–197
18. Wang JYJ, Queen C, Baltimore D (1982) Expression of an Abelson murine leukemia virus-encoded protein in *Escherichia coli* causes extensive phosphorylation of tyrosine residues. J Biol Chem 257:13 181–13 184
19. Witte ON, Rosemberg N, Paskind M, Shields A, Baltimore D (1978) Identification of an Abelson murine leukemia virus-encoded protein present in transformed fibroblasts and lymphoid cells. Proc Natl Acad Sci USA 75:2488–2492

Haematology and Blood Transfusion Vol. 29
Modern Trends in Human Leukemia VI
Edited by Neth, Gallo, Greaves, Janka

Regulin, a Cytoskeleton-Associated Protein Affecting Phosphorylation–Dephosphorylation *

G. Kramer, E. Wollny, S. Fullilove, J. Tipper, W. Kudlicki, and B. Hardesty

Translational regulation at the molecular level has been studied intensively with components from mammalian reticulocytes. Since the discovery of translational control by phosphorylation–dephosphorylation of initiation factor eIF-2 [1–3] and possibly 40 *S* ribosomal subunits [4–7], relevant protein kinases and recently counteracting phosphatases have become targets of research. The extent of phosphorylation of a given protein depends on a dynamic equilibrium between the activities of the protein kinase and phosphatase. This equilibrium reaction is schematically depicted for eIF-2 in Fig. 1.

Potentially, the equilibrium can be shifted by activation or inhibition of either the kinase or the phosphatase. Regulation of the protein kinases and phosphatases involved in translational control is poorly understood. It appears that both types of enzyme occur in latent forms in vivo. The mechanisms of activation of the heme-regulated eIF-2α kinase in reticulocytes or of the double-stranded RNA-dependent eIF-2α kinase in interferon-sensitive cells are still unclear. Almost nothing is known about the inactive form and occurrence of protein phosphatases in intact cells. In vitro, phosphatases generally can be activated by high, nonphysiologic concentrations of Mn^{2+} [8–12], by protease treatment [13, 14], or by denaturing agents [15].

* Clayton Foundation Biochemical Institute, Department of Chemistry, The University of Texas at Austin, Austin, Texas 78712, USA

We have partially purified and characterized a 76 000 daltons phosphatase from reticulocytes that counteracted the heme-controlled eIF-2α kinase [11], and recently isolated to homogeneity a 56 000 daltons, Mn^{2+}-dependent phosphatase that is most active with phosphorylated 40 *S* ribosomal subunits [12]. Using monoclonal antibodies, we have identified a 230 000 daltons, protease-sensitive protein, which we have named regulin, that stimulates the activity of this phosphatase [16]. Figure 2 shows that regulin extracted from the membrane fraction with spectrin is distinct from the 220 000 and 240 000 daltons α- and β-spectrin subunits. Regulin can be separated from spectrin by ion exchange chromatography in urea, followed by antibody affinity chromatography using monoclonal antibodies against the regulatory

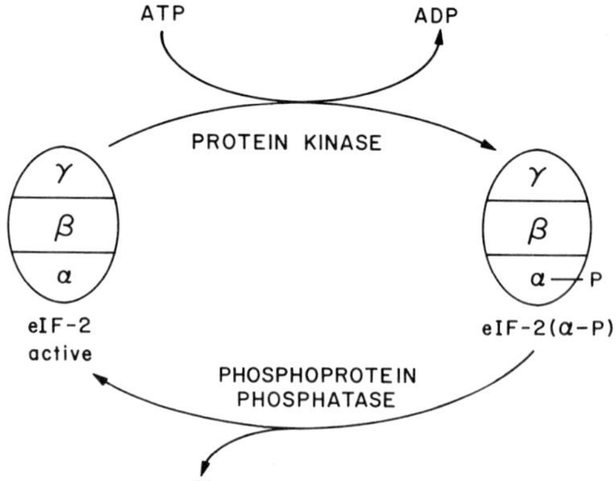

Fig. 1. Phosphorylation–dephosphorylation of eIF-2

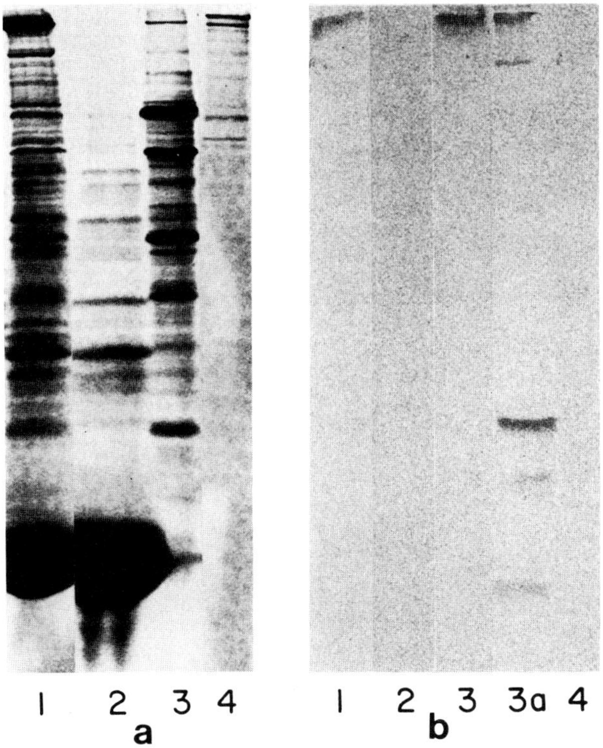

Fig. 2a, b. Separation of regulin from spectrin. Peptides of a crude spectrin preparation extracted from the reticulocyte membrane (*lane* 1) or fractions derived from it (*lanes* 2–4) were separated on 15% polyacrylamide gels in SDS and either stained with Coomassie Blue (**a**) or transferred electrophoretically to nitrocellulose, then incubated with monoclonal anti-regulin antibodies (**b**) as described [16]. Antigen peptides were visualized by dianisidine (cf. [17]). The spectrin preparation was made 6 *M* in urea, then loaded on a DEAE–cellulose column equilibrated in 40 m*M* Tris-HCl (pH 7.5), 25 m*M* KCl, 5 m*M* β-mercaptoethanol, and 6 *M* urea. The wash fraction (*lane* 2) contained mostly hemoglobin. Then proteins were eluted stepwise with the same solution, but containing 100 m*M* (*lane* 3) and 300 m*M* KCl (*lane* 4). *Lane* 3 contains regulin, *lane* 4 mostly spectrin. Lane 3a (100 m*M* KCl fraction) is from an identical preparation from which protease inhibitors were omitted

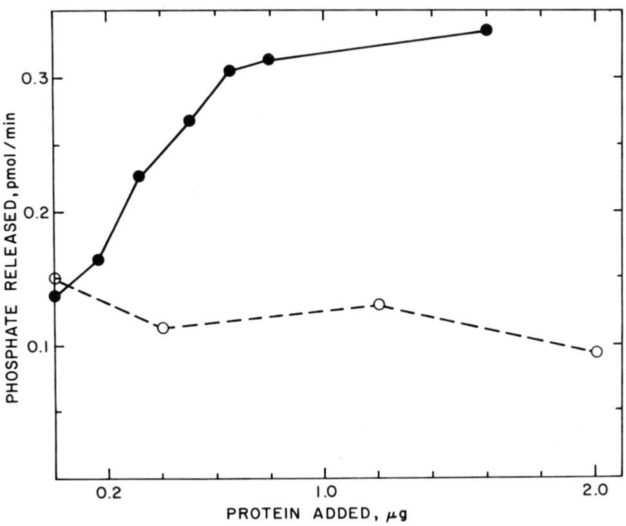

Fig. 3. Stimulation of phosphatase activity by regulin. The 56 000 daltons phosphatase was isolated and its enzymatic activity determined as described [12]. Regulin (*full circles*) or spectrin (*open circles*) were added in amounts indicated on the abscissa

protein. Regulin peptides are identified after separation of peptides by SDS–gel electrophoresis followed by Western blotting and ELISA with monoclonal antibodies (cf. [16]). The antigen–antibody complex is detected by a second antibody to which peroxidase is linked using dianisidine and H_2O_2 as substrate (cf. [17]). Regulin is a 230 000 daltons peptide that is very sensitive to proteolysis. If the cells are lysed in the absence of protease inhibitors, regulin is quickly degraded (Fig. 2B, lane 3a). It is

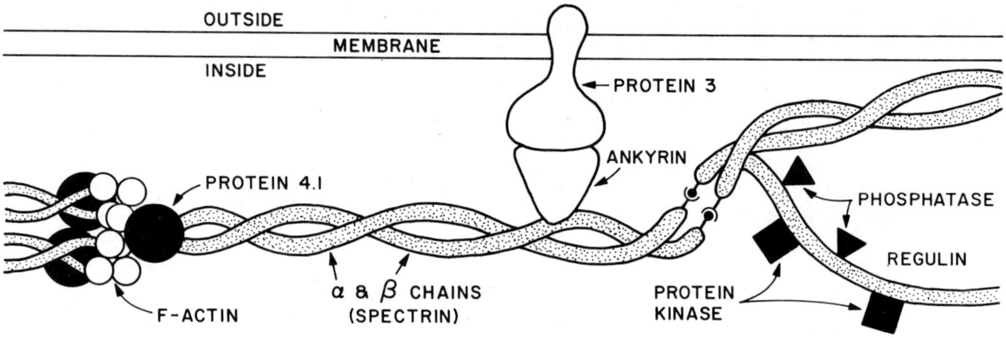

Fig. 4. Model for the association of regulin with spectrin in the red cell cytoskeleton. Illustration of the membrane-associated proteins is modified from [19]

not established whether or not this proteolytic processing of regulin has a physiologic function such as activation of protein kinase or phosphatase by extracellular stimuli that are transmitted through membrane receptors.

After reticulocytes are lysed and fractionated, regulin and its degradation products are found in part in the postribosomal supernatant and appear to copurify through most chromatographic steps with the phosphoprotein phosphatase and the heme-controlled eIF-2α kinase activities. Highly purified regulin – but not spectrin – stimulates the enzymatic activity of the homogeneous 56 000 daltons phosphatase as shown in Fig. 3.

Based on the results here and elswhere [12, 16], we suggest the model depicted in Fig. 4, indicating membrane–cytoskeleton interaction in red cells. It shows regulin associated with spectrin in the cytoskeleton and functioning to organize and modulate the activity of heme-regulated eIF-2α kinase and the protein phosphatase involved in translational control. Evidence has been presented which indicates that mRNA and polysomes active in protein synthesis also are bound to subcellular cytoskeletal structures, as reviewed recently by Trachsel and co-workers [18]. Thus, it appears likely that these elements for protein synthesis, as well as the factors that control their activity, are also organized on the cytoskeleton in intact cells.

Acknowledgments. This research was supported in part by National Institutes of Health Grant CA16608 and National Cancer Institute Grant T32-CA09182. E.W. is the recipient of a fellowship from the Deutsche Forschungsgemeinschaft.

References

1. Farrell JP, Balkow K, Hunt T, Jackson R, Trachsel H (1977) Cell 11:187–200
2. Kramer G, Cimadevilla JM, Hardesty B (1976) Proc Natl Acad Sci USA 73:3078–3082
3. Levin D, Ranu R, Ernst V, London IM (1976) Proc Natl Acad Sci USA 73:3112–3116
4. Duncan R, McConkey EH (1982) Eur J Biochem 123:539–544
5. Rosen OM, Rubin CS, Cobb MH, Smith CJ (1981) J Biol Chem 256:3630–3633
6. Wettenhall REH, Chesterman CN, Walker T, Morgan FJ (1983) FEBS Lett 162:171–176
7. Burkhard SJ, Traugh JA (1983) J Biol Chem 258:14 003–14 008
8. Antoniw JF, Cohen P (1976) Eur J Biochem 68:45–54
9. Li HC, Hsiao KJ, Chan W (1978) Eur J Biochem 84:215–225
10. Brautigan DL, Picton C, Fischer EH (1980) Biochemistry 19:5787–5794
11. Grankowski N, Lehmusvirta D, Kramer G, Hardesty B (1980) J Biol Chem 255:310–316
12. Wollny E, Watkins K, Kramer G, Hardesty B (1984) J Biol Chem 259:2484–2492
13. Lee EYC, Silberman SR, Ganapathi MK, Petrovic S, Paris H (1980) In: Greengard P, Robison GA (eds) Advances in cyclic nucleo-

tide research vol 13. Raven, New York, pp 95–131
14. Brautigan DL, Ballou LM, Fischer EH (1982) Biochemistry 21:1977–1982
15. Brandt H, Kapulong ZL, Lee EYC (1975) J Biol Chem 250:8038–8044
16. Fullilove S, Wollny E, Stearns G, Chen S-C, Kramer G, Hardesty B (1984) J Biol Chem 259:2493–2500
17. Towbin H, Staehelin T, Gordon J (1979) Proc Natl Acad Sci USA 76:4350–4354
18. Nielsen P, Goelz S, Trachsel H (1983) Cell Biol Int Reports 7:245–254
19. Lux SE (1982) In: Marchesi VT, Gallo RC (eds) Differentiation and function of hematopoietic cell surfaces. Liss, New York, pp 197–206

Haematology and Blood Transfusion Vol. 29
Modern Trends in Human Leukemia VI
Edited by Neth, Gallo, Greaves, Janka

Viruses as Tumor Initiators and Tumor Promoters

H. zur Hausen [1]

The role of specific viral genes in the induction of malignant tumors is well established in viral infections by papovaviruses and adenoviruses (e.g. review by zur Hausen 1980). In these infections viral DNA may integrate into the host cell genome, and continuous expression of a viral function is a prerequisite for the maintenance of the transformed state.

Chemical and physical carcinogens, on the other hand, introduce transient modifications in the DNA (e.g., DNA adducts, cross-links, single-stranded breaks), which subsequently result in mutational events and also in selective DNA amplification (SDA) in most systems investigated thus far (Lavi 1981; Heilbronn et al. 1985). It appears that "permanent" hereditable changes induced in initiated cells result mainly from the latter events (Heilbronn et al. 1985). No consistent exposure to the damaging event is required for the induction of malignant growth.

In recent years there has been some investigation of the question as to whether specific viral infections may lead to initiator-like effects by modifying the host cell genome similarly and by inducing cell transformation without persistence and continued expression of viral genome functions. This question was raised first when herpes simplex virus DNA, which transforms rodent cells (Duff and Rapp 1973) and has been suspected of playing a role in human cervical cancer (Rawls et al. 1968), was not detected in transformed cells and human cervical cancer biopsies (zur Hausen et al. 1974; zur Hausen 1975, Skinner 1976). Subsequently, experimental data were provided that revealed initiator-like properties of herpes simplex virus infections: The virus was shown to induce mutations within the host cell genome (Schlehofer and zur Hausen 1982) and very efficiently induced SDA in infected cells (Schlehofer et al. 1983).

At least one of the enzymes responsible for inducing these last changes was identified as herpes-specific DNA polymerase (Matz et al. 1984). This enzyme shares functional properties with host cell DNA polymerase alpha, which was recently identified as the key enzyme in SDA induced by chemical and physical carcinogens (Heilbronn et al. 1985).

Thus, herpes simplex viruses at least share properties with initiators under specific conditions they may possibly interact with host cell DNA as chemical and physical carcinogens do. It will be interesting to determine whether additional members of the herpes-virus group, such as cytomegalovirus or Epstein-Barr virus, possess similar properties.

Tumor promotion is not yet defined at the molecular level. Promoting chemicals, if applied for prolonged periods of time to initiated cells, lead to papillomatous proliferations which convert into malignant tumors. Promotors do not act as carcinogens, but they interact with carcinogen-pretreated cells, ultimately resulting in carcinomatous growth. It is tempting to speculate that

1 Deutsches Krebsforschungszentrum, Im Neuenheimer Feld 280, 6900 Heidelberg, FRG

promoters induce expression of amplified "initiated" genes.

There is one group of viruses which, upon infection of susceptible cells, shows a remarkable functional resemblance to tumor promoters: the papillomaviruses (zur Hausen et al. 1984). It appears that in the majority of specific infections with these viruses leading to malignant conversion additional interaction with chemical and physical carcinogens is required. The molecular mechanism of this interaction is presently not understood. Preliminary data suggest, however, that events favoring integration of the otherwise episomal papillomavirus DNA into the host cell genome may contribute to this process (Schwarz et al. 1985). It appears that additional changes, possibly affecting the host cell genome, are also involved.

Thus, interaction of specific types of papillomavirus infections with chemical and physical carcinogens suggests a promoter-like activity of these agents.

This is further underlined by observations revealing the effectiveness of a potent inhibitor of chemical promotion, retinoic acid, in the treatment of clinical warts and experimental papillomas (Lutzner and Blanchet-Bardon 1980; Jablonska et al. 1981; Ito 1981).

At present it is very difficult to correlate these effects with promotion at the molecular level. It is suggestive, however, that papillomaviruses represent suitable models for analysis of the process of promotion.

We can therefore conclude that viruses, in particular herpes simplex virus and specific papillomavirus types, may lead to intracellular events resembling effects exerted by chemical and physical carcinogens and tumor promoters. The availability of these agents and the accurate study of their gene organization and gene expression may render them suitable models for use in work that will expand our understanding of basic processes in carcinogenesis.

References

Duff R, Rapp F (1973) Oncogenic transformation of hamster embryo cells after exposure to inactivated herpes simplex virus type 1. J Virol 12:209–217

Heilbronn R, Schlehofer JR, Yalkinoglu AÖ, zur Hausen H (1985) Selective DNA-amplification induced by carcinogens (initiators): evidence for a role of proteases and DNA polymerase alpha. Int J Cancer (in print)

Ito Y (1981) Effect of an aromatic retinoic acid analog (Ro 10-9359) on growth of virus-induced papilloma (Shope) and related neoplasia of rabbits. Eur J Cancer 17:35–42

Jablonska S, Obalek S, Wolska H, Jarzabek-Chorzelska M (1981) Ro 10-9359 in epidermodysplasia verruciformis. In: Ofanos CE et al. (eds) Retinoids, advances in basic research and therapy. Springer, Berlin Heidelberg New York, pp 401–405

Lavi S (1981) Carcinogen-mediated amplification of viral DNA sequences in SV40-transformed Chinese hamster embryo cells. Proc Natl Acad Sci USA 78:6144–6148

Lutzner MA, Blanchet-Bardon C (1980) Oral retinoid treatment of human papillomavirus type 5-induced epidermodysplasia verruciformis. N Engl J Med 302:1091

Matz B, Schlehofer JR, zur Hausen H (1984) Identification of a gene function of herpes simplex virus type 1 essential for amplification of simian virus 40 sequences in transformed Chinese hamster cells. Virology 134: 328–337

Rawls WE, Tompkins WAF, Figueroa ME, Melnick JL (1968) Herpes virus type 2: association with carcinoma of the cervix. Science 161:1255–1256

Schlehofer JR, zur Hausen H (1982) Induction of mutations within the host genome by partially inactivated herpes simplex virus type 1. Virology 122:471–474

Schlehofer JR, Gissmann L, zur Hausen H (1983) Herpes simplex virus induced amplification of SV40 sequences in transformed Chinese hamster embryo cells. Int J Cancer 32:99–103

Schwarz E, Freese UK, Gissmann L, Mayer W, Roggenbuck B, Stremlau A, zur Hausen H (1985) Structure and transcription of human papillomavirus sequences in cervical carcinoma cells. Nature (in press)

Skinner GRB (1976) Transformation of primary hamster embryo fibroblasts by type 2 herpes simplex virus: evidence for a "hit and run" mechanism. Br J Exp Pathol 51:361–376

zur Hausen H (1975) Oncogenic herpesviruses. Biophys Biochim Acta 417:25–53

zur Hausen H (1980) The role of viruses in human tumors. Adv Cancer Res 33:77–107

zur Hausen H (1984) Similarities of papillomavirus infections with tumor promoters. In: Fujiki H, Hecker E, Moore RE, Sugimura T, Weinstein IB (eds) Cellular interactions by environment tumor promoters. Japan Scientific Societies Press, Tokyo, pp 147–152

Haematology and Blood Transfusion Vol. 29
Modern Trends in Human Leukemia VI
Edited by Neth, Gallo, Greaves, Janka

Endemic and Sporadic Cases of Epstein-Barr Virus-Positive Burkitt's Lymphoma: Immunological Characterization of Derived Cell Lines

C. M. Rooney[1], M. Rowe[1], A. B. Rickinson[1], G. M. Lenoir[2], D. M. Moss[3], and M. A. Epstein[4]

A. Introduction

Burkitt's lymphoma (BL) is a tumour which is endemic in regions of Africa and New Guinea where temperature and rainfall are high and malaria is holoendemic. BL also occurs worldwide (sporadic BL), but at a much lower incidence, and showing no association with specific climatic or geographical features. Some 98% of endemic tumours carry multiple copies of the Epstein-Barr (EB) virus genome, and it is possible that this virus has a causal relationship with BL. However, only 20% of sporadic cases are associated with the EB virus, and this would suggest that the endemic and sporadic forms of the disease may differ in pathogenesis.

In this work we have compared tumour cell lines established from endemic cases of BL with lines established from EB virus genome-positive sporadic tumours. The differences apparent between them suggest that the two diseases, even when both are EB virus-associated, may be distinct in terms of the cell of origin, and therefore in terms of pathogenesis.

New BL cell lines have been established from patients located in regions of Africa (seven cases), and New Guinea (two cases) where the tumour is endemic. Simultaneously, lymphoblastoid cell lines (LCL) were established from the normal, circulating B cells of these same patients, by in vitro infection with EB virus. BL/LCL pairs have likewise been established from sporadic cases of the disease arising in Algeria, France and La Réunion.

B. Phenotypic Analysis of Endemic and Sporadic BL Lines

In every case, BL cells were distinct from the autologous LCL cells, in being monoclonal in immunoglobulin expression, in showing specific chromosomal translocations, and in terms of cell surface phenotype and morphology [1]. More importantly there were interesting differences between individual BL lines (Table 1).

All nine BL lines of endemic origin initially grew as single cell suspensions, and, using a selected panel of monoclonal antibodies, they showed a characteristic pattern of reactivity which showed no resemblance to that shown by LCL. Endemic BL did not bind two "lymphoblastoid-specific" antibodies, AC2 and MHM6, nor two antibodies with known reactivity with Sternberg-Reed cells, Ki1 and Ki24, but they did show strong reactivity with J5, an antibody with specificity for the common acute lymphoblastic leukemia antigen (cALLA). This phenotype was called group 1. Only 2/9 sporadic BL expressed a group 1 phenotype, while the remaining 7 lines were reactive not only with J5, but also with Ki24, and showed a variable pattern of reactivity

1 Dept of Cancer Studies, University of Birmingham Medical School B15 2TJ UK
2 IARC, Lyons France
3 QIMR, Queensland, Australia
4 Dept Pathology, University of Bristol Medical School, UK

Table 1. Phenotypic analysis of endemic and sporadic BL cells

Cell line type	Patient	Early passage							Later passage						
		Growth pattern	Monoclonal antibody binding					Group	Growth pattern	Monoclonal antibody					Group
			MHM6	AC2	Ki1	Ki24	J5			MHM6	AC2	Ki1	Ki24	J5	
Endemic BL	WEW 2	Single cells	0	0	0	0	+++	I	Single cells	0	0	0	0	+++	I
	WAN	Single cells	0	0	0	0	+++	I	Single cells	0	0	0	0	+++	I
	CHEP	Single cells	0	0	0	0	+++	I	Single cells	0	0	0	0	+++	I
	MAK	Single cells	0	0	0	0	+++	I	Small clumps	0	0	0	+	+++	II
	LIV	Single cells	0	0	0	0	+++	I	Single cells	0	0	0	++	+++	II
	MUK	Single cells	0	0	0	0	+++	I	Small clumps	+	0	0	++	+++	II
	ELI	Single cells	0	0	0	0	+++	I	Small clumps	0	+	0	+++	++	II
	KYU	Single cells	0	0	0	0	+++	I	Small clumps	0	+++	++	+++	+++	II
	WEW 1	Single cells	0	0	0	0	+++	I	Small clumps	0	+	+++	+++	+++	II
Sporadic BL	LAT	Single cells	0	0	0	0	+++	I	Single cells	0	0	0	0	+++	I
	TOL	Single cells	0	0	0	0	+++	I	Single cells	0	0	0	0	+++	I
	MON	Single cells	0	0	0	+++	+++	II	Small clumps	0	0	0	+++	+++	II
	OUS	Large clumps	+	+	0	++	+++	II	Large clumps	+	+	0	+++	+++	II
	Ls32	Large clumps	++	+++	++	+++	+++	II	Large clumps	+++	+++	+	+++	0	III
	Ls92	Large clumps	++	+	++	++	+++	II	Large clumps	+++	++	++	++	0	III
	PUY	Large clumps	++	++	+	+++	+++	II	Large clumps	+	+++	++	+++	0	III
	LOU	Large clumps	+	+	0	++	++	II	Large clumps	+	++	++	+++	0	III
	BOC	Large clumps	+	+++	++	+++	+	II	Large clumps	+	+++	+++	+++	0	III
Endemic and sporadic LCL	All patients	Large clumps	+++	+++	++/+++	++/+++	0		Large clumps	+++	+++	++/+++	++/+++	0	

Table 2. Endemic and sporadic BL cells differ in their immunogenicity to NK cells, and to allospecific cytotoxic T cells

Cell line type	Patient	Group	NK activation	Susceptibility to NK cells	Allo activation	Susceptibility to allo-killing
Endemic BL	WEW 1	1	BL≪LCL	BL<LCL	BL≪LCL	BL<LCL
	WEW 2	1	BL≪LCL	BL≪LCL	BL≪LCL	BL≪LCL
	WAN	1	BL≪LCL	BL=LCL	BL≪LCL	BL<LCL
	MAK	1	ND	BL<LCL	BL≪LCL	BL<LCL
	CHEP	1	ND	BL=LCL	ND	ND
	LIV	1	BL≪LCL	BL=LCL	ND	ND
	MUK	2	BL=LCL	BL=LCL	BL<LCL	BL<LCL
	ELI	2	BL</≪LCL	BL=LCL	BL<LCL	BL<LCL
Sporadic BL	LAT	1	BL<LCL	BL=LCL	BL≪LCL	BL≪LCL
	TOL	1	ND	ND	ND	ND
	MON	2	ND	ND	ND	ND
	OUS	2	BL<LCL	BL<LCL	BL>LCL	BL>LCL
	PUY	2	BL=LCL	BL>LCL	BL>LCL	BL=LCL
	Ls32	3	BL=LCL	BL>LCL	BL<LCL	BL<LCL
	Ls92	3	BL=LCL	BL=LCL	BL<LCL	BL<LCL
	Lou	3	BL=LCL	BL>LCL	BL>LCL	BL>LCL
	BOC	3	BL=LCL	BL=LCL	BL<LCL	BL=LCL

with Ki1, AC2 and MHM6. These lines were classified as group 2.

Within 20 in vitro passages, a number of lines were seen to change both in morphology and in phenotype: 6/9 endemic BL acquired a group 2 phenotype, and began to grow in small clumps, individual cells being less uniformly spherical. This growth pattern was quite distinct from that of the sporadic lines in group 2. Group 2 sporadic lines grew as large tight clumps, and although this growth pattern remained unaltered, with subsequent passage they lost their reactivity with J5, thus acquiring a group 3 phenotype, which was more similar to that of LCL.

Differences in growth pattern, and in quantitative expression of the monoclonal antibodies MHM6, AC2 and Ki1, suggest that the stable group 2 into which the endemic group 1 BL lines progress, is probably distinct from the unstable group 2 in which sporadic BL can arise. Thus, BL appears to arise in at least two separate B cell subsets; endemic BL is restricted to just one of these subsets, while sporadic BL may arise in a range of B cell differentiation states.

C. Immunological Analysis of Endemic and Sporadic BL Lines

Endemic and sporadic cell lines in groups 1, 2 and 3 are being characterized in terms of their performance in a number of immunological assays (Table 2). First, in their ability to induce "activated NK" cells, and in their susceptibility to "activated NK" cell-mediated cytolysis. Induction of "activated NK" cells was achieved after 4–6 days of coculture of γ-irradiated BL or LCL cells, with unfractionated mononuclear cells from seronegative donors, at a low responder: stimulator ratio of 4:1. Effector cells were harvested and tested for killer activity against chromium-labelled target cells (Table 2).

Cell lines in group 1, either sporadic or endemic, were poor inducers of activated NK cell activity in comparison with LCL, or with sporadic BL lines in group 2 or group 3. Only 1/4 endemic lines which had progressed into group 2 was capable of inducing NK cell activity which was comparable to that induced by LCL. There was little difference in the sensitivity of cell lines in any one group, and LCL to NK cell-mediated cytolysis.

Second, the BL lines were tested for their ability to induce alloantigen-specific cytotoxic T cells (CTL), and for their susceptibility to lysis by these allospecific CTL. Allospecific CTL were induced by 9–10 days coculture of γ-irradiated BL or LCL cells, at a responder: stimulator ratio of 40:1. T cells were isolated by rosetting with sheep red blood cells, and soon after, a T cell growth factor-dependent cell line was established. These effector cells were tested in 5-h chromium release assays, against HLA-matched and mismatched target cell lines.

All seven endemic lines tested were poor inducers of allospecific CTL activity in comparison with the autologous LCL: BL $<$ LCL, two pairs (group 2); BL $\ll$ LCL, four pairs (two in group 1, and two in group 2). One sporadic line in group 1 was tested, and this line was a very poor inducer of allospecific CTL. However, the activity of sporadic lines in groups 2 and 3 was more comparable to that of LCL: BL $<$ LCL, 3/6 pairs; BL $\leqq$ LCL 3/6 pairs. Generally the susceptibility of each line to allospecific cytotoxicity reflected its capacity for alloactivation.

Currently, the susceptibility of these lymphoma lines to EB virus-specific T cell-mediated cytotoxicity is being tested. The outgrowth of virus-infected tumour cells in BL may be due, either to a failure of the patient's immune responses, or to a lack of sensitivity of the tumour cells to cell-mediated immune lysis. The latter hypothesis may be important in endemic cases of BL, while a depressed immune response may be a factor in most sporadic cases. Further studies of the immune responses of BL patients are required to answer these questions.

Reference

1. Rowe M, Rooney CM, Rickinson AB, Lenoir GM, Rupani H, Moss DJ, Stein H, Epstein MA (1985) Int J Cancer 35/4

Haematology and Blood Transfusion Vol. 29
Modern Trends in Human Leukemia VI
Edited by Neth, Gallo, Greaves, Janka

Herpesvirus HVMA: A New Representative in the Group of the EBV-like B-Lymphotropic Herpesviruses of Primates *

B. A. Lapin, V. V. Timanovskaya, and L. A. Yakovleva

Isolation of EBV from an African baby with malignant lymphoma in 1964 was followed by a series of investigations resulting in the establishment of antibodies to viral capsid antigen (VCA EBV) in blood sera of different African and Asian monkey species [1–7].

Detection of VCA EBV antibodies that did not differ in different lymphotropic herpesviruses, as was established later, resulted in the notion that EBV was a ubiquitous virus and that monkeys could serve as a natural reservoir of the virus being the source of human infection.

B-lymphotropic herpesvirus HVP, antigenically and biologically related but not identical to EBV and sharing only 40% DNA homology with the latter, was isolated in our laboratory in 1973–1974 from lymphomatous hamadryas baboons [8–14]. Isolation of the virus HVP has been the basis for the idea on the existence of a family of the EBV-like B-lymphotropic herpesviruses of primates (human beings and different Old World monkey species). This idea has been confirmed by subsequent isolations of lymphotropic herpesviruses of chimpanzees [15], orangoutangs [16], gorillas [17], vervets [18], and macaques [19] by other investigators. The above viruses were produced in lymphoid cell suspension cultures established both from normal and (rarely) from sick monkeys with malignant lymphoma. It can be suggested that EBV-like B-lymphotropic herpesvirus would be revealed in other representatives of the Old World primates.

The present report describes isolation of a new lymphotropic herpesvirus of *M. arctoides* produced by lymphoid cell culture MAL-1, which has been established from *M. arctoides* peripheral blood lymphocytes.

A large number of cytoplasmatic IgM were detected in MAL-1 culture cells. This meant it was impossible to investigate them in an indirect immunofluorescent test using polyspecific anti-Ig-FITC conjugate. Antigens crossreacting with EA and VCA HVP were identified in MAL-1 cells by a direct immunofluorescence test using labeled FITC globulins of anti-VCA + EA + HVP-positive serum of hamadryas baboons. The percentage of EA + VCA + cells in MAL-1 culture varied depending on the period after passage (> 1%–4%). The maximum of antigen-positive cells was noted 48–72 h after the passage (Fig. 1).

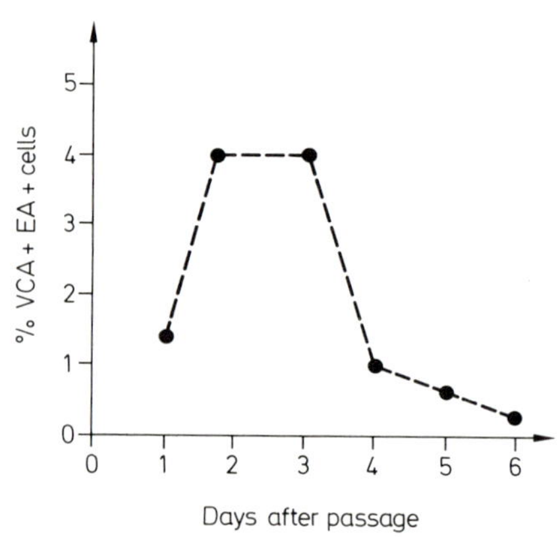

* Institute of Experimental Pathology and Therapy, USSR Academy of Medical Sciences, Sukhumi, USSR

Electronmicroscopic investigation of ultrathin sections of MAL-1 cells has revealed herpesvirus particles. Molecularbiological investigations have shown moderate DNA homology of the isolated virus with the DNA of baboon herpesvirus (30%) and the DNA of the Epstein-Barr virus (20%).

Thus, the group of B-lymphotropic herpesviruses has been replenished with a new virus of *M. arctoides* monkeys, which has been named HVMA (herpesvirus *M. arctoides*).

References

1. Gerber P, Birch SM (1967) Complement-fixing antibodies in sera of human and non-human primates to viral antigen derived from Burkitt's lymphoma cells. Proc Natl Acad Sci USA 58:478–484
2. Gerber P, Rosenblum EN (1968) The incidence of complement-fixing antibodies to herpes simplex and herpes-like viruses in man and rhesus monkey. Proc Soc Exp Biol Med 128:541–546
3. Goldman M, Landon JC, Reischer J (1968) Fluorescent antibody and gel diffusion reactions of human and chimpanzee sera with cells cultured from Burkitt's tumours and normal chimpanzee blood. Cancer Res 28:2489–2495
4. Chu CT, Yang CS, Kawamura A (1971) Antibodies to Epstein-Barr virus in a Burkitt's lymphoma cell line in Taiwan monkeys (*M. cyclopis*). Appl Environ Microbiol 21:539–540
5. Dunkel VC, Pry TW, Henle G, Henle W (1972) Immunofluorescence tests for antibodies to Epstein-Barr virus with sera of lower primates. J Natl Cancer Inst 49:435–440
6. Kalter SS, Heberling RL, Ratner JJ (1973) EBV antibody in monkeys and apes. Bibl Haematologica 39:871–875
7. Landon JC, Malan L (1971) Seroepidemiologic studies of Epstein-Barr virus antibody in monkeys. J Natl Cancer Inst 46:881–884
8. Lapin BA (1975) Possible ways viral leukemia spreads among hamadryas baboons of the Sukhumi monkey colony. In: Ito Y, Dutcher RM (eds) Comparative leukemia research. University of Tokyo Press, Tokyo/Karger, Basel, pp 75–84
9. Agrba VZ, Yakovleva LA, Lapin BA, Sangulija IA, Timanovskaya VV, Markaryan DS, Chuvirov GN, Salmanova EA (1975) The establishment of continuous lymphoblastoid suspension cell culture from hematopoietic organs of baboon (*P. hamadryas*) with malignant lymphoma. Exp Pathol 10:318–332
10. Falk L, Deinhardt F, Nonoyama M, Wolfe LG, Bergholz C (1976) Properties of a baboon lymphotropic herpesvirus related to Epstein-Barr virus. Int J Cancer 18:798–807
11. Djatchenko AG, Kakubava VV, Lapin BA, Agrba VZ, Yakovleva LA, Samilchuk EI (1976) Continuous lymphoblastoid suspension cultures from cells of haematopoietic organs of baboons with malignant lymphoma: Biological characterization and biological properties of the herpesvirus associated with culture cells. Exp Pathol 12:163–168
12. Rabin H, Neubauer RH, Hopkins RF, Dzhikidze EK, Shevtsova ZV, Lapin BA (1977) Transforming activity and antigenicity of an Epstein-Barr-like virus from lymphoblastoid cell lines of baboons with lymphoid disease. Intervirology 8:240–249
13. Deinhardt F, Deinhardt J (1979) Comparative aspects: Oncogenic animal herpesvirus. In: Epstein MA, Achong BG (eds) Epstein-Barr virus. Springer, Berlin Heidelberg New York, pp 373–415
14. Kokosha LV, Agrba VZ, Lapin BA, Yakovleva LA, Arshba NN, Markova TP, Timanovskaja VV (1977) Continuous lymphoblastoid suspension cultures from cells of haematopoietic organs of baboons with malignant lymphoma. Exp Pathol 13:247–254
15. Landon JC, Ellis LB, Leve VH, Fabrizio DP (1968) Herpes-type virus in cultured leukocytes from chimpanzees. J Natl Cancer Inst 40:181–192
16. Rasheed S, Rongey RW, Brunzweski J, Nelson-Rees WA, Rabin H, Neubauer RH, Esra G, Gardner MB (1977) Establishment of a cell line with associated Epstein-Barr-like virus from a leukemic orangutan. Science 198:407–409
17. Neubauer RH, Rabin H, Strnad BC, Nonoyama M, Nelson-Rees WA (1979) Establishment of a lymphoblastoid cell line and isolation of an Epstein-Barr-related virus of gorilla origin. J Virol 31:845–848
18. Böcker JF, Tiedemann KH, Bornkamm GW, zur Hausen H (1980) Characterization of an EBV-like virus African green monkey lymphoblasts. Virology 101:291–295
19. Reitz BA, Bieber CP, Pennock JL (1982) Cyclosporin A and lymphoma in non-human primates. In: White DJG (ed) Cyclosporin A. Elsevier Biomedical Press, Amsterdam

Haematology and Blood Transfusion Vol. 29
Modern Trends in Human Leukemia VI
Edited by Neth, Gallo, Greaves, Janka

Tumors Induced in Hairless Mice by DNA from Human Malignant Cells

F. L. Kisseljov[1], L. Z. Topol[1], A. G. Tatosyan[1], N. G. Nalbandyan[1], E. S. Revasova[1] and M. Grofova[2]

The development of a transfection technique which is based on the transfer of foreign genetic material into permissive cells allows one to isolate and identify the transformed genes in tumors of different etiology [1]. The results which have been obtained in the last few years lead to the conclusion that primary effects in human tumors during their progression are connected with the activation of different genetic elements, among which oncogenes may play an important role [2]. The main aim of this work is the elaboration of an experimental model for the analysis of human tumors and human genome DNA fragments which participate in the process of malignant cell transformation.

The following human cell lines adapted for growth in vitro were analyzed: osteosarcoma U-393 OS; sinovial sarcoma U-4 SS; malignant glioma U-251 MG [3, 4]; fibrosarcoma B-6 FS [5], and bladder carcinoma T 24 [6]. Two primary human tumors were also included: stomach carcinoma; and testis carcinoma. DNA from tumors and cells was isolated by the SDS–phenol extraction method. The transfection of high molecular weight DNA was made according to well-known methods [7]. For the selection of transformed clones we used two methods: cultivation in vitro as described by Wigler et al. [8]; and a second method including the injection of the whole pool of transfected cells in hairless mice (2×10^6 cells per mouse) on the seventh day after transfection before any indication of morphological changes in cell phenotype.

As a result, we obtained around 30 DNA preparations from the foci of transformed cells and hairless mice tumors which were analyzed by the blot hybridization technique in the presence of *Alu* sequences, as a marker of human genome [9, 10]. Among these DNA preparations including T 24 DNA (which was used as a positive control), only ten were *Alu* positive and were used for further rounds of transfection. These *Alu*-positive DNA were again transfected in NIH 3T3 cells with further implantation in hairless mice. Results presented in Table 1 show that these DNA-induced tumors appeared in mice after a shorter period of time in comparison with the first round. The development of tumors having biologically inactive DNA in further cycles of transfection may be connected with the high background of spontaneous transformation observed in the clone of NIH 3T3 cells used for experiments.

The analysis of *Alu* sequences in DNA of murine tumors shows that after EcoR1 digestion, discrete bands of human genome were obtained. The pattern of these fragments, which arose after implantation of NIH 3T3 cells transfected with DNA from the malignant glioma cell line U-251 MG, was different after each round of transfection (Fig. 1a, lanes 1, 2, 3). So, after the second cycle, *Alu* sequences are associated with the bands of 3.2 megadaltons and after the third cycle 4.0 and 4.5 megadaltons. It indicates that, during DNA transfers from donor to recipient cells, structural re-

1 Cancer Research Center, Moscow, USSR
2 Cancer Research Institute, Bratislava

Table 1. Analysis of tumors in hairless mice, occurring after implantation of NIH 3T3 cells transfected with various human DNA

Number	DNA origin	Material	First round		Second round		Third round	
			Tumor appearance (days)	Alu sequences	Tumor appearance (days)	Alu sequences	Tumor appearance (days)	Alu sequences
1	Osteosarcoma	U-393 OS	35	+	–	–	–	–
2	Osteosarcoma	U-2 OS	35	+	–	–	–	–
3	Sinovial sarcoma	U-4 SS	33	+	22	+	20	+
4	Malignant glioma	U-251 MG	34	+	15	+	18	+
5	Fibrosarcoma	B-6 FS	20	+	12	N.T.[a]		
6	Bladder carcinoma	T 24	15	+	12	N.T.		
7	Stomach carcinoma	SC	35	+	–	–	–	–
8	Testis carcinoma	TC 87	72	–	–	–	–	–
9	Normal stomach tissue		–	–	–	–	–	–
10	NIH 3T3 cells		80	–	–	–	–	–

[a] N.T. not tested

arrangements of human genetic material may occur.

For tumors induced by U-4 SS DNA after the second round of transfection and EcoR1 DNA digestion, the main *Alu* band occurred at 4.5 megadaltons and diffuse low molecular weight bands were also visible (Fig. 1a, lane 5). It is necessary to note that in tumors which developed after the first round, cell transfectants of the B-6 FS cell line *Alu*-specific sequences occurred as discrete bands at 13.7 and 4.5 megadaltons (Fig. 1a, lane 8) although it is well known that, for the first round of transfectants, the diffuse distribution of *Alu* sequences is more typical [11].

Earlier it was shown that transformation of NIH 3T3 cells with DNA from tumors of different origin, including human bladder carcinoma, was accompanied by the transfer of the *ras* oncogene family and it was suggested that these genes may qualify as transforming genes of these tumors [12–14]. Therefore, the *ras* gene was chosen for analysis of the murine tumor genome. The results of these experiments are presented in Fig. 1b. In all cases we observe hybridization with *ras*-specific probe and at the same time the main hybridizing fragments have the same mobilities as *Alu* fragments which testify to the human origin of these *ras*-specific sequences. Some additional bands which do not comigrate with *Alu* fragments where also observed. We suggest that they may represent either independent human *ras* sequences which are not linked with neighboring *Alu* sequences, or endogenous *ras* gene, for example, the 8.0 megadaltons fragment, which is also detected in NIH 3T3 cells (Fig. 1b, lane 9). Densitometric scanning of autoradiograms of *Ha-ras* blots shows that, in every round of transfection, both the increase and decrease of integrated material may have occurred (it is well documented for the second and third rounds in U-251 MG cells).

In summary, we can conclude that the transfection of the DNA from human tumor cell lines U-251 MG, U-4 OS, and B-6 FS in NIH 3T3 cells with further implantation of these cells in hairless mice was accompanied by transfer of discrete regions of human genome which contains *ras* oncogene and highly repeated *Alu* sequences, both of which may undergo structural and qualitative changes, including amplification.

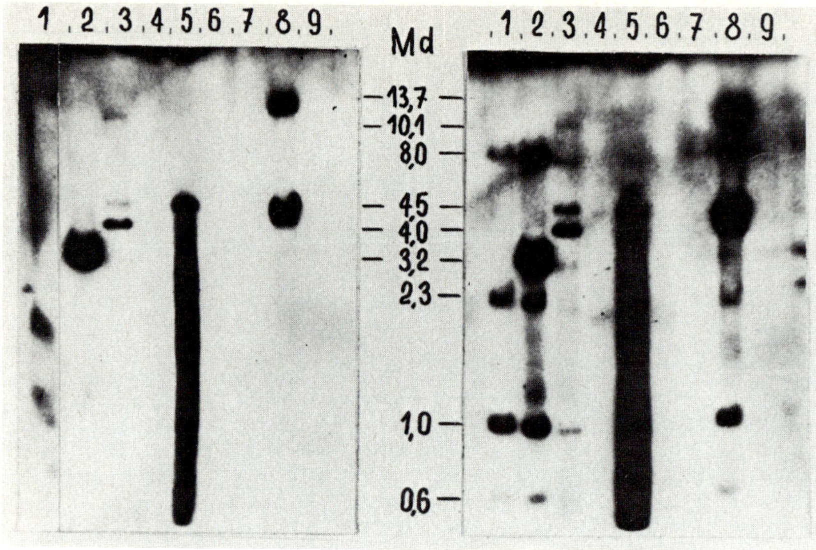

Fig. 1 a, b. Comparative analysis of hairless mice tumor genomes induced by implantation of NIH 3T3 cells transfected with various human DNA. **a** with *Alu*-specific probe, **b** with *Ha-ras*-specific probe. Human DNA for transfection was isolated from: 1, 2, 3 U-251 MG (malignant glioma) cell line (first, second, and third round of transfection, respectively), 4 testis carcinoma (first round); 5 U-4 SS (sinovial sarcoma) cell line (second round); 6 kidney of hairless mice; 7 tumor of hairless mice, induced by spontaneously transformed NIH 3T3 cells; 8 B-6 FS (fibrosarcoma) cell line (first round); 9 NIH 3T3 cells

References

1. Cooper G (1982) Science 217:801–806
2. Land H, Parada L, Weinberg R (1983) Science 222:771–778
3. Ponten J (1975) In: Human tumor cells in vitro. Plenum, New York, pp 175–178
4. Ponten J, Saksela E (1967) Int J Cancer 2:434–437
5. Thurso V, Popovic M, Matuska J, Grofova M (1976) Neoplasma 23:577–581
6. Bubenik J, Baresova M, Villicky V (1973) Int J Cancer 11:765–769
7. Graham FL, Van der Eb JA (1973) Virology 52:456–461
8. Wigler M, Sweet R, Sim GK (1979) Cell 16: 777–785
9. Southern EM (1975) J Mol Biol 98:503–507
10. Houck CM, Renehart FP, Schmid CW (1979) J Mol Biol 132:289–293
11. Peruchio M, Goldfarb M, Wigler M (1981) Cell 27:467–476
12. Shih C, Padhy LC, Murray M, Weinberg RA (1981) Nature 290:261–266
13. Krontiris TG, Cooper GM (1981) Proc Natl Acad Sci USA 78:1181–1184
14. Murray MJ, Shilo BZ, Shih C, Weinberg RA (1981) Cell 25:355–360

Haematology and Blood Transfusion Vol. 29
Modern Trends in Human Leukemia VI
Edited by Neth, Gallo, Greaves, Janka

The Human T-Cell Leukemia Virus Family, Adult T Cell Leukemia, and AIDS *

R. C. Gallo, M. G. Sarngadharan, M. Popovic, J. Schupbach, P. Markham, S. Z. Salahuddin, G. Shaw, F. Wong-Staal, and M. S. Reitz Jr

A. Introduction

Human T cell leukemia virus (HTLV) is the name by which we have designated a family of related retroviruses from humans. HTLV type I (HTLV-I) is the name we gave the first human retrovirus isolate. HTLV-I is endemic at low rates in different parts of the world, including southern Japan, the Caribbean, South and Central America, the southeastern United States, and especially in Africa. Seroepidemiologic studies show that HTLV-I is the primary etiologic agent of an aggressive form of adult T cell leukemia/lymphoma (ATLL). Infection with HTLV-I in vivo occurs preferentially with $OKT4^{+}$ T cells and results in immortalization of the infected cells as well as abrogation of various immune functions of the infected cells, in keeping with its role in the etiology of ATLL. A second related but distinct virus, HTLV type II (HTLV-II), was identified by us in collaboration with D. Golde and colleagues after type I, in material from a patient with hairy cell leukemia. HTLV-II shares many features with HTLV-I, including in vitro transforming activity, but it has been isolated only rarely and has not yet been associated with any disease. A third virus, HTLV type III (HTLV-III), has been isolated many times from individuals who have acquired immunodeficiency syndrome (AIDS) or are at risk for this disease. HTLV-III shares some antigenic cross-reactivity with I and II, as well as some general features, including an $OKT4^{+}$ T cell tropism. The virus is more highly infectious than I or II, however, and has so far shown only cytopathic and not immortalizing effects. Seroepidemiologic data show that HTLV-III is the cause of AIDS.

B. HTLV-I and Adult T Cell Leukemia/Lymphoma

The first human retrovirus isolates were obtained from malignant T cell lines established with the use of T cell growth factor (TCGF), a protein present in the media of peripheral blood cells stimulated with phytohemagglutinin [1, 27, 40]. The T cell lines were established from black patients in the United States with what were diagnosed as unusually aggressive variants of cutaneous T cell lymphoma [28, 29, 35]. The virus, which we called HTLV-I, has typical retrovirus morphology (Fig. 1) and, like other retroviruses, contains both a reverse transcriptase and high-molecular-weight polyadenylated genomic RNA. HTLV-I was shown to be unique by the criteria of protein serology [14, 37, 38] and nucleic acid hybridization [35], and to be exogenous to man [35]. Transmission is horizontal and does not occur genetically [9, 54].

The isolation of HTLV-I made it possible to make antibodies to the viral proteins. These antibodies were then used to test

* Laboratory of Tumor Cell Biology, Developmental Therapeutics Program, Division of Cancer Treatment, National Cancer Institute, Bethesda, MD 20205, USA

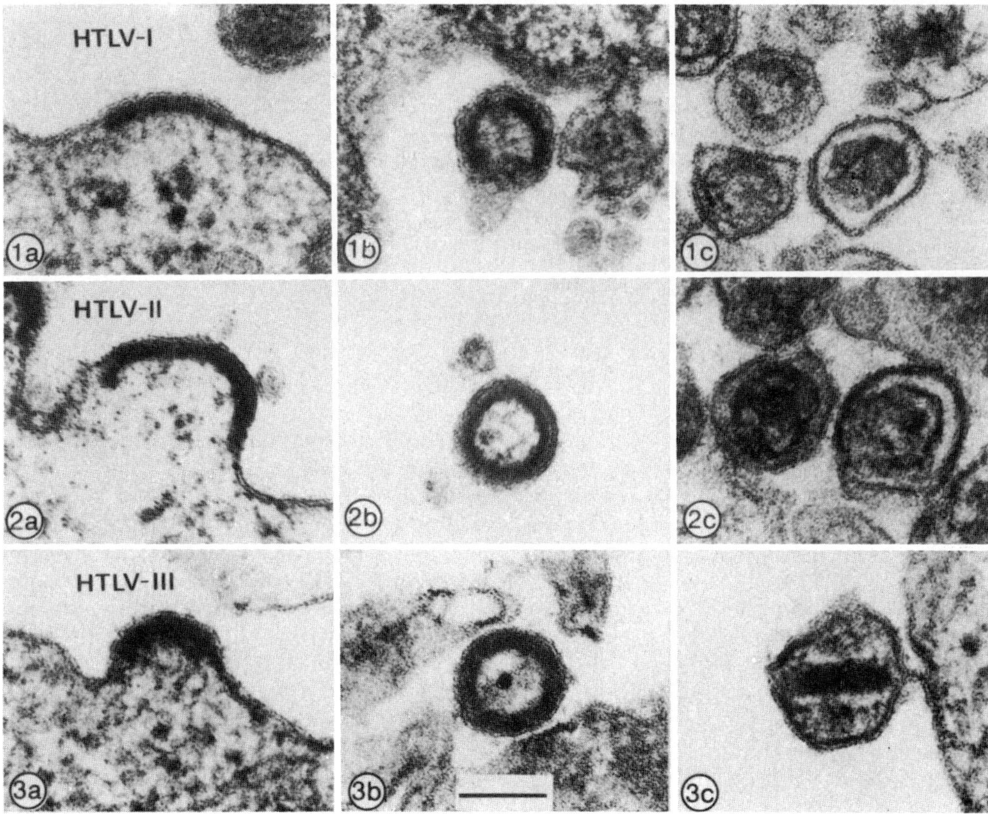

Fig. 1. Electron microscopy of HTLV-I, II, and III. Shown are budding (*panels a*), immature (*panels b*), and mature (*panels c*) virions of the three types of HTLV. The *bar* in *3b* equals 100 nm

serum samples for the presence of HTLV-I. Most persons in the United States were negative for this virus, including patients with many types of leukemia and lymphoma. HTLV-I was detected in a small fraction of persons from the United States with cutaneous T cell leukemia or lymphoma, most of whom were blacks in the southeastern United States or of Caribbean origin [4, 30]. Even most of these patients were negative.

Two regions of the world were identified, however, in which there were endemic diseases which clinically resembled those from which the first two isolates of HTLV-I were obtained. These regions were the Caribbean [5] and southwestern Japan [51]. The disease in the Caribbean was called lymphosarcoma cell leukemia, and that in Japan was called adult T cell leukemia; both were found to be closely associated with the presence of HTLV-I by seroepidemiology [3, 13, 39]. Both diseases are now regarded as the same clinical entity, and are collectively called adult T cell leukemia/lymphoma (ATLL).

Similar results have been reported by investigators in Japan, who also isolated retroviruses from ATLL cell lines [25, 54]. These retroviruses are now known to be isolates of HLTV-I [52]. Sporadic occurrences of both HTLV-I and ATLL have been noted in many other areas of the world [10], and most recently parts of Africa have also been shown to be endemic [43].

As is true for the naturally occurring animal leukemia viruses, only a small fraction of HTLV-I-infected people develop leukemia [50]. It thus appears as though other

Table 1. Relatedness of HTLV-I, II, and III

Property	Subgroup of HTLV		
	I	II	III
1. General infectivity	Lym	Lym	Lym
2. Particular tropism	T4	T4	T4
3. RT size	λ100K	λ100K	λ100K
4. RT divalent cation	Mg^{2+}	Mg^{2+}	Mg^{2+}
5. Major core	p24	p24	p24
6. Common envelope epitope	+	+	+
7. Common p24 epitope	+	+	+
8. Nucleic acid homology to I (stringent)		±	–
9. Nucleic acid homology to I (moderate stringency)		+ +	+
10. Homology to other retroviruses	0	0	0
11. pX	+	+	+
12. Produces giant multinucleated cells	+	+	+
13. African origin	Likely	?	Likely

factors, such as the host immune response, age at exposure, virus dose, or route of infection, may be important factors in determining the end result of infection.

C. In Vitro Biological Effects of HTLV-I

HTLV-I was first shown by Miyoshi et al. to transform T cells [26], but the target cells were not shown to be initially free of virus. Subsequently, transformation was achieved using target T cells shown to be HTLV-I negative [31, 32].

HTLV-I is tropic for T cells of the $OKT4^+$ phenotype both in vivo [9] and in vitro [19, 31, 32]. Transmission is achieved easily by co-cultivation with killed virus-producing cells, but only with difficulty when cell-free virus is used. The infected cells take on many of the properties of transformed ATLL cells, including altered morphology, increased growth rate, the tendency to grow in clumps, reduced dependence on TCGF, expression of high levels of the TCGF receptor and HLA-Dr antigens on the cell surface, and (usually) immortalization in culture [22, 23, 31, 32]. In vitro transformation by HTLV-I seems to be much more rapid and efficient than leukemogenesis in vitro.

Infection with HTLV-I of functional T cells results in the loss of some or all of their immune functions. For example, a T cell line which was cytotoxic for autologous tumor cells was established from one (rare) long-term survivor of ATLL [22]. These cells were themselves infectable with HTLV-I, and one clone of infected cells was shown to have lost the ability to kill its target cells. Instead, the cell would stop dividing and die when presented with the target [23]. Various other functional losses after infection with HTLV-I have been reported in addition [24, 34]. HTLV-I also infects bone marrow cells in vitro, giving rise to T cell lines of different phenotypes, including $OKT4^+T8^-$, $OKT4^-T8^+$, and $OKT4^-8^-$.

D. HTLV-II

HTLV-II was originally isolated from a patient with hairy cell leukemia [16]. Although it shares antigenic determinants of the major *gag* protein, p24, and the envelope proteins [16, 18] of HTLV-I, it is readily distinguishable by both protein serology [17] and nucleic acid hybridization [36]. It has many common biochemical properties with HTLV-I (see Table 1), including the ability to transform T cells in vitro and to mediate a loss of immune functions [34]. It has been isolated only twice, and in spite of its biological activity in vitro it is not clear at this time with what disease, if any, it is associated.

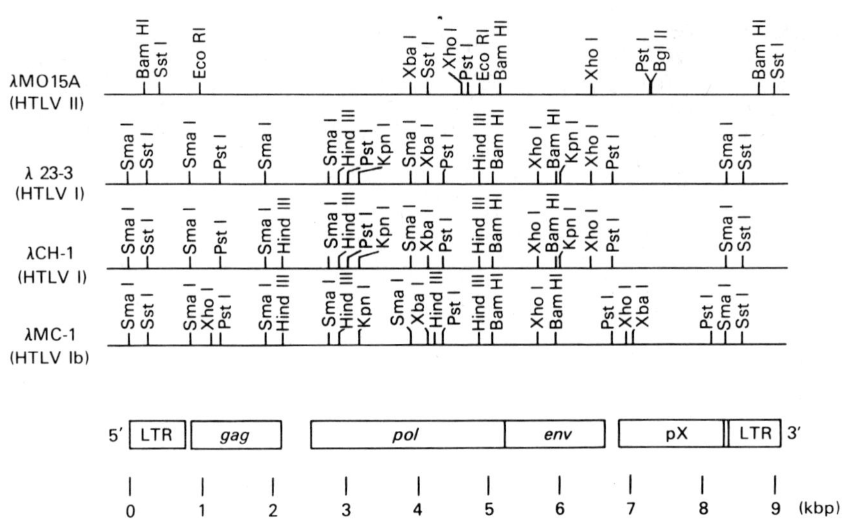

Fig. 2. Genomes and restriction maps of HTLV-I and II. λMO15A is an example of HTLV-II, λ23-3 and λCH-1 are examples of HTLV-1, and λMC-1 is HTLV-Ib. Genomic regions corresponding to LTR, *gag, pol, env,* and pX are drawn to scale according to the published nucleotide sequence of an HTLV-I isolate. Two BglII sites in the 5′ end of λMO15A are not shown

E. Genomes of HTLV-I and HTLV-II

The genome of HTLV-I has been completely sequenced [45]. HTLV-I contains two large terminal repeat (LTR) sequences, in common with other retroviruses, which contain transcriptional control signals. There are fairly typical *gag, pol,* and *env* genes, although the *gag* gene seems to code for three proteins rather than four. In addition, there is an extensive stretch of DNA 3′ to the *env* gene, which contains several potential open reading frames capable of coding for proteins. This is called the pX region, and does not seem to be necessary for viral replication. It may be important in cell transformation, as discussed below, but it is not a cell-derived *onc* gene, since it has no homology with host cell DNA. The structure of the HTLV-I genome is shown in Fig. 2.

The HTLV-II genome also contains a pX region, and has the same gene order as HTLV-I [46]. Heteroduplex analyses using relaxed hybridization conditions indicate that the two viruses are at least distantly related over the length of their genomes. The 3′ portion of pX region seems to be the most closely conserved part of the genome. The HTLV-II pX has been recently sequenced [23], and the 3′ part of this sequence has a large open reading frame which has the coding potential for a protein of at least 38 kilodaltons. The close homology with the analogous region of the HTLV-I genome suggests that the product for which these regions code is important for the biological activity of these viruses.

The *env* gene sequence of HTLV-II has also been recently reported [47], and it also shows significant homology with the HTLV-I *env* gene, except for the extreme 3′ and 5′ termini. The LTRs of the two viruses are markedly different over most of their length [49], but small regions near the RNA cap site, the primer binding site, and a 21-base pair sequence present at four copies in the HTLV-II LTR and three copies in the HTLV-I LTR are highly homologous. These last sequences could represent RNA transcriptional enhancers.

How do HTLV-I and II transform T cells? One puzzling aspect of the molecular biology of HTLV-I and II is that although transformation of infected cells is rapid, the viral genome does not contain a typical (i.e., cell-derived) *onc* gene. Moreover, leukemogenesis appears to be relatively inefficient and to involve a long latent period, as with the chronic animal leukemia viruses.

A second puzzling feature of transformation is that the proviral integration site in fresh leukemic blood cells, leukemic cell lines, and cord blood T cell lines transformed in vitro is nearly always mono- or oligoclonal [23, 53–55], suggesting that only a few of the infected cells become transformed. There does not, however, seem to be a preferential integration site common to different leukemic patients or cell lines [53, 55], suggesting that a specific integration site is not required for transformation, and that the viral genome itself contains all the necessary information.

What is the reason for these apparent paradoxes? It has been shown that the activities of the HTLV-I and II RNA polymerase promoters are strongly influenced by the cell type in which they are present [6, 48], and are far more active in T cells than in other cells. Activity is higher in cells already infected with HTLV than in uninfected cells. This has been interpreted as indicative of the presence of a *trans*-acting factor present in HTLV-infected cells, which strongly activates the HTLV promoter. Sodroski et al. [48] suggest that this factor may in fact be the pX product. If this were the case, and if it had the ability to affect the promoters of cellular genes necessary for T cell function and growth, it could help to explain both rapid transformation by HTLV without the requirement for a specific integration site and a cytopathic or dysfunctional effect on infected T cells. It does not explain, however, the monoclonality of transformed cell populations with respect to the viral integration site.

F. HTLV-III and AIDS

Acquired immunodeficiency syndrome (AIDS) is a recently recognized, generally fatal disease involving helper T cell depletion and multiple opportunistic infections and/or malignancies. It is prevalent among certain high-risk groups, including promiscuous homosexuals, intravenous drug abusers, hemophiliacs, Haitians, and infants born to members of high-risk groups. Because epidemiologic data suggested involvement of a transmissible agent and because of the involvement of $OKT4^+$ T cells in the disease, it seemed possible that an HTLV-like retrovirus might be involved. Essex et al. reported the presence of an antibody present in a large percentage of AIDS victims and high-risk populations which reacted against a cell surface protein of HTLV-I-infected cells [7, 8].

Recently, we reported on a cell line permissive for the growth of a retrovirus from AIDS and pre-AIDS patients [33]. More than 90 isolates from this group of viruses have been obtained [11; P. Markham et al., in preparation]. Based on morphology, biochemical properties of reverse transcriptase [33], antigenic determinants of *env* and *gag* proteins [44], and demonstration of distant but significant nucleic acid homology in the *gag-pol* region, this new virus is distantly related to HTLV-I and II, and has been designated HTLV-III. A more detailed characterization of HTLV-III is given by Wong-Staal et al. (this volume).

The distant relatedness of these viruses suggests that the antibody activity described by Essex and his colleagues reflected crossreactivity of HTLV-I antigen with antibodies to HTLV-III. We have isolated HTLV-III from a majority of pre-AIDS patients and a large number of actual AIDS patients [11], but isolation from the normal population is rare. Almost all AIDS and pre-AIDS patients have antibodies to HTLV-III [42]. A typical Western blot is shown in Fig. 3. The major reactivity is against a 41K protein, which is probably the *env* antigen of HTLV-III. The most recent data show that the prevalence of such antibodies in these patients is virtually 100% [41]. The association is so striking as to overwhelmingly suggest that this virus is the cause of AIDS. Recent evidence indicates that the virus called ALV or IDAV, detected previously by Barré-Sinoussi et al. [2], is a member of the same HTLV subgroup.

These accumulated data indicate that there is a group of related human retroviruses with disparate effects on the same target cell, the $OKT4^+$ T cell. It will be interesting to see whether there are

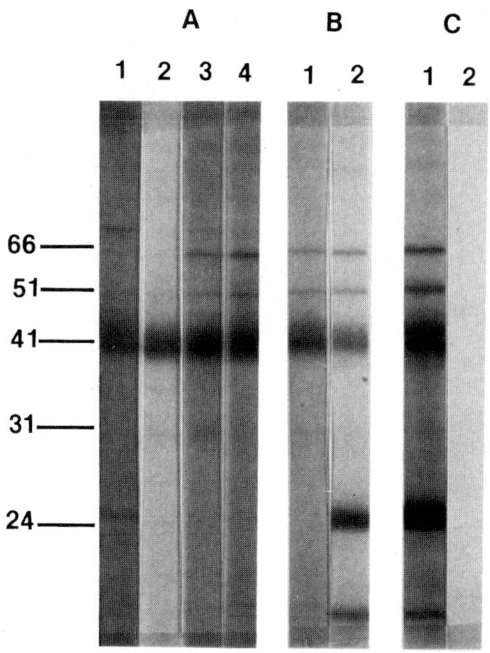

Fig. 3. Analysis of sera for antibodies to HTLV-III by Western blot. *A*, Sera from AIDS patients; *B* sera from lymphadenopathy patients; *C* a positive and a negative serum from homosexual subjects. *Numbers* refer to the molecular weight in kilodaltons

other similar viruses that have yet to be discovered. The identification of the present members of this group gives us opportunities to study T cell biology, as well as the potential to intervene in certain now fatal (and at least in the case of AIDS, increasingly prevalent) T cell diseases.

References

1. Arya SK, Gallo RC, Hahn BH, Shaw GM, Popovic M, Salahuddin SZ, Wong-Staal F (1984) Homology of genome of AIDS-associated virus (HTLV-III) with genomes of human T-cell leukemia viruses (HTLV-I and HTLV-II). Science 225:927–930
2. Barré-Sinoussi F, Chermann JC, Rey F, Nugeyre MT, Chamaret S, Gruest J, Dauguet C, Axler-Blin C, Véinet-Brun F, Rouzioux C, Rosenbaum W, Montagnier L (1983) Isolation of a T-lymphotropic retrovirus from a patient at risk for acquired immune deficiency syndrome (AIDS). Science 220:868–870
3. Blattner WA, Kalyanaraman VS, Robert-Guroff M, Lister TA, Galton DAG, Sarin PS, Crawford MH, Catovsky D, Greaves M, Gallo RC (1982) The human type-C retrovirus, HTLV, in Blacks from the Caribbean region, and relationship to adult T-cell leukemia/lymphoma. Int J Cancer 30:257–264
4. Blayney DW, Blattner WA, Robert-Guroff M, Jaffe ES, Fisher RI, Bunn PA Jr, Patton MG, Rarick HR, Gallo RC (1983) The human T-cell leukemia-lymphoma virus in the southeastern United States. JAMA 250:1048–1052
5. Catovsky D, Greaves MF, Rose M, Galton DAG, Goolden AWG, McCluskey DR, White JM, Lampert I, Bourikas G, Ireland R, Brownell AI, Bridges JM, Blattner WA, Gallo RC (1982) Adult T-cell lymphoma-leukaemia in blacks from the West Indies. Lancet I:639–643
6. Chen ISY, McLaughlin J, Golde DW (1980) Long terminal repeats of human T-cell leukemia virus II genome determine target cell specificity. Nature 309:276–280
7. Essex M, McLane MF, Lee TH, Falk L, Howe CWS, Mullins JI, Cabradilla C, Francis DP (1983a) Antibodies to cell membrane antigens associated with human T-cell leukemia virus in patients with AIDS. Science 220:859–862
8. Essex M, McLane MF, Lee TH, Tachibana N, Mullins JI, Kreiss J, Kasper CK, Poon M-C, Landay A, Stein SF, Francis DP, Cabradilla C, Lawrence DN, Evatt BL (1983b) Antibodies to human T-cell leukemia virus membrane antigens (HTLV-MA) in hemophiliacs. Science 221:1061–1063
9. Gallo RC, Mann D, Broder S, Ruscetti FW, Maeda M, Kalyanaraman VS, Robert-Guroff M, Reitz MS (1982) Human T-cell leukemia-lymphoma virus (HTLV) is in T- but not B-lymphocytes from a patient with cutaneous T-cell lymphoma. Proc Natl Acad Sci USA 79:4680–4684
10. Gallo RC, Kalyanaraman VS, Sarngadharan MG, Sliski A, Vonderheid EC, Maeda M, Nakao Y, Yamada K, Ito Y, Gutensohn N, Murphy S, Bunn PA Jr, Catovsky D, Greaves MF, Blayney DW, Blattner W, Jarrett WFH, zur Hausen H, Seligmann M, Brouet JC, Haynes BF, Jegasothy BV, Jaffe E, Cossman J, Broder S, Fisher RI, Golde DW, Robert-Guroff M (1983) Association of the human type C retrovirus with a subset of adult T-cell cancers. Cancer Res 43:3892–3899
11. Gallo RC, Salahuddin SZ, Popovic M, Shearer GM, Kaplan M, Haynes BF, Palker TJ, Redfield R, Oleske J, Safai B, White G,

Foster P, Markham PD (1984) Frequent detection and isolation of cytopathic retroviruses (HTLV-III) from patients with AIDS and at risk for AIDS. Science 224: 500–503

12. Hahn BH, Shaw GM, Arya SK, Popovic M, Gallo RC, Wong-Staal F (submitted) Molecular cloning and characterization of the virus associated with AIDS (HTLV-III)
13. Haseltine WA, Sodroski J, Patrarca R, Briggs D, Perkins D, Wong-Staal F (1984) Structure of the 3′ terminal region of type II human T-lymphotropic virus: Evidence for a new coding region. Science 225:419–421
14. Kalyanaraman VS, Sarngadharan MG, Poiesz BJ, Ruscetti FW, Gallo RC (1981) Immunological properties of a type C retrovirus isolated from cultured human T-lymphoma cells and comparison to other mammalian retroviruses. J Virol 38:906–915
15. Kalyanaraman VS, Sarngadharan MG, Nakao Y, Ito Y, Aoki T, Gallo RC (1982a) Natural antibodies to the structural core protein (p24) of the human T-cell leukemia (lymphoma) retrovirus found in sera of leukemia patients in Japan. Proc Natl Acad Sci USA 79:1653–1657
16. Kalyanaraman VS, Sarngadharan MG, Robert-Guroff M, Miyoshi I, Blayney D, Golde D, Gallo RC (1982b) A new subtype of human T-cell leukemia virus (HTLV-II) associated with a T-cell variant of hairy cell leukemia. Science 218:571–573
17. Kalyanaraman VS, Jarvis-Morar M, Sarngadharan MG, Gallo RC (1984) Immunological characterization of the low molecular weight *gag* gene proteins p19 and p15 of human T-cell leukemia-lymphoma virus (HTLV) and demonstration of human natural antibodies to them. Virology 132:61–70
18. Lee TH, Coligan JE, McLane MF, Sodroski JG, Popovic M, Wong-Staal F, Gallo RC, Haseltine W, Essex M (in press) Serologic cross-reactivity between envelope gene products of type I and type II human T-cell leukemia virus. Proc Natl Acad Sci USA
19. Mann DL, Popovic M, Murray C, Neuland C, Strong DM, Sarin P, Gallo RC, Blattner WA (1983a) Cell surface antigen expression of newborn cord blood lymphocytes infected with HTLV. J Immunol 131:2021–2024
20. Mann DL, Popovic M, Sarin PS, Murray C, Reitz MS, Strong DM, Haynes BF, Gallo RC, Blattner WA (1983b) Cell lines producing human T-cell lymphoma virus show altered HLA expression. Nature 305:58–60
21. Markham PD, Salahuddin SZ, Macchi B, Robert-Guroff M, Gallo RC (1984) Transformation of different phenotypic types of human bone marrow T-lymphocytes by HTLV-I. Int J Cancer 33:13–17
22. Mitsuya H, Matis LA, Megson M, Bunn PA, Murray C, Mann DL, Gallo RC, Broder S (1983) Generation of an HLA-restricted cytotoxic T-cell line reactive against cultured tumor cells from a patient infected with human T-cell leukemia/lymphoma virus. J Exp Med 158:994–999
23. Mitsuya H, Guo H-G, Megson M, Trainor CD, Reitz MS, Broder S (1984) Transformation and cytopathic effect in an immune T-cell clone infected by human T-cell leukemia-lymphoma virus (HTLV). Science 223:1293–1295
24. Mitsuya H, Guo H-G, Cossman J, Megson M, Reitz M, Broder S (1984) Functional properties of antigen-specific T-cells infected by human T-cell leukemia/lymphoma virus (HTLV-I). Science 225:1484–1486
25. Miyoshi I, Kubonishi I, Yoshimoto S, Akagi T, Ohtsuki Y, Shiraishi Y, Nagato K, Hinuma Y (1981a) Type C virus particles in a cord T-cell line derived by co-cultivating normal human cord blood leukocytes and human leukemic T-cells. Nature 294:770–771
26. Miyoshi T, Yoshimoto S, Kubonishi I, Tagushi H, Shiraishi Y, Ohtsuki Y, Akagi T (1981b) Transformation of normal human cord lymphocytes by co-cultivation with a lethally irradiated human T-cell line carrying type C virus particles. Gann 71:155–156
27. Morgan DA, Ruscetti FW, Gallo RC (1976) Selective in vitro growth of T-lymphocytes from normal human bone marrow. Science 193:1007–1008
28. Poiesz BJ, Ruscetti FW, Gazdar AF, Bunn PA, Minna JD, Gallo RC (1980) Detection and isolation of type C retrovirus particles from fresh and cultured lymphocytes of a patient with cutaneous T-cell lymphoma. Proc Natl Acad Sci USA 77:7415–7419
29. Poiesz BJ, Ruscetti FW, Reitz MS, Kalyanaraman VS, Gallo RC (1981) Isolation of a new type-C retrovirus (HTLV) in primary uncultured cells of a patient with Sézary T-cell leukemia. Nature 294:268–271
30. Posner LE, Robert-Guroff M, Kalyanaraman VS, Poiesz BJ, Ruscetti FW, Fossieck B, Bunn PA Jr, Minna JD, Gallo RC (1981) Natural antibodies to the human T cell lymphoma virus in patients with cutaneous T cell lymphomas. J Exp Med 154: 333–346
31. Popovic M, Lange-Wantzin G, Sarin PS, Mann D, Gallo RC (1983a) Transformation of human umbilical cord blood T cells by human T-cell leukemia/lymphoma virus. Proc Natl Acad Sci USA 80:5402–5406

32. Popovic M, Sarin PS, Robert-Guroff M, Kalyanaraman VS, Mann D, Minowada J, Gallo RC (1983 b) Isolation and transmission of human retrovirus (human T-cell leukemia virus). Science 219:856–859
33. Popovic M, Sarngadharan MG, Read E, Gallo RC (1984) Detection, isolation, and continuous production of cytopathic retroviruses (HTLV-III) from patients with AIDS and pre-AIDS. Science 224:497–500
34. Popovic M, Flomenberg N, Volkman DJ, Mann D, Fauci AS, Dupont B, Gallo RC (1984) Alteration in T-cell functions by infection with HTLV-I or HTLV-II. Science 226:459–462
35. Reitz MS, Poiesz BJ, Ruscetti FW, Gallo RC (1981) Characterization and distribution of nucleic acid sequences of a novel type C retrovirus isolated from neoplastic human T lymphocytes. Proc Natl Acad Sci USA 78: 1887–1891
36. Reitz MS Jr, Popovic M, Haynes BF, Clark SC, Gallo RC (1983) Relatedness by nucleic acid hybridization of new isolates of human T-cell leukemia-lymphoma virus (HTLV) and demonstration of provirus in uncultured leukemic blood cells. Virology 126:688–692
37. Rho HM, Poiesz BJ, Ruscetti FW, Gallo RC (1981) Characterization of the reverse transcriptase from a new retrovirus (HTLV) produced by a human cutaneous T-cell lymphoma cell line. Virology 112:355–360
38. Robert-Guroff M, Ruscetti FW, Posner LE, Poiesz BJ, Gallo RC (1981) Detection of the human T-cell lymphoma virus p19 in cells of some patients with cutaneous T-cell lymphoma and leukemia using a monoclonal antibody. J Exp Med 154:1957–1964
39. Robert-Guroff M, Nakao Y, Notake K, Ito Y, Sliski A, Gallo RC (1982) Natural antibodies to human retrovirus HTLV in a cluster of Japanese patients with adult T cell leukemia. Science 215:975–978
40. Ruscetti FW, Morgan DA, Gallo RC (1977) Functional and morphological characterization of human T-cells continuously grown in vitro. J Immunol 119:131–138
41. Safai B, Sarngadharan MG, Groopman J, Arnett K, Popovic M, Sliski A, Schupbach J, Gallo RC (1984) Seroepidemiological studies of human T-lymphotropic retrovirus type III in acquired immunodeficiency syndrome. Lancet 1:1438–1440
42. Sarngadharan MG, Popovic M, Bruch L, Schupbach J, Gallo RC (1984) Antibodies reactive with human T-lymphotropic retroviruses (HTLV-III) in the serum of patients with AIDS. Science 224:506–508
43. Saxinger WC, Blattner WA, Levine PH, Clark J, Biggar R, Hoh M, Moghissi J, Jacobs P, Wilson L, Jacobson P, Crookes R, Strong M, Ansari AA, Dean AG, Nkrumah FH, Mouvali N, Gallo RC (1984) Human T-cell leukemia virus (HTLV-I) antibodies in Africa. Science 225:1473–1476
44. Schupbach J, Popovic M, Gilden RV, Gonda MA, Sarngadharan MG, Gallo RC (1984) Serological analysis of a subgroup of human T-lymphotropic retroviruses (HTLV-III) associated with AIDS. Science 224:503–504
45. Seiki M, Hattori S, Hirayama Y, Yoshida M (1983) Human adult T-cell leukemia virus: complete nucleotide sequence of the provirus genome integrated in leukemia cell DNA. Proc Natl Acad Sci USA 80:3618 –3622
46. Shaw GM, Gonda MA, Flickinger GH, Hahn BH, Gallo RC, Wong-Staal F (1984) The genomes of evolutionarily divergent members of the human T-cell leukemia virus family (HTLV-I and HTLV-II) are highly conserved, especially in pX. Proc Natl Acad Sci USA 81:4544–4548
47. Sodroski JG, Patarca R, Perkins D, Briggs D, Lee TH, Essex M, Coligan J, Wong-Staal F, Gallo RC, Haseltine WA (1984 a) Sequence of the envelope glycoprotein gene of type II human T lymphotropic virus. Science 225: 421–424
48. Sodroski JG, Rosen CA, Haseltine WA (1984 b) *Trans*-acting transcriptional activation of the long terminal repeat of human T-lymphotropic viruses in infected cells. Science 225:381–385
49. Sodroski JG, Trus M, Perkins D, Patarca R, Wong-Staal F, Gelmann E, Gallo R, Haseltine WA (in press) Repetitive structure in the long terminal repeat element of type II human T cell leukemia virus. Proc Natl Acad Sci USA
50. Tajima K, Tominaga S, Suchi T, Kawagoe T, Komoda H, Hinuma Y, Oda T, Fujita K (in press) Epidemiological analysis on distribution of antibody to adult T-cell leukemia-virus-associated antigen (ATLA): possible horizontal transmission of adult T-cell leukemia virus. Gann
51. Takatsuki K, Uchiyama J, Sagawa K, Yodoi J (1977) Adult T-cell leukemia in Japan. In: Seno S, Takaku F, Irino S (eds) Topics in hematology. Excerpta Medica, Amsterdam, pp 73–77
52. Watanabe T, Seiki M, Yoshida M (1984) HTLV type I (U.S. isolate) and ATLV (Japanese isolate) are the same species of human retrovirus. Virology 133:238–241
53. Wong-Staal F, Hahn B, Manzari V, Colombini S, Franchini G, Gelmann EP, Gallo RC (1983) A survey of human leukaemia for se-

quences of a human retrovirus, HTLV. Nature 302:626–628
54. Yoshida M, Miyoshi I, Hinuma Y (1982) Isolation and characterization of retrovirus from cell lines of human adult T-cell leukemia and its implication in the disease. Proc Natl Acad Sci USA 79:2031–2034
55. Yoshida M, Seiki M, Yamaguchi K, Takatsuki K (1984) Monoclonal integration of human T-cell leukemia provirus in all primary tumors of adult T-cell leukemia suggests causative role of human T-cell leukemia virus in the disease. Proc Natl Acad Sci USA 81:2534–2537

Haematology and Blood Transfusion Vol. 29
Modern Trends in Human Leukemia VI
Edited by Neth, Gallo, Greaves, Janka

Molecular Studies of Human T Cell Leukemia/Lymphotropic Retroviruses

Flossie Wong-Staal[1]

A. Introduction

Human T cell leukemia/lymphoma virus (HTLV), a name originally used to designate a retrovirus associated with a form of mature T cell malignancy, namely adult T cell leukemia (ATL), now stands for a family of human retroviruses isolated in nature, which preferentially infect a subset of T lymphocytes [20]. In addition to their common cell tropism, viruses of this family share other biological, physiochemical, and biochemical properties. However, one major difference in the biological properties of these viruses is directly reflected in their different disease spectrums and transforming capabilities. The virus associated with ATL, renamed HTLV-I, transforms T cells efficiently in culture. A second virus, HTLV-II, which was obtained initially from culture T cells of a patient with hairy cell leukemia, also has the capacity to transform T cells in vitro. A third virus subgroup, HTLV-III, lacks transforming activity but is instead highly cytopathic. HTLV-III has been unambiguously shown to be the etiological agent of the acquired immunodeficiency syndrome (AIDS) [4, 9, 11, 12].

Almost all exogenous, pathogenic animal retroviruses belong to one of two categories: the chronic leukemia viruses are replication competent, require a long latency period for disease induction, and lack transforming activity in vitro. Their genomes contain only the three structural genes (*gag, pol,* and *env*) that are necessary for virus replication. The acute leukemia or sarcoma viruses are usually replication defective, induce disease rapidly in vivo, and transform appropriate target cells efficiently in vitro. They also carry a cell-derived gene which codes for a product necessary for the initiation and usually also maintenance of the transformed phenotype. Members of the HTLV family form a third distinct category. They are replication competent, their genomes containing all three replicative genes. In addition, HTLV-I and HTLV-II contain nucleotide sequences between the *env* gene and the 3′ LTR which contain a long open reading frame (LOR). The LOR sequences are not derived from conserved cellular genes, in contrast to retroviral oncogenes. Even though HTLV-I appears to induce ATL only after long latency periods, along with HTLV-II it can transfrom T lymphocytes rapidly and efficiently in vitro. The LOR product of HTLV-I and HTLV-II is believed to be important in initiating transformation by these viruses. The definition of a LOR gene of HTLV-III is less clear. Other retroviruses that fit into this category are the distantly related bovine leukemia virus (BLV) and a simian retrovirus (STLV-I), which is closely related to HTLV-I. Table 1 summarizes comparisons of leukemogenic/transforming properties of viruses in these three categories.

1 Laboratory of Tumor Cell Biology, Developmental Therapeutics Program, Division of Cancer Treatment, National Cancer Institute, Bethesda, MD 20205, USA

Table 1. Properties of the three classes of leukemia viruses

	Acute	Chronic	(HTLV/BLV)
Disease induction	Rapid	Slow	Slow
Presence of *onc* genes	Yes	No	No
Presence of gene coding for nonvirion structural protein	Yes	No	Yes
Clonality of tumor cells	Polyclonal	Monoclonal	Monoclonal
Provirus integration site	Random	Specific	Random
Transformation in vitro	Yes	No	Yes
Mechanism of action	*trans*	*cis*	(*trans*)

B. The Genomes of HTLV-I and HTLV-II

The complete nucleotide sequence of one isolate of HTLV-I [13] and partial sequences of other HTLV-I isolates (unpublished) as well as one of HTLV-II [7, 16, 18] have been determined. Some unusual features in common among HTLV-II and the several nearly identical isolates of HTLV-I have been revealed by these studies. First, the long terminal repeat (LTR) is unusually long compared with other retroviruses, with the extra length attributed to the R and U5 sequences. Second, a long, noncoding sequence with multiple-stop codons separates the *gag* and *pol* genes. Third, there is a region of about 1.6 kb between the carboxy terminus of the *env* gene and 3′ LTR, which contains several open reading frames. This region, initially referred to as the pX region [13], is not closely homologous to cellular sequences of vertebrate cells [1] and therefore is not a typical retroviral oncogene. Deletions and substitutions within the first 0.6 kb of pX found in a variant, HTLV-Ib, obtained from an African ATL patient did not affect the transforming capacity of this virus [6 a] (unpublished work with L. Ratner). Comparison of the pX of HTLV-I and that of HTLV-II revealed that the first 0.6 kb is nonconserved, but the following 1.0 kb is highly conserved, and contains a single long open reading frame, LOR [7, 14]. Splice acceptor consensus sequences are present 5′ to LOR, which does not initiate with the ATG codon [7]. Therefore, the LOR protein product is likely to be a fused protein containing amino acid residues coded by *gag* or *env*. The HTLV-I LOR sequence predicts a protein product of at least 38 kd. Sera of patients positive for HTLV-I recognize a 40- to 42-kd protein expressed in all HTLV-transformed cells, including nonproducer cells that do not synthesize virus or virion structural proteins. Amino acid analysis of cyanogen bromide cleavage fragments of this protein suggests that it is coded at least in part by the LOR sequences [8]. Sequence analysis of the BLV genome also reveals the presence of an open reading frame similar in size to HTLV-I LOR in the corresponding region [10].

C. Possible Mechanism of Transformation and Leukemogenesis by HTLV-I and HTLV-II

Cells infected by HTLV-I and HTLV-II in vitro are initially polyclonal and go through a growth crisis within 4–6 weeks. Predominantly clonal cells then emerge as immortalized cells (unpublished data). Often, these cells become independent of T cell growth factor (TCGF) and their morphology resembles that of the primary leukemic cells [3]. Although the transformed cells are clonal, the site of provirus integration is variable in different clones. The lack of a conserved integration site suggests that these viruses act by a *trans*-mechanism in cellular transformation, i.e., a diffusible viral protein product is directly involved. By analyzing expression of different viral structural proteins at different time intervals after infection and clones of trans-

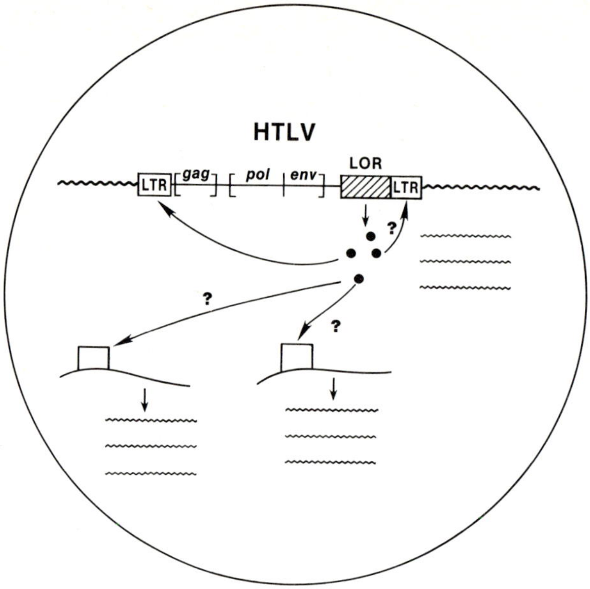

Fig. 1. Transcriptional activation of viral and cellular genes by the LOR protein: A model for the mechanism of transformation by HTLV

formed cells containing defective proviruses, we have ruled out the expression of *gag, pol,* and *env* proteins as a prerequisite for the initiation of transformation (unpublished data). The only remaining candidate is the LOR protein, especially in view of the high degree of conservation of this gene between the two transforming HTLVs. Studies on the promoter-enhancer activity of LTRs of HTLV-I and HTLV-II showed that transcription of LTR-linked genes is elevated manifold in infected cells, indicating a *trans*-acting transcriptional activation phenomenon via a viral protein [17]. There is indirect evidence that the LOR protein is responsible for this enhancing activity. Based on these studies, one can construct a model in which the LOR protein can also regulate cellular promoter-enhancer function at distant sites and the cellular genes regulated are associated with T cell proliferation. Therefore, the mechanism of transformation by HTLV is more similar to certain DNA tumor viruses than to other retroviruses. Several genes have already been identified that are activated by infection with HTLV-I and HTLV-II, and all these have been linked to T cell proliferation (Fig. 1). Therefore, it is possible to test directly whether the LOR protein binds to the enhancer-promoter sequences of these genes.

Unlike the in vitro-transformed cells, fresh ATL cells frequently contain no detectable viral mRNA or proteins, including LOR [2]. In addition, although each of these ATL cell samples is monoclonal, the integration sites of these proviruses vary. So the virus does not seem to function in *cis* or *trans* in maintaining the leukemic state. We speculate a two-stage leukemogenesis event, with the early stage being analogous to the in vitro transformation process, resulting in immortalization and enhanced proliferation of the infected cells. This in turn increases the chance of a mutation or gene rearrangement which leads to the progression of the disease. At this late stage, the virus has done its damage and is no longer needed.

D. Molecular Biology of the HTLV-III, the Etiological Agent of AIDS

A novel member of the HTLV family designated as HTLV-III has recently been identified as the etiological agent of AIDS, a disease characterized by depletion of the OKT4+ helper T cells (Gallo et al., this volume). We have cloned the genomes of several isolates of HTLV-III [5, 15]. Nucleotide sequence analysis of two of these clones revealed many structural similarities to HTLV-I and HTLV-II, particularly in the presence of extra, non-cell derived genes. Recent experiments have indicated that HTLV-III infected cells contained factors that activate transcription of HTLV-III LTR-linked genes [19], suggesting that the HTLV-III has a similar gene in *trans*-acting transcriptional activation. Either HTLV-III "LOR" activates a different set of cellular genes from LOR of HTLV-I or -II to account for the cytopathic, rather than immortalizing, effect of the virus, or HTLV-III has a transforming activity which is masked by its profound cytopathic effect.

The HTLV-III genome is completely exogenous and does not carry a conserved cellular gene. Integrated provirus can be detected in infected cell cultures as well as peripheral blood lymphocytes and lymph node tissue of AIDS and pre-AIDS patients [15]. The infected cells are polyclonal with respect to provirus integration, as expected for a virus that induces cell death rather than clonal expansion of the target cells. Furthermore, a large amount of unintegrated viral DNA persists in both the long-term cultured cells and patient tissues [15], a feature that seems to be characteristic of other cytopathic retroviruses. We also found that very few (less than 1 in 100) cells were infected in a population of lymphocytes from AIDS and pre-AIDS patients, and virus information is not detectable in several Kaposi tumor tissues examined. These results suggest that HTLV-III does not have a direct role in the proliferation of lymphocytes in lymphadenopathy of pre-AIDS patients or in the clonal expansion of endothelial cells of Kaposi tumors. These are secondary syndromes that develop as a consequence of the depletion or impaired function of the helper-inducer T-lymphocytes infected by HTLV-III.

One salient feature emerging from analyses of the genomes of different HTLV-III isolates is the extent of polymorphism among different isolates. So far, all isolates can be distinguishable from each other based on the analyses with five or six restriction enzymes. There is a whole spectrum with respect to the degree of similarity among different isolates. An isolate from a Haitian patient has practically no correspondence of restriction enzyme sites except in the LTR regions [6 b] and probably represents one end of the spectrum. This degree of genetic diversity is not seen with different HTLV-I and HTLV-II isolates, and may be due to immunoselection or to the highly replicative nature of HTLV-III as opposed to the cryptic state of the HTLV-I and HTLV-II proviruses in vivo. It will be important to determine whether changes in the HTLV-III genomes cluster in any particular regions and whether they are significant enough to alter the immunological reactivities of the different isolates.

References

1. Franchini G, Wong-Staal F, Gallo RC (1984) Molecular studies of human T-cell leukemia virus and adult T-cell leukemia. J Invest Dermatol 83:63 s–66 s
2. Franchini G, Wong-Staal F, Gallo RC (1984) Human T-cell leukemia virus (HTLV-I) transcripts in fresh and cultured cells of patients with adult T-cell leukemia. Proc Natl Acad Sci USA 81:6207–6211
3. Gallo RC (1984) Human T-cell leukaemia-lymphoma virus and T-cell malignancies in adults. In: Franks LM, Wyke LM, Weiss RA (eds) Cancer surveys. Oxford University Press, Oxford, pp 113–159
4. Gallo RC, Salahuddin SZ, Popovic M, Shearer GM, Kaplan M, Haynes BF, Palker TJ, Redfield R, Oleske J, Safai B, White F, Foster P, Markham PD (1984) Frequent detection and isolation of cytopathic retroviruses (HTLV-III) from patients with AIDS and at risk for AIDS. Science 224:500–503
5. Hahn BH, Shaw GM, Arya SK, Popovic M, Gallo RC, Wong-Staal F (1984) Molecular cloning and characterization of the HTLV-III virus associated with AIDS. Nature 212:166–169

6a. Hahn BH, Shaw GM, Popovic M, LoMonico A, Gallo RC, Wong-Staal F (1984) Molecular cloning and analysis of a new variant of human T-cell leukemia virus (HTLV-Ib) from an African patient with adult T-cell leukemia-lymphoma. Int J Cancer (in press)

6b. Hahn BH, Gonda M, Shaw GM, Popovic M, Hoxie JA, Gallo RC, Wong-Staal F (1985) Genomic diversity of the AIDS virus HTLV-III: Different viruses exhibit greatest

divergence in their envelope genes. Proc Natl Acad Sci (in press)
7. Haseltine WA, Sodroski J, Patarca R, Briggs D, Perkins D, Wong-Staal F (1984) Structure of 3′ terminal region of type II human T lymphotropic virus: evidence for new coding region. Science 225:419–421
8. Lee TH, Coligan JE, Sadroski JG, Haseltine WA, Salahuddin SZ, Wong-Staal F, Gallo RC, Essex M (1984) Identification of the putative transforming protein of the human T-cell leukemia viruses HTLV-I and HTLV-II. Science 226:57–61
9. Popovic M, Sarngadharan MG, Reed E, Gallo RC (1984) Detection, isolation, and continuous production of cytopathic retroviruses (HTLV-III) from patients with AIDS and pre-AIDS. Science 24:497–500
10. Rice N, Stephens RM, Couez D, Deschamp J, Keltmann R, Burny A, Gilden R (1984) The nucleotide sequence of the *env* gene and post-*env* region bovine leukemia virus. Virology (in press)
11. Sarngadharan MG, Popovic M, Bruch L, Schupbach J, Gallo RC (1984) Antibodies reactive with human T-lymphotropic retroviruses (HTLV-III) in the serum of patients with AIDS. Science 224:506–508
12. Schupbach J, Sarngadharan MG, Gallo RC (1984) Antigens on HTLV-infected cells recognized by leukemia and AIDS sera are related to HTLV viral glycoprotein. Science 224:607–610
13. Seiki M, Hattori S, Hirayama Y, Yoshida M (1983) Human adult T-cell leukemia virus: complete nucleotide sequence of the provirus genome integrated in leukemia cell DNA. Proc Natl Acad Sci USA 80:3618–3622
14. Shaw GM, Gonda MA, Flickinger GH, Hahn BH, Gallo RC, Wong-Staal F (1984a) Genomes of evolutionarily divergent members of the human T-cell leukemia virus family (HTLV-I and HTLV-II) are highly conserved, especially in pX. Proc Natl Acad Sci USA 81:4544–4548
15. Shaw GM, Hahn BH, Arya SK, Groopman G, Gallo RC, Wong-Staal F (1984b) Molecular characterization of human T-cell leukemia (lymphotropic) virus type III in the acquired immunodeficiency syndrome. Science 226:1165–1171
16. Shimotohno K, Golde DW, Miwa M, Sugimura T, Chen ISY (1984) Nucleotide sequence analysis of the long term repeat of human T-cell leukemia virus type II. Proc Natl Acad Sci USA 81:1079–1083
17. Sodroski JG, Rosen CA, Haseltine WA (1984a) *Trans*-acting transcriptional activation of the long terminal repeat of human T lymphotropic viruses in infected cells. Science 225:381–385
18. Sodroski J, Trus M, Perkins D, Patarca R, Wong-Staal F, Gelmann E, Gallo RC, Haseltine WA (1984b) Repetitive structure in the long-terminal-repeat element of a type II human T-cell leukemia virus. Proc Natl Acad Sci USA 81:4617–4621
19. Sodroski J, Rosen C, Wong-Staal F, Popovic M, Arya SK, Gallo RC, Haseltine WA (1984c) Trans-active transcriptional regulation of the human T-cell leukemia virus type III long terminal repeat. Science (in press)
20. Wong-Staal F, Gallo RC (1985) The family of human I-lymphotropic leukemia viruses (HTLV): HTLV-I as the cause of adult T-cell leukemia and HTLV-III as the cause of AIDS. Blood 65:253–263

Haematology and Blood Transfusion Vol. 29
Modern Trends in Human Leukemia VI
Edited by Neth, Gallo, Greaves, Janka

The Molecular Biology of Human T Cell Leukemia Virus and its Roles in Leukemogenesis of Adult T Cell Leukemia *

M. Yoshida and M. Seiki

A. Introduction

Adult T cell leukemia (ATL) is a unique T cell malignancy proposed by Takatsuki and his colleagues [1]; it is endemic in the south-western part of Japan [1, 2] and has been found in the Caribbean [3]. Human T cell leukemia virus (HTLV) was isolated by Gallo and his colleagues [4] from a patient with cutaneous T cell lymphoma, and subsequently adult T cell leukemia virus (ATLV) was isolated by us [5]. We have molecularly cloned the provirus genome [6] and determined the total nucleotide sequence of the ATLV provirus genome [7]. Based on the structural analysis, we recently reported that ATLV and HTLV type I are the same virus species [8, 9]. After these characterizations, we use the term HTLV-I for the virus previously reported as ATLV. HTLV is exogenous for humans [5, 10], distinct from known animal retroviruses [6, 7], and is closely associated with ATL [2, 5, 11]. In this chapter, we summarize our studies on the mechanism of leukemogenesis of ATL and identification of the viral proteins.

* Department of Viral Oncology, Cancer Institute, Kami-Ikebukuro, Toshima-ku, Tokyo 170, Japan

B. HTLV Plays Causative Roles in ATL Development

Structural analysis of HTLV genome [7] showed that it contains *gag*, *pol*, *env*, and an extra sequence of *pX* which can code for some proteins (Fig. 1). Since none of them showed sequence homology with uninfected human DNA, it was concluded that HTLV has no typical *onc* gene derived from a cellular sequence [7]. Thus, the following question was raised: is HTLV involved directly in leukemogenesis of ATL?

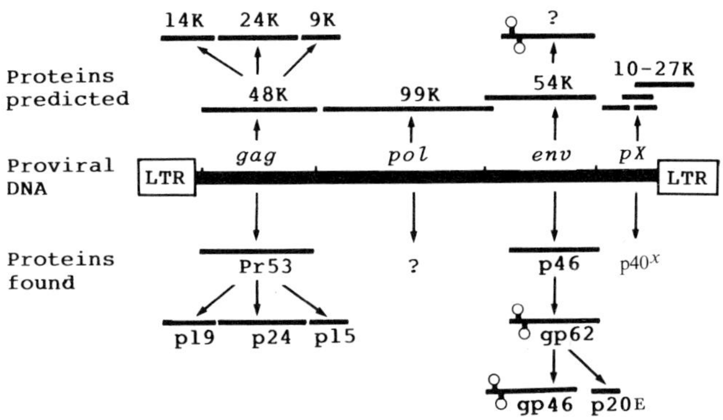

Fig. 1. Summary of provirus genome and proteins of HTLV. The *thick bar* in the middle represents the provirus genome of HTLV-I and *boxes* at the ends are LTR. Proteins above the genome are predicted from DNA sequences and those below the genome have actually been identified in HTLV-infected cells

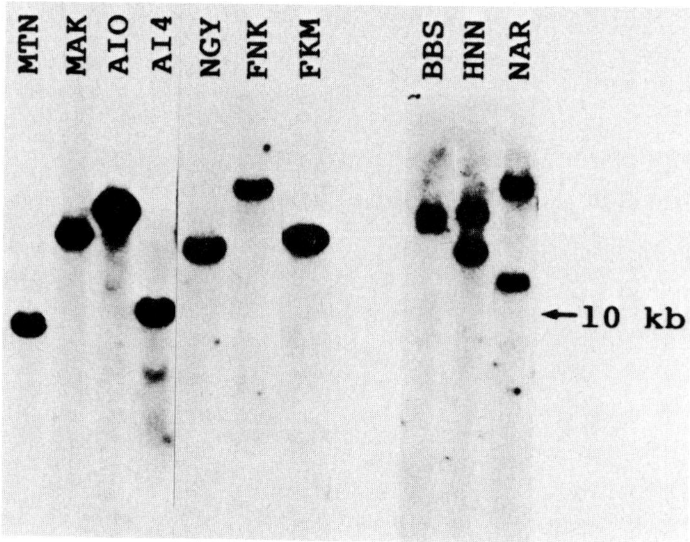

Fig. 2. Detection of HTLV provirus sequences in fresh leukemic cell DNA. Lymphocyte DNA samples from ATL patients were digested with EcoRI, which does not cleave the provirus sequence, and subjected to blotting analysis. ^{32}P-labeled DNA of cloned HTLV-I was used as a representative probe in this analysis

To solve this question, we surveyed the provirus integration in fresh tumor cells of 122 cases of ATL. Only fresh tumor cells were used in this study. Cellular DNA isolated from fresh lymphocytes was digested with EcoRI, which does not cleave the proviral genome, and analyzed by the blotting procedure. By this assay, the provirus sequence integrated monoclonally was detected as a discrete band. All 122 patients with typical ATL were infected with HTLV and the provirus sequences were detected as one or two discrete bands as shown in Fig. 2 [12]. These results clearly indicate that the leukemic cells were monoclonal, originating from a single cell infected with HTLV, because integration of HTLV genome in nonleukemic cell DNA was random [13, 14]. The monoclonal expansion of infected cells as tumor cells in all 122 cases strongly suggests that HTLV directly infects the target cell which becomes leukemic, thus implying that HTLV has causative roles in ATL development [12, 13]. If viral involvement was indirect, for example, mediated by one or more factors released by infected cells, some cases should have leukemic cells in which the provirus genome is absent or is integrated at multiple sites.

C. No Specific Integration Site in Leukemic Cell DNA

As described, HTLV plays causative roles in ATL development [12, 13], although the virus has no typical *onc* gene [7]. Consequently, one of the most probable mechanisms of ATL leukemogenesis was insertional mutagenesis in which the proviruses are integrated into a few specific loci on the chromosomal DNA and then activate an adjacent cellular *onc* gene [15].

In order to test this possibility, cellular sequences of fresh leukemic cells of a patient which were flanked to the integrated provirus were cloned and used as probes to detect DNA rearrangements induced by provirus integration at the same locus in other patients. Two sets of probes were isolated from independent patients and each set of the probes could detect an approximately 30 kilobases region of cellular DNA. These probes detected rearranged DNA fragments in the control DNA from which the probes were isolated, but did not detect such rearranged fragments in the other 35 ATL patients [16]. These observations indicate that HTLV has no common site for integration into leukemic cell DNA.

We further analyzed the specificity of provirus integration at the chromosomal

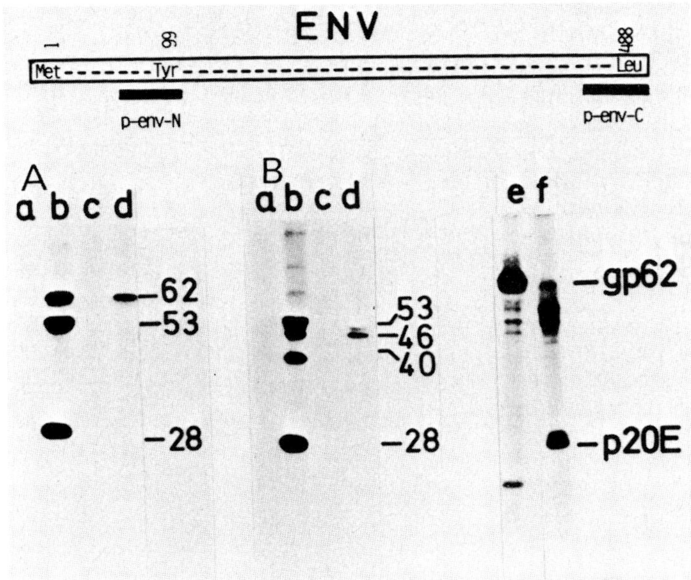

Fig. 3. Identification of *env* gene products. Decapeptide of the COOH terminus of the predicted *env* polypeptide (*top*) was synthesized and antiserum was prepared in a rabbit. MT-2 cells were labeled with cysteine ^{35}S for 1 h with (*B*) or without (*A*) tunicamycin treatment and extracts were treated with: normal human serum (*lane a*); serum from an ATL patient (*lane b*); normal rabbit serum (*lane c*); and anti-*env*-C peptide (*lane d*). Pulse-labeled MT-2 cells (*lane e*) were chased with excess cold cysteine (*lane f*) and both cell extracts were treated with anti-*env*-C peptide

level by using the human × mouse somatic cell hybrid strategy. The hybrid cells were analyzed for two probes isolated from cellular flanking sequences as described and it was found that one probe cosegregated with chromosome 7 and the other cosegregated with chromosome 17 [16]. Thus, the absence of a common integration site for HTLV was confirmed at the chromosomal level. These results do not support the simple activation of a specific cellular *onc* gene by HTLV LTR.

D. Identification and Characterization of *env* Gene Products

The absence of a common integration site in primary tumor cells [16] does not support a *cis*-acting function of the integrated proviruses. Thus, proteins coded by HTLV genome are suspected to be involved in ATL development as *trans*-acting factors. The identification and characterization of the viral proteins are also important to establish the systems for diagnosis and prevention of HTLV infection.

Monospecific antiserum against the synthetic peptide which is the COOH terminus of the predicted *env* gene product was used to identify the products. This antiserum detected a protein of 62 kilodaltons in HTLV-producing cell lines [17, 18] (Fig. 3). When the cell lines were pretreated with tunicamycin, the same antiserum detected 46 kilodaltons protein as a major band instead of 62 kilodaltons. These results indicate that the *env* gene product is 46 kilodaltons which is then glycosylated into gp62. To test the possible processing of gp62, the pulse-labeled (lane e) cells were chased with cold cysteine (lane f). Antiserum against the peptide now detected a protein of 20 kilodaltons. Thus, the COOH terminal portion of gp62 was processed into 20 kilodaltons protein (p20E) [18].

For detection of the other matured *env* gene product derived from the NH_2 terminal half of gp62, we produced a hybrid protein composed of the *env* polypeptide and β-galactosidase in *Escherichia coli* as follows. Two fragments of HTLV *env* gene were inserted into expression vectors pORF1 and pORF2, respectively [19]. *E. coli* transformed with these plasmids produced new proteins with expected sizes as much as 10%–20% of the total proteins [20]. The hybrid proteins produced were found to cross-react with sera from ATL patients, indicating that these hybrid proteins conserved antigenic sites in the native *env* gene products. Using antiserum against these *env* β-galactosidases, two diffuse bands of gp46 and gp62 were identified as *env* gene products [18]. In summary, the *env* gene codes for 46 kilodaltons precursor which is glycosylated into gp62, and the gp62 is further processed into gp46 and p20E. The proteins so far identified and the gene locations are summarized in Fig. 1 [17, 18].

Finally, we have recently established an EIA system for diagnosis of HTLV infection, detecting *env*-specific antibodies in human sera [20]. Since these hybrid proteins can be produced on a large scale and are free from any possible contamination by human proteins, the system should be widely useful.

References

1. Uchiyama T, Yodoi J, Sagawa K, Takatsuki K, Uchino H (1977) Blood 50:481–492
2. Hinuma Y, Nagata K, Hanaoka M, Nakai M, Matsumoto T, Kinoshita K, Shirakawa S, Miyoshi I (1981) Proc Natl Acad Sci USA 78:6476–6480
3. Blattner WA, Kalyanaraman VS, Robert-Guroff M, Lister TA, Galton DAG, Sarin PS, Crawford MH, Catovsky D, Greeves M, Gallo RC (1982) Int J Cancer 30:257–264
4. Poiesz BJ, Ruscetti FW, Gazdar AF, Bunn PA, Minna JD, Gallo RC (1980) Proc Natl Acad Sci USA 77:7415–7419
5. Yoshida M, Miyoshi I, Hinuma Y (1982) Proc Natl Acad Sci USA 79:2031–2035
6. Seiki M, Hattori S, Yoshida M (1982) Proc Natl Acad Sci USA 79:6899–6902
7. Seiki M, Hattori S, Hirayama Y, Yoshida M (1983) Proc Natl Acad Sci USA 80:3618–3622
8. Watanabe T, Seiki M, Yoshida M (1983) Science 222:1178
9. Watanabe T, Seiki M, Yoshida M (1984) Virology 133:238–241
10. Reitz MS, Poiesz BJ, Ruscetti FM, Gallo RC (1981) Proc Natl Acad Sci USA 78:1887–1891
11. Kalyanaraman VS, Sarngadhara MG, Nakao Y, Ito Y, Aoki T, Gallo RC (1982) Proc Natl Acad Sci USA 79:1653–1657
12. Yoshida M, Seiki M, Yamaguchi K, Takatsuki K (1984) Proc Natl Acad Sci USA 81:2534–2537
13. Yoshida M, Seiki M, Hattori S, Watanabe T (1984) In: Gallo RC, Essex ME, Grass L (eds) Human T-cell leukemia-lymphoma viruses. Cold Spring Harbor Laboratory, New York, pp 141–148
14. Yoshida M (1983) Gann 74:777–789
15. Hayward WS, Neel BG, Astrin SM (1981) Nature 290:475–480
16. Seiki M, Eddy R, Shows RB, Yoshida M (1984) Nature 309:640–642
17. Hattori S, Imagawa K, Shimizu F, Hashimura E, Seiki M, Yoshida M (1983) Gann 74:790–793
18. Hattori S, Kiyokawa T, Imagawa K, Shimizu F, Hashimura E, Seiki M, Yoshida M (1984) Virology 136:338–347
19. Weinstock GM, AP Rhys C, Berman ML, Hampar E, Jackson D, Silhavy TJ, Weisemann J, Zweig M (1983) Proc Natl Acad Sci USA 80:4432–4436
20. Kiyokawa T, Hattori S, Seiki M, Yoshida M (1984) Proc Natl Acad Sci USA 81:6202–6206

Haematology and Blood Transfusion Vol. 29
Modern Trends in Human Leukemia VI
Edited by Neth, Gallo, Greaves, Janka

HTLV-I Antibodies Associated with Cutaneous T Cell Lymphoma in Denmark *

G. Lange Wantzin, C. Saxinger, and K. Thomsen

A. Introduction

The first isolation and characterization of a human retrovirus was done by Gallo and co-workers from patients with aggressive cases of adult T cell leukemia/lymphoma in the United States [15, 16]. This virus, named human T cell leukemia/lymphoma virus (HTLV-I) is a T cell-tropic retrovirus [8, 9], initially found sporadically among United States cases of adult T cell leukemias and lymphomas (ATLL) with cutaneous manifestations resembling aggressive variants of mycosis fungoides. Subsequently, HTLV-I was specifically linked to adult T cell malignancies in Japan and the Caribbean [8]. A second human retrovirus, HTLV-II, which is related to but distinct from all previous HTLV-I isolates, was identified and isolated from a patient with hairy cell leukemia [12]. Recently, a third retrovirus, HTLV-III has been isolated and is a probable etiologic agent in the acquired immune deficiency syndrome (AIDS) [4–7].

In early studies, HTLV-I was identified in less than 1% of cutaneous T cell lymphoma (CTCL) patients and therefore was not considered a likely agent in these malignancies [8]. Because of several clinical similarities between CTCL and the HTLV-positive ATLL cases, we have used a more sensitive indirect ELISA microtest for HTLV antibodies [19] for the presence of HTLV antibodies in patients with CTCL.

* Laboratory of Tumor Cell Biology, National Institutes of Health, Bethesda, Maryland 20205, USA

B. Materials and Methods

A total of 167 serum samples from 104 patients were studied. Of these, 68 patients had CTCL. There were 5 with Sézary syndrome, 4 with mycosis fungoides tumor stage (MFIII), 15 with mycosis fungoides plaque stage, diagnostic histology (MFII), 40 with mycosis fungoides plaque stage, nondiagnostic histology (MFI), and 4 with lymphomatoid papulosis. The remaining control group of 36 contained patients with skin infiltrates of non-T cell malignancies as well as cutaneous infiltrates of benign T cells.

An ELISA assay for detection of HTLV antibodies in human sera has been developed and presented in detail earlier [19]. An additional confirmatory neutralization test was used, also described earlier in detail [19]. A suppression of the ELISA value by 50% in the sample exposed to the unlabeled anti-HTLV, relative to a standard normal human serum, was considered positive, indicated by + (confirmatory result for the presence of anti-HTLV).

C. Results and Comments

Of the 68 patients with CTCL, 10 patients were found to be HTLV antibody positive although with low titers [21]. The distribution of these HTLV antibody-positive patients among the different subgroups of CTCL is given in Table 1. The data demonstrate that positive HTLV antibody sera were found in the earliest prediagnostic stage, MFI, where tumor cells are not rec-

Table 1. Number of HTLV antibody-positive sera from 68 patients with cutaneous T cell lymphoma

Diagnosis	HTLV antibody-positive
Sézary syndrome	0/5
Mycosis fungoides (tumor stage)	2/4
Mycosis fungoides (plaque stage, diagnostic histology)	0/15
Mycosis fungoides (plaque stage, nondiagnostic histology)	7/40
Lymphomatoid papulosis	1/4
Total	10/68

ognizable in the plaque lesions as well as the later stages, MFIII, where tumor cells are histologically diagnosed and skin lesions have progressed to tumor stage. Of interest, one of the four patients with lymphomatoid papulosis had positive HTLV antibody sera. (Lymphomatoid papulosis is characterized by remittent hemorrhagic papules on the skin that in 10% of cases may progress to malignancy.) Sequential studies of at least 1 year were performed on six of the patients and, to summarize, HTLV antibody status remained constant throughout this period during which three of the patients changed from relapse to remission stages. In the control group consisting of 31 non-CTCL patients and 5 CTCL family members, all but 1 were negative in the ELISA assay for HTLV-I antibody. The positive patient had Kaposi's sarcoma.

Since the discovery, isolation, and characterization of HTLV-I in the United States, a series of epidemiologic studies have identified a particular form of aggressive T cell malignancies: adult T cell leukemias/lymphomas which are closely related to HTLV-I infection in different parts of the world [1–3, 10, 11, 13, 14, 17, 18, 20, 22, 23]. Other, much less aggressive T cell lymphomas or CTCL include mycosis fungoides, Sézary syndrome, and lymphomatoid papulosis which in past studies were HTLV negative with rare exceptions [8]. However, by more sensitive serum antibody assay [19] and a careful subtyping of patients with CTCL, we have found that positive HTLV-I antibody sera are found in cases of CTCL, including the very early clinically and nonhistologically confirmed stages, at an overall rate (15%) not previously reported or generally expected. The detection of relatively low HTLV-I antibody titers in the CTCL diseases may be explained by a restricted level of virus replication, an earlier transitory infectious stage, or only partial cross-reactivity with HTLV-I proteins used in the assay, i.e., a virus closely related to, but immunologically distinct from HTLV-I may be involved. In summary, the present data suggest that exposure to HTLV-I or a related virus exists in Denmark, that an elevated frequency of low titer antibody occurs in some cases of CTCL in the early histologically nondiagnostic (plaque) stage and also in later malignant stages, and finally that the presence of antibody is independent of the clinical status of these patients, if they are in remission or relapse.

References

1. Blattner W, Kalyanaraman V, Robert-Guroff M, Lister R, Galton D, Sarin P, Crawford M, Catovsky D, Greaves M, Gallo RC (1982) The human type-C retrovirus, HTLV, in Blacks from the Caribbean region, and relationships to adult T-cell leukemia/lymphoma. Int J Cancer 30:257–264
2. Blattner WA, Gibbs WN, Saxinger C, Robert-Guroff M, Clark J, Lofters W, Hanchard B, Campbell M, Gallo RC (1983) Human T-cell leukeamia/lymphoma virus-associated lymphoreticular neoplasia in Jamaica. Lancet II:61–64
3. Catovsky D, Greaves MF, Rose M, Galton DAG, Goolden AWG, McCluskey DR, White JM, Lampert I, Bourikas G, Ireland R, Brownell AI, Bridges JM, Blattner WA, Gallo RC (1982) Adult T-cell lymphoma-leukemia in blacks from the West Indies. Lancet I:639–642
4. Popovic M, Sarngadharan MG, Read E, Gallo RC (1984) Detection, isolation, and continuous production of cytopathic retroviruses (HTLV-III) from patients with AIDS and pre-AIDS. Science 224:297–500
5. Gallo RC, Salahuddin SZ, Popovic M, Shearer GM, Kaplan M, Haynes BF, Palker

TJ, Redfield R, Oleske J, Safai B, White G, Foster P, Markham PD (1984) Frequent detection and isolation of cytopathic retroviruses (HTLV-III) from patients with AIDS and at risk for AIDS. Science 224:500–503
6. Schüpbach J, Popovic M, Gilden RV, Gonda MA, Sarngadharan MG, Gallo RC (1984) Serological analysis of a subgroup of human T-lymphotropic retroviruses (HTLV-III) associated with AIDS. Science 224:503–505
7. Sarngadharan MG, Popovic M, Bruch L, Schüpbach J, Gallo RC (1984) Antibodies reactive with human T-lymphotropic retroviruses (HTLV-III) in the serum of patients with AIDS. Science 224:506–508
8. Gallo RC, Kalyanaraman VS, Sarngadharan MG, Sliski A, Vonderheid EC, Maeda M, Nakao Y, Yamada K, Ito Y, Gutensohn N, Murphy S, Bunn PA Jr, Catovsky D, Greaves MF, Blayney DW, Blattner WA, Jarret WFH, zur Hausen H, Seligmann M, Grouet JC, Haynes BF, Jegasothy BV, Jaffe E, Cossman J, Broder S, Fisher RI, Golde DW, Robert-Guroff M (1983) Association of the human type C retrovirus with a subset of adult T-cell cancers. Cancer Res 43:3892–3899
9. Gallo RC, Mann D, Broder S, Ruscetti FW, Maeda M, Kalyanaraman VS, Robert-Guroff M, Reitz MS (1982) Human T-cell leukemia-lymphoma virus (HTLV) is in T but not B lymphocytes from a patient with cutaneous T-cell lymphoma. Proc Natl Acad Sci USA 79:5680–5683
10. Hinuma Y, Komoda H, Chosa T, Kondo T, Kohakura M, Takenada T, Kikuchi M, Ichimaru M, Unoki K, Sato I, Matuo R, Takichi Y, Uchino H, Hanaoka M (1982) Antibodies to adult T-cell leukemia-virus-associated antigen (ATLA) in sera from patients with ATL and controls in Japan: A nationwide sero-epidemiologic study. Int J Cancer 29: 631–635
11. Kalyanaraman VS, Sarngadharan MG, Nakao Y, Ito Y, Aoki T, Gallo RC (1982) Natural antibodies to the structural core protein (p24) of the human T-cell leukemia (lymphoma) retrovirus found in sera of leukemia patients in Japan. Proc Natl Acad Sci USA 79:1653–1657
12. Kalyanaraman VS, Sarngadharan MG, Robert-Guroff M, Miyoshi I, Blayney D, Golde D, Gallo RC (1982) A new subtype of human T-cell leukemia virus (HTLV-II) associated with a T-cell variant of hairy cell leukemia. Science 218:571–573
13. Miyoshi I, Kubonishi I, Yoshimoto S, Akagi T, Ohtsuki Y, Shiraishi Y, Nagata K, Hinuma Y (1981) Type C virus particles in a cord T-cell line derived by cocultivating normal human cord leukocytes and human leukaemia T-cells. Nature 294:770–771
14. Popovic M, Sarin PS, Robert-Guroff M, Kalyanaraman VS, Mann D, Minowada J, Gallo RC (1983) Isolation and transmission of human retrovirus (human T-cell leukemia virus). Science 219:856–859
15. Poiesz BJ, Ruscetti FW, Gazdar AF, Bunn PA, Minna JD, Gallo RC (1980) Detection and isolation of type-C retrovirus particles from fresh and cultured lymphocytes of a patient with cutaneous T-cell lymphoma. Proc Natl Acad Sci USA 77:7415–7419
16. Poiesz BJ, Ruscetti FW, Reitz MS, Kalyanaraman VS, Gallo RC (1981) Isolation of a new type-C retrovirus (HTLV) in primary uncultured cells of a patient with Sézary T-cell leukemia. Nature 294:268–271
17. Robert-Guroff M, Nakao Y, Notake K, Ito Y, Slisky A, Gallo RC (1982) Natural antibodies to human retrovirus HTLV in a cluster of Japanese patients with adult T cell leukemia. Science 215:975–978
18. Robert-Guroff M, Schupbach J, Blayney D, Kalyanaraman V, Merino F, Sarngadharan M, Clark J, Saxinger WC, Blattner WA, Gallo RC (1984) Sero-epidemiological studies on HTLV-I. In: Gallo RC, Essex ME, Gross L (eds) Human T-cell leukemia viruses. Cold Spring Harbor Laboratory, New York
19. Saxinger C, Gallo RC (1983) Application of the indirect enzyme-linked immunosorbent assay microtest to the detection and surveillance of human T-cell leukemia-lymphoma virus. Lab Invest 49:371–377
20. Saxinger WC, Lange Wantzin G, Thomsen K, Lapin B, Yakovleva L, Li Y-W, Guo H-G, Robert-Guroff M, Blattner WA, Ito Y, Gallo RC (1984) HTLV and PTLV: A diverse family of related exogenous retroviruses of humans and Old World primates. In: Gallo RC, Essex ME, Gross L (eds) Human T-cell leukemia-lymphoma viruses. Cold Spring Harbor Laboratory, New York
21. Saxinger WC, Lange Wantzin G, Thomsen K, Mei Hoh MS, Gallo RC (1985) Occurrence of HTLV-I antibodies in Danish patients with cutaneous T-cell lymphoma. Scand J Haematol (in press)
22. Tajima K, Tominaga S, Kuroishi T, Shimizu H, Such T (1979) Geographical features and epidemiological approach to endemic T-cell leukemia/lymphoma in Japan. Jpn J Clin Oncol 9 [Suppl]:495–504
23. Williams CKO, Saxinger C, Alabi GO, Junaid TA, Blayney DW, Greaves MF, Gallo RC, Blattner WA (1984) HTLV-associated lymphoproliferative disease: a report of 2 cases in Nigeria. Br Med J (in press)

Haematology and Blood Transfusion Vol. 29
Modern Trends in Human Leukemia VI
Edited by Neth, Gallo, Greaves, Janka

Presence of Antibodies to the Human T-Cell Leukemia Virus HTLV I in German Patients with Symptoms of AIDS *

D. Wernicke, M. Born, K. von der Helm, and F. Deinhardt

A. Introduction

The incidence of the acquired immune deficiency syndrome (AIDS) in North America has increased steadily since 1979. This syndrome has been recognized mainly in male homosexuals in the Western hemisphere, in intravenous drug users, and occasionally in hemophiliacs and inhabitants of some tropical areas (Caribbean, Central Africa).

The human T-cell leukemia virus HTLV I is a type-C retrovirus isolated in North America initially from a patient with a malignant variant form of mycosis fungoides [1] and independently in Japan from a patient with T-cell leukemia [2]. Many additional isolates have since been identified, primarily from patients with clinical manifestations of adult T-cell leukemia-lymphoma (ATLL).

HTLV II, which is also associated with T-cell malignancies, has so far only been isolated once from a patient with hairy-cell leukemia [3]. A newly discovered subgroup of the human T-cell leukemia virus family, designated HTLV III, has been described recently [4, 5]. The virus has been isolated in North America and France from more than one-third of patients with AIDS or the lymphadenopathy syndrome.

Antibodies to HTLV III have been found in 90%–100% of American AIDS patients; antibodies against HTLV I had been found in about 30% of North and Middle American AIDS patients [6].

During a study of the presence of HTLV I in the Federal Republic of Germany we examined serum samples of patients from Munich with symptoms of AIDS (11 sera) or the lymphadenopathy syndrome (LAS) (20 sera) for the presence of antibodies to viral antigens of HTLV I.

B. Material and Methods

I. Cells and Virus Purification

HTLV-I-producing MT-2 cells, which have a OKT^{4+} phenotype [7], were donated by Dr. Hinuma. The cells were grown in RPMI 1640 medium supplemented with 10% fetal calf serum. Culture fluids were harvested daily and concentrated at 40 000 *g* for 12 h. Virus pellets were resuspended in 0.02 *M* Tris hydrochloride (pH 7.5), 0.1 *M* NaCl, and 1 m*M* ethylenediaminetetraacetate (EDTA), and were further purified by sucrose gradient centrifugation. Fractions with a density of 1.14–1.17 g/cm³ were pooled and subjected to a second run of density gradient centrifugation, from which fractions were pooled in a range of density corresponding to 1.15–1.16 g/cm³.

II. Enzyme-Linked Immunoadsorbent Assay

Sera were screened by enzyme-linked immunoadsorbent assay (ELISA) for antibodies to antigens derived from virus prep-

* Max von Pettenkofer-Institute of the University of Munich, FRG

arations of MT-2 cells. Briefly, microtiter plates were coated overnight at room temperature with aliquots of sonified, highly purified virus in 0.1 *M* carbonate buffer, pH 9.5. The plates were rinsed with phosphate-buffered saline (PBS) and incubated with 200 µl/well swine skin gelatin (Sigma) at a concentration of 5 mg/ml for 1 h at room temperature. Aliquots of test sera, diluted 1:100 with PBS containing 3% Tween 20 and 2% sheep serum, were added in duplicates and incubated for 2 h at room temperature. The plates were washed once with swine skin gelatin, twice with PBS + Tween 20, and three times with PBS. Peroxidase-conjugated rabbit immunoglobulin against human IgG (gamma-chains) in PBS + Tween 20, containing 2% sheep serum, were then added and incubated for 2–4 h at room temperature. After thorough washing, 100 µl substrate solution (0.001% H_2O_2 and 0.1% orthophenylenediamine in 0.1 *M* phosphate buffer, pH 6.0) was added to each well. The reaction was allowed to proceed for 10 min at 37 °C in the dark and then stopped by addition of 100 µl 1 *N* HCl/well. Absorbance of each well was determined at 486 nm. Specimens with a threefold higher absorbance than negative control sera were further analyzed in the radioimmunoassay.

III. Immunoprecipitation

MT-2 cells were harvested and exposed to [^{35}S]cysteine (100 µCi/ml; specific activity 1000 Ci/mmol, Amersham, Buckinghamshire, England) for 3–5 h. A soluble cell lysate was obtained after disruption with lysis buffer (0.01 *M* Tris hydrochloride, pH 7.5, 0.05 *M* NaCl, 0.5% Triton X-100, 0.5% sodium deoxycholate, 0.1% sodium dodecyl sulfate) and centrifuged for 15 min at 18 000 *g*. Aliquots of the lysate supernatant were reacted with 8–12 µl patient's sera preabsorbed with protein A beads. Immunoprecipitates were eluted in electrophoresis sample buffer by boiling for 3 min and analyzed in a 12.5% acrylamide resolving gel with 3.5% stacking gel according to Laemmli [8]. Dried gels were exposed to Kodak x-Omat film with an intensifying screen.

C. Results

Two different procedures have been used to survey serum samples for evidence of exposure to HTLV I. These include [1] an enzyme immunoassay (ELISA), with highly purified virus as antigen, and (2) radioimmunoassays with the use of solubilized [^{35}S]cysteine-labeled MT-2 cells.

1. Five of the 31 patient's sera tested by ELISA were positive for antibodies against viral antigens of HTLV I with a factor of more than 3 over the negative control (Table 1). None of the 34 sera from healthy donors contained detectable antibodies against HTLV I. The five positive sera were further examined in the radioimmunoassay.

2. Three of the five sera which showed a positive reaction in the ELISA precipitated the viral envelope antigen gp68 (Fig. 1, lanes 2–4); one serum of the three also precipitated p28 (lane 3). Also samples from ELISA-negative patients were reacted in the radioimmunoassay and none showed a positive reaction for HTLV I (data not shown).

Table 1. Results of ELISA and immunoprecipitation examinations

	AIDS	LAS	Healthy homosexuals	Others
ELISA				
Total sera tested	11	20	7	27
Sera positive	5	0	0	0
Immunoprecipitation				
Total sera tested	5	0	0	3
Sera positive	3			0

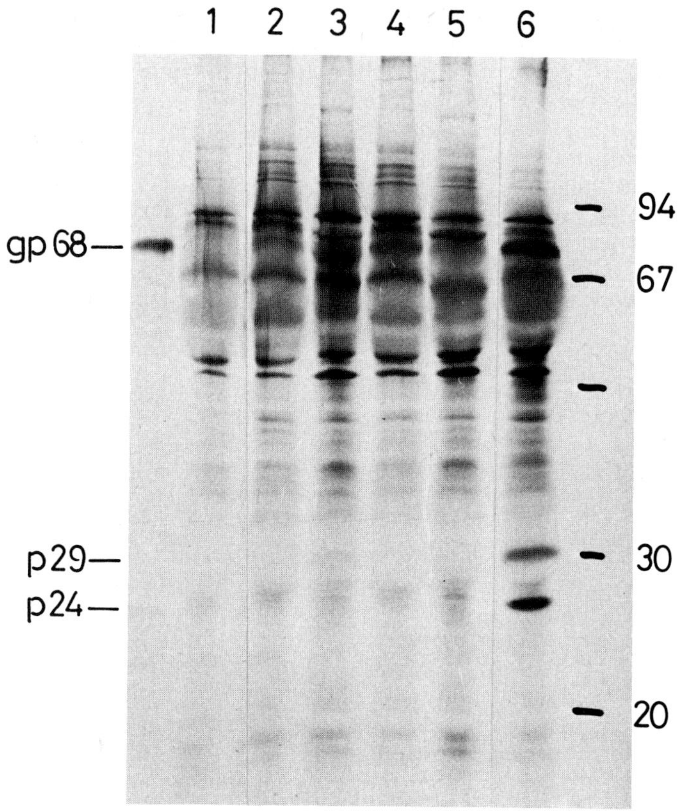

Fig. 1. Immunoprecipitation of radiolabeled HTLV-III-producing MT-2 cells. *Lanes 1–5,* ELISA-positive patient sera; *lane 6,* positive reference serum

D. Discussion

We describe here the presence of antibodies to HTLV I in five of 31 sera from patients with AIDS or LAS. Two of the five sera showing a positive reaction in the ELISA possibly represent false-positive results, probably due to nonspecific fractions with protein contaminations of the antigen preparation. Our results are compatible with the finding that 20%–30% of AIDS patients from North America are positive for antibodies to HTLV I. Not all of the 31 patients tested here were suffering from a clearly diagnosed AIDS, but all belonged to high-risk groups. Eleven patients had symptoms specific for AIDS, including opportunistic infections, Kaposi sarcoma, and altered immunological status; 20 patients suffered from lymphadenopathy syndrome (LAS). The three sera which were able to precipitate HTLV I gp68, as well as the two sera found positive only in the ELISA, came from typical AIDS patients.

Recently the detection of HTLV III as the probable cause of AIDS has been reported [4, 5]. HTLV III is a member of the HTLV family with antigens related to but distinguishable from HTLV I and II. Our findings that some sera from AIDS patients react with antigens from HTLV I are compatible with the reports of Schüpbach et al. and Sarngadharan et al. [9, 10] that AIDS sera with high titers against envelope antigens of HTLV III frequently also recognize the HTLV I envelope antigen.

The gp68 of HTLV I recognized by our three positive sera is known to be a precursor to the viral gp46 envelope protein, which is antigenically related to the gp41 of HTLV III. We thus assume that at least our three positive sera might have high titer antibodies against envelope antigens of HTLV III which cross-react with the envelope antigens of HTLV I. Our results suggest that at least some of the AIDS patients in the Federal Republic of Germany became infected with a member of the HTLV I group and produced antibodies against it.

Postscript. During the preparation of this manuscript, we tested sera from AIDS patients for antibodies against HTLV III antigens. Seventy percent of these sera were positive for Anti-HTLV III antibodies, two sera also showing a reactivity against HTLV I antigens.

References

1. Poiesz BJ et al. (1981) Nature 294:268–271
2. Hinuma Y et al. (1981) Proc Natl Acad Sci USA 78:6476–6480
3. Kalyanaraman VS et al. (1982) Science 218: 571–573
4. Popovic M et al. (1984) Science 224:497–500
5. Gallo RC et al. (1984) Science 224:500–502
6. Essex M et al. (1983) Science 220:859–862
7. Miyoshi I et al. (1981) Nature 294:770–772
8. Laemmli UK (1970) Nature 227:680–685
9. Schüpbach J et al. (1984) Science 224:503 –505
10. Sarngadharan MG et al. (1984) Science 224: 506–508

Haematology and Blood Transfusion Vol. 29
Modern Trends in Human Leukemia VI
Edited by Neth, Gallo, Greaves, Janka

Roles of HTLV-I p19 and Natural Antibody to HTLV-I in Host Immune Responses

T. Aoki [1], C. Hamada [2], S. Ohno [1], H. Miyakoshi [1], Y. Kaneko [3], M. Robert-Guroff [4], R. C. Ting [5], and R. C. Gallo [4]

A. Introduction

Since the discovery of human T cell leukemia/lymphoma virus type I (HTLV-I) [5], the immune status of HTLV-I-infected hosts, including patients with adult T cell leukemia (ATL), has not yet been sufficiently investigated [2–4]. As the first step in this kind of study, we have studied the nonspecific activity of peripheral mononuclear cells (PMNC) from ATL patients and seropositive HTLV-I carriers and the role of HTLV-I p19 antigen and HTLV-I-producing cell surface antigens in the host immune responses to HTLV-I.

B. Nonspecific Immunity

In ATL patients, the spontaneous DNA synthesis of PMNC increased significantly whereas the mitogen- (PHA, staphage lysate = SPL, or Con-A)-induced DNA synthesis and NK activity of PMNC against human myeloid K562 cells dropped tremendously (Table 1). In most seropositive healthy HTLV-I carriers, the spontaneous DNA synthesis of PMNC relatively increased, but the mitogen-induced DNA synthesis and NK activity were within the normal range. Of course, PMNC from seronegative healthy persons showed completely normal reactions for these functions. These results indicate that PMNC from ATL patients were abnormally changed in all their nonspecific functions tested by both HTLV-I infection and malignant transformation, and that PMNC from HTLV-I carriers showed partial dysfunction, but maintained some functions at normal levels. Thus, it may be concluded that PMNC from HTLV-I carriers were enhanced only in spontaneous DNA synthesis by HTLV-I infection, and that the other functions remained almost normal in HTLV-I infection without malignant transformation.

C. Specific Immunity

By means of immunofluorescence microscopy (IFM) and immunoelectron microscopy (IEM) using viable HTLV-I-producing cells, the presence of HTLV-I p19 on both the cell surface and the viral envelope was observed as spots or small sectors by reaction with mouse monoclonal antibody to HTLV-I p19 [1, 2]. This expression of HTLV-I p19 was quite specific for HTLV-I-producing cells. In the light of the presence of HTLV-I p19 in the periphery of acetone-fixed HTLV-I-producing cells as shown by IFM and on the surface of both the virions and HTLV-I-producing cells by

1 Research Division, Shinrakuen Hospital, 1-27 Nishiariakecho, Niigata 950-21, Japan
2 Department of Virology, Niigata University School of Medicine, 1 Asahimachi, Niigata 951, Japan
3 Pharmaceutical Department, Ajinomoto Company, 1-5-8 Kyobashi, Chuoku, Tokyo 104, Japan
4 Laboratory of Tumor Cell Biology, National Cancer Institute, NIH, Bethesda, Md, USA
5 Department of Cell Biology, Biotech Research Laboratory, Rockville, Md, USA

Table 1. DNA synthesis and natural killer (NK) activity of peripheral mononuclear cells (PMNC) from patients with adult T cell leukemia (ATL) and from seropositive or seronegative healthy persons

PMNC donors	DNA synthesis		NK activity
	Mitogen-induced	Spontaneous	
ATL patients	Lowered	Heightened	Negative
Seropositive carriers	Normal	Heightened	Normal
Seronegative healthy persons	Normal	Normal	Normal

Table 2. Antibody-dependent cellular cytotoxicity by peripheral mononuclear cells from patients with adult T cell leukemia (ATL) and from seropositive or seronegative healthy persons

Attacker cell donors	Antibody to HTLV-I	Cytolysis			
		HTLV-I-producing cells		HTLV-I-non-producing cells	
		Cultured	Fresh	Cultured	Fresh
ATL patients	+	–	–	–	–
	–	–	–	–	–
Seropositive carriers	+	+	–	–	–
	–	–	–	–	–
Seronegative healthy persons	+	+	–	–	–
	–	–	–	–	–

IEM, it seems most likely that HTLV-I p19 is an internal antigen of HTLV-I with part of its structure protruding from the viral and cellular membrane. Accordingly, this antigen might be involved in the surface immune reaction of HTLV-I-producing cells. However, the mouse monoclonal antibody to HTLV-I p19 did not induce antibody-dependent cellular cytotoxicity (ADCC) with PMNC from either seropositive HTLV-I carriers or seronegative healthy donors. This monoclonal antibody also failed to induce complement-dependent cytotoxicity (CDC). Therefore, HTLV-I p19 does not contribute to any cytotoxicity.

Regardless of the PMNC donors who are seropositive or seronegative for HTLV-I, PMNC from healthy donors clearly revealed ADCC against HTLV-I-producing cells in the presence of serum containing antibodies to HTLV-I-related antigens (Table 2). No differences in the ADCC effects were detected between the antibody-positive sera from healthy donors and from ATL patients. By contrast, the PMNC showed no ADCC in the presence of either antibody-negative serum or fetal calf serum. In addition, PMNC from ATL patients revealed extremely low ADCC or none at all. This may be explained by concluding that; (a) these PMNC became dysfunctional by malignant transformation; (b) the absolute number of effector cells decreased; and/or (c) the relative number of effector cells in this assay diminished according to an increase in malignant cells. Moreover, since cytotoxicity of PMNC was appreciably lowered by incubation with a mixture of anti-Leu 7 monoclonal antibody and rabbit serum as a complement source, the effector cells of ADCC may be K cells. Although NK cells also express Leu 7 antigen, NK activity of PMNC did not contribute to this ADCC because of the necessity of anti-HTLV-I antibody.

When rabbit serum was added as a complement source to a mixture of antibody-positive serum and cultured HTLV-I-producing cells, CDC distinctly occurred

Table 3. Complement-dependent cytotoxicity by sera from patients with adult T cell leukemia (ATL) and from seropositive or seronegative healthy persons in the presence of rabbit serum as a complement source

Serum sources	Cytolysis			
	HTLV-I-producing cells		HTLV-I-non-producing cells	
	Cultured	Fresh	Cultured	Fresh
ATL patients	+	–	–	–
Seropositive carriers	+	–	–	–
Seronegative healthy persons	+	–	–	–

(Table 3). No other complement sources such as human serum and guinea pig serum induced CDC. When fresh malignant cells from ATL patients were used as target cells instead of cultured malignant T cells, no CDC was recognized at all.

D. Remarks

Although PMNC from seropositive carriers were partially dysfunctional in nonspecific immune activities, they clearly showed ADCC against cultured HTLV-I-producing cells in the presence of antibody-positive serum from either seropositive carriers or ATL patients, but no ADCC against fresh malignant T cells from ATL patients. This suggests that fresh malignant T cells do not exhibit any HTLV-I-associated antigens on the surface of these cells, or that the amount of these antigens may be too small to induce ADCC. It has been proven that masked HTLV-I-associated antigens appeared on the cell surface after in vitro culture. The same phenomenon can be adapted to CDC. Thus, in ATL patients or seropositive carriers, malignant T cells can grow constantly without any interference by ADCC and/or CDC. Even the injection of rabbit serum as a complement source may not induce CDC for the same reason.

Is there any difference in the quality of antibodies in sera from ATL patients and HTLV-I carriers? According to the results of the Western blot method using disrupted HTLV-I and cell extracts as antigens, the titer of antibody to p68–70 of HTLV-I-producing cells appeared to be slightly lower in sera from healthy seropositive carriers than in sera from ATL patients (Miyakoshi and Aoki 1984). However, this difference in antibodies of sera does not provide any definite evidence to explain why ATL develops in some seropositive carriers or why carriers can prevent ATL development. The mechanisms of ATL in HTLV-I-infected hosts should be a central problem of future studies.

References

1. Aoki T, Hamada C, Ohno S, Miyakoshi H, Koide H, Robert-Guroff M, Ting RC, Gallo RC (1984) Location of human T-cell leukemia virus (HTLV) p19 antigen on virus-producing cells. Int J Cancer 33:161–165
2. Aoki T, Hamada C, Ohno S, Miyakoshi H, Koide H, Robert-Guroff M, Ting RC, Gallo RC (1984) Location of human T-cell leukemia viral (HTLV) p19 antigen and a role of natural antibody-dependent cell-mediated cytotoxicity of HTLV-producing cells. In: Gallo RC, Essex ME, Gross L (eds) Human T-cell leukemia-lymphoma viruses, Cold Spring Harbor Laboratory, New York, pp 307–312
3. Miyakoshi H, Koide H, Aoki T (1984) *In vitro* antibody-dependent cellular cytotoxicity against human T-cell leukemia/lymphoma virus (HTLV)-producing cells. Int J Cancer 33:287–291
4. Miyakoshi H, Aoki T (1984) Immunological study of HTLV-I-infected hosts. In: Aoki T, Tsubura E, Urushizaki I (eds) Manipulation of host defence mechanisms. Excerpta Medica, Amsterdam, pp 152–161
5. Poiesz BJ, Ruscetti FW, Gazdar AF, Bunn PA, Minna JD, Gallo RC (1980) Detection and isolation of type C retrovirus particles from fresh and cultured lymphocytes of a patient with cutaneous T-cell lymphoma. Proc Natl Acad Sci USA 77:7415–7419

Haematology and Blood Transfusion Vol. 29
Modern Trends in Human Leukemia VI
Edited by Neth, Gallo, Greaves, Janka

Antibodies to Human T-Cell Leukemia Virus-Membrane Antigens in Macaques with Malignant Lymphoma

P. J. Kanki [1,2], T. Homma [1], T. H. Lee [1], N. W. King Jr. [2], R. D. Hunt [2], and M. Essex [1]

A. Introduction

Gallo and co-workers first described human T-cell leukemia virus (HTLV), a type C retrovirus isolated from an aggressive case of cutaneous T-cell lymphoma [27, 28]. Cases of adult T-cell leukemia/lymphoma (ATLL), a unique mature T-cell malignancy, have also yielded numerous other isolates of HTLV [23, 7, 17, 35, 10, 29]. ATLL is seen at increased levels in southwestern Japan and the Caribbean, where seroepidemiologic studies have linked this tumor with HTLV type I. In such endemic regions, natural antibodies can be demonstrated in 4%–37% of the healthy adults whereas more than 90% of patients with ATLL have antibodies to HTLV (11, 31, 1, 32, 5, 20]. The prevalence of HTLV antibodies in healthy individuals is less than 1% in nonendemic areas [12, 6, 5, 20, 3, 4].

Miyoshi and his colleagues set the precedent for the nonhuman primate studies in 1982, when they demonstrated the presence of antibodies to HTLV in Japanese macaques (*Macaca fuscata*) by fixed-cell immunofluorescence [24]. Numerous studies since that time have identified antibodies to HTLV in other species of the genus *Macaca* as well as many African Old World primates. However, serological surveys by several investigators have not detected antibodies in New World primates or prosimians (lower primates) [24, 8, 14, 16, 34, 25, 9].

Macaque studies have shown rates of seropositivity ranging from 9% to 44% in healthy individuals [8, 14, 16, 34, 25, 9]. Familial clustering and an age dependence on the presence of HTLV antibodies have been demonstrated [25, 9]. Studies in Indonesia and Japan with wild-caught *Macaca fascicularis* and *Macaca fuscata*, respectively, show geographic clustering of seropositive individuals [8, 9, 25]. However, the geographic clustering of seropositive macaques in Japan does not appear to correlate to that seen in human populations [25, 9], suggesting that these closely related viruses have arisen independently. The studies to date have been conducted on apparently healthy macaques and there has been no disease or malignancy previously linked with this HTLV-related agent.

B. Methods

Serum samples from three species of captive macaques at the New England Regional Primate Research Center (NERPRC), Southborough, MA, were collected. In addition to sera from healthy macaques, serum samples from animals with the diagnosis of lymphoma or lymphoproliferative disorder (LPD) were included in this survey [13] (Table 1). These included: (a) *Macaca fascicularis*, the cynomologus macaque, 31 healthy controls and 5 with malignant lymphoma; (b) *Macaca mulatta*, the rhesus macaque, 30 healthy controls

1 Department of Cancer Biology, Harvard School of Public Health, Boston, MA
2 New England Regional Primate Research Center, Harvard Medical School, Southborough, MA

Table 1. Serum samples from three species of captive macaques at the NERPRC

	Diagnosis	Principle sites	Cell type
M. fascicularis M 10 yrs	ML	Mandible	Undifferentiated
M. fascicularis F 9+yrs	ML	Retro-orbital	Undifferentiated
M. fascicularis F 11 yrs	ML	Generalized	Lymphocytic
M. mulatta M 12 yrs	ML	Generalized	Lymphoblastic
M. mulatta F. 9 yrs	ML	Generalized	Lymphoblastic
M. mulatta F 10 yrs	ML	Intestine	Lymphoblastic
M. mulatta F 9+yrs	ML	Generalized	Histiocytic
M. mulatta F 4 yrs	ML	Generalized	Lymphoblastic
M. cyclopis F 4 yrs	LPD	Salivary gland, kidney, bone marrow	Lymphocytic
M. cyclopis F 4 yrs	LPD	Kidney	Lymphocytic
M. cyclopis F 3 yrs	LPD	Pancreas, kidney	Lymphocytic
M. cyclopis F 7 yrs	LPD	Bone marrow	Lymphocytic
M. mulatta F 4 yrs	LPD	Lung, salivary gland, kidney, bone marrow, bladder, muscle	Lymphocytic

M, male; F, female; ML, malignant lymphoma; LPD, lymphoproliferative disorder

Table 2. Antibodies to HTLV-MA in macaques

Health status	Cynomologus macaque *M. fascicularis*	Rhesus macaque *M. mulatta*	Taiwanese macaque *M. cyclopis*	Total
Healthy	2/30 (6.7%)	1/31 (3.2%)	2/14 (14.3%)	5/75 (6.7%)
Lymphoproliferative disorder	–	1/1 (100%)	3/4 (75%)	4/5 (80%)
Malignant lymphoma	3/3 (100%)	4/5 (80%)	–	7/8 (87.5%)

( ), percentage of seropositive macaques. Difference between healthy and malignant lymphoma/lymphoproliferative disorder significant at $P < 9.42 \times 10^{-9}$, Fisher's exact statistic

and 5 with lymphoma and 1 with LPD; and (c) *Macaca cyclopis,* the Taiwanese macaque, 14 healthy controls and 4 cases of LPD.

Reports of spontaneous lymphoid malignancies in macaques are not common [26, 22]. There have been instances where multiple cases of lymphoma have occurred over a brief time interval, at least suggestive of a transmissible agent [15, 33, 19].

Malignant lymphoma and lymphoproliferative disorders have been observed in macaques at this colony over the past 12 years, and these malignancies are believed to be part of the macaque immunodeficiency syndrome previously described [15, 18]. A type change from C to D retrovirus has been isolated from macaques at this facility with this syndrome [2]; however, none of the macaques in this study were positive for the type D-New England virus. Complete autopsies were performed on all cases of lymphoma or LPD. Lymphoma cases varied in organ distribution, cell type, and degree of metastasis. LPD has been described, and is characterized by mature lymphocytic aggregates in the liver, pancreas kidney, and bone marrow [18].

The method for detecting antibodies to membrane antigens of HTLV-infected cells (HTLV-MA) has been described [3, 4, 20]. Antibodies to two glycoproteins, gp61 and gp45, encoded by the *env* gene of HTLV are detected in this assay. In addition, representative serum samples were subjected to radioimmunoprecipitation and sodium

Table 3. Presence of antibodies to HTLV-specific proteins[a]

Class of serum	*env*		*gag*	
	gp61	gp45	p24	p19
Human immunofluorescent antibody +, ATLL case	+	+	+	+
Human immunofluorescent antibody –	–	–	–	–
Macaque malignant lymphoma/lymphoproliferative disorder immunofluorescent antibody +	+	+	+	+
Macaque healthy immunofluorescent antibody +	+	+	+	+
Macaque healthy immunofluorescent antibody –	–	–	–	–

[a] Determined by radioimmunoprecipitation and SDS-PAGE of Hut 102 cell lysate

dodecyl sulfate-polyacrylamide gel electrophoresis (SDS-PAGE) as described earlier [20, 3, 4]. Whole-cell lysate of Hut 102 cells was used as the antigenic source since the major *env* and *gag* proteins have been established in this line.

C. Results

Table 2 gives the results of the indirect immunofluorescence assays in three species of macaques. Two of 30 healthy *M. fascicularis* had antibodies to HTLV-MA, whereas 3 of 3 macaques with malignant lymphoma were seropositive. Of 31 healthy *M. mulatta* only 1 macaque was seropositive in contrast to 4 of 5 with malignant lymphoma and 1 seropositive macaque with LPD. Of 14 healthy *M. cyclopis,* 2 macaques were seropositive whereas 3 of 4 with LPD had antibodies to HTLV-MA. In total, 11 of 13 macaques with malignant lymphoma or LPD were seropositive as compared with 5 of 75 healthy controls ($P < 9.42 \times 10^{-9}$, Fisher's exact test).

Table 3 indicates the HTLV-specific proteins immunoprecipitated by various sera analyzed. Human reference serum positive for antibody to HTLV-MA immunoprecipitates four major HTLV-specific proteins, with sizes of 19 000 (p19), 24 000 (p24), 45 000 (gp45), and 61 000 daltons (gp61), as has been described previously [20, 3, 4]. These proteins were not precipitated by human reference-negative serum. Immunofluorescent antibody-positive serum from a macaque with malignant lymphoma also immunoprecipitated the same HTLV-specific proteins. Similarly, an immunofluorescent antibody-positive serum from a healthy macaque precipitated the same size proteins. These same sera when subjected to lentil-lectin chromatography precipitated two proteins presumed to be gp45 and gp61, migrating at the expected position for the *env*-gene-encoded proteins, and these were not precipitated by immunofluorescent-negative macaque sera.

D. Discussion and Conclusions

Studies of the seroepidemiology and viral-related proteins of HTLV in humans conducted by our laboratory and others illustrate many common features with the non human primate studies. Macaque sera positive for antibodies to HTLV-MA recognize the same two HTLV-specific proteins, gp61 and gp45, most frequently recognized by human HTLV-MA-positive sera. Lee and co-workers have shown these to be surface glycoproteins and at least in part encoded by the *env* gene [20]. A high proportion of human antibodies reactive to HTLV-I-infected cells also react to HTLV-II C3-44/MO cells on membrane immunofluorescence and radioimmunoprecipitation. The HTLV-II gp67 is in part encoded by the *env* gene and comparison of the deduced NH_2 terminus amino acid sequences of type I and type II shows 65% homology in the first 40 amino acids. Thus, despite apparent divergence between two members of the HTLV family the major *env* gene products show conservation in their deduced amino acid sequence and this is compatible with their serologic cross-reactivity [21]. It is therefore not unlikely that the simian member of the HTLV family might also show such conservation in its *env* gene products.

There is strong evidence that HTLV plays an etiologic role in its association with ATLL [6, 7, 35, 30]. Seroepidemiologic studies in people have shown that virtually all individuals with this tumor also have antibody to HTLV whereas the prevalence of seropositive healthy individuals is significantly lower. We have observed a similar pattern in the seroepidemiology of macaque lymphoma and lymphoproliferative disorder. Malignant lymphoma is not a common tumor of macaques; however, the incidence of this tumor at this particular colony has been high compared with non-lymphoid malignancies. Furthermore, successful transmission of malignant lymphoma from two of the macaques included in this study has been recently reported [15]. Our results indicate that an agent similar to HTLV type I is present in this colony, where it appears that the presence of antibodies to HTLV is associated with increased risk for the development of lymphoproliferative disorders or malignancies.

References

1. Blattner WA, Blayney DW, Robert-Guroff M, Sarngadharan MG, Sarin PS, Jaffe ES, Gallo RC (1983) Epidemiology of human T-cell leukemia/lymphoma virus. J Infect Dis 148:406–416
2. Daniel MD, King NW, Letvin NL, Hunt RD, Sehgal PK, Desrosiers RC (1984) A new type D retrovirus isolated from macaques with an immunodeficiency syndrome. Science 223: 602–605
3. Essex M, McLane MF, Lee TH, Falk L, Howe CWS, Mullins JI, Cabradilla C, Francis DP (1983) Antibodies to cell membrane antigens associated with human T-cell leukemia virus in patients with AIDS. Science 220:859–862
4. Essex M, McLane MF, Lee TH, Tachibana N, Mullins JI, Kreiss J, Kasper CK, Poon M-C, Landay A, Stein SF, Francis DP, Cabradilla C, Lawrence DN, Evatt BL (1983) Antibodies to human T-cell leukemia virus membrane antigens (HTLV-MA) in hemophiliacs. Science 221:1061–1064
5. Essex M, McLane MF, Tachibana N, Francis DP, Lee TH (1984) Seroepidemiology of human T-cell leukemia virus in relation to immunosuppression and the acquired immunodeficiency syndrome. In: Gallo RC, Essex M, Gross L (eds) Human T-cell leukemia viruses. Cold Spring Harbor Laboratory, Cold Spring Harbor, pp 355–362
6. Gallo RC et al. (1982) Association of the human type C retrovirus with a subset of adult T-cell cancers. Cancer Res 43:3892–3899
7. Gallo RC, Mann D, Broder S, Ruscetti FW, Maeda M, Kalyanaraman VS, Robert-Guroff M, Reitz MS (1982) Human T-cell leukemia-lymphoma virus (HTLV) is in T- but not B-lymphocytes from a patient with cutaneous T-cell lymphoma. Proc Natl Acad Sci USA 79:5680–5683
8. Hayami M, Ishikawa K, Komuro A, Kawamoto Y, Nozawa K, Yamamoto K, Ishida T, Hinuma Y (1983) ATLV antibody in cynomologus monkeys in the wild. Lancet 2:620
9. Hayami M, Komuro A, Nozawa K, Shotake T, Ishikawa K, Yamamoto K, Ishida T, Honjo S, Hinuma Y (1984) Prevalence of antibody to adult T-cell leukemia virus associated antigens (ATLA) in Japanese monkeys and other non-human primates. Int J Cancer 33:179–183
10. Haynes BF, Miller SE, Palker TJ, Moore JO, Dunn PH, Bolognesi DP, Metzgar RS (1983) Identification of human T-cell leukemia virus in a Japanese patient with adult T-cell leukemia and cutaneous lymphomatous vasculitis. Proc Natl Acad Sci USA 80:2054–2058
11. Hinuma Y, Nagata K, Hanaoka M, Nakai M, Matsumoto T, Kinoshita K-I, Shirakawa S, Miyoshi I (1981) Adult T-cell leukemia: antigen in an ATL cell line and detection of antibodies to the antigen in human sera. Proc Natl Acad Sci USA 78:6476–6480
12. Hinuma Y, Komoda H, Chosa T, Kondo T, Kohakura M, Takenaka T, Kikuchi M, Ichimaru M, Yunoki K, Sato I, Matsuo R, Takinuchi Y, Uchinao H, Hanaoka M (1982) Antibodies to adult T-cell leukemkia-virus-associated antigen (ATLA) in sera from patients with ATL and controls in Japan: a nation-wide seroepidemiologic study (1982) Int J Cancer 29:631–635
13. Homma T, Kanki PJ, King NW, Hunt RD, O'Connell MJ, Letvin NL, Daniel MD, Desrosiers RC, Yang CS, Essex M (1984) Lymphoma in Macaques: association with virus of human T-lymphotrophic family. Science 225:716–718

14. Hunsmann G, Schneider J, Schmitt J, Yamamoto N (1983) Detection of serum antibodies to adult T-cell leukemia virus in non-human primates and in people from Africa. Int J Cancer 32:329–332
15. Hunt RD, Blake BJ, Chalifoux LV, Sehgal PK, King NW, Letvin NL (1983) Transmission of naturally occurring lymphoma in macaque monkeys. Proc Natl Acad Sci USA 80: 5085–5089
16. Ishida T, Yamamoto K, Kaneko R, Tokita E, Hinuma Y (1983) Seroepidemiological study of antibodies to adult T-cell leukemia virus-associated antigen (ATLA) in free-ranging Japanese monkeys (*Macaca fuscata*). Microbiol Immunol 27(3):297–301
17. Kalyanaraman VS, Sarngadharan MG, Robert-Guroff M, Miyoshi I, Blayney D, Golde D, Gallo RC (1982) A new sub-type of human T-cell leukemia virus (HTLV-II) associated with a T-cell variant of hairy cell leukemia. Science 218:571–573
18. King NW, Hunt RD, Letvin NL (1983) Histopathologic changes in macaque monkeys with an acquired immune deficiency syndrome (AIDS). Am J Pathol 113:382–388
19. Lapin B (1973) The epidemiologic and genetic aspects of leukemia among hamadrayas baboons of the Sukhumi monkey colony. In: Dutcher RM, Chieco-Bianchi L (eds) Unifying concepts of leukemia. Bibl Haematologica 39:263–268, Karger, Basel
20. Lee TH, Coligan JE, Homma T, McLane MF, Tachibana N, Essex M (1984) Human T-cell leukemia virus-associated membrane antigens: identity of the major antigens recognized after virus infection. Proc Natl Acad Sci USA 81:3856–3858
21. Lee TH, Coligan JE, McLane MF, Sodroski JG, Popovic M, Wong-Staal F, Gallo RC, Haseltine W, Essex M (1984) Serological cross-reactivity between envelope gene products of Type I and Type II human T-cell leukemia virus. Proc Natl Acad Sci USA (in press)
22. Manning JRS, Griesemer RA (1974) Spontaneous lymphoma of the non-human primate. Lab Anim Sci 24:204–210
23. Miyoshi I, Kubonishi I, Yoshimoto S, Akagi T, Ohtsuki Y, Shiraishi Y, Nagata K, Hinuma Y (1981) Type C virus particles in a cord T-cell line derived by co-cultivating normal human cord leukocytes and human leukaemia T-cells. Nature 294:770–771
24. Miyoshi I, Yoshimoto S, Fujishita M, Taguchi H, Kubonishi I, Niiya K, Minezawa M (1982) Natural adult T-cell leukaemia virus infection in Japanese monkeys. Lancet 2:658
25. Miyoshi I, Fujishita M, Taguchi H, Matsubayashi K, Miwa K, Tanioka Y (1983) Natural infection in non-human primates with adult T-cell leukemia virus or a closely related agent. Int J Cancer 32:333–336
26. O'Gara RW, Adamson RH (1972) Spontaneous and induced neoplasms in non-human Primates. In: Fiennes RNTW (ed) Pathology of simian Primates. Karger, Basel, pp 190–238
27. Poiesz BJ, Ruscetti FW, Gazdar AF, Bunn PA, Minna JD, Gallo RC (1980) Detection and isolation of type C retrovirus particles from fresh and cultured lymphocytes of a patient with cutaneous T-cell lymphoma. Proc Natl Acad Sci USA 77:7415–7419
28. Poiesz BJ, Ruscetti FW, Reitz MW, Kalyanaraman VS, Gallo RC (1981) Isolation of a new type C retrovirus (HTLV) in primary uncultured cells of a patient with Sezary T-cell leukemia. Nature 294:268–271
29. Popovic M, Sarin PS, Robert-Guroff M, Kalyanaran VS, Mann D, Minowada J, Gallo RC (1983) Isolation and transmission of human retrovirus (human T-cell leukemia virus). Science 219:856–859
30. Reitz MS, Kalyanaraman VS, Robert-Guroff M, Popovic M, Sarngadharan MG, Sarin PS, Gallo RC (1983) Human T-cell leukemia/lymphoma virus: the retrovirus of adult T-cell leukemia/lymphoma. J Infect Dis 147:339–403
31. Robert-Guroff M, Nakao Y, Notake K, Ito Y, Sliski A, Gallo RC (1982) Natural antibodies to the human retrovirus, HTLV, in a cluster of Japanese patients with adult T-cell leukemia. Science 215:975–978
32. Schupbach J, Kalyanaraman VS, Sarngadharan MG, Blattner WA, Gallo RC (1983) Antibodies against three purified proteins of the human type-C retrovirus, human T-cell leukemia-lymphoma virus, in adult T-cell leukemia-lymphoma patients and healthy blacks from the Caribbean. Cancer Res 43:886–891
33. Stowell RC, Smith EK, Espana C, Nelson VG (1971) Outbreak of malignant lymphoma in rhesus monkeys. Lab Invest 25: 476–479
34. Yamamoto N, Hinuma Y, zur Hausen H, Schneider J, Hunsmann G (1983) African green monkeys are infected with adult T-cell leukemia virus or a closely related agent. Lancet 1:240–241
35. Yoshida M, Miyoshi I, Hinuma Y (1982) Isolation and characterization of retrovirus from cell lines of human adult T-cell leukemia and its implications in the disease. Proc Natl Acad Sci USA 79:2031–2035

Cellbiology

Haematology and Blood Transfusion Vol. 29
Modern Trends in Human Leukemia VI
Edited by Neth, Gallo, Greaves, Janka

Normal Regulators of Growth and Differentiation and the Reversal of Malignancy in Leukemia

L. Sachs[1]

A. Cloning and Clonal Differentiation of Normal Hematopoietic Cells in Culture

The cloning and clonal differentiation of normal hematopoietic cells in culture made it possible to study the controls that regulate growth (multiplication) and differentiation of different hematopoietic cell types; see [63–68]. We first showed [17, 59], as was then confirmed by others [4], that normal mouse myeloid precursor cells cultured with a feeder layer of other cell types can form clones of granulocytes and macrophages in culture. We also found that the formation of these clones is due to secretion by cells of the feeder layer of specific inducers that induce the formation of clones and the differentiation of cells in these clones to macrophages or granulocytes in mice [26, 59, 60] and in humans [57]. After we first detected their presence in culture supernatants [26, 60], these protein inducers have been referred to by a number of names and I shall use the name macrophage and granulocyte inducers (MGI) (Table 1). These proteins can be produced and secreted by various normal and malignant cells in culture and in vivo [63]. Their production can be induced by a variety of compounds [10, 12, 41, 80] and some cells produce these proteins constitutively [1, 26, 31, 34, 71]. MGI are a family of proteins that exist in a number of molecular forms that have different biologic activities. This cell culture approach has led to the cloning and isolation of growth factors for all the different types of hematopoietic cells, including different types of lymphocytes.

1 Department of Genetics, Weizmann Institute of Science, Rehovot 76100, Israel

B. Normal Growth- and Differentiation-Inducing Proteins

The family of MGI proteins include some proteins that induce cell growth (multiplication) and others that induce differentiation. Those that induce growth, which are also required for normal cell viability, we now call MGI-1. These include proteins that induce the formation of macrophage clones (MGI-1M) [26, 48, 71], granulocyte clones (MGI-1G) [26, 48, 54], or both types of clones (MGI-1GM) [6, 31, 34]. MGI-1 has previously been referred to as mashran gm [27], colony-stimulating factor (CSF) [51], colony-stimulating activity (CSA) [1], and MGI [31] (Table 1). The existence of an antibody that does not react with all forms of MGI-1M or MGI-1G has shown that there can be different antigenic sites on molecules that belong to the same form of MGI-1 [47, 48]. The other main type of MGI, which we now call MGI-2 [33, 48, 66], induces the differentiation of myeloid precursor cells, either leukemic [14] or normal [33, 66], without inducing colony formation. This differentiation-inducing protein [13, 14] has also been referred to as MGI [14], D factor [49, 82], and GM-DF [5]. It has been suggested that there are different forms of MGI-2 for differentiation to macrophages or granulocytes [33]. The regulation of MGI-1 and MGI-2 appears to be

Table 1. In vitro cloning and clonal differentiation of normal hematopoietic cells

Cloning and differentiation in liquid medium (mast cells and granulocytes) [17]
Cloning and differentiation in agar (macrophages) [59]
Inducer for cloning and differentiation secreted by cells [59]
Inducer in conditioned medium from cells (for marcrophages and granulocytes) [26, 60]
Different inducer for macrophage and granulocyte clones [26]
Cloning and differentiation of macrophages and granulocytes in methylcellulose [26]
Confirmation of cloning and differentiation in agar [4]
Production of inducer for cloning by some leukemic cells [56]
Cloning and differentiation of human cells [57, 58]
Protein inducer of differentiation that does not induce cloning [13]
Terminology used for proteins that induce cloning and differentiation of normal macrophages and granulocytes
Mashran gm [27]
Colony-stimulating factor (CSF) [51]
Colony-stimulating activity (CSA) [1]
Macrophage and granulocyte inducers (MGI) [31]
MGI-1 (=mashran gm, CSF, CSA) for cloning; MGI-2 (=D factor, DF) for differentiation [33, 44, 48, 66]

under the control of different genes [10]. Differentiation-inducing protein MGI-2, but not growth-inducing protein MGI-1, is a DNA-binding protein [79].

These macrophage and granulocyte inducers can be proteins or glycoproteins, depending on the cells in which they are produced, and the presence of carbohydrates does not appear to be necessary for their biologic activity [31]. Their molecular weights are mostly around 23 000 or multiples of this number [48, 55, 64, 65], and MGI-2 activity is more sensitive to proteolytic enzymes and high temperature than MGI-1 activity [31]. MGI-2 has a shorter half-life in serum than MGI-1 [43]. The ready separability of the different forms of MGI seems to depend on the cells from which they are derived [48]. Further studies should determine whether different forms of MGI are derived from a common precursor, and whether tumor cells with the appropriate gene rearrangements, and possibly even normal cells under certain conditions, may produce hybrid molecules of different forms of MGI, including hybrid molecules with MGI-1 and MGI-2 activity [33].

C. Control of Growth and Differentiation in Leukemia

Normal myeloid precursor cells isolated from bone marrow [37] require an external source of MGI-1 for cell viability and growth. There are, however, myeloid leukemic cells that no longer require MGI-1 for viability and growth, so that these leukemic cells can then multiply in the absence of MGI-1 [64, 66]. This gives the leukemic cells a growth advantage over the normal cells when there is a limiting amount of MGI-1. Starting with a decreased requirement for MGI-1, this eventually leads to a complete loss of this requirement. Other myeloid leukemic cells constitutively produce their own MGI-1 [54, 56] and these leukemic cells also have a growth advantage compared with normal cells that require an external source of MGI-1 (Fig. 1). A change in the requirement of MGI-1 for growth, either a partial or complete loss of this requirement, or the constitutive production of MGI-1, thus both give a growth advantage to leukemic cells.

The existence of myeloid leukemic cells that either no longer require MGI-1 for viability and growth or constitutively produce their own MGI-1, raises the question

Type of myeloid cells	Requirement of MGI-1 for growth
Normal	External source
Leukemic	Decrease ⟶ no requirement or Constitutive production

Fig. 1. Differences in MGI-1 requirement for growth in normal and leukemic myeloid cells

whether these leukemic cells can still be induced to differentiate to mature cells by the normal differentiation-inducing protein MGI-2. This question has been answered by showing that there are clones of myeloid leukemic cells that no longer require MGI-1 for growth, but can still be induced to differentiate normally to mature macrophages and granulocytes by MGI-2 via the normal sequence of gene expression; see [64–68]. These mature cells are then no longer malignant in vivo [11, 43, 47]. Injection of these myeloid leukemic cells into embryos has shown that after such injection the leukemic cells can participate in hematopoietic differentiation in apparently healthy adult animals [18, 78].

Injection of MGI-2 into animals, or in vivo induction of MGI-2 by a compound that induces the production of this differentiation-inducing protein, results in an inhibition of leukemia development in animals with such leukemic cells [43, 47]. There are also myeloid leukemic cells that constitutively produce their own MGI-1 and that can be induced to differentiate by MGI-2. Our results indicate that induction of normal differentiation in myeloid leukemic cells by MGI-2 can be an approach to therapy based on the induction of normal differentiation in malignant cells [14, 40, 43, 46, 47, 57]. There are various forms of MGI-2 which differ in their ability to induce differentiation in different clones of myeloid leukemic cells [40, 43, 46, 47].

Leukemic clones that can be induced to differentiate to mature cells by MGI-2 have been found in different strains of mice [5, 14, 15, 25, 28, 38]. They are referred to as MGI$^+$D$^+$ (MGI$^+$ to indicate that they can be induced to differentiate by MGI-2; D$^+$ for differentiation to mature cells). MGI$^+$D$^+$ leukemic cells have specific chromosome changes compared with normal cells [2, 19]. These chromosome changes thus seem to involve changes in genes other than those involved in the induction of normal differentiation. There are other clones of myeloid leukemic cells that can also grow without adding MGI-1, but that are either partly (MGI$^+$D$^-$) or almost completely (MGI$^-$D$^-$) blocked in their ability to be induced to differentiate by MGI-2 [15, 21, 23, 28, 48, 69, 70]. These differentiation-defective clones have specific chromosome changes compared with MGI$^+$D$^+$ cells [2, 19].

There are a variety of compounds, other than MGI-2, that can induce differentiation in MGI$^+$D$^+$ clones. Not all these compounds are active on the same MGI$^+$D$^+$ clone, and they do not all induce the same differentiation-associated properties. The inducers include certain steroids, lectins, polycyclic hydrocarbons, tumor promoters, lipopolysaccharides, X-irradiation, and compounds used in cancer chemotherapy [42, 64].

The existence of clonal differences in the ability of X-irradiation and cancer chemotherapeutic chemicals to induce differentiation may help to explain differences in response to therapy in different individuals [64]. As a result of these experiments, we have suggested that it may be possible to introduce a form of therapy based on induction of differentiation [14, 40, 42, 43, 57, 63–65]. This would include prescreening in culture to select for the most effective compounds, and using these compounds for a low dose chemotherapy protocol aimed at inducing cell differentiation [42]. Since different myeloid leukemic clones respond differently to MGI-2 and other compounds, such differences will also occur in leukemic cells from different patients. Based on these suggestions [63, 64], some encouraging clinical results have been obtained with the use of low dose cytosine arabinoside [3, 24, 52].

D. Alternative Pathways of Differentiation

Some of the compounds that induce differentiation in susceptible clones of $MGI^{-}D^{+}$ leukemic cells, including lipopolysaccharide, phorbol ester tumor promoters such as 12-*O*-tetradecanoylphorbol-13-acetate (TPA), and nitrosoguanide, can induce the production of MGI-2 in these clones. These compounds thus induce differentiation by inducing in the leukemic cells the endogenous production of the normal differentiation-inducing protein MGI-2 [10, 41, 80]. Other compounds such as the steroid dexamethasone, can induce differentiation in $MGI^{+}D^{+}$ clones without inducing MGI-2 [10]. This steroid induces differentiation by other pathways of gene expression than MGI-2 [7, 38]. The same applies to dimethylsulfoxide (DMSO).

Induction of differentiation in some myeloid leukemic clones requires combined treatment with different compounds [30, 39, 41, 74, 75]. In these cases, one compound induces changes not induced by the other, so that the combined treatment results in new gene expression. This complementation of gene expression can occur both at the level of mRNA production and mRNA translation [22]. With the appropriate combination of compounds, we have been able to induce all our $MGI^{-}D^{-}$ leukemic clones for some differentiation-associated properties [74, 75]. It will be interesting to determine whether the same applies to differentiation of erythroleukemic cells [16, 50]. It is possible that all myeloid leukemic cells no longer susceptible to the normal differentiation-inducing protein MGI-2 by itself, can be induced to differentiate by choosing the appropriate combination of compounds to give the required complementation. This can include the use of hormones such as steroids [35, 36], or insulin [73, 74], and different nonphysiologic compounds [64], with or without MGI-2.

E. Coupling of Growth and Differentiation in Normal Cells

We have developed a simple procedure for isolating normal myeloid precursor cells from the bone marrow [37]. Incubation of isolated normal myeloid precursors with MGI-1, either MGI-1M or MGI-1G [48], induces the viability and growth of these normal precursors, and results in cell differentiation to macrophages or granulocytes, even without adding the differentiation-inducing protein MGI-2. The incubation of normal myeloid precursors with MGI-1 also results in the induction of MGI-2 [33, 44, 45, 66]. This induction of MGI-2 can be detected as early as 6 h after the addition of MGI-1 [44]. This induction of MGI-2 by MGI-1 can thus account for the induction of differentiation after adding MGI-1 to the normal cells. The induction of differentiation-inducing protein MGI-2 by growth-inducing protein MGI-1 thus appears to be an effective control mechanism for coupling growth and differentiation in the normal cells.

It has been shown that the receptor for epidermal growth factor has tyrosine-specific protein kinase activity [76]. This has also been found for receptors for other growth factors such as insulin [29] and presumably also applies to the receptor for the myeloid cell growth-inducing protein MGI-1. The myeloid differentiation-inducing protein MGI-2, but not MGI-1, can bind to cellular DNA [79]. This shows that growth and differentiation in normal myeloid cells are coupled by induction of a differentiation-inducing, DNA-binding protein by a growth-inducing protein. This mechanism for coupling growth and differentiation may also apply to other types of cells. Differences in the time of the switch-on of the differentiation inducer would produce differences in the amount of multiplication before differentiation. The platelet-derived growth factor is structurally related to the simian sarcoma virus oncogene *sis* [9, 77]. It will be interesting to determine whether MGI-1 and MGI-2 are structurally related to any of the known oncogenes.

The multiplication of normal cells is regulated at two control points. The first control is that which requires MGI-1 to produce more cells that can then differentiate by the MGI-2 induced by MGI-1. The second control is the stopping of cell multiplication that occurs as part of the program of terminal differentiation to mature cells induced by MGI-2. There is thus a coupling of growth and differentiation in normal cells at both these points.

F. Uncoupling of Growth and Differentiation in Leukemia

As pointed out already, there are MGI^+D^+ clones of myeloid leukemic cells that no longer require MGI-1 for growth, but can still be induced to differentiate normally by MGI-2. These leukemic cells have thus uncoupled the normal requirement for growth from the normal requirement for differentiation. Experiments on the properties of these cells after induction of differentiation by MGI-2 have shown that the normal requirement for MGI-1 for cell viability and growth is restored in the differentiating leukemic cells [13, 44, 45]. MGI-1 added to normal myeloid precursors induces the production of MGI-2, so that the cells can then differentiate by the endogenously produced MGI-2. However, in these leukemic cells, MGI-1 did not induce the production of MGI-2 even though, like normal cells, they again required MGI-1 for viability and growth. There was therefore no induction of differentiation after adding MGI-1 [44, 45]. There is another type of leukemic cell that constitutively produces its own MGI-1 and can also show this lack of induction of MGI-2 by MGI-1, so that the cells do not differentiate [72]. The absence of induction of MGI-2 by MGI-1 therefore uncouples growth and differentiation in these leukemic cells. The lack of requirement of MGI-1 for growth and the absence of induction of the differentiation-inducing protein MGI-2 by the growth-inducing protein MGI-1, are thus mechanisms that uncouple growth and differentiation in MGI^+D^+ leukemic cells [44, 45, 66, 72].

In leukemic cells with constitutive production of MGI-1, changes in specific components of the culture medium can result in an autoinduction of differentiation owing to the restoration of the induction of MGI-2 by MGI-1, which then restores the normal coupling of growth and differentiation (Fig. 2). These changes in the culture medium include the use of mouse or rat serum instead of horse or calf serum, serum-free medium, and removal of transferrin from serum-free medium [72]. Autoinduction of differentiation in this type of leukemic cell may also occur under certain conditions in vivo.

This coupling of growth and differentiation in normal cells is regulated at two control points. The uncoupling of growth and differentiation in MGI^+D^+ leukemic cells is at the first control point, but the coupling at the second control in normal cells, between the induction of differentiation by MGI-2 and the stopping of multiplication in the mature cells, is maintained. There are differentiation-defective MGI^+D^- leukemic cells, that, like the MGI^+D^+ leukemic cells, no longer require addition of MGI-1 for growth. However, in these cells MGI-2 induces only a partial differentiation, mature cells are not produced, and the cells do not stop multiplying. In addition to uncoupling growth and differentiation at the first control point, MGI^+D^- leukemic cells thus show a second uncoupling between the initiation of differentiation by MGI-2 and the stopping of cell multiplication that occurs as part of the normal program of terminal differentiation. It has been suggested that leukemia originates by uncoupling the first control and

Type of myeloid cells	Requirement of MGI-1 for growth	Induction of MGI-2 by MGI-1	Differentiation
Normal	+	Production of MGI-2 →	+
Leukemic	+ or −	No production of MGI-2	−
	Constitutive production MGI-1	Production of MGI-2 →	+ *

* Autoinduction of differentiation under specific conditions

Fig. 2. Differences in induction of differentiation-inducing protein MGI-2 by growth-inducing protein MGI-1 in normal and leukemic myeloid cells

that uncoupling of the second control then results in a further evolution of leukemia [64, 66].

G. Constitutive Gene Expression in Malignancy

Since there are leukemic cells which, unlike normal myeloblasts, no longer require MGI-1 for cell viability and growth, the molecular changes required for viability and growth that have to be induced in the normal cells are constitutive in these leukemic cells. This also applies to leukemic cells that constitutively produce their own MGI-1. This suggests that the origin of myeloid leukemia can be due to a change from an induced to a constitutive expression of genes that control cell viability and growth [64, 66].

Studies on changes in the synthesis of specific proteins in normal myeloblasts, MGI^+D^+, MGI^+D^-, and MGI^-D^- leukemic clones at different times after adding MGI-1 and MGI-2, using two-dimensional gel electrophoresis [32], have directly shown that there have been changes from inducible to constitutive gene expression in the leukemic cells. The results also indicate a relationship between constitutive gene expression and uncoupling of the induction of differentiation by MGI-2 and the stopping of multiplication in the mature cells. The results indicate that changes from an induced to a constitutive expression of certain genes are associated with the uncoupling of growth and differentiation, both at the control which requires MGI-1 to produce more cells and at the control of the stopping of cell multiplication that occurs in the formation of mature cells.

The protein changes during the growth and differentiation of normal myeloblasts seem to be induced by MGI-1 and MGI-2 as a series of parallel multiple pathways of gene expression [32]. It can be assumed that the normal developmental program that couples growth and differentiation in normal cells requires synchronous initiation and progression of these multiple parallel pathways. The presence of constitutive gene expression for some pathways can be expected to produce asynchrony in the coordination required for the normal development program. Depending on the pathways involved, this asynchrony could then result in an uncoupling of the controls for growth and differentiation and produce different blocks in the ability to be induced for the differentiation process and to terminate it.

We have been able to treat MGI^-D^- leukemic cells so as to induce the reversion of specific proteins from the constitutive to the nonconstitutive state. This reversion was then associated with a gain of inducibility by MGI-2 for various differentiation-associated properties. Reversion from the constitutive to the nonconstitutive state in these cells thus restored the synchrony required for induction of differentiation [75].

The suggestion derived from these results [32, 64, 66] is, therefore, that myeloid leukemia originates by a change that produces certain constitutive pathways of gene expression, so that cells no longer require MGI-1 for growth or constitutively produce MGI-1 without inducing MGI-2. These leukemic cells can, however, still be induced to differentiate normally by MGI-2 added exogenously or induced in the cells in other ways. The differentiation program induced by MGI-2 can thus proceed normally when it is uncoupled from the growth program induced by MGI-1. This can be followed by constitutive expression of other pathways, resulting in the uncoupling of other controls and an asynchrony that interferes with the normal program of terminal differentiation. These second changes then result in the further evolution of leukemia [66].

H. Reversal of Malignancy by Induction of Differentiation in Various Types of Tumors

These conclusions on the origin and evolution of myeloid leukemia may be applicable to malignant tumors derived from other types of cells whose viability, growth, and differentiation are induced by other physiologic inducers. Identification of the physiologic inducers of growth and differentiation for different cell types would be a crucial requirement in extending these conclusions to those other tumors. However, even in the absence of such identifications, it appears likely that teratocarcinoma cells [8, 53] may be comparable to $MGI^{+}D^{+}$ myeloid leukemic cells. The presence of fetal proteins in certain tumors may also be due to constitutive gene expression in the tumor of a protein that is induced by the physiologic inducer during the developmental program in the normal fetus [66]. There are probably a variety of tumors in which: (a) the original malignancy has a normal differentiation program and the cells are malignant because of uncoupling of the requirement for growth from the requirement for differentiation by changing the gene expression required for growth from inducible to constitutive; and (b) where the further evolution of the tumor results from changes from inducible to constitutive of other pathways of gene expression that produce asynchrony in the normal differentiation program, so that mature nondividing cells are not formed by the physiologic inducer of differentiation. However, even these tumors may still be induced to differentiate to form nonmalignant cells by treatment with compounds that can reverse the constitutive to the nonconstitutive state or induce the differentiation program by other pathways. In some tumors, such as sarcomas, reversal of malignancy can be obtained by specific changes in the karyotype [20, 61–63, 81]. But the stopping of cell division in mature cells by inducing differentiation induces a reversion of malignancy by bypassing the genetic changes that produce the malignant phenotype.

Acknowledgments. This research is now being supported by a contract with the National Foundation for Cancer Research, Bethesda, and by grants from the Jerome A. and Estelle R. Newman Assistance Fund, and the Julian Wallerstein Foundation.

References

1. Austin PE, McCulloch EA, Till JE (1971) Characterization of the factor in L cell conditioned medium capable of stimulating colony formation by mouse marrow cells in culture. J Cell Physiol 77: 121–134
2. Azumi J, Sachs L (1977) Chromosome mapping of the genes that control differentiation and malignancy in myeloid leukemic cells. Proc Natl Acad Sci USA 74: 253–257
3. Baccarani M, Tura S (1979) Correspondence, differentiation of myeloid leukemic cells: new possibilities for therapy. Br J Haematol 42: 485–487
4. Bradley TR, Metcalf D (1966) The growth of mouse bone marrow in vitro. Aust J Exp Biol Med Sci 44: 287–300
5. Burgess AW, Metcalf D (1980) Characterisation of a serum factor stimulating the differentiation of myelomonocytic leukemic cells. Int J Cancer 26: 647–654
6. Burgess AW, Camakaris J, Metcalf D (1977) Purification and properties of colony-stimulating factor from mouse lung conditioned medium. J Biol Chem 252: 1998–2003
7. Cohen L, Sachs L (1981) Constitutive gene expression in myeloid leukemia and cell

competence for induction of differentiation by the steroid dexamethasone. Proc Natl Acad Sci USA 78:353–357

8. Dewey MJ, Martin DW Jr, Martin GR, Mintz B (1977) Mosaic mice with teratocarcinoma-derived mutant cells deficient in hypoxanthine phosphoribosyltransferase. Proc Natl Acad Sci USA 74:5564–5568
9. Doolittle RF, Hunkapiller MW, Hood LE, Devare SG, Robbins KC, Aaronson SA (1983) Simian sarcoma virus onc gene, v-sis, is derived from the gene (or genes) encoding a platelet-derived growth factor. Science 221:275–277
10. Falk A, Sachs L (1980) Clonal regulation of the induction of macrophage and granulocyte inducing proteins for normal and leukemic myeloid cells. Int J Cancer 26:595–601
11. Fibach E, Sachs L (1974) Control of normal differentiation of myeloid leukemic cells. IV. Induction of differentiation by serum from endotoxin treated mice. J Cell Physiol 83: 177–185
12. Fibach E, Sachs L (1975) Control of normal differentiation of myeloid leukemic cells. VIII. Induction of differentiation to mature granulocytes in mass culture. J Cell Physiol 86:221–230
13. Fibach E, Sachs L (1976) Control of normal differentiation of myeloid leukemic cells. XI. Induction of a specific requirement for cell viability and growth during the differentiation of myeloid leukemic cells. J Cell Physiol 89:259–266
14. Fibach E, Landau T, Sachs L (1972) Normal differentiation of myeloid leukemic cells induced by a differentiation-inducing protein. Nature New Biol 237:276–278
15. Fibach E, Hayashi M, Sachs L (1973) Control of normal differentiation of myeloid leukemic cells to macrophages and granulocytes. Proc Natl Acad Sci USA 70:343–346
16. Friend C (1978) The phenomenon of differentiation in murine erythroleukemic cells. Harvey Lectures 72. Academic, New York, pp 253–281
17. Ginsburg H, Sachs L (1963) Formation of pure suspension of mast cells in tissue culture by differentiation of lymphoid cells from the mouse thymus. J Natl Cancer Inst 31:1–40
18. Gootwine E, Webb CG, Sachs L (1982) Participation of myeloid leukaemic cells injected into embryos in haematopoietic differentiation in adult mice. Nature 299:63–65
19. Hayashi M, Fibach E, Sachs L (1974) Control of normal differentiation of myeloid leukemic cells. V. Normal differentiation to aneuploid leukemic cells and the chromosome banding pattern of D^+ and D^- clones. Int J Cancer 14:40–48
20. Hitosumachi S, Rabinowitz Z, Sachs L (1971) Chromosomal control of reversion in transformed cells. Nature 231:511–514
21. Hoffman-Liebermann B, Sachs L (1978) Regulation of actin and other proteins in the differentiation of myeloid leukemic cells. Cell 14:825–834
22. Hoffman-Liebermann B, Liebermann D, Sachs L (1981) Control mechanisms regulating gene expression during normal differentiation of myeloid leukemic cells. Differentiation defective mutants blocked in mRNA production and mRNA translation. Dev Biol 81:255–265
23. Hoffman-Liebermann B, Liebermann D, Sachs L (1981) Regulation of gene expression by tumor promoters. III. Complementation of the developmental program in myeloid leukemic cells by regulating mRNA production and mRNA translation. Int J Cancer 26:615–620
24. Housset M, Daniel MT, Degos L (1982) Small doses of Ara-C in the treatment of acute myeloid leukemia: differentiation of myeloid leukemia cells? Br J Haematol 51: 125–129
25. Ichikawa Y (1969) Differentiation of a cell line of myeloid leukemia. J Cell Physiol 74: 223–234
26. Ichikawa Y, Pluznik DH, Sachs L (1966) *In vitro* control of the development of macrophage and granulocyte colonies. Proc Natl Acad Sci USA 56:488–495
27. Ichikawa Y, Pluznik DH, Sachs L (1967) Feedback inhibition of the development of macrophage and granulocyte colonies. I. Inhibition by macrophages. Proc Natl Acad Sci USA 58:1480–1486
28. Ichikawa Y, Maeda N, Horiuchi M (1976) *In vitro* differentiation of Rauscher virus induced myeloid leukemic cells. Int J Cancer 17:789–797
29. Kasuga M, Fujita-Yamaguchi Y, Blithe DL, Kahn CR (1983) Tyrosine-specific protein kinase activity is associated with the purified insulin receptor. Proc Natl Acad Sci USA 80: 2137–2141
30. Krystosek A, Sachs L (1976) Control of lysozyme induction in the differentiation of myeloid leukemic cells. Cell 9:675–684
31. Landau T, Sachs L (1971) Characterization of the inducer required for the development of macrophage and granulocyte colonies. Proc Natl Acad Sci USA 68:2540–2544
32. Liebermann D, Hoffmann-Liebermann B, Sachs L (1980) Molecular dissection of differentiation in normal and leukemic myelo-

blasts: separately programmed pathways of gene expression. Dev Biol 79:46–63
33. Liebermann D, Hoffman-Liebermann B, Sachs L (1982) Regulation and role of different macrophage and granulocyte proteins in normal and leukemic myeloid cells. Int J Cancer 29:159–161
34. Lipton J, Sachs L (1981) Characterization of macrophage and granulocyte inducing proteins for normal and leukemic myeloid cells produced by the Krebs ascites tumor. Biochim Biophys Acta 673:552–569
35. Lotem J, Sachs L (1974) Different blocks in the differentiation of myeloid leukemic cells. Proc Natl Acad Sci USA 71:3507–3511
36. Lotem J, Sachs L (1975) Induction of specific changes in the surface membrane of myeloid leukemic cells by steroid hormones. Int J Cancer 15:731–740
37. Lotem J, Sachs L (1977a) Control of normal differentiation of myeloid leukemic cells. XII. Isolation of normal myeloid colony-forming cells from bone marrow and the sequence of differentiation to mature granulocytes in normal and D^+ myeloid leukemic cells. J Cell Physiol 92:97–108
38. Lotem J, Sachs L (1977b) Genetic dissection of the control of normal differentiation in myeloid leukemic cells. Proc Natl Acad Sci USA 74:5554–5558
39. Lotem J, Sachs L (1978a) Genetic dissociation of different cellular effects of interferon on myeloid leukemic cells. Int J Cancer 22:214–220
40. Lotem J, Sachs L (1978b) *In vivo* induction of normal differentiation in myeloid leukemic cells. Proc Natl Acad Sci USA 75:3781–3785
41. Lotem J, Sachs L (1979) Regulation of normal differentiation in mouse and human myeloid leukemic cells by phorbol esters and the mechanism of tumor promotion. Proc Natl Acad Sci USA 76:5158–5162
42. Lotem J, Sachs L (1980) Potential prescreening for therapeutic agents that induce differentiation in human myeloid leukemic cells. Int J Cancer 25:561–564
43. Lotem J, Sachs L (1981) *In vivo* inhibition of the development of myeloid leukemia by injection of macrophage and granulocyte inducing protein. Int J Cancer 28:375–386
44. Lotem J, Sachs L (1982) Mechanisms that uncouple growth and differentiation in myeloid leukemia: restoration of requirement for normal growth-inducing protein without restoring induction of differentiation-inducing protein. Proc Natl Acad Sci USA 79:4347–4351
45. Lotem J, Sachs L (1983a) Coupling of growth and differentiation in normal myeloid precursors and the breakdown of this coupling in leukemia. Int J Cancer 32:127–134
46. Lotem J, Sachs L (1983b) Control of *in vivo* differentiation of myeloid leukemic cells. III. Regulation by T lymphocytes and inflammation. Int J Cancer 32:781–791
47. Lotem J, Sachs L (1984) Control of *in vivo* differentiation of myeloid leukemic cells. IV. Inhibition of leukemia development by myeloid differentiation-inducing protein. Int J Cancer 33:147–154
48. Lotem J, Lipton J, Sachs L (1980) Separation of different molecular forms of macrophage and granulocyte inducing proteins for normal and leukemic myeloid cells. Int J Cancer 25:763–771
49. Maeda M, Horiuchi M, Numa S, Ichikawa Y (1977) Characterization of a differentiation stimulating factor for mouse myeloid leukemic cells. Gann 68:435–447
50. Marks P, Rifkind RA (1978) Erythroleukemic differentiation. Ann Rev Biochem 47: 419–448
51. Metcalf D (1969) Studies on colony formation in vitro by mouse bone marrow cells. I. Continuous cluster formation and relation of clusters to colonies. J Cell Physiol 74:323–332
52. Michalewicz R, Lotem J, Sachs L (1984) Cell differentiation and therapeutic effect of low doses of cytosine arbinoside in human myeloid leukemia. Leuk Res (in press)
53. Mintz B, Illmensee K (1975) Normal genetically mosaic mice produced from malignant teratocarcinoma cells. Proc Natl Acad Sci USA 72:3585–3589
54. Moore MAS (1982) G-SCF: its relationship to leukemia differentiation-inducing activity and other hemopoietic regulators. J Cell Physiol [Suppl] 1:53–64
55. Nicola NA, Burgess AW, Metcalf D (1979) Similar molecular properties of granulocyte-macrophage colony stimulating factors produced by different organs. J Biol Chem 24:5290–5299
56. Paran M, Ichikawa Y, Sachs L (1968) Production of the inducer for macrophage and granulocyte colonies by leukemic cells. J Cell Physiol 72:251–254
57. Paran M, Sachs L, Barak Y, Resnitzky P (1970) *In vitro* induction of granulocyte differentiation in hematopoietic cells from leukemic and non-leukemic patients. Proc Natl Acad Sci USA 67:1542–1549
58. Pike B, Robinson WA (1970) Human bone marrow growth in agar gel. J Cell Physiol 76:77–84
59. Pluznik DH, Sachs L (1965) The cloning of normal "mast" cells in tissue culture. J Cell Comp Physiol 66:319–324

60. Pluznik DH, Sachs L (1966) The induction of clones of normal "mast" cells by a substance from conditioned medium. Exp Cell Res 43:553–563
61. Rabinowitz Z, Sachs L (1968) Reversion of properties in cells transformed by polyoma virus. Nature 220:1203–1206
62. Rabinowitz Z, Sachs L (1970) Control of the reversion of properties in transformed cells. Nature 225:136–139
63. Sachs L (1974) Regulation of membrane changes, differentiation, and malignancy in carcinogenesis. Harvey Lectures 68. Academic, New York, pp 1–35
64. Sachs L (1978a) Control of normal cell differentiation and the phenotypic reversion of malignancy in myeloid leukemia. Nature 274:535–539
65. Sachs L (1978b) The differentiation of myeloid leukemia cells. New possibilities for therapy. Br J Haematol 40:509–517
66. Sachs L (1980) Constitutive uncoupling of pathways of gene expression that control growth and differentiation in myeloid leukemia: a model for the origin and progression of malignancy. Proc Natl Acad Sci USA 77:6152–6156
67. Sachs L (1982a) Control of growth and differentiation in leukemic cells: regulation of the developmental program and restoration of the normal phenotype in myeloid leukemia. J Cell Physiol [Suppl] 1:151–164
68. Sachs L (1982b) Normal developmental programmes in myeloid leukemia: regulatory proteins in the control of growth and differentiation. Cancer Surveys 1:321–342
69. Simantov R, Sachs L (1978) Differential desensitization of functional adrenergic receptors in normal and malignant myeloid cells. Relationship to receptor mediated hormone cytoxicity. Proc Natl Acad Sci USA 75:1805–1809
70. Simantov R, Shkolnik T, Sachs L (1980) Desensitization of enucleated cells to hormones and the role of cytoskeleton in control of a normal hormonal response. Proc Natl Acad Sci USA 77:4798–4802
71. Stanley ER, Heard PM (1977) Factors regulating macrophage production and growth. Purification and some properties of the colony stimulating factor from medium conditioned by mouse L cells. J Biol Chem 252: 4305–4312
72. Symonds G, Sachs L (1982a) Autoinduction of differentiation in myeloid leukemic cells: restoration of normal coupling between growth and differentiation in leukemic cells that constitutively produce their own growth-inducing protein. EMBO J 1:1343–1346
73. Symonds G, Sachs L (1982b) Cell competence for induction of differentiation by insulin and other compounds in myeloid leukemic clones continuously cultured in serum-free medium. Blood 60:208–212
74. Symonds G, Sachs L (1982c) Modulation of cell competence for induction of differentiation in myeloid leukemic cells. J Cell Physiol 111:9–14
75. Symonds G, Sachs L (1983) Synchrony of gene expression and the differentiation of myeloid leukemic cells: reversion from constitutive to inducible protein synthesis. EMBO J 2:663–667
76. Ushiro H, Cohen S (1980) Identification of phosphotyrosine as a product of epidermal growth factor-activated protein kinase in A-431 cell membranes. J Biol Chem 225: 8363–8365
77. Waterfield MD, Scrace GT, Whittle N, Stroobant P, Johnsson A, Wasteson A, Westermark B, Heldin CH, Huang JS, Deuel TF (1983) Platelet-derived growth factor is structurally related to the putative transforming protein $p28^{sis}$ of simian sarcoma virus. Nature 304:35–39
78. Webb CG, Gootwine E, Sachs L (1984) Developmental potential of myeloid leukemia cells injected into mid-gestation embryos. Dev Biol 101:221–224
79. Weisinger G, Sachs L (1983) DNA-binding protein that induces cell differentiation. EMBO J 2:2103–2107
80. Weiss B, Sachs L (1978) Indirect induction of differentiation in myeloid leukemic cells by lipid A. Proc Natl Acad Sci USA 75:1374–1378
81. Yamamoto T, Rabinowitz Z, Sachs L (1973) Identification of the chromosomes that control malignancy. Nature (New Biol) 243:247–250
82. Yamamoto Y, Tomida M, Hozumi M (1980) Production by spleen cells of factors stimulating differentiation of mouse myeloid leukemic cells that differ from colony stimulating-factor. Cancer Res 40:4804–4809

Haematology and Blood Transfusion Vol. 29
Modern Trends in Human Leukemia VI
Edited by Neth, Gallo, Greaves, Janka

Self-Renewal of Haemopoietic Stem Cells: The Roles of the Environment, of Growth Factors and of the *src* Oncogene

T. M. Dexter [1], D. Boettiger [2], and E. Spooncer [1]

A. Introduction

Haemopoietic stem cells are derived early in embryogenesis, are relatively few in number, but persist throughout adult life by virtue of their ability to undergo self-renewal. This ability to undergo self-renewal is a characteristic and essential property of stem cells: in the absence of self-renewal the haemopoietic system would rapidly decline, while excessive and persistent self-renewal (in the absence of death or differentiation) would lead to a dramatic reduction in the production of mature cells and an increase in primitive cells, i.e. a leukaemia [24, 35]. It follows, then, that an investigation of self-renewal and differentiation is an over-riding problem in the understanding of growth control in normal tissues as well as the lack of growth control which occurs during tumourigenesis. In this context, the role of tissue and cell lineage-restricted growth factors and of oncogenes (and their products) is assuming more and more importance [16, 48]. In this communication, the role of one such growth factor (haemopoietic cell growth factor), the stromal cell milieu, and the *src* oncogene are discussed in relation to self-renewal and differentiation of haemopoietic cells.

1 Department of Experimental Haematology, Paterson Laboratories, Christie Hospital & Holt Radium Institute, Withington, Manchester M20 9BX, England
2 Department of Microbiology, University of Pennsylvania, Pennsylvania, USA

B. The Role of the Marrow Stroma in Haemopoiesis

Haemopoietic cell development in the adult occurs mainly in the bone marrow, where the developing blood cells are found in intimate association with a stromal cell network [26, 49]. Evidence indicates that the stromal cells supply the extracellular matrix and cell–cell interactions necessary for the proliferation of stem cells [40] as well as their differentiation and development into the various myeloid lineages. For example, the stromal cells present in long-term marrow cultures produce factors which specifically (and reversibly) stimulate or inhibit DNA synthesis in CFU-S [46, 53, 54]: thus, changes in the respective concentrations of these opposing activities act to modulate proliferative activity of the stem cells. However, within the long-term cultures (and in marrow in vivo), the population size of stem cells is strictly controlled, such that in normal steady state conditions the number of CFU-S remains fairly constant [45]. This control can operate at two levels. First, at the level of stem cell proliferation where an increased demand for CFU-S (following partial ablation with cytotoxic chemicals) is met by increased proliferative activity [19, 52] (associated with increased production of the CFU-S "stimulator" alluded to earlier). Second, at the level of stem cell differentiation, a process which is an enigma at present, but which generates a series of lineage-restricted progenitor cells such as granulocyte/macrophage colony-forming cells (GM-CFC), erythroid colony forming cells

(BFU-E) and so on. Most, if not all, of these committed progenitor cells can be recognised by their ability to undergo clonal expansion in soft gel systems to produce colonies containing mature cells of the appropriate cell lineages [13, 28]. The development of the cells *within these soft gel systems* requires the continuous presence of appropriate growth factors such as granulocyte/macrophage colony-stimulating factor (GM-CSF), burst-promoting activity (BPA), etc. However, the development of the progenitor cells *in long-term marrow cultures* occurs in association with the marrow stromal cells and does *not* require the presence of added stimulatory molecules [12, 50].

Indeed, it is difficult to detect the presence of molecules such as GM-CSF or BPA in medium conditioned by the growth of marrow stromal cells in vitro, and for this reason we believe that such molecules are normally produced by the stromal cells and stimulate progenitor cells *locally,* where an effective concentration of the growth factor can be maintained [14, 18, 37, 51]. In other words, the haemopoietic system may be best viewed as consisting of a series of stromal cell niches facilitating stem cell proliferation/differentiation or promoting progenitor cell development. This view is supported by our observation that specific stromal cell–haemopoietic cell interactions occur during erythroid cell development and that similar but different stromal cell–haemopoietic cell interactions occur during granulocyte development [1, 2, 11]. The net result of these complex interactions is the maintenance of homeostasis such that for every one CFU-S there are about ten progenitor cells and for every one GM-CFC, there are between 500 and 1000 mature cells being produced. These ratios are highly consistent and are found both in marrow in vivo and in long-term cultures in vitro. Obviously, an increase or a decrease in the self-renewal probability of the stem cells may have a profound effect upon the production of mature cells – leading either to an aplasia or a hyperplasia.

C. The Role of Growth Factors in Self-Renewal

Several haemopoietic growth factors have now been purified to homogeneity, partial amino acid sequence determined and, in at least two cases, molecularly cloned [8, 10, 20, 29, 33, 42, 55] and A.W. Burgess, personal communication). One of these growth factors is GM-CSF, purified from mouse lung cell-conditioned medium. This factor stimulates the development of GM-CFC to produce colonies in vitro containing neutrophils and macrophages [8]. In this case, however, little or no self-renewal occurs: after several days' growth, the GM-CFC give rise to colonies containing only mature cells [4, 7, 30]. Because of this, it was once thought that GM-CSF was a *lineage-restricted* regulatory molecule. Recently, however, it has been shown that multipotential stem cells can also respond to this molecule, which acts as a proliferative signal as well as facilitating differentiation of the multipotential cells to lineage-restricted progenitor cells [31]. Thus, GM-CSF may have a wider range of "target" cells than initially thought. Despite this, there is no evidence that GM-CSF is acting as a *self-renewal* stimulus for multipotential cells or GM-CFC; rather, it appears to be involved in facilitating development of the stem and progenitor cells in the absence of self-renewal. A similar role can also be ascribed to the molecule which selectively stimulates granulocyte development from the GM-CFC [29, 33] (so-called granulocyte colony-stimulating factor, or G-CSF) and to the molecule which preferentially stimulates macrophage development from the GM-CFC [42] (macrophage colony- stimulating factor, M-CSF or CSF-1). Similarly, the hormone erythropoietin (which acts on the terminal stages of erythropoiesis) has so far not been shown to act as a self-renewal-inducing molecule (E. Spooncer, unpublished work). Consequently, the role of lineage-restricted regulatory molecules seems to be one of facilitating development rather than self-renewal.

In contrast to this is the action of the molecule which we have recently purified to homogeneity from WEHI-3 cell-conditioned medium. This molecule, which we term haemopoietic cell growth factor [4] (or HCGF) is a glycoprotein of ~25 kilodaltons with a polypeptide core of 15 kilodaltons, and is almost certainly the same molecule as that known as IL-3, BPA, PSF, mast cell growth factor or multi-CSF [9, 22, 23, 32, 36, 56].

The widespread interest in this molecule arises from the observation that it can "immortalise" granulocyte precursor cells and mast cells, i.e. it will allow such cells to self-renew continuously in vitro [15, 21, 44]. It will also promote proliferation and self-renewal of CFU-S in short-term liquid culture [27, 47] and L. Dorssers, personal communication), as well as proliferation and development of multipotential stem cells and the various types of myeloid committed progenitor cells [4]. In other words, HCGF appears to be a "master control" molecule influencing the earliest stages of haemopoiesis. This does not mean that the lineage-restricted molecules (such as CSF-1 and erythropoietin) do not have a role to play in haemopoietic cell development. Rather, they may best be seen as the "fine tuners" in the system, modulating cell production to meet the demand existing at any one time.

Of major interest is that, unlike the molecules such as GM-CSF, M-CSF, G-CSF and erythropoietin, HCGF *cannot* be detected in the serum of mice, although it is readily produced in vitro from lectin-stimulated T cells [9]. Our proposition is that the in vivo production of this molecule is probably very stringently controlled, being normally produced only in areas where self-renewal is required. Obviously, excessive or systemic production of HCGF may be expected to have a dramatic effect on haemopoiesis. Indeed, it could be that the WEHI-3 leukaemic cells (a potent source of HCGF) are leukaemic by virtue of their ability to produce HCGF and are thus "autostimulated" for self-renewal.

D. Enhanced Self-Renewal in Response to the *src* Oncogene

From the previous discussion, it is clear that the maintenance of homeostasis requires a delicate balance between cell–cell interactions and diffusible regulatory molecules (growth factors). The products of certain oncogenes, i.e. the oncogenes associated with leukaemic transformation such as *abl, myc, myb, erb,* presumably alter this balance in such a way that increased self-renewal occurs at the expense of differentiation [6]. How they do this is unclear, although the evolutionary conservation of cellular oncogenes suggests an important role for their products in *normal* cell growth and differentiation [17, 38, 43].

Recently, we have been investigating the effects of the *src* oncogene (which codes for a product called $pp60^{src}$), an oncogene which is associated with the production of sarcomas in chickens [5]. Using molecular recombination techniques, the avian *src* has been placed under the influence of an amphotropic murine virus promoter sequence [3], and this virus, *src* (MoMuLV), has been used to infect murine long-term marrow cultures [7, 41]. The effect was dramatic.

I. Effects on the Stroma

Little change was seen in the gross morphology or organisation of the stromal elements for several weeks. However, the cultures were infected with the *src* (MoMuLV) between 5 and 8 weeks after initiation of the cultures – a time at which little proliferative activity is occurring in the stromal cells, hence to initial lack of effect is not unexpected. However, within 8–10 weeks after infection there occurred a progressive overgrowth of "transformed" fibroblasts and macrophages which, at later times in culture, were released from the adherent layer and were found admixed with haemopoietic cells in the growth medium [7].

II. Effects on Haemopoietic Cells

Following infection with *src* (MoMuLV) there was a progressive increase in the concentration and in the absolute number of stem cells (CFU-S) and committed progenitor cells (GM-CFC) released into the growth medium. The increases in the con-

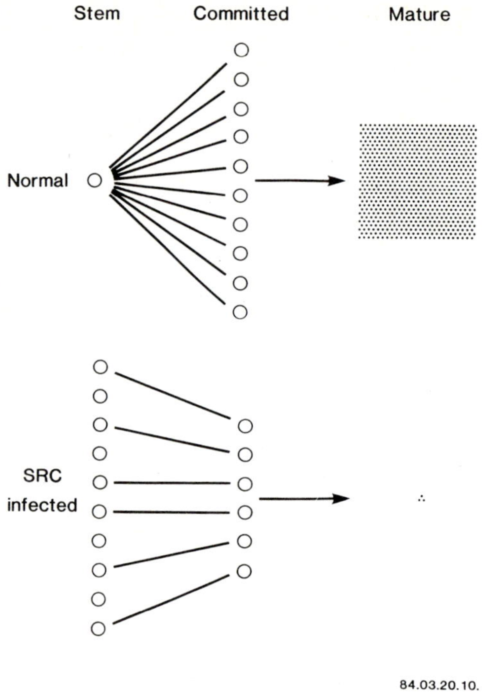

Fig. 1. Schematic illustration of the influence of *src* (MoMuLV) infection of long-term cultures on the development expansion of haemopoietic cells

centration of CFU-S and GM-CFC (which are 50–100 times the level seen in the control) reflected an absolute increase of 10–20 times the number seen in the corresponding control cultures. At the same time, however, the number of mature haemopoietic cells produced fell dramatically. In control cultures, between 400 and 1000 mature cells were present per GM-CFC. In infected cultures, on the other hand, the level of mature cells progressively declined to reach a level of about 5–10 mature cells per GM-CFC [7]. In other words, *src* (MoMuLV) infection of long-term marrow cultures led to an inversion of the developmental hierarchies seen during normal haemopoiesis. The effects are schematically described in Fig. 1.

III. Are the Haemopoietic Cells Leukaemic?

Notwithstanding the effects seen on developmental transitions described earlier, we repeatedly found that (irrespective of the time since infection) injection of the cells into immunocompromised or potentially lethally irradiated recipients did *not* lead to the development of a leukaemia [7, 41]. In fact, the spleen colonies produced from the CFU-S present in *src* (MoMuLV)-infected cultures were normal in all aspects examined, the cells would protect mice from the effects of a lethal dose of radiation, and the reconstituted animals lived a normal life span without the emergence of leukaemic disease [41]. In these reconstituted animals a slight anaemia was occasionally observed, but no evidence of a gross block in differentiation was seen – as happened in the original *src* (MoMuLV)-infected long-term cultures. We conclude, therefore, that the haemopoietic cells produced in the *src*-infected cultures are essentially normal (at least in terms of differentiation ability) and the developmental block seen in the infected long-term culture is due primarily to an effect of *src* on the supportive stromal cell elements.

IV. Infection with *src* (MoMuLV) is Associated with Changes in the Self-Renewal Capacity of Haemopoietic Cells

While the CFU-S in the *src*-infected cultures are apparently normal in their ability to produce spleen colonies and to reconstitute irradiated mice, we did detect a profound change in their self-renewal ability. For example, when normal CFU-S are serially transferred in vivo in irradiated recipients, they rapidly lose their ability to produce more CFU-S or to reconstitute haemopoiesis in such mice, after the second or third transfer [25, 34, 39]. Similarly, if normal CFU-S are serially passaged in vitro on the irradiated *stromal cell layer* of a long-term marrow culture, they likewise rapidly lose their ability to self-renew and establish haemopoiesis [34].

CFU-S from the *src* (MoMuLV)-infected cultures, however, can be repeatedly passaged in vivo or in vitro without any apparent decline in their ability to produce CFU-S or to establish apparently normal haemopoiesis. Thus, these data argue that while the cells are not leukaemic, they have

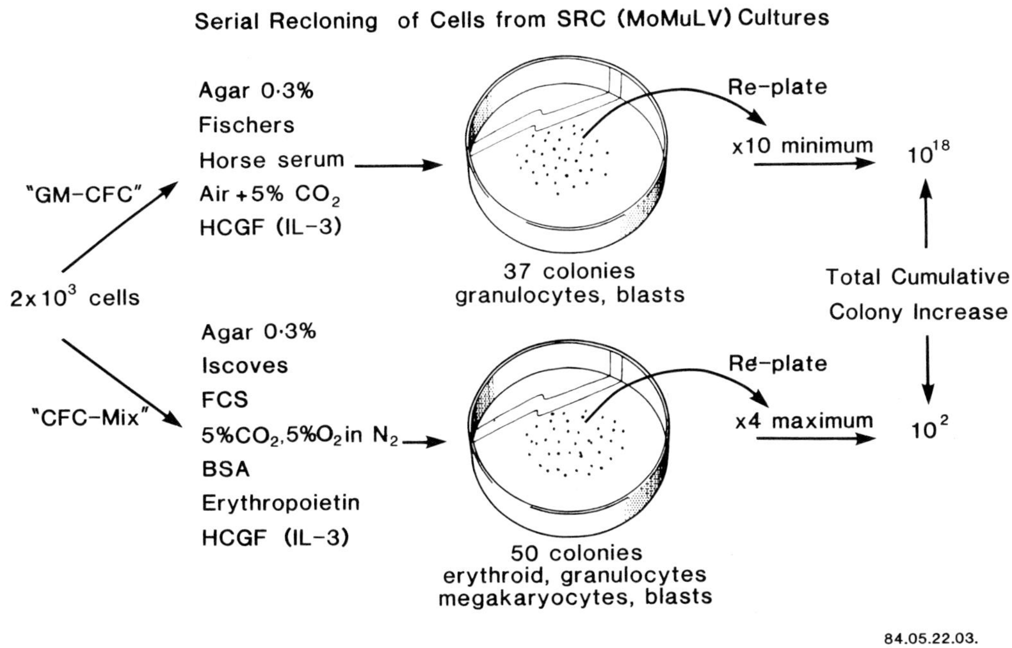

Fig. 2. Scheme of serial recloning of cells from *src* (MoMuLV)-infected long-term cultures in the GM-CFC and CFC-mix assay conditions. The primary colonies grown from the long-term cultured cells are replated into fresh medium at 7-day intervals

been changed or selected in some way for the characteristic of extended self-renewal ability in situations which are unfavourable for self-renewal of normal stem cells [7, 41].

This ability to undergo extended self-renewal is found not only for the CFU-S, in association with the stroma of marrow cultures, but also for cells which form colonies in soft gel media in vitro in the absence of stroma [7, 41]. For example, when normal cells are plated in a clonogenic assay system developed for the growth of GM-CFC, using HCGF as the stimulus for development, little or no self-renewal occurs and the cells undergo terminal maturation [4, 7, 41]. When similar studies were performed using cells from *src*-infected cultures, we found that after 7 or 14 days' growth the developing colonies contained not only mature cells, but a high proportion of blast cells as well [7, 41]. When these cells were replated in fresh agar gels, they produced more colonies which in turn could be replated again. Thus far, we have continued this replating for at least ten serial passages and have obtained a potential cumulative colony increase of up to 10^{18} colony-forming cells (Fig. 2). Of some importance is that this serial recloning in the absence of stromal cells can *only* be performed in the presence of HCGF – the lineage-restricted molecules such as CSF-1 do not facilitate this self-renewal [41]. From these data, therefore, we can conclude: (a) that *src* (MoMuLV) infection of long-term cultures has in some way given rise to a population of HCGF-responsive cells with considerably enhanced self-renewal ability; and (b) that this increased self-renewal ability is a property intrinsic to the haemopoietic cells, since the enhanced replating ability occurs in the absence of stroma provided that the cells are supplied with an exogenous supply of HCGF.

V. Increased Self-Renewal of Multipotential Stem Cells In Vitro in the Absence of Stroma

The colonies developing in the agar culture system described previously have been analysed for their developmental potential. To do this, colony cells at various transfer numbers, i.e. between one and ten serial in vitro reclonings, were plated in growth medium facilitating the development of multipotential cells [41]. We consistently found that in these conditions, between 30% and 50% of the colonies produced contained cells of more than one myeloid lineage, including erythroid cells. It seems, then, that the serial recloning ability of the cells in vitro (in a GM-CFC assay system) is associated with self-renewal of multipotential stem cells (CFC-mix). However, when these mixed myeloid colonies were tested for *their* ability to undergo further serial recloning in vitro, the results were uniformly poor (Fig. 2). From these data, we conclude that the self-renewal observed is in part a reflection of the differentiation pressure imposed by the different culture conditions. The results are schematically described in Fig. 2 [41].

VI. The Development of Continuously Growing, Multipotential Stem Cell Lines

Individual colonies developing in the GM-CFC assay system (Fig. 2) were picked out and the cells resuspended in Fischer's medium supplemented with 20% horse serum and WEHI-3 cell-conditioned medium (10% vol/vol) as a source of HCGF. Of 75 individual colonies isolated in this way, all grew and formed continuously growing cell lines in liquid culture. The growth of these cells was absolutely dependent upon HCGF; in its absence, the cells died. The cell lines produced have a primitive morphology and resemble other growth factor-dependent cell lines (FDC-P). However, all the clones so far examined possess an ability to produce mixed myeloid colonies (erythroid cells plus one other lineage) when plated in soft agar. A more detailed examination of one clone FDC/Mx1 has demonstrated that the cells will grow in the absence of HCGF provided they are cultured on a marrow stromal cell layer (E. Spooncer and T. M. Dexter, in preparation). In this respect, the cells are unlike other FDC-P cells, which do not retain this ability. Furthermore, the FDC/Mx1 cells "infiltrate" the marrow stromal cells and form foci of haemopoiesis. As these foci grow and develop, mature granulocytes and (in appropriate conditions) mature red cells are produced for many months. In this respect, therefore, the FDC/Mx1 cells are like normal stem cells which also have the ability to infiltrate marrow stromal cell layers and establish haemopoiesis (E. Spooncer and T. M. Dexter, to be published). Thus far, these detailed studies have only been performed with one clone of cells, FDC/Mx1. However, preliminary data suggests that this retention of stem cell character applies to all the clones isolated. Furthermore, injection of the cells in vivo has thus far not given rise to any leukaemias. Thus, the original infection of the long-term cultures with *src* (MoMuLV) has led to the eventual development of continuously growing, nonleukaemic, multipotential stem cell lines which require the presence of HCGF for their growth in liquid cultures, but where the HCGF can be replaced by marrow stromal cells. These cells should provide a powerful system for investigating the processes of self-renewal and differentiation in normal haemopoiesis and leukaemogenesis.

VII. The Role of the *src* Oncogene

Infection of long-term marrow cultures with other "helper" or rapidly transforming RNA tumour viruses has not led to the effects observed after infection with the *src* (MoMuLV) virus [6]. Therefore, it seems reasonable to conclude that the haemopoietic changes and generation of HCGF-dependent multipotential stem cell lines is directly or indirectly associated with *src* gene expression. Indeed, previous results have clearly demonstrated high levels of $pp60^{src}$, measured by its kinase activity, in both the adherent (mainly stromal) and in the nonadherent (mainly haemopoietic) cell populations of infected long-term cultures [7]. However, the continuously growing cell lines do not produce infectious *src* (MoMuLV) nor do they express high levels of *src* kinase activity (J. Wyke and A. Stoker, personal communication), although such cells clearly have an extended capacity for self-renewal compared with their normal counterparts. Thus, the role of pp60^{src} remains an enigma. Obviously several possibilities are raised by this finding. First, that *src* (MoMuLV) infection of the long-term cultures "selected" for cells with a greater self-renewal ability. If this is the case, however, it is difficult to understand how the phenotype is maintained after prolonged growth in vitro in the absence of stroma. Other possible explanations include "hit and run" events, initial expression and subsequent repression of pp60^{src}, or the integration of provirus adjacent to some important regulatory gene. However, these must be highly frequent events to account for the ease with which *src* (MoMuLV)-infected cultures undergo transformation and the ease with which continuously growing multipotential stem cell lines can be established from such cultures. These possibilities are being explored at present. Nonetheless, the effects observed indicate the complex events which determine self-renewal of the stem cells, the importance of the cellular environment, of the different growth factors and the effects that oncogene expression can have on these processes.

Acknowledgments. This work was supported by the Cancer Research Campaign (UK) T.M. Dexter is a Cancer Research Campaign Fellow.

References

1. Allen TD, Dexter TM (1982) Ultrastructural aspects of erythropoietic differentiation in long-term bone marrow culture. Differentiation 21:86–94
2. Allen TD, Dexter TM (1983) Long term bone marrow cultures: an ultrastructural review. Scan Electron Microsc 4:1851–1866
3. Anderson SM, Scolnick EM (1983) Construction and isolation of a transforming murine retrovirus containing the src gene of Rous sarcoma virus. J Virol 46:594–605
4. Bazill GW, Haynes M, Garland J, Dexter TM (1983) Characterization and partial purification of a haemopoietic cell growth factor in Wehi-3 cell conditioned medium. Biochem J 210:747–759
5. Beard JW (1963) Avian virus growths and their etiologic agents. Adv Cancer Res 7:1–127
6. Boettiger DB, Dexter TM (1984) Long-term marrow cultures in the analysis of viral leukemogenesis. Clin Haematol 13:349–370
7. Boettiger DB, Anderson S, Dexter TM (1984) Effect of src infection on long-term marrow cultures: Increased self-renewal of hemopoietic progenitor cells without leukemia. Cell 36:763–773
8. Burgess AW, Camakaris J, Metcalf D (1977) Purification and properties of colony-stimulating factor from mouse lung conditioned medium. J Biol Chem 252:1998–2003
9. Burgess AW, Metcalf D, Russel SHM, Nicola NA (1980) Granulocyte/macrophage-megakaryocyte-, eosinophil-, and erythroid-colony-stimulating factors produced by mouse spleen cells. Biochem J 185:301–314
10. Das SK, Stanley ER (1982) Structure-function studies of a colony stimulating factor (CSF-1). J Biol Chem 257: 13 579 – 13 684
11. Dexter TM (1982) Stromal cell associated haemopoiesis. J Cell Physiol [Suppl] 1:87–94
12. Dexter TM, Shadduck RK (1980) The regulation of haemopoiesis in long-term bone marrow cultures. I. Role of L-cell CSF. J Cell Physiol 102:279–286
13. Dexter TM, Testa NG (1980) *In vitro* methods in haemopoiesis and lymphopoiesis. J Immunol Methods 38:177–190
14. Dexter TM, Allen TD, Lajtha LG (1977) Conditions controlling the proliferation of haemopoietic stem cells *in vitro.* J Cell Physiol 91:335–344
15. Dexter TM, Garland J, Scott D, Scolnick E, Metcalf D (1980) Growth of factor dependent haemopoietic precursor cell lines. J Exp Med 152:1036–1047
16. Downward J, Yarden Y, Mayes F, Scrau G, Totty N, Stockwell P, Ullrich A, Sclessinger J, Waterfield MD (1984) Close similarity of epidermal growth factor receptor and V-erb-B oncogene protein sequences. Nature 307: 521–527
17. Duesberg PH (1983) Retroviral transforming genes in normal cells. Nature 304:219–226
18. Eliason JF, Dexter TM, Testa N (1982) The regulation of hemopoiesis in long-term bone marrow cultures III. The role of burst-promoting activity. Exp Hemat 10:444–450
19. Frindel E, Croizat H, Vassart F (1976) Stimulating factors liberated by treated bone marrow: *In vitro* effect on CFU kinetics. Exp Hemat 4:56–61
20. Fung MC, Hapel AJ, Ymer S, Cohen DR, Johnson RM, Campbell HD, Young IG (1984) Molecular cloning of cDNA for murine interleukin-3. Nature 307:233–237

21. Greenberger JS, Eckner RJ, Sakakeeny M, Marks P, Reid D, Nabel G, Hapel A, Ihle JN, Humphries KC (1983) Interleukin 3-dependent hematopoietic progenitor cell lines. Fed Proc 42:2762–2771
22. Ihle JN, Keller J, Oroszlan S, Henderson LE, Copeland TD, Fitch F, Prystowsky MB, Goldwasser E, Schrader JW, Palaszynski E, Dy M, Lebel B (1983) Biologic properties of homogeneous interleukin 3. J Immunol 131: 282–287
23. Iscove NN, Roitch CA, Williams N, Guilbert LJ (1982) Molecules stimulating early red cell, granulocyte/macrophage, and megakaryocyte precursors in culture: similarity in size, hydrophobicity and charge. J Cell Physiol [Suppl] 1:23–30
24. Lajtha LG (1979) Stem cell concepts. Differentiation 4:23–34
25. Lajtha LG, Schofield R (1971) Regulation of stem cell renewal and differentiation: possible significance in ageing. In: Strehler BL (ed) Advances in gerontological research. Academic, New York, pp 131–146
26. Lictman MA (1981) The ultrastructure of the hemopoietic environment of the marrow: A review. Exp Hematol 9:391–410
27. Lowenberg B, Dicke KA (1977) Induction of proliferation of haemopoietic stem cells in culture. Exp Hematol 5:314–331
28. Metcalf D (1977) Hemopoietic colonies. Springer, Berlin Heidelberg New York, p 227
29. Metcalf D, Nicola NA (1983) Proliferative effects of purified granulocyte colony-stimulating factor (G-CSF) on normal mouse haemopoietic cell. J Cell Physiol 116:198–206
30. Metcalf D, Johnson GR, Mandel TE (1979) Colony formation in agar by multipotential hemopoietic cells. J Cell Physiol 98:401–424
31. Metcalf D, Johnson GR, Burgess AW (1980) Direct stimulation by purified GM-CSF of the proliferation of multipotential and erythroid progenitor cells. Blood 55:138–147
32. Nabel G, Galli SJ, Dvorak AM, Dvorak HF, Cantor H (1981) Inducer T-lymphocytes stimulate a factor that stimulates proliferation of cloned mast cells. Nature 291:332–334
33. Nicola NA, Metcalf D, Matsumoto M, Johnson GR (1983) Purification of a factor inducing differentiation in murine myelomonocyte leukemia cells. J Biol Chem 258:9017–9023
34. Schofield R, Dexter TM (1984) Studies on the self-renewal ability of CFU-S which have been serially transferred in long-term culture or *in vivo*. Leuk Res (in press)
35. Schofield R, Lajtha LG (1983) Determination of the probability of self-renewal in haemopoietic stem cells: a puzzle. Blood Cells 9:467–473 (1983)
36. Schrader JW, Clark-Lewis I (1982) A T-cell derived factor stimulating multipotential hemopoietic stem cells: molecular weight and distinction from T-cell growth factor and T-cell derived granulocyte macrophage colony-stimulating factor. J Immunol 129: 30–35
37. Shadduck RK, Waheed A, Greenberger JS, Dexter TM (1983) Production of colony-stimulating factor in long-term bone-marrow cultures. J Cell Physiol 114:88–92
38. Shilo B, Weinberg RA (1981) DNA sequences homologous to vertebrate oncogenes are conserved in Drosophila melanogaster. Proc Natl Acad Sci USA 78:6789–6792
39. Siminovitch L, Till JE, McCulloch EA (1964) Decline in colony-forming ability of marrow cells subjected to serial transplantation into irradiated mice. J Cell Comp Physiol 64:23–31
40. Spooncer E, Gallagher JT, Krizsa F, Dexter TM (1983) Regulation of haemopoiesis in long term bone marrow cultures. IV. Glycosaminoglycan synthesis and the stimulation of haemopoiesis by β-D-xylosides. J Cell Biol 96:510–514
41. Spooncer E, Boettiger DB, Dexter TM (1984) Continuous *in vitro* generation of clonogenic multipotential stem cells from src infected cultures. Nature (in press)
42. Stanley ER (1979) Colony stimulating factor (CSF) radioimmunoassay: Detection of a CSF subclass stimulating macrophage production. Proc Natl Acad Sci USA 76:2969–2973
43. Tatchell K, Chaleff DT, Defeo-Jones D, Scolnick EM (1984) Requirement of either of a pair of ras-related genes of saccharomyces cerevisiae for spore viability. Nature 309: 523–527
44. Tertian G, Yung TP, Guy-Grand D, Moore MAS (1981) Long term *in vitro* culture of murine mast cells. I. Description of a growth factor-dependent culture technique. J Immunol 127:788–794
45. Toksoz D (1980) Ph.D. Thesis, University of Manchester
46. Toksoz D, Dexter TM, Lord BI, Wright EG, Lajtha LG (1980) The regulation of hemopoiesis in long-term bone marrow cultures. II. Stimulation and inhibition of stem cell proliferation. Blood 55:931–936
47. Wagemaker G, Peters MF (1978) Effects of human leukocyte conditioned medium on mouse haemopoietic progenitor cells. Cell Tissue Kinet 11:45–56

48. Waterfield MD, Scrace GT, Whittle N, Stroobart D, Johnsson A, Wasterson A, Westermark B, Heldin CM, Huang JS, Duel TF (1983) Platelet derived growth factor is structurally related to the putative transforming protein of p28 sis of Simian sarcoma virus. Nature 304:35–39
49. Weiss L (1981) Haematopoiesis in mammalian bone marrow. In: Porter R, Whelan J (eds) Cell interactions in haemopoietic differentiation. Ciba Foundation Symposium 84. Pitman Medical, Tunbridge Wells, pp 1–4
50. Williams N, Burgess AW (1980) The effect of mouse lung granulocyte macrophage colony stimulating factors and other colony stimulating activities on the proliferation and differentiation of murine bone marrow cells in long-term cultures. J Cell Physiol 102:287–295
51. Williams N, Jackson H, Rabellino E (1977) Proliferation and differentiation of normal granulopoietic cells in continuous bone marrow cultures. J Cell Physiol 93:435–440
52. Wright EG, Lord BI (1977) Regulation of CFU-S proliferation by locally produced endogenous factors. Biomed Express 27:215–218
53. Wright EG, Garland JM, Lord BI (1980) Specific inhibition of haemopoietic stem cell proliferation: characterization of inhibitor producing cells. Leuk Res 4:537–545
54. Wright EG, Ali AM, Riches AC, Lord BI (1982) Stimulation of haemopoietic stem cell proliferation: characteristics of stimulator producing cells. Leuk Res 6:531–539
55. Yokota T, Lee F, Rennick D, Hall C, Arai N, Mosmann T, Nabel G, Cantor H, Arai K (1984) Isolation and characterization of a full-length cDNA for mast cell growth factor from a mouse T-cell clone: expression in monkey cells. Proc Nat Acad Si USA 81: 1070–1074
56. Yung YP, Eger R, Tertian G, Moore MAS (1981) Long-term *in vitro* culture of murine mast cells. II. Purification of a mast cell growth factor and its dissociation from TCGF. J Immunol 127:794–799

Haematology and Blood Transfusion Vol. 29
Modern Trends in Human Leukemia VI
Edited by Neth, Gallo, Greaves, Janka

Coordinated Expression of c-*myc* Gene and a Multigenic Set May Modulate the Malignant Phenotype in Human Haemopoietic Cell Lines*

J. Harel, N. Hanania, D. Shaool, D. Zeliszewski, and M. Castagna

A. Introduction

We previously showed that about 2000 non repeated DNA sequences of 3 Kbs each, designated as tumor-activated DNA (TaDNA), are transcriptionally activated in human neoplasias [1, 2]. A growing body evidence supports the concept that oncogenic transformation may depend on abnormal activation of cellular oncogenes (see general reviews [3, 4]), resulting in gene amplification, chromosomal rearrangements [5], or point mutations [6] and possibly involving cooperative oncogenes [7].

The aim of the present study was to search for possible correlations between tumor-activated DNA (TaDNA) activation and abnormal activation of oncogenes. For that purpose, we investigated the effects of various differentiation inducers in three lines of malignant hemopoietic cells characterized by translocation and/or abnormal expression of c-*myc*.

B. Cell Cultures and Treatment with Different Inducers

Raji and Namalwa cells (two Burkitt's lymphoma-derived lines), Epstein-Barr virus (EBV)-immortalized normal lymphocytes, the Priess cells, and HL-60 cells (a myeloid leukemia-derived cell line) were grown in suspension in conditions already described [1, 2]. They were seeded at cell concentrations of $2.5–3 \times 10^5$ cells/ml, treated with different inducers 24 h after seeding, and collected 24 h later for measuring the levels of TaDNA or *myc*-transcripts, or at different times for analysis of cell multiplication and differentiation. The HEL cells (normal skin fibroblasts) were cultured in monolayers and treated before attaining confluence. We used various agents known to be efficient differentiation inducers for HL-60 cells: DMSO, retinoic acid, mezerein, TPA [8, 9] and teleocidin [10]. Phorbol esters induce macrophage characteristics whereas DMSO or retinoic acid favor the appearance of granulocytic or megakaryocytic cells [8, 9]. TPA is of particular interest because this potent tumor promoter for skin cancer can modulate cell phenotypes in opposite directions, depending on the cell line studied [9]. In particular, TPA can induce various different markers in Burkitt's lymphoma lines or, in normal cells, provoke pleiotropic changes which mimic those associated with oncogenic conversion. A chemical analog of TPA, 4α-phorbol-12,13-didecanoate (4α-PDD) which is almost devoid of activity [10] was used as control.

I. Hybridizations Liquid

Cellular RNA and Raji cell DNA were prepared as described [1]. A single-stranded DNA fraction, greatly enriched in transcribing sequences, was labeled with ^{125}I, and depleted of sequences shared with Priess cells by successive cycles of hybridization with RNA from Priess and Raji cells,

* Institut Gustave-Roussy, 39–53, Rue Camille Desmoulins, F-94805 Villejuif

both cells proliferating with similar growth rates [11]. Centrifugations in cesium sulfate gradients allowed the separation of DNA–RNA hybrids from nonhybridized DNA sequences [1, 2].

II. Dot Blot Hybridizations

Dot blot hybridizations were performed following Thomas [12]. The c-*myc* probe, consisting of a cloned 1.5 kilobases Sac I restriction fragment containing most of the two exons (plasmid obtained from Dr. D. Stehelin) was nick-translated as described by Maniatis et al. [13] with ^{32}P-labeled dCTP (NEN) (3000 Ci/mmol) to obtain specific activities in the range of $5–8 \times 10^8$ cpm/μg.

C. Results

I. Cell Differentiation

When treated with potent inducers like TPA in the range of 15–20 n*M*, 80%–90% of the HL-60 cells became attached to the plastic support and the activities of two enzymatic markers (an esterase and an acid phosphatase) were increased four- to sixfold. The same treatment in Raji or Namalwa cells caused a significant decrease in the amounts of two antigenic markers (cALL and HLAdr) of the lymphoid precursor cells.

II. Cell Multiplication

Similar growth rates, at least for 48 h after seeding, were observed in all hemopoietic cell lines studied. Low concentrations (15–20 n*M*) of TPA, mezerein, or teleocidin caused an almost complete arrest of multiplication of malignant cells, but did not affect that of Priess cells. Greater concentrations of DMSO (1.3% = 60 n*M*) and retinoic acid (0.1–1 μ*M*), which are known to induce the differentiation of HL-60 cells, resulted in a 50%–55% reduction in the multiplication rates. In control assays, 4α-PDD (10–100 n*M*) had no effect on cell differentiation and growth rates.

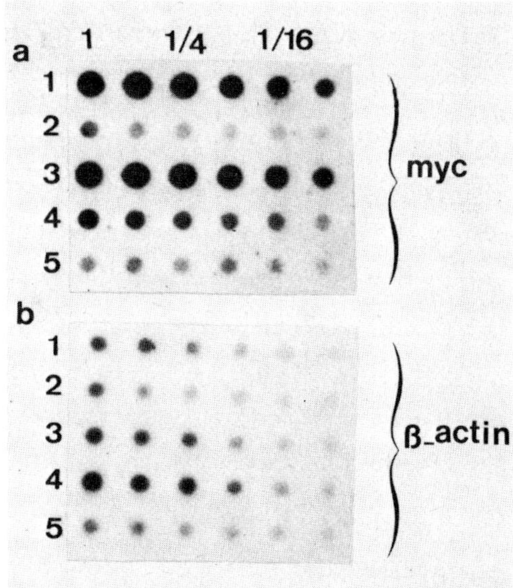

Fig. 1 a, b. Dot blot hybridizations showing the level of c-*myc* RNA in HL-60 cells treated with various agents. From left to right, the dots contained decreasing amounts (by half) of total cellular RNA: 2.5 μg, 1.25 μg, etc. *Row* 1: no treatment; *row* 2: 15 n*M* mezerein; *row* 3: 20 n*M* 4α-PDD; *row* 4: 20 n*M* teleocidin; *row* 5: 1 μ*M* retinoic acid. **a** the blots were prehybridized overnight at 42 °C in 50% formamide (v/v), 0.75 *M* NaCl–0.075 Na-citrate–0.05 *M* Na-phosphate buffer pH 6.5, containing 125 μg/ml sonicated, denatured salmon sperm DNA and 0.02% each of bovine serum albumin, Ficoll, and polyvinylpyrrolidone. They were thereafter hybridized for 24 h with the c-*myc*-specific probe (10^6 cpm/ml) in the same medium, **b** internal controls: the same blots were dehybridized (by boiling 30 min in 0.015 *M* NaCl, 0.0015 *M* Na-citrate, 0.1% SDS) and rehybridized with *β*-actin-specific recombinant DNA probe (obtained from Dr. A. J. Mirty, Institut Pasteur, Paris)

III. Effects on TaDNA Transcripts

The percentages of TaDNA forming DNA–RNA hybrids at saturation levels, with an excess of total RNA from the various treated or untreated cells are summarized in Table 1. It is clear that, in malignant cells, the various differentiation inducers caused a roughly dose-dependent reduction in the population of TaDNA transcripts. It was also noticed that a tenfold higher concentration of mezerein than TPA is required to

Table 1. Summary of TaDNA-RNA hybridization data

Chemical agent	Concentration	Percentage TaDNA hybridized[a] to RNA from				
		Malignant cells			Normal cells	
		HL-60	Raji	Namalwa	Priess	HEL
None		74±3	81±5	76±4	5±1.5	5±2
4α-PDD	20 nM	70	76	73	–	–
	3 nM	51	44.5	46	–	–
	16 nM	10.5	14	15.5	31	42.5
TPA	50 nM	–	–	–	40.5	58
	160 nM	–	–	–	58	–
	1.6 μM	–	–	–	85	–
Teleocidin	4 nM	48	–	42.5	–	–
	20 nM	13	–	13	–	–
Mezerein	15 nM	68	–	–	–	–
	150 nM	11.5	–	–	28.5	–
	1.5 μM	9	–	–	45	–
Retinoic acid	400 nM	40	–	–	–	–
	1 μM	12	–	–	22.5	–
	10 μM	–	–	–	35	–
DMSO	60 mM	16	–	–	–	–

[a] The percentages indicated are those obtained by the use of S1 nuclease at apparent saturation levels [1, 2]. In some crucial experiments, isopyknic centrifugation (in cesium sulfate gradient) confirmed that the S1 nuclease-resistant molecules exclusively consisted of DNA-RNA duplexes [1, 2]

obtain the same level of inhibition of TaDNA activity, although these agents are equipotent differentiation inducers. On the contrary, in normal cells TPA treatment caused the occurrence of RNA species, hybridizable up to 85% of the Raji cell TaDNA, in a dose- dependent manner, whereas only 4%–5% of the latter could form hybrids with RNA from untreated normal cells. At much higher concentrations, mezerein and retinoic acid produced partial enhancing effects.

IV. Effects on c-*myc* RNA

The treatment of HL-60 cells with optimal amounts of each differentiation inducer resulted in a drastic reduction (at least tenfold) in the level of c-*myc* RNA (Fig. 1). This reduction in the level of c-*myc* RNA was also found in Namalwa cells treated with TPA whereas this level was not modified in Priess cells treated with higher amounts of TPA (not shown). We have established with an actin gene-specific probe that none of the agents studied caused a significant reduction in the level of actin-specific RNA.

D. Conclusions

We have shown that the treatment of three distinct malignant cell lines, characterized by translocation and/or abnormal activation of the c-*myc* gene, with several chemically unrelated differentiation inducers, produces a drastic reduction in the levels of both d-*myc* RNA and TaDNA-specific RNA. This cannot be simply due to the cell growth inhibition caused by the differentiation inducers, for several reasons, in particular because the majority of TaDNA sequences, which were silent in normal lymphoid cells and in normal fibroblasts, both growing exponentially, became transcriptionally active within 24 h of treatment with TPA which did not change their proliferation rates. These opposite effects of TPA suggest that this agent (and probably other agents as well) may operate either as a tumor promoter or a differentiation inducer through a common control mechanism of the TaDNA transcripts. Finally, our results suggest that TaDNA corresponds to a multigenic set which modulates the malignant phenotype, possibly in cooperation with c-*myc* or other oncogenes implicated in the initiation and genotypic maintenance of cancer. If one considers that TaDNA corresponds to a common genomic domain consisting of many distinct transcription units which are coordinated in their activation or regulation, it is unlikely, although not impossible, that the unique role of this domain is to control the cancer phenotype. The same is true for cellular oncogenes and, in fact, recent data support the hypothesis of normal functions for oncogens. This is the case for c-*myc* which appears to be involved in control of the cell cycle (for example see [14]). It is tempting to assume that TaDNA is normally implicated at early stages of embryogenesis or in the regulation of certain differentiation pathways. Further advances in the understanding of TaDNA must await the construction of a library of TaDNA sequences which is under way in our laboratory.

References

1. Hanania N, Shaool D, Poncy C, Harel J (1981) Proc Natl Acad Sci USA 78:6504–6508
2. Hanania N, Shaool D, Harel J, Wiels J, Tursz T (1983) EMBO J 2:1621–1624
3. Cooper GM (1982) Science 218:801–807
4. Weinberg RA (1982) Adv Cancer Res 36:149–163
5. Klein G (1983) Cell 32:311–315
6. Sukamar S, Notario V, Martin-Zanca D, Barbacid M (1983) Nature 306:658–661
7. Tabin JG et al. (1982) Nature 300:143–149
8. Collins ST, Ruscetti SW, Gallagher RE, Gallo RC (1978) Proc Natl Acad Sci USA 75:2458–2461
9. Rovera G, O'Brien TG, Diamond L (1979) Science 204:868–870
10. Fisher PB et al. (1982) Cancer Res 42:2829–2835
11. Hanania N, Shaool D, Poncy C, Tapiero H, Harel J (1977) Cell Biol Int Rep 1:309–315
12. Thomas P (1980) Proc Natl Acad Sci USA 76:5201–5205
13. Maniatis T, Kee SG, Efstradiatis A, Kafatos FC (1975) Proc Natl Acad Sci USA 1154–1158
14. Kelly K, Cochran BH, Leder P (1983) Cell 35:603–610

Haematology and Blood Transfusion Vol. 29
Modern Trends in Human Leukemia VI
Edited by Neth, Gallo, Greaves, Janka

Proliferation In Vivo and In Vitro of Haemopoietic Progenitor Cells Induced by AF-1, a New *ras*-Containing Retrovirus

G. R. Johnson [1], W. Ostertag [2], and N. A. Nicola [1]

A. Introduction

Many studies have been performed on the effects of murine retrovirus infection upon the haematopoietic system. In some instances following a variable period after in vivo infection transplantable tumours or continuous cell lines have been developed [1, 2]. The cell lines appear to proliferate independently of haemopoietic growth factors, although the possibility remains that the transformed cells are able to produce their own growth factors. In most cases of transformation of haemopoietic cells and production of continuous cell lines by retroviruses the target cell for viral transformation remains unknown.

Although several in vitro infection systems have been developed [3, 4], these contain both haemopoietic and non-haemopoietic cells and thus make the interpretation of target cell type impossible. The present experiments were performed to answer some of these questions using a newly isolated murine retrovirus AF-1. AF-1 is a replication defective retrovirus derived from passage of cloned F-MuLV through newborn BALB/c mice [5]. It contains a *ras* oncogene related to that of Ha-*ras* [5]. Infected animals develop a rapid splenomegaly, associated with increased levels of splenic haemopoietic progenitor cells and a histiocytosis [5]. Cell lines derived from AF-1-infected spleen cells are capable of producing G-CSF and GM-CSF but not multi-CSF (IL-3) (W. Ostertag, G. W. Johnson, unpublished observations).

B. Results

I. Growth of "Factor-Independent Colonies" from AF-1-Infected Spleen and Bone Marrow

DBA mice were infected with AF-1 and 14 days later spleen and bone marrow cells were cultured in semisolid agar medium [6]. Cells in half of the cultures were stimulated by the addition of pokeweed mitogen-stimulated spleen-cell-conditioned medium (SCM) [7]. When scored at 7 days, the frequency and distribution of colony types in stimulated infected bone marrow cultures did not differ significantly from control non-infected cultures. Infected spleen-cell cultures when stimulated contained an approximately tenfold higher frequency of colonies than control cultures. Cultures of infected spleen or bone marrow cells without stimulus displayed cell dose-dependent "factor-independent" colony formation. Thus with spleen cells cultured at 1, 2 and 4×10^5 cells, 0, 7 ± 1 and 56 ± 2 colonies were obtained (control cultures of 1×10^5 cells stimulated with SCM contained 121 ± 19 colonies) including macrophage, neutrophil, erythroid and multipotential colonies (see Table 1). Sequential "factor-independent" colonies were removed from

1 Developmental Haematopoiesis Laboratory, Walter and Eliza Hall Institute of Medical Research, P.O. Royal Melbourne Hsopital, 3050, Melbourne, Australia
2 Heinrich-Pette-Institut für Experimentelle Virologie und Immunologie an der Universität Hamburg, Martinistrasse 52, 2000 Hamburg 20, FRG

Table 1. Colony types producing cell lines

Colony source		Number of colonies transferred	Number of colonies with proliferating cells
Bone marrow	Macrophage	24	3
	Neutrophil-macrophage	20	9
	Macrophage-blast-mast	1	0
	Erythroid-macrophage	2	0
	Macrophage-erythroid-blast	2	0
Spleen	Macrophage	29	14
	Neutrophil-macrophage	12	4
	Neutrophil	1	0
	Blast	1	0
	Neurophil-macrophage-erythroid	2	0
	Neutrophil-macrophage-blast-mast	2	1

Colonies isolated from 7-day cultures of 1×10^5 cells obtained from CBA or DBA mice infected with AF-1 14 days previously. Proliferation of colony cells determined at 14 days and in all cases consisted of elongated adherent cells

spleen and bone marrow cultures and half of each colony was recultured in 200 µl medium to determine the ability for continued proliferation of colony cells. The remaining cells from each colony were smeared and stained to determine colony morphology. The results of one experiment are shown in Table 1. Continued proliferation of colony cells was observed from macrophage and neutrophil-macrophage colonies and occasional multipotential colonies (Table 1). After 14 days, medium from wells containing proliferating colony cells was assayed and found to contain no detectable GM-CSF, G-CSF or multi-CSF. Cells continued to proliferate until the experiment was terminated at 8 weeks after initial colony-cell transfer and at no stage were any haemopoietic growth factors detected in supernatants from the proliferating cells. Cells from all factor-independent colonies induced foci in cocultures with indicator fibroblasts, indicating the presence of virus.

II. Effect of AF-1 on Single Haemopoietic Progenitor Cells

To determine whether the effect of AF-1 on haemopoietic progenitor cells was direct or indirect single cells obtained from fractions highly enriched for colony-forming cells and purified from CBA fetal liver as described previously [8] were cultured in microtitre wells in the presence of virus. The results of these experiments are shown in Table 2. Single cells were transferred to wells containing medium alone or SCM, SCM plus AF-1 and AF-1 alone. When scored 7 days later, as expected no cells were present in medium-alone controls and over 20% of wells with SCM contained proliferating cells. The addition of the supernatant containing dialyzed AF-1 to SCM cultures markedly inhibited proliferation. AF-1 supernatant alone was able to induce limited proliferation from single cells but after 14 days all proliferation had ceased in these wells (Table 2).

C. Discussion

Mice infected with AF-1 show marked splenomegaly and elevation of splenic haematopoietic progenitor cells. The present experiments suggest that this may in part be a direct proliferative effect of the virus complex upon progenitor cells. However, a more significant effect, at least during the

Table 2. Effect of AF-1 on single haemopoietic progenitor cells

Addition to well	Medium	SCM	SCM + AF-1	AF-1
Proliferating clones per number of single cells transferred	0/120	27/119	9/96	6/95
Cell number per clone at 7 days (range)	0	9–560	2–16	4–74

Single cells from progenitor-cell-enriched fraction (CFC fraction, see [8]) micromanipulated into 200 μl medium alone or containing SCM and/or AF-1

early stages of infection, may be mediated by the activation of accessory-cell-derived haemopoietic growth factor synthesis. This would be in agreement with the observation of cell-number-dependent colony formation in spleen or bone marrow cultures from which SCM was omitted. The non-linearity of colony formation coupled with the fact that less than 50% of the colonies contained cells capable of further proliferation suggests that non-proliferating cells are producing the stimuli required for proliferation.

The continued proliferation of colony cells from macrophage and neutrophil-macrophage colonies suggests that granulocyte-macrophage progenitor cells (GM-CFC) may be the primary target cell for AF-1-induced transformation. The presence of virus-inducing fibroblast transformation in all "factor-independent" colonies probably indicates that all cells can be infected with AF-1. Furthermore, the continued proliferation of cells from one multipotential colony (containing neutrophils, macrophages, blast cells and mast cells) together with the association of proliferation with macrophage differentiation may suggest that infection of all cell types can occur, but that commitment to macrophage differentiation may be important for transformation and continued proliferation of cells.

Although accessory cells probably play a role in AF-1-induced haemopoietic proliferation the experiments with single cells suggest that the AF-1 viral complex itself may be able to induce limited proliferation directly. Further experiments with more purified viral preparations are required to clarify this point although in the experiments reported here the viral supernatants were passaged through membranes to exclude molecules of less than 300 000 daltons and were shown to be negative for haemopoietic growth factors by bioassay. This latter treatment is important as most fibroblasts used for the maintenance of cloned virus preparations produce growth factors [9] (G. R. Johnson and W. Ostertag, unpublished observations).

In summary, the experiments reported here suggest that the AF-1 virus complex is able to induce haemopoietic-cell proliferation by both direct and indirect means and that factor-independent cell proliferation may be related to macrophage differentiation. Further experiments are required to determine the role of the AF-1 ras gene on these processes.

Acknowledgments. Part of this work was supported by the Carden Fellowship Fund of the Anti-Cancer Council of Victoria, the J. D. and L. Harris Cancer Fund, the National Health and Medical Research Council, Canberra, and the National Institutes of Health, Bethesda, Grant No. CA-25972. Another part (W. O.) was funded by the Deutsche Forschungsgemeinschaft and by the UICC. The Heinrich-Pette-Institut is supported by Freie und Hansestadt Hamburg and Bundesministerum für Jugend, Familie und Gesundheit. – The excellent technical assistance of Misses E. Viney and U. Bergholz is gratefully acknowledged.

References

1. Friend C, Scher W, Holland JG, Sato T (1971) Proc Natl Acad Sci USA 68:378–382
2. Ostertag W, Melderis H, Steinheider G, Kluge N, Dube S (1972) Nature New Biol 239:231–234
3. Liao SK, Axelrad AA (1975) Int J Cancer 15: 467–482

4. Hankins WD, Kost TA, Koury MJ, Krantz SB (1978) Nature 276:506–508
5. Franz T, Löhler J, Fusco A, Pragnell IB, Nobis P, Padua R, Ostertag W (to be published)
6. Johnson GR (1980) J Cell Physiol 103:371–383
7. Metcalf D, Johnson GR (1978) J Cell Physiol 96:31–42
8. Nicola NA, Johnson GR (1982) Blood 60:1019–1029
9. Koury MJ, Pragnell IB (1982) Nature 299: 638–640

Haematology and Blood Transfusion Vol. 29
Modern Trends in Human Leukemia VI
Edited by Neth, Gallo, Greaves, Janka

Cloning and Expression of the Gene for Murine Granulocyte-Macrophage Colony-Stimulating Factor

N. M. Gough [1], J. Gough [1], D. Metcalf [2], A. Kelso [2], D. Grail [1], N. A. Nicola [2] and A. R. Dunn [1]

A. Introduction

It has become apparent from studies in vitro that the survival, proliferation and differentiation of progenitor cells and functional activation of the various mature cell types of the haemopoietic system are controlled by a group of glycoprotein regulators, notably erythropoietin, T cell growth factor (IL2) and the colony-stimulating factors (CSFs) [1, 2]. Four CSFs with distinct biochemical and biological properties have been purified: M-CSF is a selective proliferative stimulus for macrophages [3]; G-CSF for granulocytes [4]; GM-CSF for both granulocytes and macrophages [5]; while multi-CSF (also known as interleukin-3 [6], burst-promoting activity [7], P cell-stimulating factor [8], mast cell growth factor [9] and haemopoietic cell growth factor [10]) stimulates the proliferation not only of neutrophilic granulocytes and macrophages, but also eosinophils, megakaryocytes, erythroid and mast cells. GM-CSF synthesized by mouse lung tissue is a glycoprotein of molecular weight 23 000 [5] and is required continuously for the in vitro proliferation of progenitor cells of granulocytes and macrophages, controls the irreversible commitment of these progenitors to the formation of mature granulocytes and macrophages [11] and regulates the functional activity of the mature end cells. Although it has been possible to purify all four CSFs, detailed analysis of many aspects of the biology and biochemistry of these factors has been hampered by the limited quantities available. This problem can be largely circumvented by molecular cloning of the corresponding gene sequences and by using the cloned gene sequence to direct the synthesis of the corresponding factor. We have previously isolated cDNA clones containing partial copies of the GM-CSF mRNA from mouse lung [12]. In this paper we report the isolation of a cDNA clone which contains all of the information required to direct the synthesis of biologically active GM-CSF in simian COS cells [13].

B. Results

I. Cloning of Murine GM-CSF cDNA Sequences

We have recently isolated two cDNA clones complementary to the GM-CSF mRNA from the lungs of endotoxin-treated mice [12]. The structure of this mRNA is illustrated in Fig. 1. We have previously shown by Northern blot analysis that this mRNA is approximately 1200 nucleotides in length [12], of which 100–200 nucleotides are presumably contributed by the poly(A) tail. Nucleotide sequence analysis of the two cDNA clones (pGM37 and pGM38 in Fig. 1) complementary to

---

1 Melbourne Tumour Biology Branch, Ludwig Institute for Cancer Research, Post Office, Royal Melbourne Hospital, Melbourne, Vic., 3050 Australia
2 The Walter and Eliza Hall Institute for Medical Research, Post Office, Royal Melbourne Hospital, Melbourne, Vic., 3050 Australia

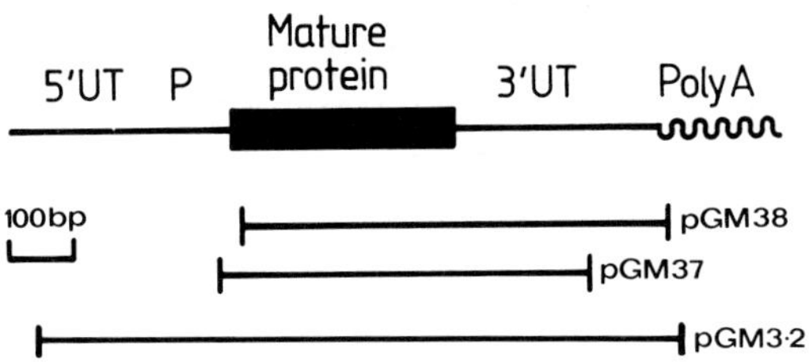

Fig. 1. Map of the murine GM-CSF mRNA. The region of the mRNA encoding the mature protein is shown as a *thick line*, the untranslated regions are designated by *UT* and the putative precursor peptide by *P*. The regions contained within clones pGM37, pGM38 and pGM3.2 are indicated with *bars*

IleIleValThrArgProTrpLysHisValGluAlaIleLysGluAlaLeuAsnLeuLeu 20

AspAspMetProValThrLeuAsnGluGluValGluValValSerAsnGluPheSerPhe 40

LysLysLeuThrCysValGlnThrArgLeuLysIlePheGluGlnGlyLeuArgGlyAsn 60

PheThrLysLeuLysGlyAlaLeuAsnMetThrAlaSerTyrTyrGlnThrTyrCysPro 80

ProThrProGluThrAspCysGluThrGlnValThrThrTyrAlaAspPheIleAspSer 100

LeuLysThrPheLeuThrAspIleProPheGluCysLysLysProSerGlnLys 118
Gly

Fig. 2. Predicted amino acid sequence of murine GM-CSF. The sequence presented is of the mature protein and is that predicted by nucleotide sequence analysis [12] of clones pGM37 and pGM38. Owing to a nucleotide sequence difference between the two clones, residue 116 could be either glycine or serine [12]

this mRNA indicated that the 3′ untranslated region of the mRNA is 319 nucleotides in length and the region encoding the mature protein is 354 nucleotides, leaving some 350 nucleotides for the putative NH_2 terminal signal peptide and the 5′ untranslated region [12]. The amino acid sequence of GM-CSF deduced from the nucleotide sequence of the mRNA is given in Fig. 2, starting with the first amino acid of the mature protein [14]. The protein is predicted to be 118 amino acids in length, with a molecular weight of 13 500. The cDNA sequence in clone pGM37 extends about 20 nucleotides 5′ to the region encoding the mature protein, into the region encoding the signal peptide, but does not extend to the translational initiation codon.

As a prelude to the direct expression of the cloned GM-CSF gene sequence in cell culture, we needed to isolate a cDNA clone containing the entire coding region of the GM-CSF mRNA, including the translational initiation codon. In order to isolate more GM-CSF cDNA clones we have made use of a cloned T lymphocyte line, LB3 [15], in which the synthesis of high levels of GM-CSF mRNA is inducible by concanavalin A (see Fig. 2 in reference [12]). We estimate the abundance of GM-CSF mRNA in con-A-stimulated LB3 RNA to be at least two orders of magnitude greater than in lung RNA. We therefore constructed a library of cDNA clones complementary to con-A-stimulated LB3 RNA, and screened this library for GM-CSF clones by colony hybridization using a fragment of DNA from pGM38 as a probe. Of 24 GM-CSF cDNA clones purified and examined, one (pGM3.2) appears to contain a substantial, if not complete, copy of the GM-CSF mRNA. The region of GM-CSF mRNA contained in this clone, determined by mapping the location of various restriction endonuclease sites, is illustrated in Fig. 1.

II. Direct Expression of GM-CSF in COS Cells

In order to be able to express eukaryotic cDNA sequences in cell culture, we have constructed a vector (pJL) which utilizes the late promoter of the simian virus SV40 to transcribe inserted DNA sequences

(Fig. 3). The vector contains the β-lactamase gene and origin of DNA replication from the bacterial plasmid pAT153 [16], the SV40 origin of DNA replication and T antigen coding sequences [17] and a "multicloning site" adjacent to the SV40 late promoter. This multicloning site contains cleavage sites for several restriction endonucleases suitable for insertion of foreign DNA sequences: *Eco*RI, *Bam*HI, *Sac*I, *Xba*I, *Sal*I and *Sma*I. When introduced into cultured simian cells, such as CV1 or COS [13], this vector is able to replicate and to transcribe any DNA sequence inserted at the multicloning site. Provided that translational start and stop codons are included, the inserted sequence will be translated.

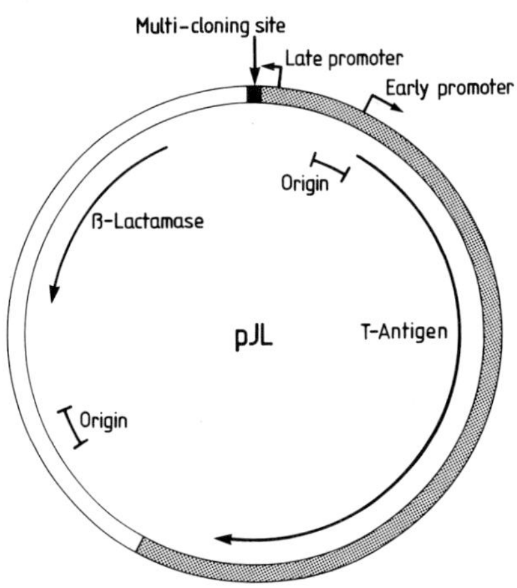

Fig. 3. Map of the expression vector pJL. The region derived from pAT153 [16] is indicated by an *open segment,* that from SV40 [17] by *stippling* and the multicloning site is *filled in*

The cDNA sequence of clone pGM3.2 has been installed in the multicloning site of pJL with the GM-CSF coding region in the same orientation as transcription from the late promoter. This recombinant was introduced into COS cells essentially as described by Dana and Sompayrac [18] and the culture medium assayed for GM-CSF activity 48 h after transfection. As negative controls, COS cells were also transfected with pJL DNA alone or with two different recombinant plasmids containing incomplete copies of the GM-CSF mRNA; COS cells which received no DNA were also assayed for GM-CSF activity. The various conditioned media were assayed for GM-CSF activity using both the FD cell line, which is absolutely dependent upon the presence of either GM-CSF or multi-CSF for growth (A. Hapel, personal communications) and the 32D CL3 cell line [19], which is responsive only to multi-CSF. As shown in Fig. 4, the medium for COS cells transfected with pGM3.2 DNA was able to support the growth of FD cells whereas media from all of the negative controls were completely inactive. As expected, the medium from pGM3.2-transfected COS cells was inactive on 32D CL3 cells (not shown), indicating that the active factor was GM-CSF rather than multi-CSF. The medium from pGM3.2-transfected COS cells also stimulated the formation of morphologically identifiable granulocyte and macrophage colonies in agar cultures containing bone marrow cells (Table 1) [5], the ratio of the three colony types being characteristic of GM-CSF at these concentrations [20]. The full range of biological ac-

Table 1. Colony formation by mouse bone marrow cells stimulated with medium from pGM3.2-transfected COS cells[a]

Total number of colonies	Colony type (%)		
	Granulocyte	Mixed granulocyte macrophage	Macrophage
33	15	19	66
23	27	27	46
24	17	17	66

[a] Medium from three separate cultures of COS cells transfected with pGM3.2 DNA were assayed in agar cultures containing 75 000 C57BL/6 bone marrow cells [5]

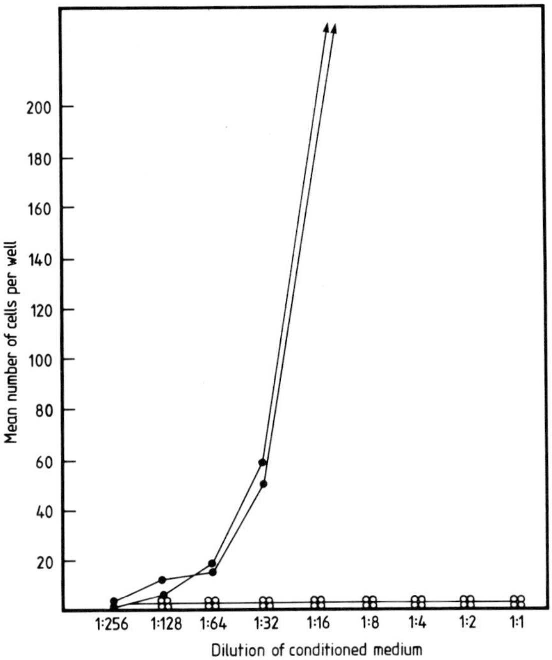

Fig. 4. Stimulation of cellular proliferation in suspension cultures of FD cells by medium from DNA-transfected COS cells. Clone pGM3.2 DNA is indicated with *full circles* and vector DNA (pJL), two clones containing partial copies of the GM CSF mRNA and COS cells which received no DNA are indicated with *open circles;* 5-μl volumes of conditioned medium were assayed in serial dilutions in 15- μl cultures containing 300 FD cells. Each point is the mean cell count from duplicate cultures after 2 days of incubation

tivities of the factor specified by this cloned gene is currently being assessed.

C. Conclusion

The molecular cloning of genes encoding the various haemopoietic growth regulators should allow the resolution of many outstanding questions and also bring to light hitherto unappreciated problems. By nucleotide sequence analysis of cloned gene sequences, the complete amino acid sequences of murine GM-CSF [12] and multi-CSF [21, 22] have been deduced – a goal that was essentially unattainable by conventional biochemical approaches. Comparison of these two sequences has now raised further intriguing issues. As we have previously discussed [12], neither the primary amino acid sequences nor the predicted secondary structures of these two factors show any significant homology, despite the similar activities that they display in stimulating the growth of granulocyte and macrophage colonies from committed progenitor cells. It should now be possible to study in more detail the interaction between these two factors and their receptors, since we can now produce both GM-CSF (this paper) and multi-CSF (N. M. Gough, unpublished work) in a clonally pure form upon introduction of the cloned gene sequences into COS cells. Moreover, by in vitro mutagenesis and expression of the mutated gene sequences it should be possible to dissect the active site (or sites) of the molecules and to ask whether their various activities are determined by the same or different active sites.

Acknowledgments. The work at the Walter and Eliza Hall Institute was supported by grants from the Carden Fellowship Fund of the Anti-Cancer Council of Victoria, the NH and MRC (Canberra) and the NIH (Bethesda) grant numbers CA 22556 and CA 25972.

References

1. Metcalf D, Moore MAS (1971) Haemopoietic cells. North Holland, Amsterdam
2. Metcalf D (1981) In: Baserga R (ed) Tissue growth factors. Springer, New York, pp 343–384

3. Stanley ER, Heard PM (1977) J Biol Chem 252:4305–4312
4. Nicola NA, Metcalf D, Matsumoto M, Johnson GR (1983) J Biol Chem 258:9017–9021
5. Burgess AW, Camakaris J, Metcalf D (1977) J Biol Chem 252:1998–2003
6. Ihle JN et al. (1982) J Immunol 129: 2431–2436
7. Iscove NN, Roitsch CA, Williams N, Guilbert LJ (1982) J Cell Physiol [Suppl] 1:65–78
8. Clark-Lewis I, Schrader JW (1981) J Immunol 127:1941–1947
9. Yung, Y-P, Eger R, Tertlan G, Moore MAS (1981) J Immunol 127:794–799
10. Bazill GW, Haynes M, Garland J, Dexter TM (1983) Biochem J 210:747–759
11. Metcalf D, Burgess AW (1982) J Cell Physiol 111:275–283
12. Gluzman Y (1981) Cell 23:175–182
13. Gough NM et al. (1984) Nature 309:763–767
14. Sparrow L et al. (1985) Proc Natl Acad Sci USA 82:292–296
15. Kelso A, MacDonald HR, Smith KA, Cerottini J-C, Brunner KT (1984) J Immunol 132: 2932–2938
16. Twigg AJ, Sherratt D (1980) Nature 283: 216–218
17. Tooze J (1980) Molecular biology of tumour viruses, part 2: DNA tumour viruses. Cold Spring Harbor Laboratory
18. Danna KJ, Sompayrac LM (1982) J Virol Methods 5:335–341
19. Greenberger JS et al. (1982) In: Baum SJ, Ledney GD, Thierfelder S (eds) Experimental haematology today 1982. Karger, Basel, pp 195–209
20. Burgess AW, Metcalf D (1977) In: Baum SJ, Ledney GD (eds) Experimental haematology today 1977. Springer, New York, pp 135–146
21. Fung MC et al. (1984) Nature 307:233–237
22. Yakota T et al. (1984) Proc Natl Acad Sci USA 81:1070–1074

Haematology and Blood Transfusion Vol. 29
Modern Trends in Human Leukemia VI
Edited by Neth, Gallo, Greaves, Janka

Partial Characterization of Murine Haematopoietic Cell Growth Factor mRNA

G. J. Cowling [1], L. Healy [2], and T. M. Dexter [2]

Specific regulatory molecules are required for the growth and development of haematopoietic cells in vitro. Some of these molecular species appear to have a broad specificity, being able to promote the proliferation and differentiation of multipotential cells, as well as megakaryocytic, erythroid and granulocytic progenitor cells. Haematopoietic cell growth factor (HCGF) is a glycoprotein of molecular weight 28 500 which is produced constitutively by WEHI-3b myelomonocytic leukaemic cells and stimulated lymphoid cell populations in vitro [1]. Comparative studies [2] have shown that HCGF may share most, if not all, of the biochemical and biological properties of factors described variously as interleukin-3 (IL3) [3], burst-promoting activity (BPA) [4], mast cell growth factor (MCGF) [5], multicolony-stimulating factor (multi-CSF) [1], P cell-stimulating factor [6], histamine-producing cell-stimulating factor [7] and Thy-l-inducing activity [8].

Fig. 1. Published murine 1L3 sequence [3]. Coding sequence is indicated by *brackets*. Oligonucleotide probes, complementary to mRNA sequences, were synthesized for those areas in boxes. Probe (121–138) (shown below) contains codon degeneracies and corresponds to the NH_2-terminus sequence of mature IL3. Such degeneracies were included to increase the probability of detecting homologous human sequences. In subsequent RNA blot experiments, an equimolor mixture of these probes was labelled using T4 polynucleotide kinase and [^{32}P]-labelled γ-ATP

```
5'GAC.ACA.CAC.CGA.TTA.ACAA3'
   T   C   T   C   T   C
       G       G       G
       T       T       T
```

```
            10         20         30         40         50         60
  1 AACCCTTGGA GGACCAGAAC GAGAACAATG GTTCTTGCCA GCTCTACCAC CAGCATCCAC
 61 ACCATGCTGC TCCTGCTCAT GCTCTTCCAC CTGGGACTCC AAGCTTCAAT CAGTGGCCGG
121 GATACCCACC TTTAACCAGA ACGTTGAATT GCAGCTCTAT TGTCAAGGAG ATTATAGGGA
181 AGCTCCCAGA ACCTGAACTC AAAACTGATG ATGAAGGACC CTCTCTGAGG AATAAGAGCT
241 TTCGGAGAGT AAACCTGTCC AAATTCGTGG AAAGCCAAGG AGAAGTGGAT CCTGAGGACA

           310        320        330        340        350        360
301 GATACGTTAT CAAGTCCAAT CTTCAGAAAC TTAACTGTTG CCTGCCTACA TCTGCGAATG
361 ACTCTGCGCT GCCAGGGGTC TTCATTCGAG ATCTGGATGA CTTTCGGAAG AAACTGAGAT
421 TCTACATGGT CCACCTTAAC GATCTGGAGA CAGTGCTAAC CTCTAGACCA CCTCAGCCCG
481 CATCTGGCTC CGTCTCTCCT AACCGTGGAA CCGTGGAATG TTAAAACAGC AGGCAGAGCA
541 CCTAAAGTCT GAATGTTCCT CATGGCCCAT GGTCAAAAGG ATTTTACATT CCTTTATGCC

           610        620
601 ATCAAATGTC TTATCAATTT ATCTA
```

1 Searle Research and Development, Lane End Road, High Wycombe, Bucks HP12 4HL, UK
2 Paterson Laboratories, Christie Hospital and Holt Radium Institute, Manchester, UK

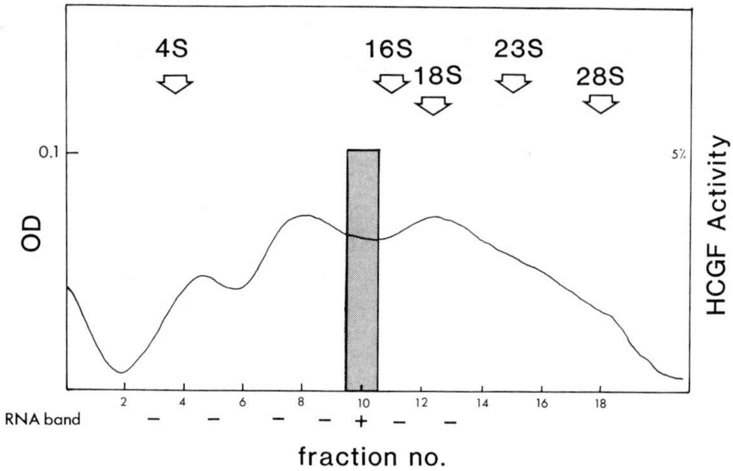

Fig. 2. Sucrose density gradient of WEHI-3b mRNA showing fractions that give HCGF activity when translated in *Xenopus* oocytes and hybridized to IL3 probes. Total RNA was prepared by cell lysis in 10 m*M* ribonucleoside–vanadyl complexes as RNase inhibitor and phenol extraction. Further purification involved oligo-dT-cellulose chromatography. RNA was applied to exponential 15%–50% sucrose gradients and centrifuged at 37 000 rpm for 18 h at 15 °C (SW41). The gradients were fractionated using an Isco UV monitor. Following ethanol precipitation, RNA from each fraction was redissolved in water (0.1 mg/ml) prior to microinjection into *Xenopus* oocytes. Secreted HCGF activity was measured using the factor-dependent cell (FDC-P) assay and shown in the *hatched area.* RNA from each fraction was also treated with glyoxal, separated by electrophoresis on 0.8% agarose gels and transferred to nitrocellulose. RNA blots were prehybridized in 6×SSC, 0.1% SDS, 5×Denharts for 48 h at 45 °C before the addition of labeled probes for a further 48 h at 45 °C. The filter was washed in 6×SSC for 10 min at 25 °C and 20 min at 45 °C

Recently cDNA sequences for IL3 [3] and MCGF [5] have been shown to be identical (Fig. 1).

Prior to cloning and expressing the cDNA gene for HCGF in *Escherichia coli,* we have partially characterized the mRNA which codes for HCGF by translation of mRNA size classes in *Xenopus* oocytes and RNA blot analysis using oligonucleotide probes to IL3 gene sequences (Fig. 2). We have also attempted to identify putative human IL3 sequences in mRNA isolated from mitogen-stimulated, lymphocyte-enriched buffy coat cells (Fig. 3).

We concluded that a 15 *S* mRNA species isolated from WEHI-3b cells is capable of coding for HCGF. Identical fractions contain a mRNA, 1100 nucleotides long, which hybridizes with murine IL3 oligonucleotide probes. These results suggest that the cDNA gene for HCGF is identical to those of IL3 and MCGF. Biological results indicate that IL3 and HCGF are the same. Recombinant IL3 (monkey COS cells/SV40 vector) displays almost identical biological behaviour to purified HCGF (T. M. Dexter, unpublished work).

In experiments designed to detect human IL3 sequences, oligonucleotide probes to the NH_2 terminus protein sequence of murine IL3 failed to hybridize to human mRNA isolated from mitogen-stimulated lymphocytes. Using the same experimental conditions and oligonucleotide probes of the same size and composition, IFN-γ and IL2 messenger RNA species of the correct size were observed. The failure of these experiments may be due to the lack of homologous sequences or its low abundance in human mRNA prepared by this mitogen regime. Cloning of the complete HCGF gene may facilitate the detection of human sequences on a genomic level.

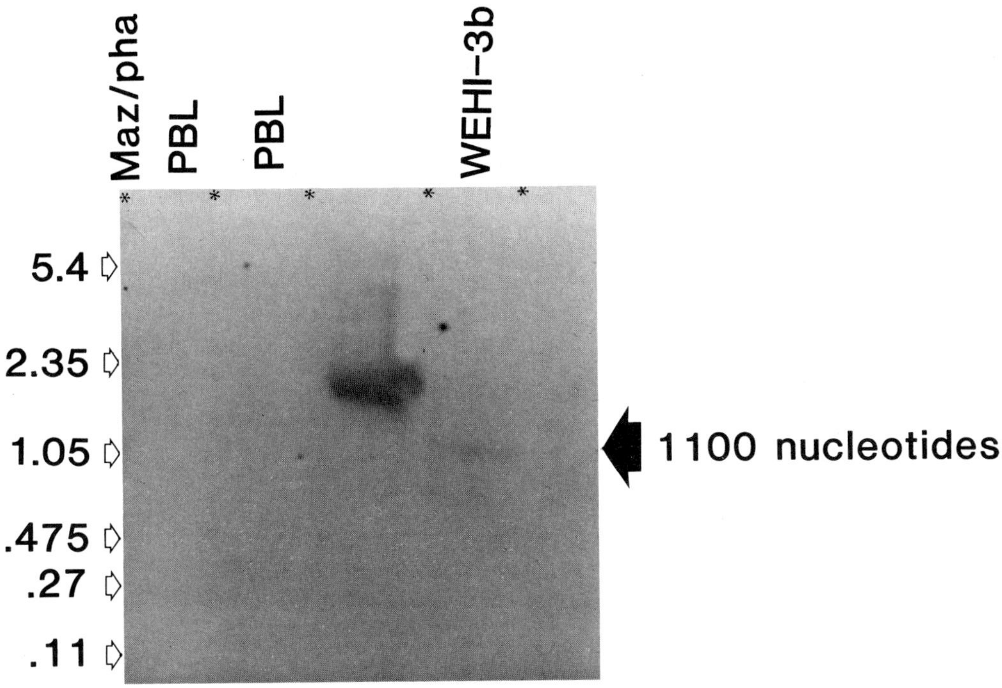

Fig. 3. RNA blot analysis of mRNA from: WEHI-3 cells; human buffy coat cells; and Mazerein/PHA-stimulated human buffy coat cells. Human mononuclear cells were isolated from buffy coats by Ficoll–Hypaque gradients. Cultures containing 5×10^6 mononuclear cells per millilitre in RPMI 1640 medium containing 1% fetal calf serum were treated with Mazerein (50 ng/ml) for 3 h at 37 °C; PHA was then added at a concentration of 10 μg/ml. The mean IFN-γ titre per induction was 3.9 $\log_{10}$ IU/ml after 24 h at 37 °C

References

1. Bazill GW, Haynes M, Garland J, Dexter TM (1983) Biochem J 210: 747–759
2. Garland JM, Dexter TM (1983) Lymphokine Research 2: 13–22
3. Fung MC, Hapel AJ, Ymer S, Cohen DR, Johnson RM, Campbell HD, Young IG (1983) Nature 307: 233–237
4. Iscove NN, Roitsch CA, Williams N, Guilbert LJ (1982) J Cell Physiol [Suppl] 1: 65–78
5. Yokota T, Lee F, Rennick D, Hall C, Arai N, Mosmann T, Nabel G, Cantor H, Arai K (1984) Proc Natl Acad Sci USA 81: 1070–1074
6. Schrader JW, Lewis SJ, Clark-Lewis I, Culvenor JG (1981) Proc Natl Acad Sci USA 78: 323–327
7. Dy M, Lebel B, Kamoun P, Hamburger J (1981) J Exp Med 153: 293–309
8. Schrader JW, Battye F, Scollay R (1982) Proc Natl Acad Sci USA 79: 4161–4165

Haematology and Blood Transfusion Vol. 29
Modern Trends in Human Leukemia VI
Edited by Neth, Gallo, Greaves, Janka

Molecular Cloning of cDNA for the Human Interleukin-2 Receptor *

W. C. Greene, J. M. Depper, G. R. Crabtree, S. Rudikoff, J. Pumphrey, R. J. Robb, M. Krönke, P. Svetlik, N. J. Peffer, T. A. Waldmann, and W. J. Leonard

A. Introduction

Interleukin-2 (IL-2 or T cell growth factor) is a 14,500 daltons glycoprotein critically involved in the development of a normal human immune response [1, 2]. Recently, cDNA for this lymphokine has been isolated and expressed in both prokaryotic and eukaryotic cells [3–5]. Further, the human IL-2 gene has been cloned, sequenced [6], and localized to chromosome 4. As with other polypeptide hormones, IL-2 exerts its biologic effects through binding to specific high affinity membrane receptors [7]. However, neither IL-2 nor IL-2 receptors are produced by resting T cells [7, 8]. Following exposure to antigen, T cells binding antigen enter a program of cellular activation leading to de novo synthesis and secretion of IL-2 and expression of IL-2 receptors. The interaction of IL-2 with its cellular receptor then triggers cellular proliferation, resulting in the growth and development of helper, suppressor, and cytotoxic T cells. Thus, induction of IL-2 receptor expression is a principal mechanism by which the specificity and magnitude of the human immune response is regulated. While IL-2 receptors are not present in most human leukemic T cell lines, these receptors are uniformly expressed in large numbers in adult T cell leukemia (ATL) cells infected with human T cell leukemia/lymphoma virus-1 (HTLV-1) [9]. Though unproven, it is possible that these receptors are involved in the malignant growth of these leukemic cells.

We have previously demonstrated that monoclonal anti-Tac antibody, prepared by Uchiyama, Broder and Waldmann [10], recognizes the human IL-2 receptor [11–13]. We have characterized the IL-2 receptor on normal activated T cells as a densely glycosylated, sulfated, and phosphorylated structure containing intrachain disulfide bonds with an apparent $M_r = 55\,000$ [12]. These receptors are composed of a peptide precursor (apparent $M_r = 33\,000$) which is cotranslationally processed by *N*-linked glycosylation to two intermediate forms (apparent $M_r = 35\,000$ and 37 000). Following export to the Golgi apparatus, these intermediate precursors undergo further posttranslational processing, involving the addition of *O*-linked carbohydrate, sialic acid, sulfate, and phosphate. We now describe the molecular cloning, sequencing, and expression of cDNA corresponding to the human IL-2 receptor isolated from HTLV-1-transformed HUT 102B2 cells.

B. Materials and Methods

HTLV-1-infected HUT 102B2 cells were used as a source of IL-2 receptor protein and RNA. mRNA was prepared from these cells using guanidine isothiocyanate and isopyknic centrifugation in cesium chloride followed by selection of poly(A^+) mRNA

* The Metabolism Branch, the Laboratory of Pathology, and the Laboratory of Genetics, National Cancer Institute, National Institutes of Health, Bethesda, MD and E. I. duPont de Nemours and Co., Glenolden, PA

with oligo(dT)-cellulose. Using approximately 5 μg HUT 102B2 mRNA, a cDNA library was constructed in λ gt10 according to the method of St. John, except that size-fractionated double-stranded cDNA was purified by absorption to glass silica mesh. The resultant cDNA library contained 2.4×10^6 recombinant phage clones with inserts ranging in size from 500 base pairs to several kilobases. Following amplification, 200 000 phage clones were screened by Benton–Davis plaque hybridization [14] with a 17 nucleotide synthetic probe based on the protein sequence of the receptor (see Sect. C). Candidate clones were evaluated by selective hybridization of mRNA [15] and complete sequencing using the dideoxy chain termination method of Sanger and Coulson in M13 bacteriophage [16]. DNA sequence data were analyzed and compared on an IBM system 370 using the program described by Queen and Korn. cDNA were expressed by ligating each into the EcoR1 site of pcEXV-1 (generously provided by Dr. James Miller and Dr. Ron Germain, NIH). This vector places the cDNA inserts under the control of the early SV40 promoter and enhancer sequences. These constructs were subsequently transfected into COS-1 cells by calcium phosphate precipitation and evaluated for IL-2 receptor expression 48–72 h later in binding assays with purified radiolabeled IL-2 and anti-Tac. Analysis of genomic DNA and mRNA in varying cell lines was performed as previously described [17, 18].

C. Results and Discussion

I. Purification of the Human IL-2 Receptor

The IL-2 receptor was purified from NP-40 detergent extracts of HUT 102B2 cells by immunoaffinity chromatography with anti-Tac antibody. The extract was first passed over a control UPC 10 monoclonal antibody column and then over the anti-Tac column. Following serial washes at varying ionic strengths, the receptor was eluted with 2.5% acetic acid. Following lyophilization, the receptor was found to retain biologic activity (capacity to bind IL-2) and was > 95% pure as judged by silver staining of SDS–polyacrylamide gels. The sequence of the NH_2 terminal 29 amino acids was determined by gas phase microsequencing (100–250 pmol per analysis) and selected positions identified or confirmed by sequencing receptor biosynthetically labeled with radioactive amino acids (Table 1).

II. Molecular Cloning of cDNA Corresponding to the Human IL-2 Receptor

Based on the protein sequence, an oligonucleotide probe 17 nucleotides in length with 64-fold degeneracy was synthesized (Table 2). This oligonucleotide probe was used to screen 200 000 recombinant phages from the amplified HUT 102B2 cDNA library. Following sequential screening, 11 candidate phage clones containing cDNA inserts which hybridized to the 17mer were identified (Fig. 1). Clone 2 (900 base pairs), clone 3 (2400 base pairs), and clone 4 (1600 base pairs) were chosen for further analysis and subcloned into pBR322. Each of these clones was evaluated for the capacity to hybridize selectively to mRNA which, when translated and immunoprecipitated, would produce the primary translation product of the IL-2 receptor. As shown in Fig. 2, each of the three clones, but not pBR327 nor filters without DNA, selectively hybridized to IL-2 receptor mRNA. These data suggested the association of these cDNA with the human IL-2 receptor.

Each of the inserts or appropriate restriction fragments from clones 2, 3, and 4 were subcloned into M13 bacteriophage and the complete DNA sequence determined. A complete listing of these sequences is reported in reference [19]. Each of the sequences contained a long open reading frame, including a region of 87 nucleotides which coded for the 29 NH_2 terminal amino acids determined by protein sequencing; thus, their relationship to the IL-2 receptor was confirmed. However, comparison of the sequences of clone 3 and 4 revealed that clone 4 lacked a 216 base pairs segment within the protein coding region which was present in clone 3. Further, this segment was flanked on either side by the sequence TTCCAGGT, indicative of a typical mRNA donor and acceptor splicing site [20]. Thus, the presence of this internally truncated cDNA suggested that an alternate pathway of mRNA processing existed for the IL-2 receptor. Since the predicted protein from the spliced cDNA (clone 4) was 72 amino acids shorter than that encoded by the unspliced cDNA (clone 3), but otherwise identical, it was unclear which cDNA corresponded to the true IL-2 receptor mRNA. To address this issue, the cDNA inserts from clone 3 and 4 were ligated into an expression vector pcEXV-1 which contains SV40 promoter and enhancer sequences. Plasmids with the cDNA in the correct orientation were then transfected into COS-1 cells by calcium phosphate precipitation and analyzed for directed synthesis of the IL-2 receptor. As shown in Fig. 3, radiolabeled binding of IL-2 and anti-Tac occurred only when the unspliced cDNA was transfected (clone 3). Further, cell surface iodination and immunoprecipitation with anti-Tac confirmed the presence of the $M_r = 50\,000$ receptor characteristic of HUT 102B2 cells. In contrast, the spliced cDNA, while effectively transcribed, did not result in the production of receptors capable of binding either IL-2 or anti-Tac. These data raise the possibility that IL-2 receptor expression may not only be regulated at the level of initiation of transcription, but also at a posttranscriptional step involving splicing of this internal segment.

Fig. 1. DNA from 12 recombinant λ gt10 phage clones selected in serial screening with the 17mer were restricted with EcoR1, electrophoresed on a 1% agarose gel, transferred to nitrocellulose, and probed with the 17mer. Inserts from 11 of the 12 phage clones hybridized to the 17mer, however, two negative phage clones (N28, N29) which contained 1 kilobase inserts did not hybridize. Phage clones 2, 3, and 4 were chosen for further analysis as they were representative of the smallest and two largest cDNA insert

Table 1. NH_2 terminal amino acid sequence of the human IL-2 receptor [a]

1 2 3 4 5 6 7 8 9 10 11
glutamic-leucine-cysteine-aspartic-aspartic-aspartic-proline-proline-glutamic-isoleucine-proline-
12 13 14 15 16 17 18 19 20 21
histidine-alanine-threonine-phenylalanine-lysine-alanine-methionine-alanine-tyrosine-lysine-
22 23 24 25 26 27 28 29
glutamic-glycine-threonine-methionine-leucine-asparagine-cysteine-glutamic

[a] The human IL-2 receptor from HUT 102B2 was sequenced by automated Edman degradation on a gas phase sequencer followed by analysis of samples by high liquid chromatography. The positions of leucine, cysteine, aspartic acid, proline, and methionine were determined or confirmed by sequencing of receptor biosynthetically labeled with the respective radioactive amino acid

Table 2. Nucleotide sequence of the synthetic oligonucleotide probes complementary to mRNA corresponding to amino acids 3–8 [a]

G-G-A/G-G-G-A/G-T-C-A/G-T-C-A/G-T-C-A/G-C-A	(Pool 1)
G-G-C/T-G-G-A/G-T-C-A/G-T-C-A/G-T-C-A/G-C-A	(Pool 2)

[a] Since the 17 nucleotide sequence for amino acids 3–8 was 64-fold degenerate, the oligonucleotides were synthesized in two separate pools each containing 32 species. Following end-labeling with ATP ^{32}P and polynucleotide kinase, both pools identified two mRNA in Northern blotting experiments and thus Benton-Davis screening of the cDNA library was performed with a mixture of both pools

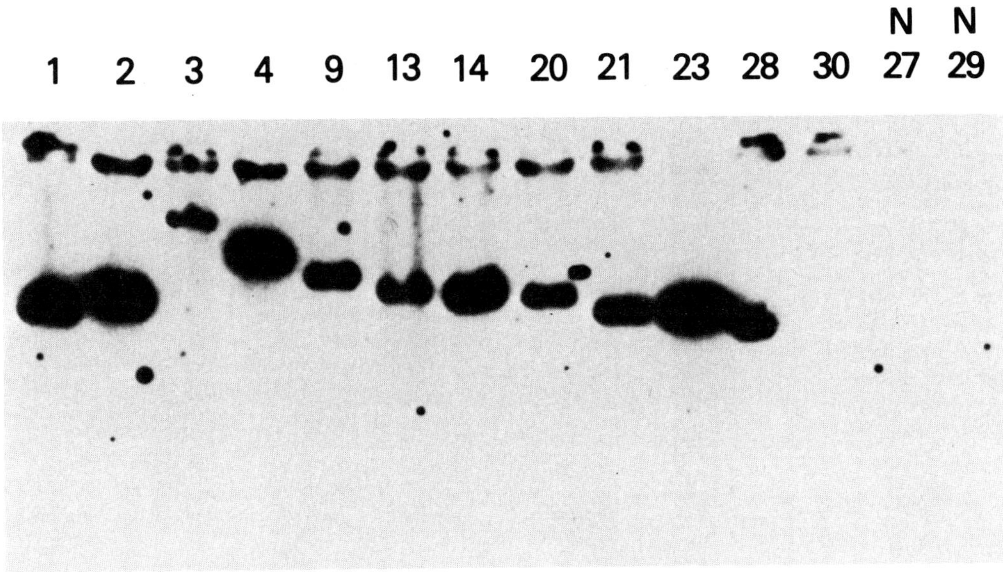

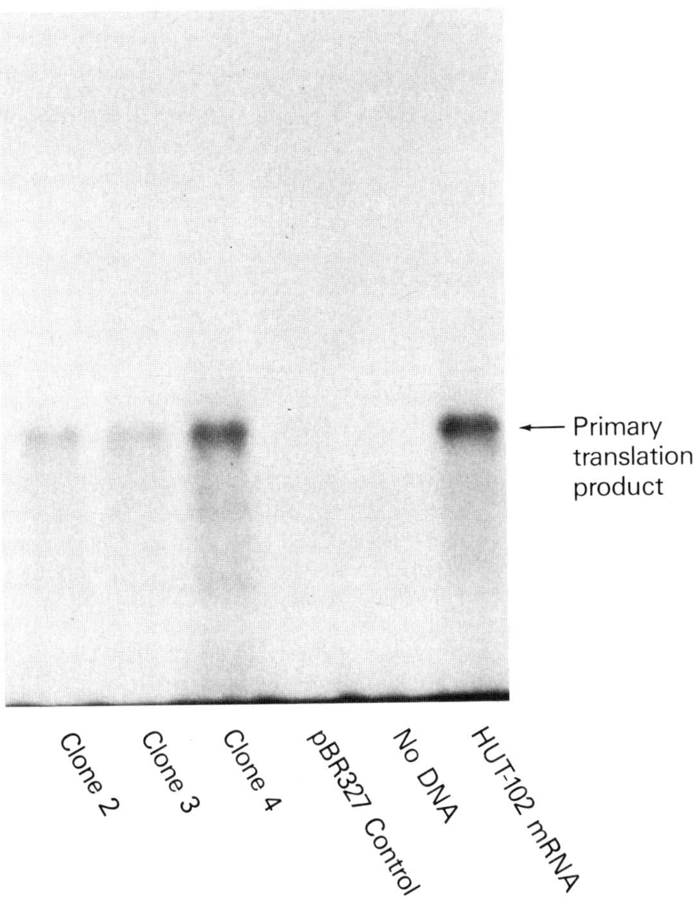

Fig. 2. Selective hybridization of IL-2 receptor mRNA. The cDNA inserts of phage clones 2, 3, and 4 were subcloned into the EcoR1 site of pBR322. Approximately 5 μg plasmid DNA containing these inserts or pBR327 were linearized with SalI and bound to nitrocellulose. Nitrocellulose filters were then hybridized with HUT 102B2 mRNA and mRNA selectively retained was eluted and translated in a wheat germ lysate cell-free translation system. Translations were immunoprecipitated with an anti-IL-2 receptor heteroantibody and analyzed by SDS–PAGE. As shown, clones 2, 3, and 4, but not pBR327 nor filters lacking DNA, selectively hybridized to mRNA which when translated generated the same primary translation product as obtained with HUT 102B2 mRNA. (This figure appears in reference [19] and is presented with the permission of the publishers of *Nature*.)

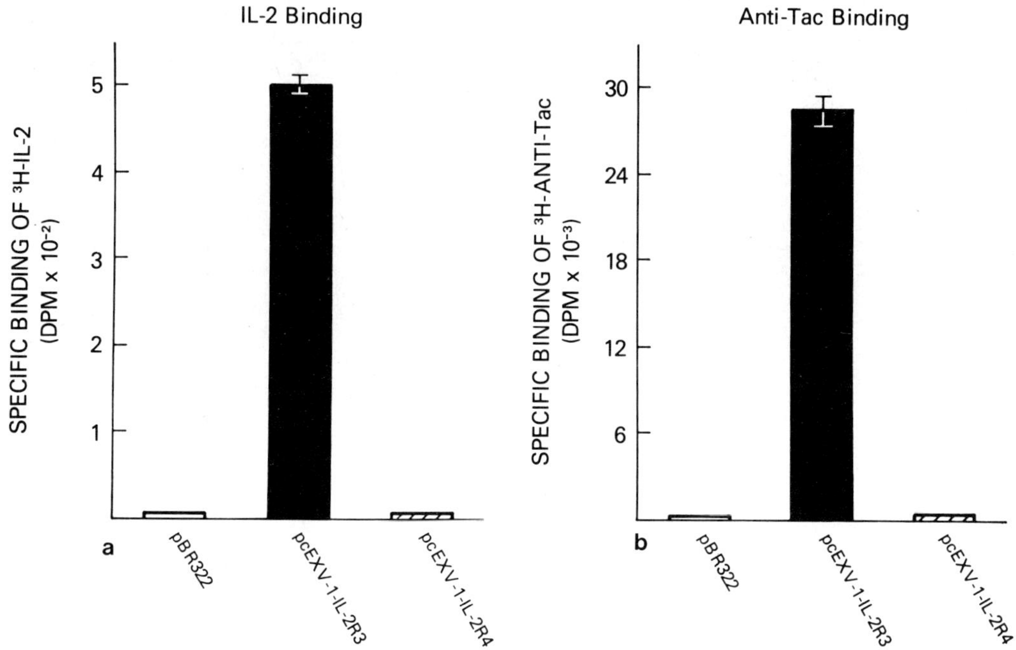

Fig. 3a, b. DNA from pcEXV-1 expression vector constructs containing clone 3 and clone 4 cDNA inserts in the proper orientation or pBR322 were transfected into COS-1 cells by calcium phosphate precipitation as described [19]. Specific binding of **a** purified radiolabeled JURKAT IL-2 and **b** purified radiolabeled anti-Tac was measured after 48 h of culture

III. Southern and Northern Blotting Studies of the IL-2 Receptor

Southern blots of EcoR1-restricted genomic DNA probed with an IL-2 receptor cDNA suggested the presence of a single structural gene rather than a multiple gene family for the human IL-2 receptor (Fig. 4). Digests with Bam H1 and HindIII also revealed simple patterns of bands, supporting a single gene for this receptor. These data however do not exclude a recent gene duplication event with preservation of these restriction endonuclease sites.

Northern blot analysis of mRNA expression from several cellular sources demonstrated the presence of two differently sized mRNA. As shown in Fig. 5, two mRNA are present in HTLV-1-transformed HUT 102B2 cells. Also, transformation of B cells with HTLV-1 resulted in the expression of IL-2 receptor mRNA production [19]. In general, acute lymphocytic leukemic T cells do not display IL-2 receptors. Consistent with this observation, JURKAT acute lymphocytic leukemic T cells do not contain detectable IL-2 receptor mRNA. However, we have previously reported that IL-2 receptor expression is induced in JURKAT and HSB-2 leukemic T cells following stimulation with PHA and phorbal myristate acetate (PMA) [21]. As shown in Fig. 5, PHA and PMA induction of JURKAT leukemic cells resulted in IL-2 receptor mRNA expression. In other studies not shown, neither non-T cells nor resting T cells contain mRNA for the IL-2 receptor. Induction of purified T cells with PHA, PMA, or combinations of these agents results in the expression of the two major mRNA species identical in size to those present in HUT 102B2 cells.

Further study of the molecular basis for the difference in size of the two mRNA has revealed that use of different polyadenylation signal sequences is involved. A proximal AATAAA sequence is apparently disregarded to generate the large mRNA

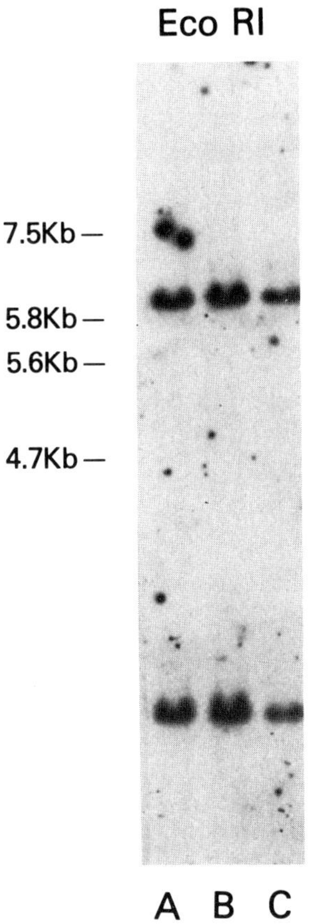

Fig. 4. Southern blot analysis of human genomic DNA restricted with EcoR1 probed with ^{32}P-labeled IL-2 receptor cDNA containing 937 bases from the 5′ end of the mRNA. DNA were isolated from human placenta (*lane A*) and human tonsil (*lanes B* and *C*). More recent blots also indicate the presence of a 10 kilobases band in EcoR1 digests seen faintly in the autoradiogram. (This figure appears in reference [19] and is presented with the permission of the publishers of *Nature*.)

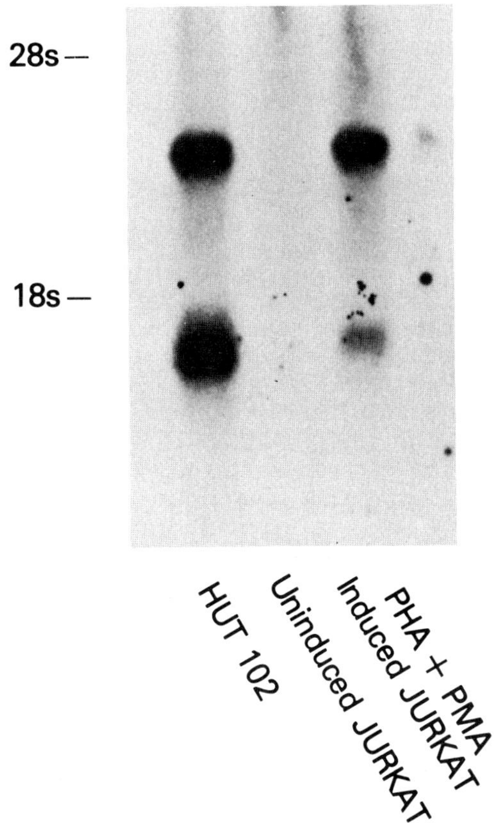

Fig. 5. Northern blot of IL-2 receptor mRNA expression in HUT 102B2 cells, JURKAT leukemic T cells, and JURKAT leukemic T cells induced for 18 h with PHA (1 μg/ml) and PMA (50 ng/ml); 10 μg oligo(dT)-selected mRNA was electrophoresed in each lane and blots were brobed with nick-translated IL-2 receptor cDNA. Migration of 28 *S* and 18 *S* ribosomal RNA is indicated

(3500 nucleotides) while the smaller mRNA (1500 nucleotides) is produced when the proximal polyadenylation signal sequence is utilized [19]. Both mRNA appear functional since size separation of HUT 102B2 mRNA on a methylmercuric hydroxide gel, translation of mRNA from different slices of the gel, and immunoprecipitation of the resultant proteins demonstrate the primary translation product for the receptor from fractions corresponding to both the small and large mRNA.

IV. Analysis of the Primary Structure of the Human IL-2 Receptor

The complete amino acid sequence of the IL-2 receptor was deduced from the cDNA sequence [19]. The receptor is composed of 272 amino acids, including a signal peptide of 21 amino acids. The length of the signal peptide has been confirmed preliminarily by sequencing the primary translation product after labeling with methionine ^{35}S (W.J. Leonard, S. Rudikoff, and W.C.

Greene, unpublished work). The protein contains 13 cysteine residues, suggesting potentially extensive intrachain disulfide bonding, confirmed in immunoprecipitates electrophoresed under reducing and non-reducing conditions [12]. Two potential *N*-linked glycosylation sites are present and multiple potential *O*-linked glycosylation sites are located in a region we believe to occur immediately extractoplasmic to the cell membrane. In pulse-chase labeling studies of the protein performed with and without tunicamycin, we have demonstrated two *N*-linked precursor forms and thus suggest that both *N*-glycosylation sites are utilized [12]. Further, we have provided evidence for *O*-linked glycosylation occurring in the Golgi apparatus [12, 22]. Hydrophobicity analysis suggests the presence of a single transmembrane domain near the COOH terminus and a short intracytoplasmic domain (13 amino acids). The intracytoplasmic domain contains several basic amino acids which form a charge cluster and presumably serves as a cytoplasmic anchoring region. Further, a serine and threonine residue are present within the putative intracytoplasmic domain and could serve as potential phosphate acceptor sites. We have previously demonstrated that this receptor is constitutively phosphorylated [22].

A second moderately hydrophobic region exists within the protein, but is removed in the spliced form of the receptor. It is unlikely that this region represents a second transmembrane crossing as this would result in the *N*-linked glycosylation sites occurring within the cytoplasm which would be without precedent. However, this region could represent a loop into the membrane. Alternatively, this segment may be involved in the binding of IL-2 which is unexpectedly rich in hydrophobic residues.

In view of the exceedingly short intracytoplasmic tail predicted by the DNA sequence, it seems unlikely that signal transduction by the receptor involves an enzymatic activity of this domain. In immunoprecipitates labeled with methionine ^{35}S, we have previously observed coprecipitation of two larger proteins ($M_r = 113\,000$ and 180 000). These proteins appear to be located on the inner face of the membrane as they are not glycosylated nor labeled with cell surface iodination techniques. However, each is constitutively phosphorylated. It is possible, though unproven, that these proteins form a receptor complex with the IL-2 receptor and thus might be involved in signal transduction following IL-2 binding.

The availability of cDNA probes to the IL-2 receptor hopefully will aid in studies relating to IL-2 receptor structure, function, and regulation. Further, these cDNA should be useful in further defining the intriguing relationship between HTLV-1-induced transformation of T cells and expression of IL-2 receptors.

References

1. Morgan DA, Ruscetti FW, Gallo RC (1976) Science 193:1007–1008
2. Smith KA (1980) Immunol Rev 51:337–357
3. Taniguchi T, Matsui H, Fujita T, Takaoka C, Kashima N, Yoshimoto R, Hamuro J (1983) Nature 302:305–310
4. Devos R, Paetinck G, Cheroute H, Simons G, Degrave W, Tavernier J, Remout E, Fiers W (1983) Nucl Acid Res 11:4307–4323
5. Clark SC, Arya SK, Wong-Staal F, Matsumoto-Kobayashi M, Kay RM, Kaufman RJ, Brown EL, Shoemaker C, Copeland T, Oroszlan S, Smith KA, Sarngadharan MG, Lindner SG, Gallo RC (1984) Proc Natl Acad Sci USA 81:2543–2547
6. Fujita T, Takeoka C, Matsui H, Taniguchi T (1983) Proc Natl Acad Sci USA 81: 1634–1638
7. Robb RJ, Munck A, Smith KA (1981) J Exp Med 154:1455–1474
8. Greene WC, Robb RJ (1984) In: Gillis S (ed) Contemporary topics in molecular immunology. Plenum, NY 10:1
9. Depper JM, Leonard WJ, Kronke M, Waldmann TA, Greene WC (1984) J Immunol 133:1691–1695
10. Uchiyama T, Broder S, Waldmann TA (1981) J Immunol 126:1393–1397
11. Leonard WJ, Depper JM, Uchiyama T, Smith KA, Waldmann TA, Greene WC (1982) Nature 300:267–269
12. Leonard WJ, Depper JM, Robb RJ, Waldmann TA, Greene WC (1983) Proc Natl Acad Sci USA 80:6957–6961
13. Robb RJ, Greene WC (1983) J Exp Med 158:1332–1337
14. Benton WD, Davis RW (1977) Science 196: 180–182

15. Maniatis T, Fritsch EF, Sambrook J (1982) In: Molecular cloning. Cold Spring Harbor Laboratory, pp 330–333
16. Sanger F, Coulson AR (1975) J Mol Biol 94:414–418
17. Southern EM (1975) J Mol Biol 98:503–517
18. Thomas PS (1980) Proc Natl Acad Sci USA 77:5201–5205
19. Leonard WJ, Depper JM, Crabtree GR, Rudikoff S, Pumphrey J, Robb RJ, Kronke M, Svetlik PB, Peffer NJ, Waldmann TA, Greene WC (1984) Nature 311:626–631
20. Breathnach R, Benoist C, O'Hare K, Gannon F, Chambon P (1978) Proc Natl Acad Sci USA 75:4853–4857
21. Greene WC, Robb RJ, Depper JM, Leonard WJ, Drogula C, Svetlik PB, Wong-Staal F, Gallo RC, Waldmann TA, Greene WC (1984) J Immunol 133:1042–1047
22. Leonard WJ, Depper JM, Robb RJ, Kronke M, Waldmann TA, Greene WC (1985) J Biol Chem 260:1872–1880

Haematology and Blood Transfusion Vol. 29
Modern Trends in Human Leukemia VI
Edited by Neth, Gallo, Greaves, Janka

Purification of Normal Human T-Cell Growth Factor to Molecular Homogeneity *

S. G. Lindner, R. Rahman, M. G. Sarngadharan, and R. C. Gallo

T-cell growth factor (TCGF), also called interleukin-2, supports proliferation of lectin- or antigen-activated T cells. It was originally discovered in the conditioned media of phytohemagglutinin-stimulated peripheral blood lymphocyte (PBL) cultures [1, 2]. It is also produced by some leukemic cell lines (e.g., Jurkat) after stimulation and, constitutively, by certain retrovirus-infected neoplastic T-cell lines [3]. TCGF produced by normal human PBL cultures has been purified to molecular homogeneity by biochemical means using a multistep procedure.

First, the lymphocyte-conditioned media (Ly-CM) were concentrated 40-fold by diafiltration using the Millipore Pellicon Cassette system. The filter used was the polysulfate filter PTGC (10 000 NMWL). Serum-containing media were further processed by anion-exchange chromatography: the concentrate was loaded onto a diethylaminoethyl-(DEAE)-sepharose column and eluted with an NaCl gradient in Tris buffer. TCGF activity of the collected fractions was determined in a [^{3}H]thymidine incorporation assay using a cloned TCGF-dependent mouse-cell line (CTLL). When starting with serum-free media anion-exchange chromatography was unnecessary.

In the next step Ly-CM concentrate or the active fractions of the DEAE-sepharose column, respectively, were adsorbed to controlled-pore glass (Electronucleonics). After overnight incubation in roller bottles the glass beads were packed into a column, washed with phosphate-buffered saline (PBS-Dulbecco) and Tris buffer, and eluted with Tris buffer containing tetramethyl-

* Laboratory of Tumor Cell Biology, National Cancer Institute, National Institutes of Health, Bethesda, Md., USA

Table 1. Purification of TCGF from lymphocyte-conditioned media

Purification step	Volume (ml)	TCGF titer	Total activity (arbitrary units)	Total protein (mg)	Specific activity (unit/mg)	Fold purification	% Recovery
Ly-CM (concentrate)	1 475.0	4 390	6.48×10^6	501.0	12.9×10^3	1.0	100.0
CPG – eluate	1 310.0	3 760	4.93×10^6	85.0	57.9×10^3	4.5	76.0
HPLC – step I	350.0	7 406	2.59×10^6	7.9	328.0×10^3	25.4	40.0
HPLC – final	2.8	1 752 000	4.91×10^6	0.089	$55\,168.0 \times 10^3$	4 277.0	75.8

The TCGF titer was determined by serial dilutions in a [^{3}H]thymidine incorporation assay. For calculation of the total activity of the different steps (see text) the titers were multiplied by the respective volumes ammonium chloride. After extensive dialyzation against Tris buffer fractions were assayed for TCGF activity.

Active fractions of the controlled-pore glass step were acidified with trifluoroacetic acid (TFA) and loaded onto a reverse-phase high-performance liquid chromatography (RP-HPLC) column. The column was washed with 30% and 50% aqueous acetonitrile acidified with TFA; then it was eluted with 65% aqueous acetonitrile. To remove remaining impurities the eluate was diluted twofold with water and reloaded onto RP-HPLC. In the final step the column was washed with 40% aqueous acetonitrile and then developed with a gradient between 40% and 65% aqueous acetonitrile. The effluent was monitored by measuring the absorbance at 214 nm. TCGF eluted as a single peak at 60% aqueous acetonitrile.

The degree of purification of the different steps and the recovery are shown in Table 1. Molecular homogeneity of the purified TCGF was proved by determination of the NH_2-terminal amino acid sequence by Edman degradation using a microprocedure [4]. Pure TCGF was able to support the long-term growth of human and murine T cells.

References

1. Morgan DA, Ruscetti FW, Gallo RC (1976) Science 193:1007–1008
2. Ruscetti FW, Morgan DA, Gallo RC (1977) J Immunol 119:134–138
3. Gootenberg JE, Ruscetti FW, Gallo RC (1982) J Immunology 129:1499–1505
4. Copeland TD, Grandgennett DP, Oroszlan S (1980) J Virol 36:115–119

Haematology and Blood Transfusion Vol. 29
Modern Trends in Human Leukemia VI
Edited by Neth, Gallo, Greaves, Janka

Purification to Apparent Homogeneity and Biochemical Characterization of Human Pluripotent Hematopoietic Colony-Stimulating Factor *

K. Welte, E. Platzer, J. L. Gabrilove, L. Lu, E. Levi, A. Polivka, R. Mertelsmann and M. A. S. Moore

A. Introduction

Colony-stimulating factors (CSFs) are a family of hematopoietic growth factors required for the proliferation and differentiation of hematopoietic progenitor cells [1, 2]. In the human system, purification to homogeneity and biochemical characterization has only been reported for macrophage-active CSF (CSF-1) [3]. However, there are many reports about highly purified human granulocyte-macrophage CSFs (e.g. [4–7]), but not about pluripotent human CSF.

Assays are available to detect human clonogenic precursors that give rise to cells of the erythroid, granulocytic, megakaryocytic, macrophage, colony-forming unit granulocytes, erythrocytes, macrophages, and megakaryocytes, CFU-GEMM, and possibly lymphoid lineages [8–10]. CSFs with activities on these pluripotential progenitor cells (pluripotent CSF) are produced by mitogen- or antigen-activated T-lymphocytes [11] and by human tumor-cell lines [12] or HTLV-transformed lymphoid cells [13].

We report in this paper the purification to homogeneity and biochemical characterization of a human pluripotent CSF, produced and released by the human bladder carcinoma-cell line 5637.

B. Assay Systems

Granulocyte-macrophage-CSF (GM-CSF), granulocyte-macrophage-erythrocyte-megakaryocyte-CSF (GEMM-CSF), and early erythroid burst-forming unit (BFU-E) activities were tested on low-density, T-cell-depleted, nonadherent human bone marrow cells as described [14–15] and detailed in another paper by Platzer et al. in this volume. For assay of differentiation induction, the method of Metcalf [16] was used, whereby pluripotent CSF was added to cultures of the murine myelomonocytic WEHI-3B(D+) or the human promyelocytic HL-60 leukemic cells and scored for differentiation on day 7 and 14 respectively.

As shown in the Results, a single protein stimulates colony formation by CFU-GEMM, BFU-E, and CFU-GM progenitor cells. We termed this protein "pluripotent CSF" or "pluripoietin". Due to the low numbers of mixed colonies per dish attainable in this assay system, titration of test samples for determination of pluripotent CSF activity presented difficulties in quantitation. Therefore, we used the GM-CSF assay as described [14, 15] to measure the GM-CSF aspect of the pluripotent CSF in the samples that supported growth of CFU-GEMM and BFU-E for calculating the specific activities throughout the purification procedure.

---

* Laboratory of Developmental Hematopoiesis and Laboratory of Molecular Hematology, Memorial Sloan-Kettering Cancer Center, New York, NY 10021
Supported by NIH grants CA 20194, CA 31780, CA 32516, CA 33873, and CA 34995, American Cancer Society grants CH 251 and CH-3GH, NCI grant K08-CA00966-01, and the Gar Reichman Foundation

Table 1. Purification of human pluripotent CSF

	Total activity (units)[a]	Total protein (mg)	Specific activity (units/mg)	Purification (-fold)	Yield (%)
Conditioned media (20 L)	12×10^6	2000	6 000	–	100
DE 52 ion exchange chromatography	5×10^6	300	16 700	1[b]	42
AcA 54 gel filtration	3.1×10^6	13.2	235 000	14[b]	26
HPLC reverse phase	0.74×10^6	0.005	1.5×10^8	9 000[b]	6.2

[a] Units of activity in the GM-CSF assay in agar, as tested on low-density normal human bone marrow cells

[b] Estimate of -fold purification based on starting activity from one selected peak of DE 52

C. Purification of Pluripotent CSF

The human bladder carcinoma-cell line 5637 has been reported to produce constitutively a GM-CSF [17] and GEMM-CSF [12]. The cells were cultured in RPMI 1640 supplemented with glutamine (2 m*M*), antibiotics, and 10% fetal calf serum (FCS). For production of pluripotent CSF used for purification cells were kept for 48–72 h in medium containing low serum (0.2% FCS). The conditioned medium from low-serum-containing cultures was harvested and used for purification. The first three steps of purification involved ammonium sulfate precipitation (80% saturation), anion-exchange chromatography [diethylaminoethanol (DEAE)-cellulose, DE 52, Whatman, Clifton, NJ], and gel filtration (AcA 54 Ultrogel, LKB Products, Inc., Rockland, MD) (Table 1). These steps were used because they were highly effective for other cytokines, notably Interleukin 2 [18] and B-cell-differentiating factor [19] and have been described in detail elsewhere [18]. Pluripotent CSF eluted from the DE 52 cellulose column between 0.075 and 0.1 *M* NaCl in 0.05 *M* Tris/HCl, pH 7.8, and from the AcA 54 column with a single peak at around 32 000 molecular weight. The final step involved chromatography on a reverse-phase high-performance liquid chromatography (HPLC) column (uBondapak C 18, Waters) and a Waters HPLC system using 1-propanol as organic solvent (20%–50% 1-propanol gradient in 2 h) and a buffer system containing 0.9 *M* acetic acid and 0.2 *M* pyridine, pH 4.0. Pluripotent CSF activity eluted as a single peak at 42% 1-propanol. The purification schedule with degree of purification of pluripotent CSF as measured by GM-CSF activity, protein content, specific activity, and yield is detailed in Table 1. We obtained a specific activity of 1.5×10^8 U/mg protein.

D. Biochemical Characterization of Pluripotent CSF

The final preparation obtained after HPLC was analyzed on a 15% sodium dodecyl sulfate polyacrylamide gel electrophoresis (SDS-PAGE) gel [20] followed by the sensitive silver staining technique (Biorad Lab., Rockville Centre, NY; Fig. 1). Only one protein band with a molecular weight of 18 000 was seen under reducing (5% 2-mercaptoethanol; Fig. 1) and nonreducing (not shown) conditions. After electrophoresis under nonreducing conditions, a parallel gel was sliced into 2-mm sections and proteins eluted from each slice into phosphate buffer. Pluripotent CSF was found to be localized in the slice number corresponding to 18 000 molecular weight (Fig. 1). Reelectrophoresis of the protein in the active slice-fraction with SDS-PAGE under reducing conditions revealed again a protein band of 18 000 molecular weight (not shown).

The purified pluripotent CSF was also subjected to isoelectrofocusing analysis in

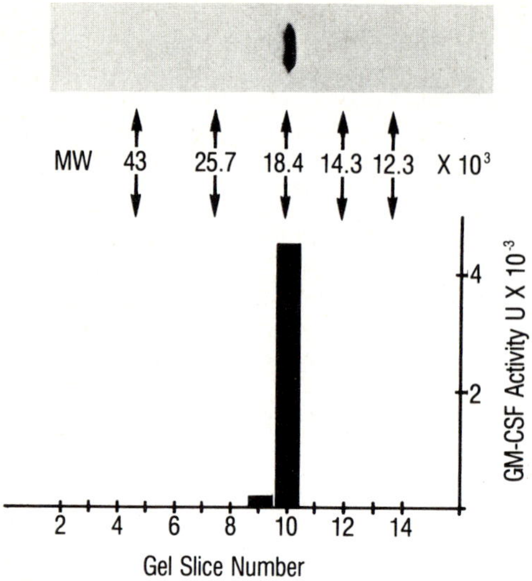

Fig. 1. *SDS-PAGE.* The pluripotent CSF eluted from the HPLC column (peak fraction) was lyophilized and treated with 1% SDS in 0.065 *M* Tris/HCl, pH 6.8, and 20% glycerol, under reducing conditions (5% 2-mercaptoethanol) for 1 h at 37 °C and then applied to a 15% polyacrylamide gel [20]. After electrophoresis, the proteins were visualized by the silver staining technique (*upper panel*). Treatment of pluripotent CSF under nonreducing conditions and subsequent electrophoresis gave the same results. For elution of biological activity pluripotent CSF was treated as above (nonreducing conditions) and after electrophoresis under the same conditions the gel was sliced into 2-mm sections and proteins from each slice were eluted into phosphate buffer (20 m*M*, pH 7.2). After 18 h eluted proteins were assayed for pluripotent activity (*lower panel;* GM-CSF activity, *black* columns). The following marker proteins (*arrows*) were used: ovalbumin (molecular weight, 43 000), chymotrypsinogen (molecular weight, 25 700), lactoglobulin (molecular weight, 18 400), lysozyme (molecular weight, 14 300), and cytochrome C (molecular weight, 12 300)

Table 2. Biochemical characteristics of human pluripotent CSF

Molecular weight (AcA 54 gel filtration)	32 000
Molecular weight (SDS-Page)	18 000
Isoelectric point	5.5
pH stability	2–9
Binding to concanavalin A-agarose	No

an IEF column (LKB 8100) [18] using ampholines with a pH range of 3.5–10. Pluripotent CSF was localized in one fraction with a pH of 5.5 (Table 2).

E. Biological Activity of Pluripotent CSF

Fifty units of GM-CSF activity of pluripotent CSF (1.8×10^{-11} *M*) supported the half-maximal cloning of CFU-GM, while 500 U/ml was needed to support the cloning of human CFU-GEMM and BFU-E. In addition pluripotent CSF at a concentration of between 500 and 1000 U/ml was capable of inducing differentiation of the leukemic cell lines HL-60 and WEHI-3B(D+). A detailed biological characterization of pluripotent CSF is described in the paper by Platzer et al. in this volume.

F. Discussion

The protein described in this paper is capable of stimulating the in vitro growth of human mixed colony progenitor cells (CFU-GEMM), early erythroid progenitor cells (BFU-E), and granulocyte-macrophage progenitors (CFU-GM) and in addition induces differentiation of the murine myelomonocytic (WEHI-3B(D+)) and the human promyelocytic (HL-60) leukemic cell lines. It has a molecular weight of 18 000 and an isoelectric point of 5.5. The specific activity is 1.5×10^8 U/mg protein. The purified protein, shown in Fig. 1, and the pluripotent CSF activity are identical because: (1) protein and activity eluted in the same fraction from the HPLC; (2) we were not able to separate biological activity and the 18 000 molecular weight protein by using additional HPLC columns (Diphenyl, C4, Hydroxylapatite) and buffer systems; (3) identical localization of protein and activity in SDS-PAGE (Fig. 1); (4) high specific activity (1.5×10^8 U/mg protein; 1 U $= 3.7 \times 10^{-13}$ *M*), which is comparable to pure murine CSF [21] and human CSF-1 [3]. Therefore, it is very unlikely that pluripotent CSF activity is not associated with the 18 000 molecular weight protein.

The availability of purified human pluripotent CSF has important and far-reaching implications for the analysis of human hematopoiesis and possibly for the understanding and management of clinical diseases involving hematopoietic derangement or failure.

Acknowledgment. We would like to thank Ms. Maureen Sullivan and Mr. John Foster for excellent technical assistance.

References

1. Burgess AW, Metcalf D (1980) The nature and action of granulocyte-macrophage colony-stimulating factors. Blood 56:947–958
2. Nicola NA, Vadas M (1984) Hematopoietic colony-stimulating factors. Immunol Today 5:76–81
3. Das SK, Stanley ER (1982) Structure–function studies of a colony stimulating factor (CSF-1). J Biol Chem 257:13 679–13 684
4. Wu MC, Yunis AA (1980) Common pattern of two distinct types of colony-stimulating factor in human tissues and cultured cells. J Clin Invest 65:772–775
5. Lusis AJ, Quon DH, Golde DW (1981) Purification and characterization of a human T-lymphocyte-derived granulocyte-macrophage colony-stimulating factor. Blood 57:13–21
6. Abboud CN, Brennan JK, Barlow GH, Lichtman MA (1981) Hydrophobic adsorption chromatography of colony-stimulating activities and erythroid-enhancing activity from the human monocyte-like cell line CGT. Blood 58:1148–1154
7. Motoyoshi K, Suda T, Kusumoto K, Takaku F, Miura Y (1982) Granulocyte-macrophage colony-stimulating and binding activities of purified human urinary colony-stimulating factor to murine and human bone marrow cells. Blood 60:1378–1391
8. Fauser AA, Messner HA (1978) Granulocyte-erythropoietic colonies in human bone marrow, peripheral blood and cord blood. Blood 52:1243–1248
9. Fauser AA, Messner HA (1979) Identification of megakaryocytes, macrophages and eosinophils in colonies of human bone marrow containing neutrophilic granulocytes and erythroblasts. Blood 53:1023–1027
10. Messner HA, Izaguirre CA, Jamal N (1981) Identification of T lymphocytes in human mixed hematopoietic colonies. Blood 58:402–405
11. Ruppert S, Lohr GW, Fauser AA (1983) Characterization of stimulatory activity for human pluripotent stem cells (CFU-GEMM). Exp Hematol 11:154–161
12. Myers CD, Katz FE, Joshi G, Millar JL (1984) A cell line secreting stimulating factors for CFU-GEMM culture. Blood 64:152–155
13. Salahuddin SZ, Markham PD, Lindner SG, Gootenberg J, Popovic M, Hemmi H, Sarin PS, Gallo RC (1984) Lymphokine production by cultured human T cells transformed by human T cell leukemia-lymphoma virus-I. Science 223:703–707
14. Broxmeyer HE, Moore MAS, Ralph P (1977) Cell-free granulocyte colony inhibitory activity derived from human polymorphonuclear neutrophils. Exp Hematol 5:87–102
15. Li L, Broxmeyer HE, Meyers PA, Moore MAS, Tzvi Thaler H (1983) Association of cell cycle expression of Ia-like antigenic determinants on normal human multipotential (CFU-GEMM) and erythroid (BFU-E) progenitor cells with regulation in vitro by acidic isoferritins. Blood 61:250–256
16. Metcalf D (1980) Clonal extinction of myelomonocytic leukemic cells by serum from mice injected with endotoxin. Int J Cancer 25:225–233
17. Svet-Modalsky GJ, Zinzer SN, Svet-Modalsky IA, Mann PE, Holland JF, Fogh J, Arlin Z, Clarkson BD (1980) CSF-producing human tumor cell lines. Lack of CSF activity of human stromal bone marrow fibroblasts. Exp Hematol 8 [Suppl] 7:76 (abstract)
18. Welte K, Wang CY, Mertelsmann R, Venuta S, Feldman S, Moore MAS (1982) Purification of human interleukin 2 to apparent homogeneity and its molecular heterogeneity. J Exp Med 165:454–464
19. Ralph P, Welte K, Levi E, Nakoinz I, Litkovsky PB, Mertelsmann R, Moore MAS (1984) Human B cell-inducing factor(s) for production of IgM, IgG and IgA: independence from IL2. J Immunol 132:1858–1862
20. Laemmli UK (1970) Cleavage of structural proteins during the assembly of the head of bacteriophage T4. Nature 227:680–685
21. Ihle JN, Keller J, Henderson L, Klein F, Palaszynski E (1982) Procedures for the purification of interleukin 3 to homogeneity. J Immunol 129:2431–2436

Haematology and Blood Transfusion Vol. 29
Modern Trends in Human Leukemia VI
Edited by Neth, Gallo, Greaves, Janka

Differentiation in Myelodysplastic, Myeloid Leukaemic and Normal Haemopoietic Cells: A New Approach Exploiting the Synergistic Interaction Between Differentiation Inducers and DNA Synthesis Inhibitors *

G. E. Francis, J. E. T. E. Guimaraes, J. J. Berney, and M. A. Wing

A. Introduction

The normal haemopoietic system behaves as if proliferation and the differentiation transitions on and between the granulocytic, erythroid and other lineages are stochastic events governed by probabilities determined by the levels of growth and differentiation stimuli [1]. Recent studies of myeloid leukaemic and myelodysplastic (AML and MDS) cells suggest that, in contrast to cell lines, there is a shift in the balance of probabilities for proliferation and differentiation rather than a maturation block at any particular stage [2]. This in turn suggests that these cells retain many of the features of normal proliferation and differentiation and that they will be accessible to the same means of altering the proliferation–differentiation balance as in normal cells. We recently proposed that physiological and pharmacological agents which enhance differentiation and maturation in vitro act by two fundamentally different routes: (a) by hastening progression through various differentiation/maturation steps; and (b) by slowing proliferation by inhibition of DNA synthesis. In order to test this thesis we looked for synergistic interaction between these two groups of agents. Combinations of differentiation-inducing agents (retinoic acid and *N*-methylformamide) with DNA synthesis inhibitors (6-mercaptopurine, cytosine arabinoside and aphidicolin) produced a differentiation-inducing effect on normal, MDS and AML cells, equivalent to that of 10-, 100- or even 1000-fold higher concentrations of single agents. Myelotoxic effects in vitro were not synergistic. The use of these highly synergistic combinations should greatly enhance the usefulness of differentiation inducers in the therapy of MDS and AML.

The myelodysplastic syndromes (MDS) [3] are a group of closely related disorders which tend to evolve to acute myeloid leukaemia (AML) [4]. They are characterised by peripheral blood cytopenias, usually in association with a hypercellular bone marrow. This suggests a defective maturation process and there is a detectable maturation delay in vitro [5, 6]. MDS cultures are reminiscent of those in which the proliferation and differentiation of normal cells has been partially uncoupled by supplying them with a source of growth stimulus relatively deficient in differentiation-inducing activity [7].

There is no generally effective therapy available for the MDS [8], but recently there has been an upsurge of interest in using differentiation-inducing agents in MDS and also in refractory AML. Retinoic acid, vitamin D3, butyrate and harringtonine have all been used in limited clinical trials [9–14]. Agents which slow DNA synthesis by a wide variety of different mechanisms have an apparently differentiation-inducing action in vitro and there have been several trials of low dose cytotoxic drug

* Academic Department of Haematology, Royal Free Hospital, Pond Street, London, NW3 2QG, England

therapy with varied results, in some cases suggestive of a cytotoxic action, in others of differentiation induction [15–18].

The first aim of this study was to determine whether DNA synthesis inhibitors have or induce differentiation-inducing activity or whether they act by some other mechanism. One possible mechanism of action is suggested by experimental evidence for the existence of a differentiation-responsive "window" in the cell cycle in or around the S-phase in both granulocyte–macrophage and erythroid cells [19–21]. If DNA synthesis inhibitors act by extending this window or any other mechanism independent of that involved in differentiation induction by other types of agent, DNA synthesis inhibitors and these differentiation inducers would be expected to interact synergistically. In the context of MDS this might be most useful because aggravated cytopenia and marrow hypoplasia is a common complication of therapy with low dose cytosine arabinoside and other DNA synthesis inhibitors [16, 17, 22].

True differentiation-inducing agents have the theoretical advantage that although they inevitably decrease the amplification of the haemopoietic system (i.e. the total number of cells produced from each stem cell committed to the differentiation pathway) they should not impair the stem cell compartment's ability to compensate for this. In contrast, DNA synthesis inhibitors, whatever their mechanism of action in enhancing differentiation, not only reduce the amplification of the system directly by slowing proliferation but also, since they are nonselective, inhibit stem cell division and thus reduce any possibility for compensation. That such a compensatory mechanism may operate in vivo is suggested by the different incidence of hypoplasia in patients receiving DNA synthesis inhibitors and conventional differentiation inducers.

The ability, demonstrated in this report, to enhance the differentiation-inducing effect of retinoic acid and *N*-methylformamide by very low doses of DNA synthesis inhibitors should prove useful in designing new and less toxic differentiation induction therapeutic protocols for the treatment of MDS patients and of AML patients unsuitable for or unresponsive to conventional AML therapy.

B. Materials and Methods

Marrow aspirates were obtained from three healthy volunteers, from three patients with MDS (FAB classification refractory anaemia with excess of blasts (RAEB), RAEB in transformation (RAEB-T), chronic myelomonocytic leukaemia (CMML) [1]) and peripheral blood blasts from one patient with AML (FAB-M4) and another with AML following MDS. With the exception of the last patient none had received cytotoxic therapy.

I. Differentiation Inducers and DNA Synthesis Inhibitors

The following freshly prepared stock solutions were used: 10^{-2} *M* retinoic acid (All *trans*) (Sigma), 0.6 *M* *N*-methylformamide (Aldrich 5×10^{-2} *M* 6-mercaptopurine (Wellcome), 10^{-2} *M* cytosine arabinoside (Upjohn), 10^{-3} *M* aphidicolin (Sigma). Diluents were absolute ethanol, tissue culture medium (McCoy's 5A, Flow), 0.1 *M* NaOH, pyrogen-free water, and propane-1,2-diol, respectively. The concentration of diluent was adjusted to the same level for all drug concentrations. The final concentration of ethanol was 1:10 000, of 0.1 *M* NaOH 1:500 and of propane-1,2-diol 1:1000 (v/v).

II. Semisolid Agar Cultures

A double-layer technique [23] was used. Target marrow cells (10^5 cells < 1.077 g/cm^{-3}) and differentiation-inducing agents were incorporated into 0.3% agar overlayers. Feeder layers contained 10^6 peripheral blood leucocytes/ml and 0.5% agar and in three experiments performed to exclude the possibility of any effect of drugs on feeder layer cells and also to ensure the growth of leukaemic cells, parallel experiments were performed using a cell-free source of gm-CSA, phytohaemagglutinin-stimulated leucocyte-conditioned medium

(5% PHA-LCM). Cultures were incubated for 7 days in 5% CO_2 in air. For morphological studies overlayers were removed and stained for nonspecific and chloroacetate esterase as previously described [7].

III. Suspension Cultures

Marrow cells (< 1.077 g/cm^{-3}) were cultured at low concentration (0.5×10^5 cells/ml) in order to limit contribution of bone marrow derived gm-CSA and thus possible indirect effects; gm-CSA was provided by 5% PHA-LCM.

IV. Nitroblue Tetrazolium Reduction

Oxygen radical generation in response to *Escherichia coli* broth (kindly supplied by Dr. G.W. Smith) was assessed by reduction of NBT to produce blue-black formazan deposits. Suspension culture cells (50 µl containing approximately 10^6 cells) were incubated for 15 min at 37 °C with 20 µl *E. coli* broth and 100 µl NBT (0.1% w/v in Hank's balanced salt solution without calcium, magnesium or phenol red), cytocentrifuged and counterstained (Diffquik).

C. Results

I. Alterations of the Proliferation–Differentiation Balance of Normal Cells

In the normal granulocyte–macrophage pathway proliferation and differentiation can be partially uncoupled and their rates varied independently [7]. This affects both the amplification of the system (since it affects the number of cell divisions occurring before end cell production intervenes) and also the proportion of mature to immature cells observed in in vitro systems and predicted for in vivo steady state conditions. Figure 1 shows the four hypothetical ways in which the proliferation–differentiation balance of normal cells can vary and the effects on the amplification of the system and the proportion of mature cells. Three of the four have been tested experimentally. In a previous study [7] we showed that the effect of reducing the differentiation rate without reducing the proliferation rate is increased amplification and a reduced proportion of mature cells. The converse of this effect is obtained with gm-CSA sources rich in differentiation-inducing activity or with pharmacological inducers of differentiation.

The effects of changes in the proliferation rate cannot be assessed readily with physiological inducers since the proliferation stimulus also conveys a differentiation stimulus. Table 1 shows the effect of reducing the proliferation rate with low levels of DNA synthesis inhibitor. Although the total number of cells produced decreased, both the proportion and the absolute number of mature cells (in this example assessed by NBT reduction) were increased. Modelling experiments based on earlier work [1] showed that this increase in mature cells is not consistent with a system in which differentiation and cell division are completely independent events and the low level of DNA synthesis has merely decreased the rate of cell division (M.F. Leaning and G.E. Francis, unpublished work). It suggests instead some special relationship between proliferation and differ-

Fig. 1. Since differentiation (*D*) and proliferation (*P*) can be partially uncoupled in normal cells the amplification of the system (*A*) can be varied: (1) by altering the rate at which cells undergo one or more differentiation/maturation transitions (*horizontal lines*); or (2) by altering the proliferation rate (shown here diagramatically as the width of the *triangles*). The proportion of mature cells (*M*) predicted for steady state conditions in vivo (and observed in vitro) also varies

Fig. 2. Synergistic interaction between DNA synthesis inhibitors (*vertical hatching*) and differentiation inducers (*horizontal hatching*) used in combination (cross hatching) in day 4–6 suspension cultures of normal marrow cells. The increased percentage NBT-reducing cells was due to an absolute increase in these cells in association with a decrease in the total number of cells formed. RET retinoic acid; N-MF *N*-methylformamide; 6-MP 6-mercaptopurine; ARA-C cytosine arabinoside; APH aphidicolin. The combination of 2 DNA synthesis inhibitors (*black column*) was not synergistic, merely additive

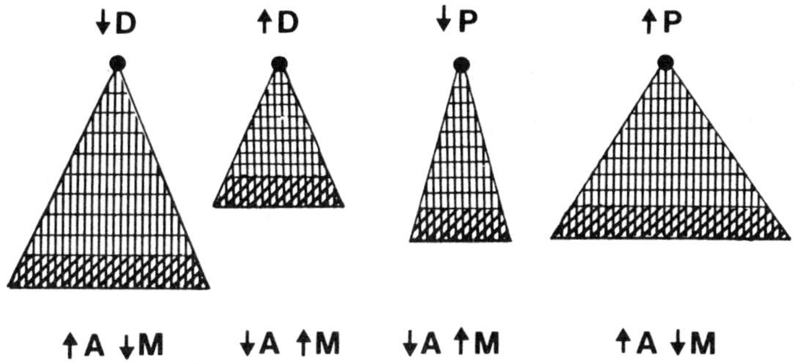
↓D
↑D
↓P
↑P
↑A ↓M
↓A ↑M
↓A ↑M
↑A ↓M

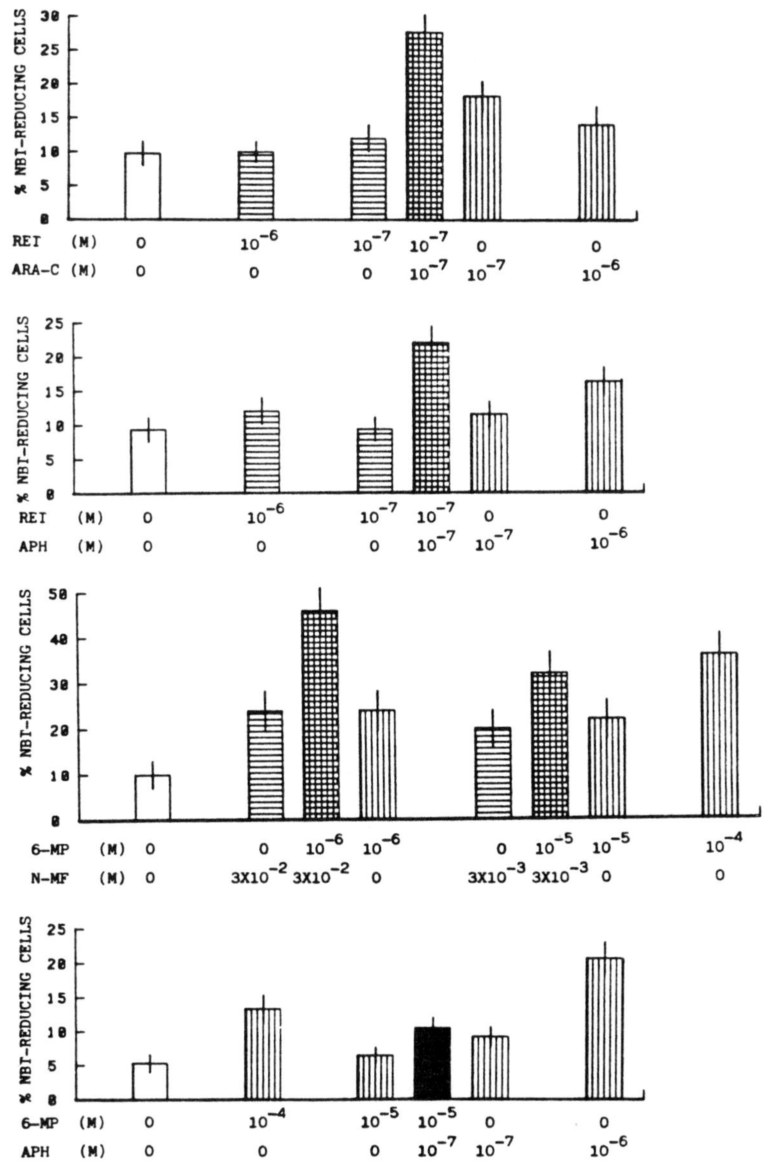
% NBT-REDUCING CELLS
RET (M) 0 10^-6 10^-7 10^-7 0 0
ARA-C (M) 0 0 0 10^-7 10^-7 10^-6
% NBT-REDUCING CELLS
RET (M) 0 10^-6 10^-7 10^-7 0 0
APH (M) 0 0 0 10^-7 10^-7 10^-6
% NBT-REDUCING CELLS
6-MP (M) 0 0 10^-6 10^-6 0 10^-5 10^-5 10^-4
N-MF (M) 0 3X10^-2 3X10^-2 0 3X10^-3 3X10^-3 0 0
% NBT-REDUCING CELLS
6-MP (M) 0 10^-4 10^-5 10^-5 0 0
APH (M) 0 0 0 10^-7 10^-7 10^-6

Table 1. The effect of DNA-synthesis inhibitors (day 6 suspension cultures of normal marrow cells)[a]

6-Mercaptopurine (*M*)	0	10^{-7}	10^{-6}	10^{-5}	10^{-4}
Nucleated cells (% control)	100	91	77	76	75
NBT-reducing cells (% total)	10	19	24	22	36
NBT-reducing cells (% control)	100	173	183	167	271

[a] Similar results were obtained with cytosine arabinoside, aphidicolin, 6-thioguanine and hydroxyurea

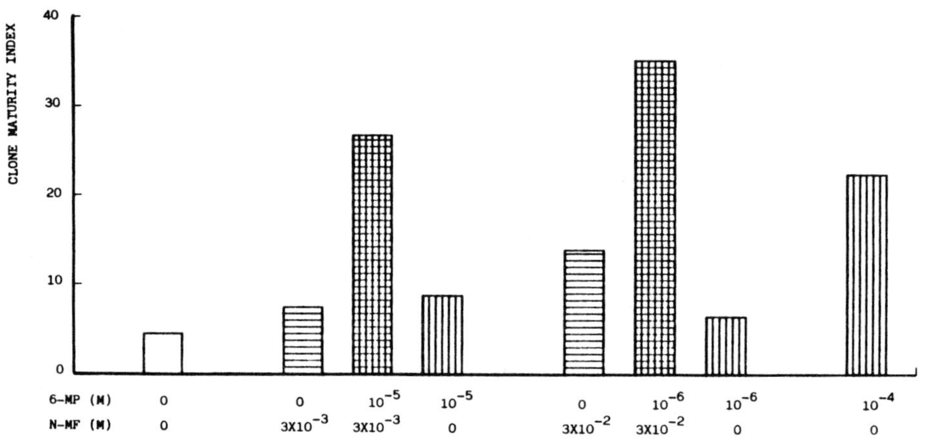

Fig. 3. Clone maturity indices (see text for definition) at day 7 based on differential counts of 90–120 consecutive clones in dual esterase-stained agar gels; marrow from an MDS (CMML) patient. Keys as in Fig. 2

entiation (such as the presence of a differentiation-responsive window already mentioned).

In order to test the thesis that DNA synthesis inhibitors enhance differentiation by a fundamentally different mechanism from that of the differentiation-inducing agents we looked for synergistic interactions between DNA synthesis inhibitors (cytosine arabinoside, 6-mercaptopurine and aphidicolin) and differentiation inducers (retinoic acid and *N*-methylformamide). Figure 2 shows the proportions of NBT reducing cells in day 4–day 6 suspension cultures. In each case there is evidence for synergistic interaction between the DNA synthesis inhibitors and the differentiation inducers. When two DNA synthesis inhibitors were added (6-mercaptopurine and aphidicolin) the effects were not synergistic, but merely additive. Similar results were obtained from dual esterase staining or proliferative capacity (assessed in secondary clonal assays) used to monitor cellular maturity in suspension cultures.

II. Synergistic Differentiation-Inducing Effects on Myelodysplastic and Leukaemic Cells

Figure 3 shows clone maturity indices in semisolid agar cultures at day 7 for a myelodysplastic marrow. In the absence of any differentiation-inducing agent the clone maturity index (defined as the percentage of clones containing mature neutrophils plus the percentage of clones containing mature macrophages divided by the percentage of clones containing blasts) at day 7 of culture was equivalent to that seen at day 4 or 5 for normal marrow cells. There was a highly synergistic interaction between *N*-methylformamide and 6-mercaptopurine such that the clone maturity index was restored to within the normal range for day 7. Figure 4 shows synergistic interactions assessed in suspension cultures by monitoring the percentage of NBT-reducing or the percentage of mature NSE- and CAE-positive cells. The myelotoxic effects assessed by inhibition of colony and cluster formation in day 7 marrow cultures

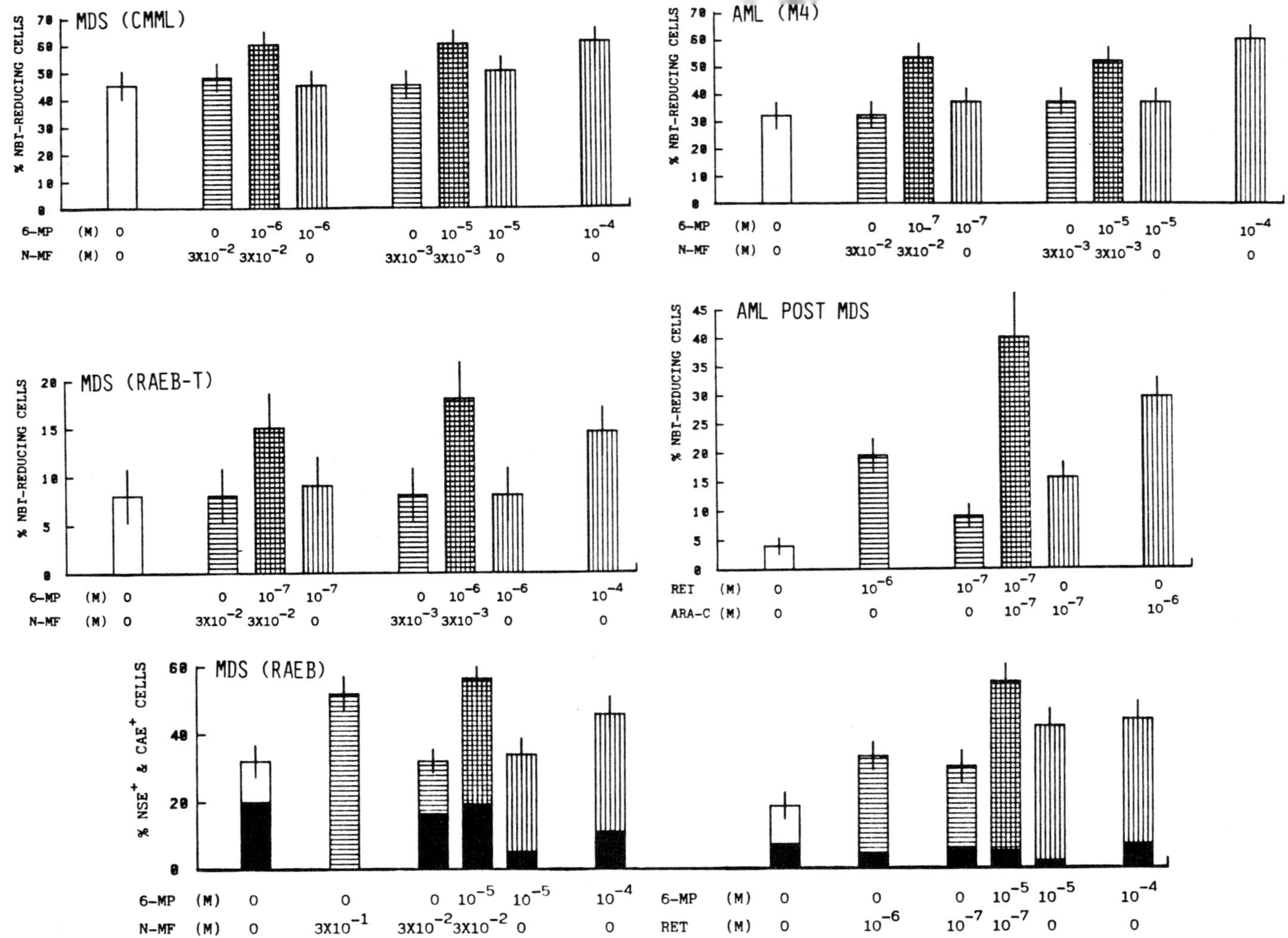

Fig. 4. Synergistic interactions were observed with cells from 3 patients with MDS (FAB classes CMML, RAEB-T, RAEB) and 2 patients with AML (FAB-M4 and post-MDS) in day 4–6 suspension cultures. Cell maturity was assessed by either NBT-reduction or by dual esterase staining for neutrophils (chloroacetate esterase$^+$; CAE$^+$) and macrophages (nonspecific esterase$^+$; NSE$^+$, the filled portion of each column)

did not show evidence of a synergistic interaction (data not shown).

D. Discussion

The results show that DNA synthesis inhibitors enhance differentiation by mechanisms which are distinct from those of the differentiation-inducing agents retinoic acid and N-methylformamide since these two groups of agents show synergistic interactions in differentiation induction. Although maturation appears arrested in acute myeloid leukaemia and differentiation-defective myeloid cell lines are plentiful, cells freshly explanted from patients retain many of the features of the normal proliferation–differentiation balance. The differentiation dose–response curves for these cells do not provide evidence for a maturation block (i.e. a maturational stage through which the cell cannot pass or can only pass with the aid of pharmacological differentiation inducers), but suggest instead that there is a shift in the probability of undergoing one or more differentiation transitions [2]. This implies that the cell is accessible (albeit with reduced sensitivity) to agents which enhance the differentiation of normal cells.

The differentiation-enhancing effect of DNA synthesis inhibitors seems unlikely to be due to any conventional differentiation-inducing activity, since agents inhibiting DNA synthesis by a wide variety of different mechanisms have this effect (e.g. not only the agents tested in this study but also hydroxyurea and 6-thioguanine). The results are, however, consistent with the accumulating evidence for the existence of a differentiation-responsive window in the cell cycle since DNA synthesis inhibitors might enhance differentiation by prolonging this window. The effect might simply be temporal or due to build-up of some receptor or enzyme important in the differentiation process during this period. Whatever the mechanism of interaction the highly synergistic effect observed for myelodysplastic and AML cells suggests that improved differentiation-inducing therapeutic protocols may be devised on this basis.

Acknowledgments. G.E.F. is a Wellcome Senior Research Fellow in Clinical Science. This study was also funded in part by the Cancer Research Campaign. M.A.W. is supported by the Leukaemia Research Fund. We wish to thank Mrs. Megan Evans for typing this manuscript.

References

1. Francis GE, Leaning MF (1984) Exp Haematol 13:92–98
2. Guimaraes JE et al. (1985) Leuk Res (in press)
3. Bennet JM et al. (1982) Br J Haematol 51:189–199
4. Francis GE, Hoffbrand AV In: Hoffbrand AV (ed) Recent advances in haematology. Churchill Livingstone, Edinburgh 1985 (in press)
5. Koeffler HP, Golde DW (1978) Blood 52: 355–361
6. Elstner E et al. (1983) In: Neth R, Gallo RC, Graves MF, Moore MAS, Winkler K (eds) Modern trends in human leukemia 5. New results in clinical and biological research including pediatric oncology. Springer, Berlin Heidelberg New York Tokyo (Haematology and blood transfusion vol 28)
7. Francis GE et al. (1982) Exp Haematol 10 [Suppl 11]: 179–193
8. Editorial (1984) Lancet i: 943–944
9. Gold EJ et al. (1983) Cancer Treat Rep 67:981–986
10. Besa EC et al. (1983) Blood 62 [Suppl 1]: 199a
11. Flynn PJ et al. (1983) Blood 62:1211–1217
12. Moore MAS et al. (1983) In: Neth R, Gallo RC, Greaves MF, Moore MAS, Winkler (eds) Modern trends in human leukemia 5. New results in clinical and biological research including pediatric oncology. Springer, Berlin Heidelberg New York Tokyo (Haematology and blood transfusion vol 28)
13. Novogrodsky A et al. (1983) Cancer 52:9–14
14. Boyd AV, Sullivan JF (1984) Blood 63:384–392
15. Griffin J et al. (1982) Exp Hematol 10:774–781
16. Tricot G et al. (1984) Br J Haematol 58: 231–240
17. Solal-Celigny et al. (1984) Blood 63:634–638
18. Housset M et al. (1982) Br J Haematol 51: 125–129
19. Boyd AW, Metcalf D (1984) Leuk Res 8:27–43
20. Tanaka M et al. (1975) Proc Natl Acad Sci USA 72:1003–1006
21. Yen A, Chiao JW (1983) Exp Cell Res 147: 87–93
22. Mufti GJ et al. (1983) N Engl J Med 309: 1653–1654
23. Pike BL, Robinson WA (1970) J Cell Physiol 76:77–84

Haematology and Blood Transfusion Vol. 29
Modern Trends in Human Leukemia VI
Edited by Neth, Gallo, Greaves, Janka

Vitamin D: Myeloid Differentiation and Proliferation

H. P. Koeffler, M. D.[1]

A. Background

The active metabolite of vitamin D ($1,25(OH)_2D_3$) is a major physiologic regulator of mineral metabolism in humans. The $1,25(OH)_2D_3$ facilitates calcium absorption from the intestine, acts to mobilize calcium from bone, and possibly stimulates renal reabsorption of calcium. In contrast to the current progress achieved in elucidating the role of $1,25(OH)_2D_3$ in mineral metabolism, the mechanism of action and biologic significance of vitamin D metabolites in the hematopoietic system are just beginning to be studied.

Early reports suggested that vitamin D-deficient rickets patients frequently had anemia, extramedullary hematopoiesis, and mononuclear phagocytes that poorly performed chemotaxis and phagocytosis. A murine myeloblastic leukemia cell line (M-1) was discovered to undergo macrophage-like differentiation in the presence of $1,25(OH)_2D_3 > 24,25(OH)_2D_3 > 25(OH)_2D_3$ [1]. Development of leukemia was inhibited or the survival time of mice prolonged after M-1 cells were injected into syngeneic mice and the mice were treated with $1,25(OH)_2D_3$.

B. Vitamin D and Differentiation of HL-60 Cells

Preliminary evidence by Miyaura et al. [9] suggested that the cells from the human promyelocytic leukemia line known as HL-60 differentiated to granulocytes when cultured with $1,25(OH)_2D_3$. Further studies by others as well as ourselves showed that the HL-60 became predominantly macrophage-like after culture with $1,25(OH)_2D_3$ [2, 7, 8]. Likewise, we have studied a variant of HL-60 (HL-60 blast) that is unable to undergo differentiation [7]. As shown in Table 1, after 7 days of treatment with as little as 10^{-10} *M* $1,25(OH)_2D_3$, significant differentiation occurred as measured by four test parameters of macrophage differentiation. In contrast, the HL-60 blast cells were unresponsive at each concentration of $1,25(OH)_2D_3$.

Morphological and functional changes began to be minimally expressed after 7 days with a $1,25(OH)_2D_3$ incubation as short as 18 h [7]. The differentiation response became more pronounced the longer the hormone remained in the culture medium, suggesting that the presence of $1,25(OH)_2D_3$ is required and must be maintained over a long period of time relative to transient events occurring at the molecular level.

The mechanism by which $1,25(OH)_2D_3$ induces differentiation is unknown. Preliminary evidence by Tanaka et al. [12] implicated the presence of cytosolic $1,25(OH)_2D_3$ receptors in HL-60 and suggested that differentiation may be occurring by a mechanism similar to that of

1 UCLA School of Medicine, Department of Medicine, Division of Hematology-Oncology, 11-240 Louis Factor Building, Los Angeles, California 90024, USA

Table 1. Functional and morphologic changes in HL-60 and HL-60 blast cells by various concentrations of $1.25(OH)_2D_3$[a]

Added concentration of $1,25(OH)_2D_3$[b] (M)	Cell line	NBT reduction (%)	Phagocytic cells (%)	Morphology: Myeloblasts and promyeloblasts (%)	Intermediate to mature[c] (%)	Nonspecific acid esterase-positive[d] (%)
0	HL-60	2± 3	2±2	99±2	1±2	2
	HL-60 blast	0	1	100	0	0
10^{-11}	HL-60	10± 2	2±3	95±3	5±4	3
	HL-60 blast	0	0	100	0	0
10^{-10}	HL-60	18±11	13±7	82±5	18±7	10
	HL-60 blast	0	0	100	0	0
10^{-9}	HL-60	37±19	20±7	66±9	34±6	25
	HL-60 blast	0	0	100	0	0
10^{-8}	HL-60	64±13	26±4	45±12	55±9	54
	HL-60 blast	0	0	100	0	0
10^{-7}	HL-60	82± 8	44±9	32±5	67±6	82
	HL-60 blast	3	5	96	4	0
10^{-6}	HL-60	86±12	60±3	27±6	78±14	98
	HL-60 blast	1	0	100	0	0

[a] HL-60 and HL-60 blast cells were cultured in the presence or absence of various concentrations of $1.25(OH)_2D_3$. After 7 days cells were assessed for the various differentiation parameters. Cell viability was >99%. All data are expressed as the percentage of total cells assayed. At least 200 cells were assessed for each parameter. The HL-60 cell data represent the mean±standard deviation of triplicate assays

[b] Basal $1,25(OH)_2D_3$ in 10% fetal bovine serum is 1.6×10^{-11} M

[c] Intermediate to mature cells include monocytes and macrophages

[d] Represents the average of two experiments

classical steroid hormone action. We reported the unqualified identification of the $1,25(OH)_2D_3$ receptor in HL-60 cells and the existence of a positive correlation between $1,25(OH)_2D_3$-induced differentiation and the occurrence of occupied $1,25(OH)_2D_3$ receptors [7].

Aliquots of high salt nuclear extracts, prepared by first labeling intact HL-60 and HL-60 blast cells with ^3H $1,25(OH)_2D_3$, were analyzed by high salt sucrose density gradient centrifugation. As illustrated in Fig. 1a, virtually all of the bound ^3H $1,25(OH)_2D_3$ migrated in a single 3.3 S peak, characteristic of $1,25(OH)_2D_3$ receptors. This peak was completely obliterated by the mercurial reagent, PCMBS (Fig. 1a), indicating dissociation of the $1,25(OH)_2D_3$ hormone–receptor complex. Finally, to confirm the 3.3 S macromolecule as the $1,25(OH)_2D_3$ receptor, monoclonal antibodies to the $1,25(OH)_2D_3$ receptor were incubated with the nuclear extract before sedimentation. The monoclonal antibody 4A5λ shifted the migration of the 3.3 S macromolecule to the 7–8 S position (Fig. 1a), a finding consistent with the sedimentation properties of the hormone–receptor–antibody complex. In contrast, the 8D3 monoclonal antibody is specific for chick intestinal receptor and therefore had no effect on the sedimentation of this 3.3 S macromolecule (Fig. 1a). Figure 1b shows a similar sedimentation pattern for the nuclear extract derived from HL-60 blast. A PCMBS-dissociable 3.3 S macromolecule that was recognized by 4A5λ (but not 8D3) antibody demonstrated the presence of a small, yet detectable, amount of $1,25(OH)_2D_3$ receptor in HL-60 blast cells.

We measured the specific uptake of ^{3}H $1{,}25(OH)_2D_3$ into intact HL-60 under conditions that are normally used to grow these cells in culture. Figure 2a demonstrates that ^{3}H $1{,}25(OH)_2D_3$ uptake by intact HL-60 cells was a specific and saturable process. Accordingly, Scatchard transformation of these data yielded an equilibrium dissociation constant for $1{,}25(OH)_2D_3$ internalization (K_{int}) of 5.4 n*M* (Fig. 2b) and extrapolation to the abscissa predicts 4000 $1{,}25(OH)_2D_3$ receptor molecules per HL-60 cell. The K_{int} (5.4 n*M*) is nearly identical to the concentration that induces 50% of HL-60 cells to differentiate. This correspondence, plus the resistance of the relatively receptor-poor HL-60 blast, strongly suggests that $1{,}25(OH)_2D_3$-induced differentiation of HL-60 cells to monocytes/macrophages is occurring via receptor-mediated events.

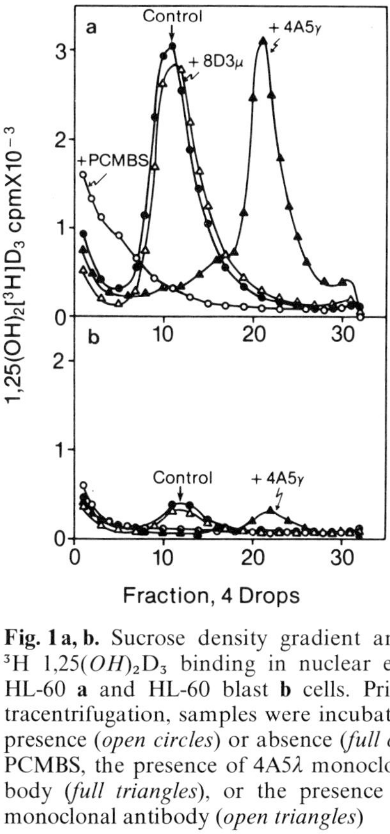

Fig. 1 a, b. Sucrose density gradient analysis of ^{3}H $1{,}25(OH)_2D_3$ binding in nuclear extract of HL-60 **a** and HL-60 blast **b** cells. Prior to ultracentrifugation, samples were incubated in the presence (*open circles*) or absence (*full circles*) of PCMBS, the presence of 4A5λ monoclonal antibody (*full triangles*), or the presence of 8D3μ monoclonal antibody (*open triangles*)

C. Effect of $1{,}25(OH)_2D_3$ and its Fluorinated Analogs on Myeloid Differentiation

I. Normal Myeloid Stem Cells

We examined the effect of $1{,}25(OH)_2D_3$ and two fluorinated analogs of $1{,}25(OH)_2D_3$ on differentiation of the normal human myeloid stem cell (GM-CFC) [6]. We studied the two fluorinated analogs of $1{,}25(OH)_2D_3$, known as 24,24-F_2-$1{,}25(OH)_2D_3$ and 26,26,26,27,27,27,-$1{,}25(OH)_2D_3$ (26,27-F_6-$1{,}25(OH)_2D_3$), because both compounds are as active or more active than $1{,}25(OH)_2D_3$ in calcium reabsorption and probably have a longer in vivo half-life than $1{,}25(OH)_2D_3$.

We found that the $1{,}25(OH)_2D_3$ and its fluorinated analogs markedly induced human myeloid GM-CFC to differentiate to colonies containing only macrophages. In the absence of $1{,}25(OH)_2D_3$, normal human bone marrow GM-CFC differentiated to approximately 55% neutrophil, 10% mix,

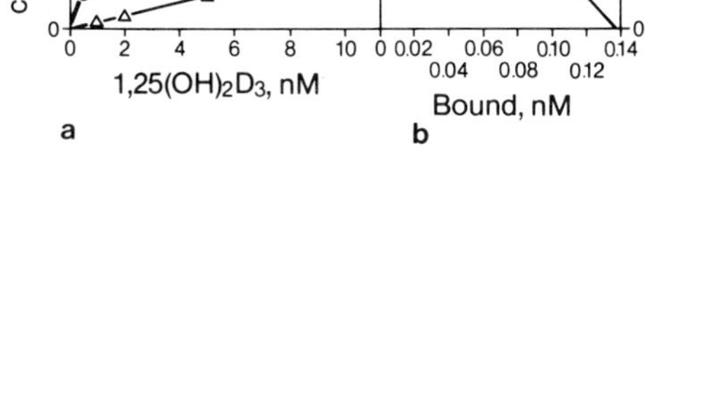

Fig. 2 a, b. Determination of the euqilibrium dissociation constant of $1{,}25(OH)_2D_3$ internalization of intact HL-60 cells. Saturation analysis **a** was determined by incubating intact cells under normal growth conditions for 4 h with 10% serum along with various concentrations of tritiated $1{,}25(OH)_2D_3$ in the presence of or absence of 100-fold excess nonradioactive $1{,}25(OH)_2D_3$. Specific binding was transformed by Scatchard analysis and the data line-fitted by linear regression, **b** to yield $K_{int} = 5.4$ n*M* (abscissa intercept = 4000 molecules per cell, $r = -0.71$)

and 25% macrophage colonies. Nearly 95% of the colonies were composed of only macrophages in culture plates containing 10^{-7}–10^{-8} M 1,25(OH)$_2$D$_3$. Some 55% of the colonies were composed of only monocytes/macrophages in plates containing 10^{-9} M 1,25(OH)$_2$D$_3$. Similar results were observed with the fluorinated analogs.

The 1,25(OH)$_2$D$_3$ and fluorinated analogs (10^{-7}–10^{-9} M) increased the absolute number of macrophage colonies, rather than merely increasing the relative proportion of macrophage colonies, by selectively inhibiting granulocytic differentiation of GM-CFC. Plates containing either 10^{-7} or 10^{-8} M 1,25(OH)$_2$D$_3$ developed approximately 75 and 90 macrophage colonies, respectively per 10^5 cultured marrow cells. Likewise, plates with 10^{-9} M 1,25(OH)$_2$D$_3$ developed about 65 macrophage colonies per 10^5 cultured marrow cells. In contrast, 35 macrophage colonies per 10^5 cultured marrow cells developed in control plates containing no 1,25(OH)$_2$D$_3$. Similar results were observed with the fluorinated analogs.

The hypothesis that 1,25(OH)$_2$D$_3$ may be a possible inducer of differentiation of GM-CFC to macrophages is appealing because of the known ability of 1,25(OH)$_2$D$_3$ to modulate bone resorption. Osteoclasts resorb bone. Evidence suggests that osteoclasts may develop from monocyte/macrophage cells [4] and one study suggested that 1,25(OH)$_2$D$_3$ may modulate the number of osteoclasts [5]. Therefore, 1,25(OH)$_2$D$_3$ might modulate bone resorption by inducing GM-CFC to differentiate to monocytes and macrophages and eventually to osteoclasts. Likewise, in vitro, the monocytes can directly resorb bone [10].

Caution must be exercised in the overinterpretation of the data. The plasma concentration of 1,25(OH)$_2$D$_3$ in humans is approximately 7.7×10^{-11} M [3]. Our studies showed that only concentrations $\geqq 10^{-9}$ M 1,25(OH)$_2$D$_3$ induced significant macrophage differentiation of myeloid progenitor cells in vitro. Therefore, 1,25(OH)$_2$D$_3$ may not have a physiologic role in the induction of differentiation of human myeloid stem cells to macrophages. Likewise, patients who received superphysiologic doses of 1,25(OH)$_2$D$_3$ have not been reported to have an increased concentration of blood monocytes [11]. The true hematopoietic role of vitamin D metabolites in vivo is unknown and will require careful experimentation.

II. Leukemic Myeloid Stem Cells

Interest has developed in attempting to induce differentiation of myeloid leukemic blast cells to functional cells that are no longer capable of proliferation (Kœffler HP, 1983). It can be shown that 1,25(OH)$_2$D$_3$, 24,24-F_2-1,25(OH)$_2$D$_3$, and 26,27-F_6-1,25(OH)$_2$D$_3$ induce macrophage differentiation of leukemic myeloid colony-forming cells (Table 2). The potency of induction of differentiation of leukemic cells by 1,25(OH)$_2$D$_3$ and the fluorinated analogs was almost equivalent – concentrations of 10^{-8} M induced about 90% of CML and 50% of AML myeloid leukemic colony-forming cells to differentiate to colonies containing macrophage-like cells. These concentrations of the agents can be achieved in patients. The CML and AML control dishes containing no 1,25(OH)$_2$D$_3$, developed only 30% and 15% macrophage colonies, respectively. The study suggests that the myeloid stem cell can be induced to undergo terminal macrophage differentiation and be removed from the proliferative pool.

D. Effect of 1,25(OH)$_2$ D$_3$ on Maturation of Human Leukemic Cells in Liquid Culture

We also examined the effect that 1,25(OH)$_2$D$_3$ would have on proliferation and differentiation in liquid culture of freshly isolated myeloid leukemic blast cells from nine patients (Fig. 3). Blast cells of two patients (1, 2) were at the early myeloblast M1 (French–American–British classification) stage of development; blast cells of three patients (3, 4, 5) were at the myeloblast (M2) stage of differentiation; blasts from two patients (6, 7) were at the myelomonoblast stage (M4); cells from patient 8 were CML myeloid blasts and cells from patient 9 were CML lymphoid blasts.

Table 2. Effects of 1,25(OH)$_2$D$_3$ and fluorinated analogs of 1,25(OH)$_2$D$_3$ on differentiation and proliferation of leukemic human myeloid colony-forming cells

Cell source	Vitamin D analog	Concentration (H)	No. of colonies (% of control)[a]	Colony morphology[b] (%) N	NM	M	B
Chronic myelogenous leukemia (4 patients)	1,25(OH)$_2$D$_3$	0	100	62±6	7±1	31±2	
		10^{-10}	98±5	66±5	4±1	30±4	0
		10^{-9}	110±6	42±2	6±1	52±5	0
		10^{-8}	101±6	5±1	3±1	92±1	0
		10^{-7}	76±7	0	0	100±1	0
Acute nonlymphocytic leukemia (4 patients)	1,25(OH)$_2$D$_3$	0	100	12±2	0	18±3	70±5
		10^{-10}	103±8	7±3	4±1	17±4	72±6
		10^{-9}	112±8	7±1	3±1	28±3	53±5
		10^{-8}	89±6	6±1	3±1	53±4	38±6
		10^{-7}	80±6	1±1	4±3	60±5	36±6
Chronic myelogenous leukemia	24,25-F_2-1,25-(OH)$_2$D$_3$	0	100	62±6	7±1	31±2	0
		10^{-10}	106±9	55±6	2±1	43±4	0
		10^{-9}	109±7	38±3	5±2	51±4	0
		10^{-8}	83±5	0	4±1	96±2	0
Acute nonlymphocytic leukemia	24,24-F_2-1,25(OH)$_2$D$_3$	0	100	12±2	0	18±3	70±5
		10^{-10}	104±8	5±2	2±1	8±1	84±4
		10^{-9}	116±6	3±1	4±1	26±3	67±3
		10^{-8}	85±7	1±1	7±1	56±4	36±3

[a] Marrow cells were obtained from 4 acute nonlymphocytic leukemia (AML) patients, and peripheral blood cells were obtained from 4 chronic myelogenous leukemia (CML) patients. The low density, nonadherent, mononuclear cells were cultured in the presence of 2.5% T lymphocyte CM (source of CSF) and various concentrations of 1,25(OH)$_2$D$_3$ and fluorinated analogs of 1,25(OH)$_2$D$_3$. The CMLV and AML cultures contained a mean of 121±7, and 31±8 (±standard error) myeloid colonies, respectively

[b] N neutrophilic colonies; NM neutrophil/macrophage mixed colonies; M monocyte/macrophage colonies; B blast cell colonies

Net cellular proliferation was examined after the blast cells (5×10^5/ml) from each of the leukemic patients were exposed for 6 days to 1,25(OH)$_2$D$_3$ or culture media alone (control). The median (range) of day 6 cell counts ($\times 10^5$/ml) in flasks containing 10^{-7} M 1,25(OH)$_2$D$_3$, 10^{-6} M 1,25(OH)$_2$D$_3$, and culture medium alone (control) was 5 (2–9), 4 (2–8), and 7 (5–9), respectively. The 1,25(OH)$_2$D$_3$ had an inhibitory effect on cellular proliferation with the higher concentration of 1,25(OH)$_2$D$_3$ (10^{-6} M) producing a significant inhibition of growth as compared with control flasks ($P < 0.05$) (Fig. 3).

The 1,25(OH)$_2$D$_3$ induced maturation of leukemia cell maturation to monocytes, macrophages, metamyelocytes, and granulocytes. At day 6, the median percentage of mature myeloid cells in flasks containing 10^{-7} M and 10^{-6} M 1,25(OH)$_2$D$_3$ or culture medium alone was 36%, 40%, and 5%, respectively. The percentage of mature myeloid cells at day 6 of culture was significantly ($P < 0.05$) higher for the flasks containing 10^{-6} M 1,25(OH)$_2$D$_3$ as compared with day 6 control flasks. Macrophages and granulocytes are able to reduce NBT, but their immature progenitors can not. We examined the ability of the leukemic cells from the nine patients to reduce NBT after culture with 1,25(OH)$_2$D$_3$ for 6 days (Fig. 3). The median percentage of NBT-reducing cells in control, 10^{-7} M, and 10^{-6} M 1,25(OH)$_2$D$_3$-containing flasks was 10%, 33%, and 49%, respectively. The number of NBT-reducing cells was significantly ($P < 0.05$) greater in the flasks containing

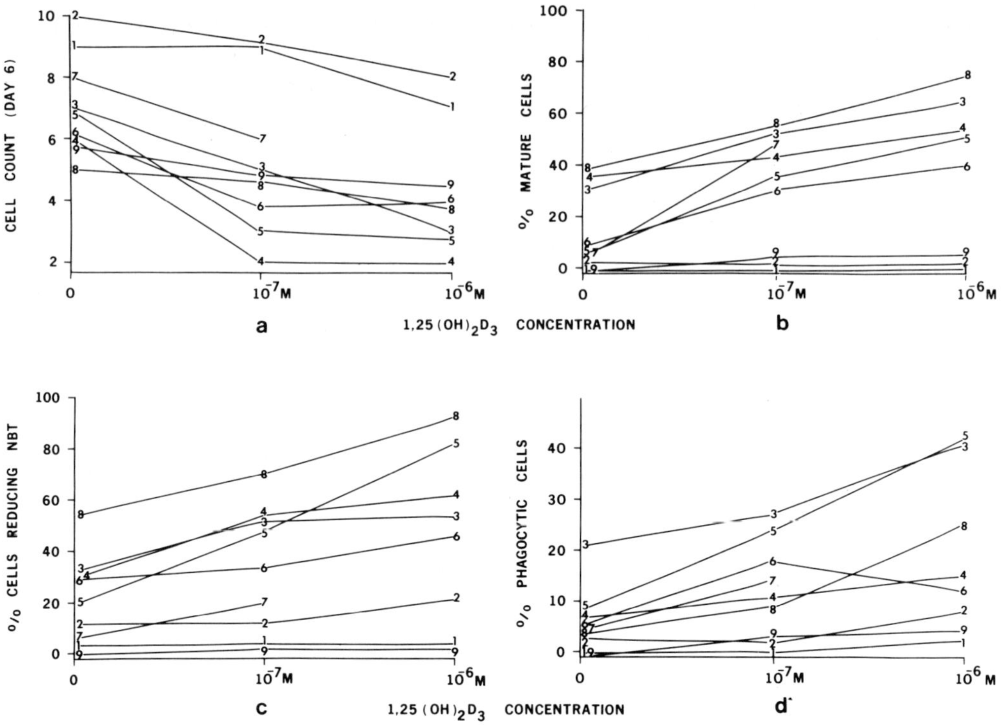

Fig. 3a–d. In vitro study of 1,25$(OH)_2D_3$ on myeloid blast cells from leukemic patients **a** effect of 1,25$(OH)_2D_3$ on proliferation of leukemic blast cells, **b** effect of 1,25$(OH)_2D_3$ on morphological maturation of leukemic blast cells; **c** effect of 1,25$(OH)_2D_3$ on NBT reduction by leukemic blast cells; **d** effect of 1,25$(OH)_2D_3$ on *Candida* phagocytosis by leukemic blast cells. Cells were cultured in media containing 0, 10^{-7}, or 10^{-6} *M* 1,25$(OH)_2D_3$, harvested on day 6, and viable cell counts, morphology, and function of the cells were determined

10^{-6} *M* 1,25$(OH)_2D_3$ as compared with control flasks.

We examined the ability of the blast cells from the leukemic patients to phagocytose *Candida* after culture with 1,25$(OH)_2D_3$ for 6 days (Fig. 3). Median percentage of blasts cells which phagocytosed *Candida* in control, 10^{-7} *M*, and 10^{-6} *M* 1,25$(OH)_2D_3$-containing flasks were 5%, 11%, and 14%, respectively. The percentage of phagocytic cells was significantly ($P < 0.05$) increased in the flasks containing 10^{-6} *M* 1,25$(OH)_2D_3$ as compared with control flasks. This study suggests that high concentrations of 1,25$(OH)_2D_3$ can induce terminal differentiation of leukemic cells in liquid culture.

E. 1,25$(OH)_2$ D_3: In Vivo Myelodysplastic Study

A group of 18 myelodysplastic patients were treated with 1,25$(OH)_2D_3$ (Table 3). All patients received weekly escalating (0.5 μg) doses of 1,25$(OH)_2D_3$ until a daily dose of 2 μg was reached. The median duration of therapy with 1,25$(OH)_2D_3$ was 12 weeks (range 4 to > 20 weeks). Tables 3, 4 and Fig. 4 show the results of treatment. During the study, the peak granulocyte, macrophage, and platelet blood concentrations increased in most patients as compared with their starting values. As a group, the peak granulocyte, macrophage, and platelet values during the study increased significantly as compared with initial and final peripheral blood cell levels (Table 3). In contrast, by the end of the trial, the pe-

Table 3. Preleukemic patients: clinical characteristics and $1,25(OH)_2$ vitamin D_3 therapeutic response

Patient	Age/sex	Time from diagnosis to treatment (months)	Duration of treatment (weeks)	Response (weeks)	Diagnosis before treatment[a]	End of treatment
1	70/F	4	13	Prog	RAEB-TR	AML (M2)
2	34/F	3	14	PR; Prog	RAEB	AML (M4)
3	51/M	30	12	Prog	RAEB	AML (M2)
4	60/M	11	12	MR; Prog	RAEB-TR	AML (M2)
5	59/M	20	12	Prog	RAEB-TR	AML (M2)
6	65/F	27	12	MR	PASA	PASA
7	36/F	10	12	MR	RAEB	RAEB
8	59/M	23	8	MR; Prog	PASA	PASA
9	66/F	6	15	MR	RAEB	RAEB
10	52/M	7	12	S	PASA	PASA
11	71/M	35	8	Prog	PASA	RAEB
12	78/F	3	12	S	RAEB	RAEB
13	74/M	18	12	S	CMML	CMML
14	79/M	5	6	MR	RAEB	RAEB
15	71/M	7	10	Prog	RAEB	AML (M1)
16	65/M	5	4	Prog	RAEB	AML (M1)
17	80/M	6	7	Prog	RAEB	Death
18	61/M	12	>20	MR	PASA	PASA

[a] RAEB refractory anemia with excess blasts; RAEB-TR RAEB in transformation; PASA primary acquired sideroblastic anemia; CMML chronic myelomonocytic leukemia; AML acute myelogenous leukemia with M subclassification according to FAB classification. Prog progression; PR partial response; MR minor response; S stable

Table 4. Treatment of myelodysplastic patients with $1,25(OH)_2D_3$[a]

	Median	Range	P[c]
Granulocytes (per microliter blood)			
Start[b]	2 300	180–11 520	
Peak	3 750	486–29 820	0.0007
End	3 110	96–24 480	0.0347
Macrophages (per microliter blood)			
Start	50	3– 8 435	
Peak	300	43–16 898	0.0022
End	80	3–10 200	0.1578
Platelets ($\times 10^3$ per microliter blood)			
Start	58	12–300	
Peak	105	23–610	0.0003
End	65	4–358	0.9622
Marrow blasts (%)			
Start	10	3–20	
End	15	4–70	0.0068
Serum calcium (mg/dl)			
Start	8.9	8.2–10.4	
Peak	10.8	9.7–17.0	0.0002
End	10.3	9.6–12.4	0.0002

[a] Results represent data from 18 preleukemic patients

[b] Start, initial value before therapy; peak, highest value during therapy; end, value on last day of therapy

[c] Wilcoxon signed rank test. Values are compared with baseline (starting) values and $p \leqq 0.05$ is significant

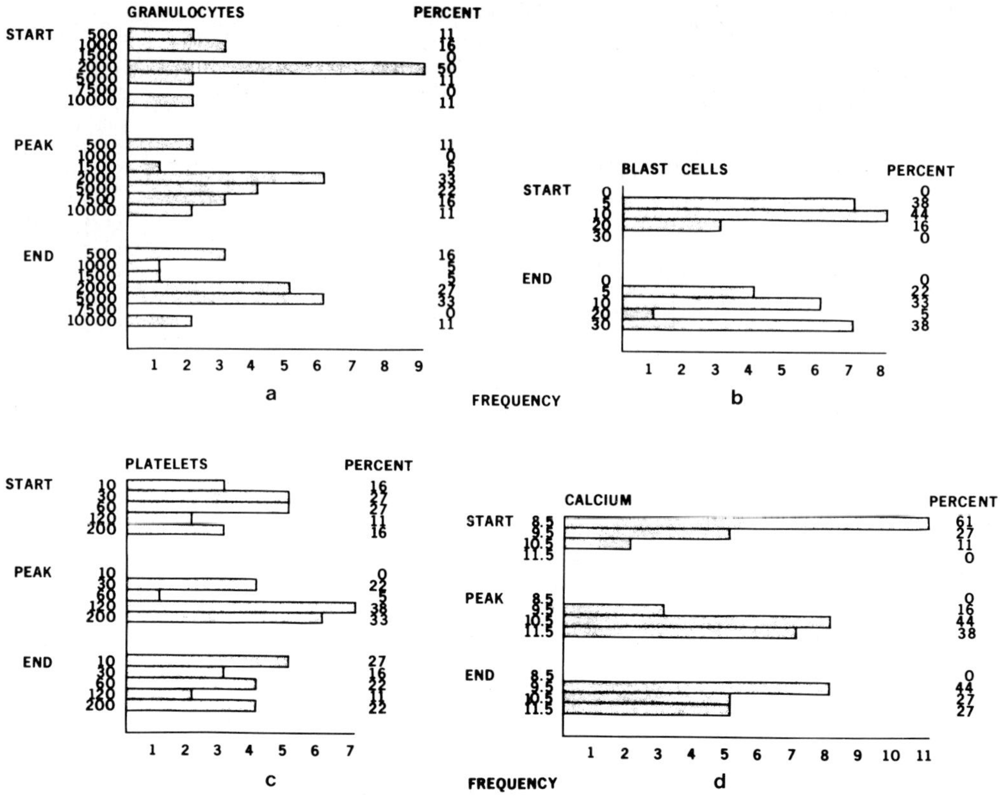

Fig. 4a–d. In vivo study of 1,25$(OH)_2D_3$ in preleukemic patients **a** effect of 1,25$(OH)_2D_3$ on peripheral blood granulocyte counts; **b** effect of 1,25$(OH)_2D_3$ on peripheral blood platelet counts; **c** effect of 1,25$(OH)_2D_3$ on percentage of bone marrow myeloblasts; **d** effect of 1,25$(OH)_2D_3$ on serum calcium concentration (mg/dl). Start, baseline value; peak, highest value during study; end, value on last day of study

ripheral blood cell values were not significantly different than at the initiation of the trial. Likewise, the percentage of marrow blasts rose from a median value of 10% (range 3%–20%) at the initiation of the study to a median value of 15% (4%–70%) by the completion of the study.

Patient 2 had a 50% improvement in absolute blood granulocyte, monocyte, and platelet counts for greater than 5 weeks of treatment (partial response, Table 3). This patient, however, developed AML on week 11 of receiving 1,25$(OH)_2D_3$. Seven patients (4, 6, 7–9, 14, 18) had an improvement of either their absolute granulocyte, monocyte, or platelet peripheral blood counts for greater than 4 weeks of treatment (minor response). However, two of these patients (4, 8), developed AML while receiving 1,25$(OH)_2D_3$. Three patients (10, 12, 13) had no change in granulocyte, monocyte, or platelet peripheral blood counts. By the conclusion of the therapeutic trial, seven patients progressed to AML with greater than 10% blast cells in the peripheral blood and greater than 30% blast cells in the bone marrow (Table 3). The serum calcium increased in each of the patients while receiving 1,25$(OH)_2D_3$. The serum calcium was a median 8.9 mg/dl (range 8.2–10.4) prior to therapy; a peak median 10.8 mg/dl (range 9.7–17) during therapy; and a median 10.3 mg/dl (range 9.6–12.4) at the end of study (Table 4, Fig. 4). Nine patients had serum calcium levels above 11 mg/dl, and six of these patients had symptoms of hepercalcemia.

We attempted to improve the peripheral blood cytopenia and bone marrow ineffective hematopoiesis in patients with myelodysplastic syndromes by having the patients ingest pharmacologic doses of $1{,}25(OH)_2D_3$. The in vivo administration of $1{,}25(OH)_2D_3$ produced only a very temporary improvement in hematopoietic parameters in a minority of the patients. Patients received 2 μg/day $1{,}25(OH)_2D_3$ which would be expected to produce serum levels of about $2 \times 10^{-10}\ M$ $1{,}25(OH)_2D_3$. This dosage of drug induced hypercalcemia in 6 of 18 patients. However, this concentration of $1{,}25(OH)_2D_3$ induced only about 20% of HL-60 cells to mature in vitro and $10^{-9}\ M$ $1{,}25(OH)_2D_3$ had only a small effect on maturation in vitro of fresh leukemic blast cells. Severalfold higher concentrations of $1{,}25(OH)_2D_3$ can not be given to patients because the drug will precipitate life-threatening hypercalcemia. The future development of vitamin D analogs that induce heamtopoietic cell differentiation without hypercalcemia might be medically useful for selected preleukemic and leukemic patients. The induction of differentiation of myeloid leukemic cells to functional end cells offers an appealing therapeutic prospect. However, the future role of biologic modifiers in the treatment of hematopoietic malignancies remains undefined at this time.

Acknowledgments. I would like to thank Hillary Merriman and Regina Simon for excellent secretarial assistance and to acknowledge the excellent collaborative studies with Dr. D. Mangelsdorf, Dr. M. Haussler, Dr. H. DeLuca, Dr. L. Itri, and Dr. A. Norman that made this report possible. This work was supported in part by National Institutes of Health grants CA 26038, CA 3273, CA 33936. The Bruce Fowler Memorial Fund, and the Jonsson Comprehensive Cancer Center. Dr. Koeffler is a scholar of the Leukemia Society of America, Incorporated, and has a Career Development Award from NIH.

References

1. Abe E, Muyayra C, Sakagami H, Takeda M, Konno K, Yamazaki T, Yoshikil S, Suda T (1981) Proc Natl Acad Sci USA 78:4990–4994
2. Abe E, Miyayra C, Tanaka H et al. (1983) Proc Natl Acad Sci 80:5583
3. Bishop JE, Norman AW, Coburn JW, Roberts PA, Henry HL (1980) Mineral J Electrolyte Metabol 3:181–189
4. Burger EH, Van der Meer JWM, Van de Gevel JS, Gribnau JC, Thesingh CW, Van Furth (1982) J Exp Med 156:1604–1614
5. Holtrop M, Cox K, Clark M, Holick M, Anast C (1981) Endocrinology 108:2293–2301
6. Koeffler HP, Amatruda T, DeLuca H (1984) (submitted)
7. Mangelsdorf D, Koeffler HP, Donaldson C, Pike J, Haussler M (1984) J Cell Biol 98: 391–398
8. McCarthy DM, San Miguel JF, Greake HC, Green PM, Zola H, Catovsky D, Goldman JM (1983) Leuk Res 7:51–55
9. Miyayra C, Abe E, Kuribayashi T et al. (1981) Biochem Biophys Res Commun 102: 937–943
10. Mundy D, Altman A, Gonder M, Bandelin J (1977) Science 196:1109–1111
11. Norman AW, Johnson RL, Okamura WH (1979) J Biol Chem 254:11 450–11 456
12. Tanaka H, Abe E, Miyayra C, Kuribayashi T, Konno K, Nishii Y, Suda T (1981) Biochem J 204:713–719

Haematology and Blood Transfusion Vol. 29
Modern Trends in Human Leukemia VI
Edited by Neth, Gallo, Greaves, Janka

Biological Activities of a Human Pluripotent Hemopoietic Colony-Stimulating Factor *

E. Platzer [1], K. Welte [2], L. Lu [2], J. L. Gabrilove [2], Y.-P. Yung [2], C. F. Nathan [3], R. Mertelsmann [2], and M. A. S. Moore [2]

A. Introduction

As described elsewhere in this volume by Welte et al., a human pluripotent hemopoietic colony-stimulating factor (CSF) was purified to apparent homogeneity from media conditioned by the human bladder carcinoma cell line, 5637. The purified material supports colony formation in vitro from human multipotential (CFU-GEMM), early erythroid (BFU-E), granulocyte and monocyte (CFU-G, M) progenitor cells [4]. A murine CSF, Interleukin 3 or multi-CSF, with similar activities on normal mouse bone marrow [1, 2], has recently been purified [3] and genetically cloned [4]. Interleukin 3 was originally detected by its ability to induce 20-alpha-OH-steroid dehydrogenase (20αSDH) in cultured spleen cells of *nu/nu* mice [5]. Later on it was discovered to have biological activities on a wide range of hemopoietic cells: progenitor cells of erythrocytes, megakaryocytes, granulocytes, monocytes and eosinophils, mast cells and their precursors, and possibly lymphocytes [2, 6–8]. Since come activities of Interleukin 3 and pluripotent CSF, or Pluripoietin, on hemopoietic progenitor cells appeared similar, we screened for additional biological effects of Pluripoietin.

Supported by NCI grant CA 32516, ACS grant CH3G, grant Pl 103/1-1 from the Deutsche Forschungsgemeinschaft, and the Gar Reichman Foundation

1 Institut f. klin. Immunologie, Krankenhausstr. 12, D-8520 Erlangen, FRG
Henry Kaplan Award for the best poster Cell-biological Session
2 Laboratory of Developmental Hematopoiesis, and Laboratory of Molecular Hematology, Memorial Sloan-Kettering Cancer Center
3 Laboratory of Cellular Physiology and Immunology, The Rockefeller University, New York, N.Y. 10021, USA
4 CFU-GEMM, colony-forming unit granulocytes, erythrocytes, macrophages, and megakaryocytes; BFU-E, burst-forming unit erythroid; CFU-G, M, colony-forming unit granulocytes and macrophages

B. Pluripoietin Supports In Vitro Development of Precursors of Colony-Forming Progenitor Cells

Normal human bone marrow cells taken from volunteers after informed consent were separated by density gradient centrifugation on Ficoll, adherence to plastic surfaces and depletion of cells rosetting at 4 °C with neuraminidase-treated sheep red blood cells. When this cell population was cultured in methylcellulose as described [9], Pluripoietin in the absence of phytohemagglutinin-stimulated lymphocyte-conditioned medium (PHA-LCM) supported colony formation from CFU-GEMM and BFU-E, suggesting that pluripotent CSF acts directly on early progenitor cells, not via macrophages or T-lymphocytes as accessory cells of hematopoiesis. In agar cultures [10], Pluripoietin induced mostly neutrophil colonies by day 7, and neutrophil, macrophage, and mixed neutrophil/macrophage colonies as well as some eosinophil clusters by day 14. Furthermore, Pluripoietin induced the development of immature precursors of colony-forming progenitor cells of granulocytes and macrophages [11]. This was studied by incubating low-density, nonadherent, and T-cell-depleted marrow cells in liquid culture in the presence of Pluripoietin for 7 days prior to agar culture, in a granulocyte-potentiating activity (ΔGPA)-type [12] or precursor of CFU-G, M progenitor cell (pre-CFU-c) [13] assay. There are no reports of Interleukin 3 tested in such assays, but it appears to have a similar effect on murine stem cells in vitro prior to transplantation [14].

C. Pluripoietin Acts on Mature Hemopoietic Cells

Normal human peripheral blood monocytes were isolated by adherence procedures as described [15]. When cultured in the presence of Pluripoietin from day 1 through 4, monocytes/macrophages showed marked spreading and an increase of adherent cell protein, suggesting increased protein synthesis as compared with untreated controls [11]. This effect was not seen when Pluripoietin was added at day 4 of culture or later, possibly because macrophages produce their own CSF. Pluripoietin did not increase the production of H_2O_2-producing enzymes or anti-*Toxoplasma* activity in macrophages when added after 3 days of culture [15]. Interleukin 3 was not reported to be active on macrophages, but its activity in supporting long-term growth in vitro of natural cytotoxic effector cells [16] and histamine-producing cells [6] may reflect activities on mature hemopoietic cells.

D. Pluripoietin Induces Differentiation in Leukemic Cell Lines

Differentiation of leukemic cell lines in vitro can be achieved by a variety of nonphysiologic [e.g., dimethylsulfoxide (DMSO), phorboldiesters] and physiologic (e.g., retinoic acid, vitamin D_3) inducers [17]. Murine granulocyte-CSF (G-CSF) is known to be a potent inducer of differentiation of WEHI-3B (D+) murine myelomonocytic leukemia cells, whereas Interleukin 3 lacks this activity (for review, see [1]). We tested Pluripoietin for leukemia-differentiating activity (GM-DF, leukemia-differentiating activity for granulocyte and macrophage pathway) in a clonal assay system described by Metcalf [18], using murine WEHI-3B (D+) and human HL-60 promyelocytic leukemia cell lines [11]. Quantitation of GM-DF was obtained by incubation of leukemic cells in agar with serial dilutions of pluripotent CSF. Pluripoietin had GM-DF activity on both cell lines. However, HL-60 required approximately fivefold higher concentrations of Pluripoietin to achieve 50% differentiated, spreading colonies versus undifferentiated tight blast-cell colonies than did WEHI-3B (D+) [11]. The human leukemia cell line KG1 (courtesy Dr. H.P. Koeffler) responded to Pluripoietin with increased colony formation in agar and increased [^{3}H]thymidine incorporation after 24–48 h in suspension culture. This might indicate that the GM-DF activity of Pluripoietin reflects the differentiating capacity of leukemia cell lines rather than an intrinsic property of the factor.

Table 1. Murine mast-cell growth factor activity of Pluripoietin

Stimulator	[^{3}H]thymidine uptake (cpm)	[^{3}H]thymidine uptake (% max)
ConA-LBRM CM		
1:4	5617± 12 [a]	100
1:8	4416±661 [a]	79
1:16	2987± 70 [a]	53
Medium	164± 64	2.9
Pluripoietin		
500 U/ml	344± 87 [b]	6.7
250 U/ml	594±153 [b]	11.5
125 U/ml	485±214 [c]	9.4
63 U/ml	380±105 [b]	7.4

Results are expressed as mean±1 standard deviation of triplicate cultures.
Significance of difference from medium control cultures (Student's *t*-test):
[a] $2P<0.001$
[b] $2P<0.05$
[c] $2P<0.1$

Table 2. Biological activities of purified human Pluripoietin and murine Interleukin 3

Activity	Pluripoietin[a]	Interleukin 3[b]
Clonal growth of hemopoietic progenitors:		
CFU-GEMM	+	+
BFU-E	+	+
CFU-G, M, GM	+	+
CFU-EOS	+	+
CFU-MEG	NT	+
pre-CFU-c (ΔGPA)	+	NT
Stem-cell multiplication (CFU-s)	[d]	+
Species cross-reactivity[c]	±	–
Leukemia-differentiating activity (GM-DF) on:		
WEHI-3B (D+)	+	–
HL60	+	–
[^{3}H]thymidine uptake in cell lines:		
KG1	+	–
FDC-P2	–	+
Murine mast-cell lines (MCGF activity)	±	+
Histamine production	NT	+
Protein synthesis of mature macrophages	+	NT
Induction of 20αSDH	[d]	+
Growth of:		
Natural cytotoxic cells	[d]	+
Pre-B-cell clones	NT	+

[a] Pluripoietin was tested on human target cells, if not noted otherwise
[b] Interleukin 3 activity on murine target cells, if not noted otherwise. Data derived from literature, except GM-DF and activity on KG1
[c] Activity on bone-marrow-derived colony formation in agar cultures
[d] No human test system available
NT, not tested

E. Pluripoietin Shows Minimal Species Cross-Reactivity on Murine Cells

Normal mouse bone marrow cells cultured in agar for 7 days in the presence of saturating concentrations of Pluripoietin formed approximately 10% of the colonies supported by WEHI-3B-conditioned media as a standard source of CSF(s). All colonies formed in the presence of Pluripoietin were of similar morphology, not staining for alpha-naphthyl-acetate esterase or Kaplow's myeloperoxidase; this suggests that only a subpopulation of murine colony-forming progenitors is responsive to Pluripoietin. Weak cross-species activity was also found on continuous murine mast-cell lines, established as described from murine long-term bone marrow cultures [19]. Five thousand cells per well of a mast-cell growth factor (MCGF)-dependent murine mast-cell line were incubated for 24 h at 37 °C in 96 well plates with serial dilutions of growth factors and then assayed for [^{3}H]thymidine uptake as described [20]. The results are given in Table 1 and demonstrate little more than 10% murine MCGF activity of Pluripoietin as compared with ConA-LBRM CM (concanavalin-A-stimulated conditioned media from LBRM murine lymphoma line), which was used as a standard preparation of murine MCGF.

The murine Interleukin-3-dependent cell line FDC-P2 (courtesy Dr. M. Dexter) did not respond with increased [^{3}H] thymidine uptake to concentrations of Pluripoietin as high as 2000 U/ml (data not shown).

F. Conclusion

Table 2 gives a summary of biological activities of Pluripoietin and Interleukin 3. Comparison is incomplete, since for some activities of Interleukin 3 on murine cells there exist no equivalent human assay systems, as for instance long-term mast-cell lines. From the results obtained so far, leukemia-differentiating activity is a most remarkable property of Pluripoietin, distinguishing it from murine Interleukin 3, which lacks this activity [1]. In addition, Pluripoietin is active on a wide range of hemopoietic cells, with respect to cell lineage and to their place in the hierarchy of stem cells to mature cells. The availability of purified human hemopoietic growth factors should facilitate future studies of complex regulatory mechanisms in hematopoiesis.

References

1. Nicola NA, Vadas M (1984) Hemopoietic colony-stimulating factors. Immunol Today 5:76–81
2. Watson JD, Prestidge RL (1983) Interleukin 3 and colony-stimulating factors. Immunol Today 4:278–280
3. Ihle JN, Keller J, Henderson L, Klein F, Palaszynski E (1982) Procedures for the purification of Interleukin 3 to homogeneity. J Immunol 129:2431–2436
4. Fung MC, Hapel AJ, Ymer S, Cohen DR, Johnson RM, Campbell HD, Young IG (1984) Molecular cloning of c-DNA for murine interleukin 3. Nature 307:233–237
5. Ihle JN, Pepersack L, Rebar L (1981) Regulation of T cell differentiation: in vitro induction of 20-alpha-steroid dehydrogenase in splenic lymphocytes is mediated by a unique lymphokine. J Immunol 126:2184–2189
6. Ihle JN, Keller J, Oroszlan S, Henderson LE, Copeland TD, Fitch F, Prystowski MB, Goldwasser E, Schrader JW, Palaszynski E, Dy M, Lebel B (1983) Biologic properties of homogeneous Interleukin 3. J Immunol 131:282–287
7. Razin E, Ihle JN, Seldin D, Mencia-Huerta JM, Katz HR, Leblanc PA, Hein A, Caulfield JP, Austen KF, Stevens RL. Interleukin 3: a differentiation and growth factor for the mouse mast cell that contains chondroitin sulfate E proteoglycan. J Immunol 132: 1479–1486
8. Palacios R, Henson G, Steinmetz M, McKearn JP (1984) Interleukin 3 supports growth of mouse pre-B-cell clones in vitro. Nature 309:126–131
9. Lu L, Broxmeyer HE, Meyers PA, More MAS, Thaler T (1983) Association of cell cycle expression of Ia-like antigenic determinants on normal human multipotential (CFU-GEMM) and erythroid (BFU-E) progenitor cells with regulation in vitro by acidic isoferritins. Blood 61:250–256
10. Broxmeyer HE, Moore MAS, Ralph P (1977) Cell-free granulocyte colony inhibitory activity derived from human polymorphonuclear neutrophils. Exp Hematol 5:87–102
11. Platzer E, Welte K, Gabrilove JL, Lu L, Nathan CF, Mertelsmann R, Moore MAS (to be published) Biological activities of a human pluripotent colony stimulating factor on normal and leukemic cells
12. Hoang T, Iscove NN, Odartchenko N (1983) Macromolecules stimulating human granulocytic colony-forming cells, precursors of these cells, and primitive erythroid progenitors: some apparent nonidentities. Blood 61:960–966
13. Jacobsen N, Broxmeyer HE, Grossbard E, Moore MAS (1979) Colony-forming units in diffusion chambers (CFU-d) and colony-forming units in agar culture (CFU-c) obtained from normal human bone marrow: a possible parent-progeny relationship. Cell Tissue Kinet 12:213–226
14. Wagemaker G, Dorssers L (1984) Properties of purified stem cell activating factor (SAF) and its use for selective multiplication of stem cells for bone marrow transplantation in mice. Exp Hematol 12:454 (abstract 247)
15. Nathan CF, Prendergast TJ, Wiebe ME, Stanley ER, Platzer E, Remold HG, Welte K, Rubin BY, Murray HW (1984) Activation of human macrophages. J Exp Med 160:600–605
16. Djeu JY, Lanza E, Pastore S, Hapel AJ (1983) Selective growth of natural cytotoxic but not natural killer effector cells in interleukin 3. Nature 306:788–791
17. Koeffler HP (1983) Induction of differentiation of human acute myelogenous leukemia cells: therapeutic implications. Blood 62:709–721

18. Metcalf D (1980) Clonal extinction of myelomonocytic leukemic cells by serum from mice injected with endotoxin. Int J Cancer 25:225–233
19. Tertian G, Yung YP, Guy-Grand D, Moore MAS (1980) Long-term culture of murine mast cells. I. Description of a growth factor dependent in vitro culture technique. J Immunol 127:788–794
20. Yung YP, Eger R, Tertian G, Moore MAS (1981) Long-term in vitro culture of murine mast cells, II. Purification of a mast cell growth factor and its dissociation from TCGF. J Immunol 12:794–799

Haematology and Blood Transfusion Vol. 29
Modern Trends in Human Leukemia VI
Edited by Neth, Gallo, Greaves, Janka

A T Lymphocyte-Derived Differentiation-Inducing Factor for Myeloid Leukemia Cells: Purification and Characterization *

I. Olsson, U. Gullberg, M. G. Sarngadharan, and R. C. Gallo

Acute myeloid leukemia (AML) is characterized by an apparent maturation arrest leading to accumulation of immature cells. Such cells obviously preserve normally transient phenotypes. Recent work also indicates that leukemic transformation does not necessarily lead to an irreversible block in cell differentiation. Leukemic cell lines which grow continuously in vitro are useful systems in the search for normal regulatory molecules which can act in leukemia. The promyelocytic HL-60 line [2] is induced into granulocytes and monocytes by incubation with a variety of agents [4]. We have concentrated our work on mechanisms of action of "physiologic" inducers of differentiation in leukemia. Nitroblue tetrazolium (NBT) reduction has been used as the parameter of induced maturation in HL-60 as well as phagocytic capacity, cell surface antigen expression detected with monoclonal antibodies, nonspecific esterase, and composition of cytoplasmic granules.

Mitogen-stimulated human mononuclear blood cells release polypeptide factors which we call differentiation-inducing factors (DIF) [5, 6]. These induce HL-60 cells to mature into phagocytizing monocyte-like cells, which can reduce NBT. Gel chromatography has showed that mitogen-stimulated cells release one or two species of DIF with apparent molecular weights of 40 000 and 25 000, depending on which mitogen was used. At least the 40 000 molecular weight species of DIF was distinct from colony-stimulating factor (CSF). It was subsequently found that the T lymphocyte leukemic cell line HUT-102, established from a patient with an adult lymphoma of mature T cells and which releases the human retrovirus called human T cell leukemia virus (HTLV), is a reliable constitutive producer of DIF [8]. Large-scale production of HUT-102 supernatants can therefore be employed to obtain enough starting material for purification of DIF.

DIF has now been purified more than 10 000-fold from HUT-102 conditioned media utilizing ion exchange chromatography on DEAE–sepharose, gel filtration on Sephadex G-75, ion exchange chromatography on Mono Q, and reverse-phase chromatography utilizing the Pharmacia Pro RPC column. DIF appeared homogeneous on gel filtration with a molecular weight of approximately 60 000 while SDS–polyacrylamide gel electrophoresis revealed a somewhat lower molecular weight. However, high resolution chromatography on an ion exchange Mono Q column using the fast pressure liquid chromatography (FPLC) system, which resulted in substantial purification, also revealed considerable charge heterogeneity. Thus, DIF eluted in three separate peaks at an ionic strength of 0.05–0.11 *M* NaCl pH 8.0. Chromatofocusing on a Mono P column confirmed the charge heterogeneity of DIF, which was eluted in the pH range 5.6–5.9. Highly purified DIF eluted from the Mono Q column was also subjected to reverse-phase chromatography using the Pro RPC Hr 5/10 column with the FPLC system.

* Lund Hospital, Research Dept. 2, S-22185 Lund

DIF was eluted with 44% acetonitrile. Substantial purification was achieved in this step, but it has not yet been possible to elute DIF with a single protein peak. DIF is protein in nature as it is destroyed by proteases. It is relatively heat stable, resisting heating to 60 °C–70 °C. It is not inactivated by periodate oxidation and shows no affinity to lectins.

DIF acts synergistically with retinoic acid (RA) to induce maturation not only of HL-60, but also of the monoblast-like cell line U-937 (measured as percentage of cells reducing NBT) [7]. The synergistic effect indicates that DIF and RA act by different mechanisms to induce differentiation. Other inducers such as dimethylsulfoxide (DMSO), 1,25-dihydroxycholecalciferol, actinomycin D, and cAMP-inducing agents like cholera toxin and PGE_2 act additively with DIF to induce maturation of HL-60. The finding of a synergistic effect between RA and DIF prompted a study on the effects of sequential treatment with these agents. Both HL-60 and U-937 could be "primed" for differentiation by treatment for 10–20 h with low concentrations of RA followed by exposure to low concentrations of DIF. Priming with RA for the inducing effect of DIF did not depend on the normal rate of protein synthesis as it occurred even better in the presence of 1 μg/ml cycloheximide, a concentration which inhibited growth completely and protein synthesis by 86%. However, the resulting maturation obtained by addition of DIF was, as expected, inhibited by cycloheximide. Our results suggest that a decrease in synthesis of some unknown protein or proteins favors maturation of the leukemic cells.

HL-60 cells have a very high self-renewal capacity. However, some spontaneous maturation occurs toward granulocytes and monocytes, which may fit a stochastic model. If probabilities for commitment to granulocyte and monocyte are P_1 and P_2, respectively, the probability for self-renewal will be $1-(P_1+P_2)$. P_1 is increased by DMSO and RA. P_2 is increased by DIF, cAMP agents, phorbol esters, and cholecalciferol. With most inducers, probabilities for commitment are very high so that self-renewal is lost and the culture terminated. The mechanism by which DIF induces maturation into monocyte-like cells is not known. Since DIF is a polypeptide, it presumably acts through a cell surface receptor. The second messenger is not cAMP, since the latter was not increased upon addition of DIF and since adenyl cyclase inhibitors did not abolish the effect. The DIF effect was not blocked by inhibitors of calmodulin. Furthermore, the DIF effect is independent of cell proliferation since it occurred equally well in the presence of polyamine inhibitors or other agents, which blocked cell proliferation completely. It is clear that different agents can act by different mechanisms, even to induce more or less identical end stage cells. Defining the mechanisms of action of several inducers may therefore help to identify regulation of differentiation in hemopoiesis and leukemia.

The relationship, if any, of HUT-102-produced DIF to other previously described lymphokine factors is not yet established. The highly purified DIF was completely devoid of CSF activity. This does not rule out that some CSF may induce differentiation of leukemic cells as described in the mouse system [1, 3]. The physiochemical properties of DIF eliminate its identity with interleukin-1, -2, or -3. Interferon-γ did not alone induce maturation of HL-60. Furthermore, a neutralizing antibody for interferon-γ did not abolish the DIF effect on HL-60. It is concluded that DIF and interferon-γ are separate molecules.

Conclusions

DIF is a polypeptide produced by mitogen-stimulated human mononuclear blood cells and constitutively by certain T lymphocyte lines such as the HUT-102 line. It induces maturation of the HL-60 cell line into monocyte-like cells. DIF is *not* identical with CSF, interleukin-1, -2, or -3, or interferon-γ. Using supernatants from the HUT-102 line, it has been purified more than 10 000-fold and its chemical properties have been defined. Its role in hemopoiesis and leukemia now remains to be determined.

References

1. Burgess AW, Metcalf D (1980) Int J Cancer 26:647–654
2. Collins SJ, Gallo RC, Gallagher RE (1977) Nature 270:347–349
3. Lotem J, Lipton JH, Sachs L (1980) Int J Cancer 25:763–771
4. Olsson I (1983) Acta Med Scand 214:261–272
5. Olsson I, Olofsson T (1981) Exp Cell Res 131:225–230
6. Olsson I, Olofsson T, Mauritzon N (1981) J Natl Cancer Inst 67:1225–1230
7. Olsson I, Breitman TR, Gallo RC (1982) Cancer Res 42:3928–3933
8. Olsson I, Sarngadharan MG, Breitman TR, Gallo RC (1984) Blood 63:510–517

Haematology and Blood Transfusion Vol. 29
Modern Trends in Human Leukemia VI
Edited by Neth, Gallo, Greaves, Janka

A Model Scheme of Hematopoietic Cell Differentiation Based on Multiple Marker Analysis of Leukemia–Lymphomas: T Cell Lineage

J. Minowada [1], H. G. Drexler [1], M. Menon [1], H. Rubinstein [1], H. Messmore [1], S. Krasnow [1], J. Takeuchi [2], and A. A. Sandberg [2]

A. Introduction

The analysis of human leukocyte differentiation antigens has been greatly facilitated by studies of leukemia and lymphoma cells [1]. Because of the two characteristics common to both leukemia and lymphoma, i.e., single clonal cell population of respective hematopoietic cell type and arrested differentiation profile in each case, studies of multiple marker analysis and in vitro induced cellular differentiation system by a variety of chemical and natural inducers have continued to provide steady progress in this area of knowledge. Furthermore, recent advances in molecular biology relative to cytogenetic nonrandom abnormalities in the hematopoietic malignancies provide further insight into pathophysiology of these diseases [2].

We have been primarily interested in characterizing both permanent leukemia–lymphoma cell lines and fresh uncultured leukemia–lymphoma cells by means of multiple marker analysis. At present, we have a total of 85 proven human leukemia–lymphoma cell lines and a couple dozen of their clonal sublines and mutants in the laboratory. These lines include T cell, B cell, lymphoid precursor, myelomonocyte, erythroid, and histiocytic lineages. Over 675 cases of patients with various types of hematopoietic malignancies have also been studied in the laboratory. Despite a continuous hope of finding a "tumor-specific" marker, all of the markers thus far studied were of normal gene products, except cytogenetic abnormalities [3]. Consequently, we have been able to propose a hypothetical differentiation scheme of human hematopoietic cells which are assumed to be reflected by the marker profiles of these tumor cells [4].

In our earlier studies [5], we were able to divide such a model scheme of T cell differentiation into five stages of maturation. The present report summarizes the results of 30 permanent T cell leukemia–lymphoma cell lines and 58 cases of patients with T cell malignancies.

B. Material and Methods

I. Cell Lines and Fresh Leukemia–Lymphomas

A total of 85 factor-independent leukemia–lymphoma cell lines were maintained in RPMI medium 1640 supplemented with 5%–10% heat-inactivated fetal calf serum at 37 °C. Details of each cell line establishment and characterization have previously been reported [4]. Mononuclear cells were prepared by Hypaque–Ficoll gradient centrifugation for the fresh leukemia–lymphoma study.

II. Multiple Marker Analysis

Multiple marker analysis of leukemia–lymphoma has been developed in our

1 Edward J. Hines, Jr. Veterans Administration Hospital, Hines, Illinois 60141 and Loyola University Stritch School of Medicine, Maywood, Illinois 60153, USA
2 Roswell Park Memorial Institute, Buffalo, N.Y. 14263, USA

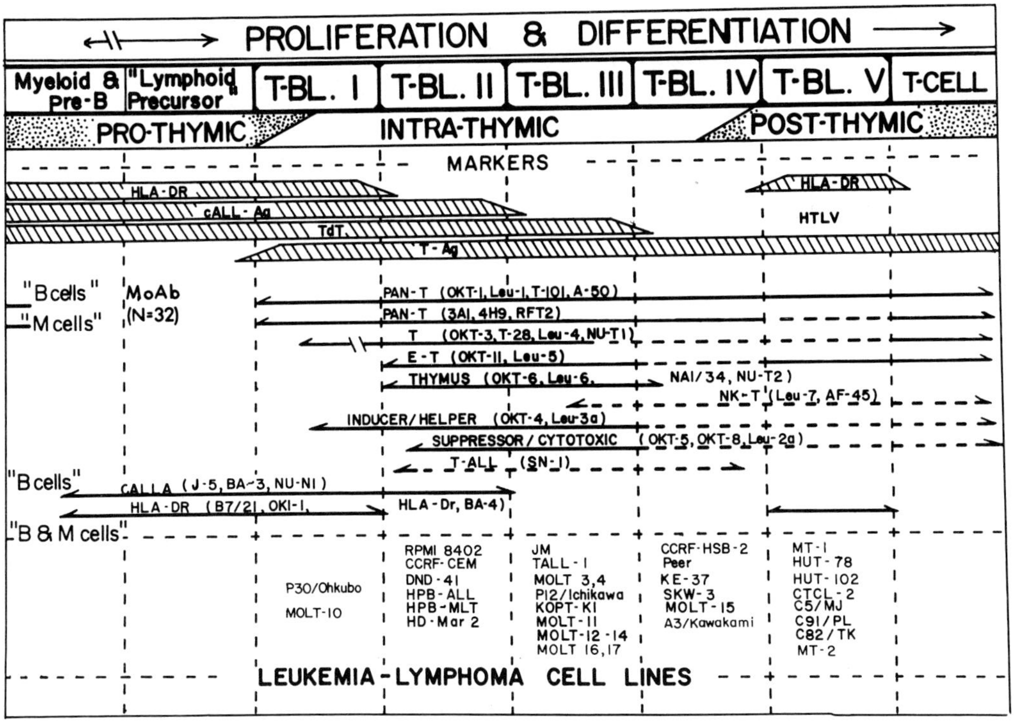

Fig. 1. T cell differentiation model. *Hatched horizontal bars* represent HLA-DR, cALL-Ag, TdT, and T-Ag detected by rabbit polyclonal antibody reagents. *Full horizontal line* represents antigen expression detected by MoAb. Portion of *broken line* in the *full line* indicates that the antigen may not be detectable on all cells within respective differentiation stages. "B cells" and "M cells" denote certain B cell and myelomonocytic cell subsets which are cross-reactive with respective MoAb

laboratory [1]. The analysis includes rosette assay, immunofluorescence assay, enzyme assay, cytochemical assay, cytogenetic assay, and certain functional assays. In the present report, in addition to the polyclonal rabbit antisera to pan-T cell antigens, HLA-DR antigens, common ALL-associated antigens, pan-myelomonocytic antigens, terminal deoxynucleotidyl transferase antigens, EB virus antigens, HTLV antigens, and immunoglobulin chains, a large battery of murine monoclonal hybridoma antibodies were also used for the immunofluorescence assay.

C. Results and Discussion

I. Five Stages of T Cell Differentiation

It is conceivable that the marker profiles of malignant T cells may be an aberrant expression of these markers, not reflecting their normal counterparts. However, this possibility has never been proved with unequivocal experimental evidence. On the contrary, these marker studies of leukemia–lymphomas have been taken as a mirror image of what normal hematopoietic differentiation should be.

Figure 1 illustrates the five stages of our T cell differentiation model. The 30 T cell leukemia–lymphoma cell lines are assigned into respective T blast stages according to individual marker profiles. The possible relationship of the T cell differentiation steps involved in the thymic environment is shown at the top of the figure. Four conventional markers as determined by polyclonal antibodies (HLA-DR, cALL-Ag, TdT-Ag, and pan-T-Ag) are the principal marker combination by which the staging

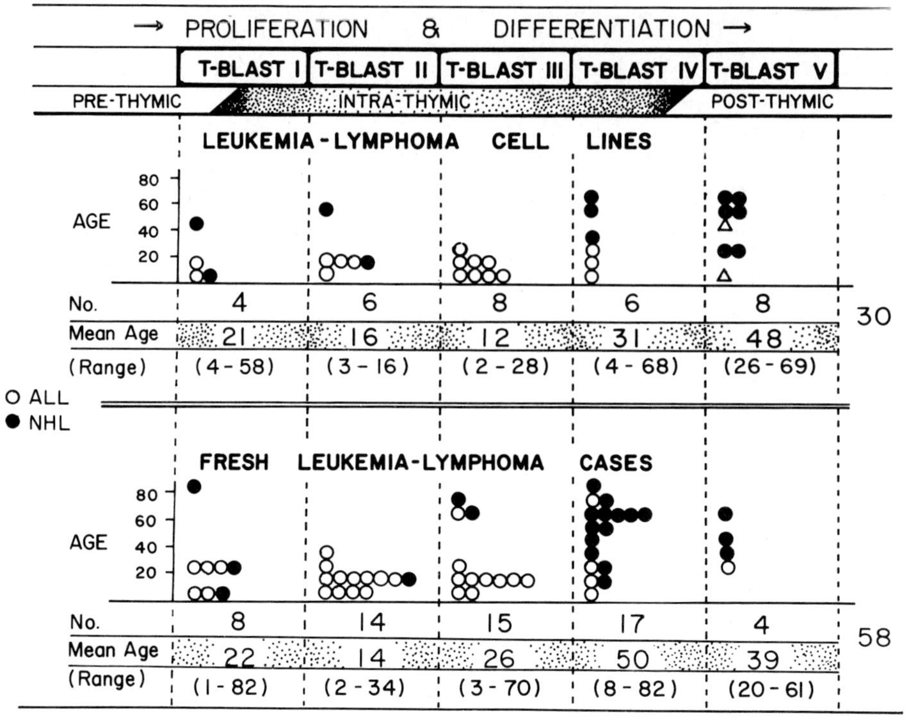

Fig. 2. Correlation among T cell malignancies of ALL or NHL manifestation, stage of differentiation arrest in T cell tumors, and patient's age

was made [5]. A total of 32 murine monoclonal antibodies (MoAb) is utilized and their expression along the T cell differentiation is also illustrated in the Fig. 1. It should be noted that no single MoAb among them fulfills the requirement of "pan-T" specificity in the strict sense. Those which are reported as pan-T MoAb are found to react with certain B cells ("B cells"), myelomonocytic cells ("M cells"), or both. Caution in the use of MoAb and choice of MoAb panel for a particular purpose is necessary. Furthermore, evidence for wider cross-reactivity of some MoAb has been documented. Nevertheless, the exquisite specificity and unlimited availability of those MoAb would enhance the importance and significance of multiple marker analysis for leukemia–lymphoma diagnosis and for basic hematology–immunology research [6–10].

II. Differentiation Arrest of T Cell Tumor Cells and Ages of Patients

As summarized in Fig. 2, there appears to be a significant correlation between the age of individual patients with T cell malignancy and the stage of differentiation arrest of malignant T cell tumor cells. Reviewing a total of 33 T cell lines for their donors' ages, it became apparent that a majority of T cell lines in T blast I, II, and III stages were derived from the patients in a younger age bracket as opposed to those of T cell lines in T blast IV and V which were mainly derived from older patients. This correlation is also related to conventional diagnosis between ALL and non-Hodgkin's lymphoma (NHL). The upper portion of Fig. 2 illustrates these observations. Two T cell lines (MT-2 and C82/TK) are excluded from the analyses for mean age and age range owing to the fact that they are in vitro-transformed normal T cells by HTLV (human T cell leukemia–lymphoma virus) (marked by triangles in Fig. 2).

Because of the tissue culture environment as a limiting as well as a selection factor, analysis was extended to fresh uncultured T cell leukemia–lymphomas. As illustrated to the lower portion of Fig. 2, a total of 58 cases of patients with T-cell tumor demonstrate essentially the same features. Neither the reasons for such a discrete differentiation arrest of T cell tumor cells relative to the host patient's age nor for the form of clinical manifestation of T cell tumor (ALL versus NHL) are known at the present time. The present study nonetheless may provide further insight into the pathophysiology of hematopoietic malignancy.

References

1. Minowada J (1982) Immunology of leukemic cells. In: Gunz FW, Henderson ES (eds) Leukemia. 4th edn, Grune and Stratton, New York, pp 119–139
2. Rowley JD (1983) Human oncogene locations and chromosome aberrations. Nature 301:290–293
3. Greaves M, Janossy G (1978) Patterns of gene expression and the cellular origins of human leukaemias. Biochim Biophys Acta 516:193–230
4. Minowada J, Sagawa K, Lok MS, Kubonishi I, Nakazawa S, Tatsumi E, Ohnuma T, Goldblum N (1980) A model of lymphoid-myeloid cell differentiation based on the study of marker profiles of 50 human leukemia-lymphoma cell lines. In: Serrou B, Rosenfeld C (eds) Symposium on new trends in human immunology and cancer immunotherapy. Doin, Paris, pp 188–199
5. Minowada J, Minato K, Tatsumi E, Sugimoto T, Nakazawa S, Ohnuma T, Kubonishi I, Miyoshi I, Frankel A, Gallo RC (1983) A model scheme for human hematopoietic cell differentiation as determined by multiple markers of leukemia-lymphomas. In: Neth R, Gallo RC, Greaves MF, Moore MAS, Winkler K (eds) Modern trends in human leukemia 5. Springer, Berlin Heidelberg New York (Haematology and Blood Transfusion vol 28), pp 348–350
6. Reinherz EL, Kung PC, Goldstein G, Levey RH, Schlossman SF (1980) Discrete stages of human intrathymic differentiation: analysis of normal thymocytes and leukemic lymphoblasts of T-cell lineage. Proc Natl Acad Sci USA 77:1588–1592
7. Greaves M, Rao J, Hariri G, Verbi W, Catovsky D, Kung R, Goldstein G (1981) Phenotypic heterogeneity and cellular origins of T-cell malignancies. Leuk Res 5:281–299
8. Bernard S, Boumsell L, Reinherz EL, Nadler LM, Ritz J, Coppin H, Richard Y, Valensi F, Dausset J, Flandrin G, Lemerle J, Schlossman SF (1981) Cell surface characterization of malignant T-cells from lymphoblastic lymphoma using monoclonal antibodies: evidence for phenotypic differences between malignant T-cells from patients with acute lymphoblastic leukemia and lymphoblastic lymphoma. Blood 57:1105–1110
9. Habeshaw JA, Bailey D, Stansfeld AG, Greaves MF (1983) The cellular content of non-Hodgkin's lymphomas: a comprehensive analysis using monoclonal antibodies and other surface marker techniques. Br J Cancer 47:327–351
10. Koziner B, Grebhard D, Denny T, McKenzie S, Clarkson BD, Miller DA, Evans RL (1982) Analysis of T-cell differentiation antigens in acute lymphatic leukemia using monoclonal antibodies. Blood 60:752–757

Haematology and Blood Transfusion Vol. 29
Modern Trends in Human Leukemia VI
Edited by Neth, Gallo, Greaves, Janka

Changes in Isoenzyme Patterns Expressed by the Erythroleukemia Cell Lines K-562 and HEL After Induction of Differentiation

H. G. Drexler[1], K. Otsuka[1], P. J. Martin[2], G. Gaedicke[3], and J. Minowada[1]

A. Introduction

Stable human leukemia–lymphoma cell lines provide model systems to study the processes involved in leukemic and normal cell differentiation [10]. Leukemic cells, arrested at a certain stage of differentiation, can be triggered to differentiate to functionally and morphologically more mature cells [7]. Both "fresh" leukemic cells and cells maintained in long-term culture are sensitive to in vitro induction of differentiation. Furthermore, cell differentiation is a novel concept in the treatment of acute leukemias and several substances such as low dose Ara-C and the physiologic compound retinoic acid have been shown to act as differentiating agents in vivo [7].

Two human erythroleukemia cell lines, K-562 [8] and HEL [9], were used to study the effects of 12-*O*-tetradecanoylphorbol-13-acetate (TPA) and of a differentiation inducing factor-(DIF)-containing medium for induction of differentiation.

B. Materials and Methods

Conditioned medium was prepared by stimulating cultured lymphocytes of the T cell line HUT-102 with TPA for 5 h. The TPA-free supernatant from the stimulated cells (harvested after 48 h) had multiple biologic activities including the DIF. A concentration of 5×10^5 cells/ml was incubated in the presence of 10^{-8}–10^{-11} *M* TPA or of 5%–10% DIF-containing medium in RPMI 1640 medium supplemented with 5% Fetal Calf Serum at 37 °C in 5% CO_2 humidified atmosphere.

Cells were harvested after 0, 24, 48, 72, and 96 h and examined for the following parameters: cell growth and viability by trypan blue dye exclusion test, morphology (cytospin preparation stained with Wright–Giemsa), nitro blue tetrazolium (NBT) reduction test, and main emphasis on isoenzyme patterns of the enzymes carboxylic esterase (Est, EC 3.1.1.1), acid phosphatase (acP, EC 3.1.3.2), hexosaminidase (Hex, β-*N*-acetylglucosaminidase, EC 3.2.1.30) and lactate dehydrogenase (LDH, EC 1.1.1.27). Enzymes were separated into isoenzymes by isoelectric focusing (IEF) on horizontal thin layer gels containing 4.8% polyacrylamide [1]. Isoenzymes were visualized by histocytochemical staining techniques as described in detail earlier [1–3].

C. Results

I. Morphology

The most striking alterations in the morphology of the HEL cells during treatment with TPA was the prominent size change. HEL cells became larger with more cyto-

1 Hines Veterans Administration Medical Center, Hines, Illinois 60141, and Loyola University of Chicago Stritch School of Medicine, Maywood, Illinois 60153, USA
2 Fred Hutchinson Cancer Research Center, Seattle, Washington 98104, USA
3 Universitäts-Kinderklinik, Abteilung Paediatrie II, 7900 Ulm/Donau, FRG

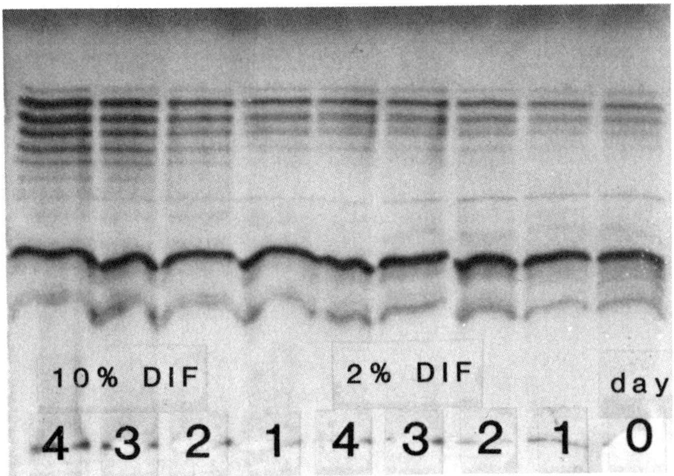

Fig. 1. Induction of differentiation of K-562 with a differentiation inducing factor (DIF). Esterase isoenzyme profiles of K-562 at day 0, 1, 2, 3, and 4 during exposure to 2% and 10% DIF in the medium. *Left side* 10% DIF; *right side* 2% DIF (*top* cathode, *bottom* anode)

plasm. Some cells were extremely large with a tendency to spread out accompanied by adherence to plastic surfaces and development of pseudopodia. In most cells the cytoplasm was vacuolated; many multinucleated cells were seen. DIF did not induce such strong cytoplasmic changes, but enlargement and vacuolization of the cytoplasm were also detected. TPA led to vacuolization and increase of cytoplasm in K-562. No change of size was found after exposure to DIF, only larger and more vacuoles were seen in K-562. K-562 cells did not show surface adherence or pseudopodia.

II. NBT Reduction

A maximum of 40% of the HEL cells became NBT positive with either 10^{-9} or 10^{-10} *M* TPA or 10% DIF. Maximally, 12% of the K-562 cells showed positivity with 10^{-9} *M* TPA.

III. Cell Growth

TPA was very cytotoxic (for HEL more than for K-562). DIF was less cytotoxic (for K-562, no effect on HEL).

IV. Isoenzymes

TPA and DIF induced the new expression and a stronger staining intensity of several Est isoenzymes in K-562 (Fig. 1). A stronger staining intensity and one new Est isoenzyme were seen in HEL with TPA. An Est isoenzyme which is specific for monocytes [2] could not be detected in K-562 or HEL after TPA or DIF treatment. TPA and DIF increased the intensity of all AcP isoenzymes in K-562, including a tartrate-resistant AcP band [1], whereas no changes in the AcP profile occurred in HEL. TPA and DIF (TPA > DIF) led to the new expression of the Hex A isoenzyme, an increase in the intensity of Hex B, and the loss of Hex I in K-562. An increase of Hex A was seen in HEL. One new isoenzyme was induced in the LDH pattern (LDH 1) in both K-562 and HEL by TPA and by DIF.

D. Discussion

Phenotypic changes could be induced by use of the chemical agent TPA and the physiologic inducer DIF in K-562 and HEL. Although not identical, the changes seen after exposure to TPA were similar to those induced by DIF. Recently, a DIF obtained from the same cell line which we used (HUT-102) has been extracted, purified, and characterized [11]. The changes seen in K-562 were quantitatively and qualitatively stronger than in HEL when compared with their original features. HEL cells differentiated mainly along the myeloid–macrophage cell lineage (morphological changes, NBT positivity, adherence to plastic surfaces, development of pseudopodia, and typical isoenzymatic alterations), but also along the erythroid cell axis as we detected the expression of hemoglobin (data not shown). K-562 cells which appear to be originally arrested at an earlier stage of differentiation than HEL cells [4–6] probably differentiated into the myeloid and erythroid series. A monocyte-specific isoenzyme [2] was not found in K-562 or HEL.

In conclusion, HEL and K-562 represent cell lines which can be induced by various agents such as TPA, DIF, hemin (data not shown), and others to differentiate along different cell lineages. Therefore, these cell lines have been termed multipotential stem cells.

References

1. Drexler HG, Gaedicke G (1983) Analysis of isoenzyme patterns of acid phosphatase in acute leukemias. Blut 47:105–113
2. Drexler HG, Gaedicke G (1983) Isoenzyme studies in human leukemia. II. Carboxylic esterase (E.C. 3.1.1.1). Leuk Res 7:599–609
3. Drexler HG, Gaedicke G (1983) Isoenzyme studies in human leukemia. III. β-hexosaminidase (E.C. 3.2.1.30). Leuk Res 7:611–619
4. Drexler HG, Gaedicke G, Minowada J (1985) Isoenzyme studies in human leukemia-lymphoma cell lines. I. Carboxylic esterase. Leuk Res 9:209–229
5. Drexler HG, Gaedicke G, Minowada J (1984) Isoenzyme studies in human leukemia-lymphoma cell lines. II. Acid phosphatase. Leuk Res (submitted for publication)
6. Drexler HG, Gaedicke G, Minowada J (1984) Isoenzyme studies in human leukemia-lymphoma cell lines. III. β-Hexosaminidase. Leuk Res (submitted for publication)
7. Koeffler HP (1983) Induction of differentiation of human acute myelogenous leukemia cells: therapeutical implications. Blood 62:709–721
8. Lozzio CB, Lozzio BB (1975) Human chronic myelogenous leukemia cell line with positive Philadelphia chromosome. Blood 45:321–334
9. Martin P, Papayannopoulou T (1982) HEL cells: a new human erythroleukemia cell line with spontaneous and induced globin expression. Science 216:1233–1235
10. Minowada J (1983) Immunology of leukemic cells. In: Gunz FW, Henderson ES (eds) Leukemia, 4th edn. Grune and Stratton, New York, pp 119–139
11. Olsson IL, Sarngadharan MG, Breitman Th, Gallo RC (1984) Isolation and characterization of a T lymphocyte derived differentiation inducing factor for the myeloid leukemic cell line HL-60. Blood 63:510–517

Haematology and Blood Transfusion Vol. 29
Modern Trends in Human Leukemia VI
Edited by Neth, Gallo, Greaves, Janka

B Cell Lineage: Part of the Differentiation Program of Human Pluripotent Stem Cells

A. A. Fauser[1], L. Kanz[2], B. A. Cooper[1], and G. W. Löhr[2]

A. Introduction

In the past, developmental methods for examining hematopoiesis began to influence concepts of studying hematologic malignancies. A new approach became possible with the establishment of cell culture procedures for committed and more recently for noncommitted hematopoietic stem cells [1–3]. These primitive progenitors (CFU-GEMMT) derived from human bone marrow can be identified in culture by their ability to form colonies containing different myeloid lineages and T cells of different phenotypes. The observation of a common progenitor of myeloid and lymphoid cells in normal and disturbed hematopoiesis led to the question whether B cells are part of the differentiation program of human stem cells. In the present study, we attempted to induce B cell differentiation of human marrow cells from healthy volunteers.

B. Material and Methods

Bone marrow samples were obtained from four consenting healthy individuals.

I. Preparation of Leukocyte-Conditioned Medium

Conditioned medium was prepared from Leu-5-positive cells of normal individuals [4]. Briefly, 10^6 Leu-5 positive cells were incubated with 1% human serum albumin, IMDM (Iscove's modified Dulbecco's medium) and 1% PHA (Wellcome HA 15). This material, Leu-5-PHA-TCM, was harvested after 4 days of incubation at 37 °C in a humidified atmosphere with 5% CO_2.

II. Preparation of Cell Suspensions

Mononuclear cells of density less than 1.077 g/ml were incubated in antibody-coated dishes using B_1, B_2 (Coulter Immunology, Hialeah), and BA_1 (Hybritech) for 20 min at 4 °C. The supernatant containing nonadherent and B cell-depleted cells was plated as outlined.

III. Colony Assay for Hematopoietic Progenitors

Mixed hematopoietic colonies (CFU-GEMMT) [1–3], erythroid bursts (BFU-E), and granulocytic colonies (CFU-C) [6] were grown as previously described. Nonadherent and B cell-depleted cells were admixed with IMDM, 30% human plasma, 0.9% methylcellulose, and 5% Leu-5-PHA-TCM. Erythropoietin (EPO) 1 U/ml (Step III, Connaught) was added on day 4 of culture. Each dish was examined after an additional 10 days of incubation for the presence of hematopoietic colonies, i.e., BFU-E, CFU-C, and CFU-GEMMT.

1 Royal Victoria Hospital, 687, Avenue des Pins Quest, Montreal, Que. H3A 1A1, Canada
2 Med. Univ.-Klinik, Hugstetterstr. 55, 7800 Freiburg, FRG

Table 1. Identification of pre-B-cells and B-cell-associated antigen-positive cells in multilineage hematopoietic colonies (CFU-GEMMT)

Patient	Cytoplasmic μ	CFU-GEMMT Positive for B cell-associated antigen B_1/BA_1	Analyzed
N.H.	4	7/3	41
K.G.	9	11/6	74
B.S.	2	3/5	33
S.C.	5	8/9	62

IV. Examination of Hematopoietic Colonies for SIg (M + D), B Cell-Associated Antigen, and Cytoplasmic μ-Positive Cells

Individual colonies (CFU-GEMMT), erythroid bursts (BFU-E), and granulocytic colonies (CFU-C) were aspirated by micropipe from the cultures and washed in NKH buffer (5 min, 300 g). Aliquots were transfered onto poly-L-lysine-coated wells on glass slides. Attached cells were fixed with glutaraldehyde (0.05% in 0.1 *M* phosphate buffer, pH 7.4) to block Fc receptors and to preserve cell morphology. Cells were stained with the monoclonal antibodies IgM and IgD (Bethesda Research Laboratories), with B_1, or with the use of a monoclonal anti-μ-chain (Miles Laboratories). Controls were performed with β_2- microglobulin and the sandwich antisera, i.e., SAR (swine anti-rabbit) and RAM (rabbit anti-mouse) [7].

C. Results

I. Surface Immunoglobulin, B Cell-Associated Antigen, and Cytoplasmic μ-Positive Cells in Multilineage Hematopoietic Colonies

Mixed hematopoietic colonies, erythroid bursts, and granulocytic colonies were grown from nonadherent and B cell-depleted marrow cells of four normal individuals in the presence of a Leu-5-PHA-TCM and EPO. A total of 211 individual mixed hematopoietic colonies were aspirated from the cultures and were examined for the coexistence of lymphopoietic progeny, i.e., pre-B cells, and B cells. Cytoplasmic μ-, B_1-, and SIg-positive cells could be identified in multilineage colonies of each individual (Table 1). The number of pre-B cells observed in the mixed colonies examined ranged from 0 to 45 cells per colony. The number of B_1-positive cells per colony ranged from 0 to 278 cells (173 ± 46, mean ± standard deviation). In contrast, cells derived from individual BFU-E and CFU-C colonies did not stain for cytoplasmic μ, B_1, or surface immunoglobulins.

D. Discussion

A culture assay for human multilineage hematopoietic progenitors has been established. These primitive precursors form mixed colonies containing lymphopoietic and myeloid cells of different lineages. Recloning experiments of multilineage colonies indicated that some fulfill criteria of stem cells [8]. The lymphopoietic component in mixed colonies consisted of T cells of various phenotypes, i.e., OKT 3, OKT 4, OKT 8, or E 2–22 [2, 3, 7]. Until recently, B cells could not be observed in mixed colonies derived from marrow cells of healthy volunteers. The availability of a Leu- 5-PHA-TCM facilitated the formation of mixed colonies containing SIg M + D, B cell-associated antigen, and cytoplasmic μ-positive cells from normal donors. In the murine system, cytogenetic evidence for the coexistence of a pluripotent stem cell capable of differentiating into myeloid and lymphoid progeny, including both B and T lymphocytes has been provided by Abramson et al. [9].

Acknowledgments. This work was supported in part by Deutsche Forschungsgemeinschaft

(FRG), and Research Institute, Royal Victoria Hospital, Montreal, Canada.

References

1. Fauser AA, Messner HA (1979) Identification of megakaryocytes, macrophages and eosinophiles in colonies of human bone marrow containing neutrophilic granulocytes and erythroblasts. Blood 53:1023
2. Messner HA, Jzaguirre CY, Jamal N (1981) Identification of T-Lymphocytes in human mixed hematopoietic colonies. Blood 58:402
3. Fauser AA, Löhr GW (1982) Recloned colonies positive for T-cell associated antigens derived from mixed hematopoietic colonies (CFU-GEMM). Proc Soc Exp Biol Med 170:220
4. Fauser AA, Kanz L, Löhr GW (1985) Interaction of 3-deaza-adenosine, a phospholipid methyltransferase inhibitor, on the production of pluripoietins from human peripheral T-cells. Exp Hem (in press)
5. Iscove NN, Sieber F, Winterhalter K (1974) Erythroid colony formation in cultures of mouse and human marrow: analysis of requirement for erythropoietin by gel filtration chromatography on agarose concanavalin. Am J Cell Physiol 83:309
6. Senn JS, McCulloch EA, Till JE (1967) Comparison of colony forming ability of normal and leukemic human marrow in cell culture. Lancet II:597
7. Fauser AA, Neumann HA, Bross KG, Kanz L, Löhr GW (1982) Cytotoxic T-cell clones derived from pluripotent stem cells (CFU-GEMM) of patients with Hodgkin's Lymphoma. Blood 60:1317
8. Messner HA, Fauser AA (1980) Culture studies of human pluripotent hemopoietic progenitors. Blut 41:327
9. Abramson S, Miller RG, Philipps RA (1977) The identification in adult bone marrow of pluripotent and restricted stem cells of the myeloid and lymphoid systems. J Exp Med 145:1567

Haematology and Blood Transfusion Vol. 29
Modern Trends in Human Leukemia VI
Edited by Neth, Gallo, Greaves, Janka

Differentiation Capacity of Null-AL(L) Cells in Culture *

A. Ganser and D. Hoelzer

A. Introduction

The cellular phenotype of the blast cells has remained unclassified in a small percentage of patients with acute leukemia (AL) (Greaves et al. 1983). Although markers are expressed on the cells, these are not sufficiently lineage specific to allow an unequivocal allocation of these null-AL cells to one of the defined myeloid and lymphoid cell lineages. We therefore investigated the differentiation potential of leukemic blast cells from patients with null-AL cells under in vivo and in vitro culture conditions to find out whether lineage-specific markers can be induced and whether differentiation is restricted to a single lineage or can occur along several lineages.

B. Patients and Methods

Five patients with newly diagnosed acute leukemia were selected because of the absence of morphological and immunological features characteristic of a particular cell lineage. Peripheral blast cells were separated on a Ficoll-Isopaque (1.077 g/cm^3) gradient. For differentiation induction the blast cells were cultured in vivo within diffusion chambers (DC) implanted into the peritoneal cavity of host mice preirradiated with 7.5 Gy (Hoelzer et al. 1977). Chamber contents were harvested after 1, 7, and 14 days of DC culture and investigated for total and differential cell counts and for the expression of immunological cell markers.

In three patients the blast cells were cultured in vitro for 1–3 days in BM-86 Wissler medium (Boehringer, Mannheim, West Germany) supplemented with 50 μM 2-mercaptoethanol and 10% heat-inactivated fetal calf serum and incubated at 37 °C in a 5% CO_2 humidified atmosphere. During suspension culture the cells were exposed continuously to 5 n*M* 12-O-tetradecanoylphorbol-13-acetate (TPA) (Sigma, Munich), or 1 unit/ml porcine platelet-derived growth factor (PDGF) (Speywood Laboratories, Nottingham, England), or 10% medium conditioned by the Burkitt cell line X-308 (X308-CM) (Heit et al. 1983), 1 μ*M* retinoic acid (RA) (Sigma), or 1 m*M* butyric acid (BA) (Sigma). Appropriate control cultures were set up in parallel.

Cells attached to poly-l-lysine coated glass slides (Morich et al. 1983) were analyzed with a panel of antibodies using an immunoalkaline phosphatase technique. The monoclonal antibodies used are listed in Table 1. Surface *μ* was determined by a polyclonal antibody (Sigma). Cytoplasmic *μ* was detected by a peroxidase-antiperoxidase method.

C. Results and Discussion

The objective of this study was to determine whether leukemic blast cells of a null-AL phenotype can differentiate in cul-

---

* Department of Hematology-Oncology, University of Ulm, Parkstr. 11, D-7900 Ulm, FRG
Supported by the Deutsche Forschungsgemeinschaft, SFB 112, Project B3

Table 1. Monoclonal antibodies used in this study

Selectivity	Designation	Reactive structure	Source
Hematopoietic progenitor cells	RFB-1		Bodger, Christchurch
Common ALL/lymphocyte progenitor associated	J 5	p100	Coulter
	BA-3	p100	Hybritech
T lineage associated			
Intrathymic subset	OKT 6		Ortho
Mature T	OKT 3	p19–29	Ortho
Helper T	OKT 4	p62	Ortho
Suppressor T	OKT 8	p76	Ortho
B lineage associated	BA-1	p30	Hybritech
	BA-2	p24	Hybritech
Granulocytic-monocytic lineage associated	82 H 5		Janowska-Wieczorek, Edmonton
	B 4.3		Lansdorp, Amsterdam
	B 13.9		Lansdorp, Amsterdam
	VIM-D5		Knapp, Vienna
	MO-2		Coulter
Erythroid lineage	VIE-G4	Glycophorin	Knapp, Vienna
Megakaryocytic lineage	C 17.28	gp IIIa	Lansdorp, Amsterdam
Pan-leukocyte	T 29/33	p200	Hybritech
Anti-transferrin receptor	B 3/25	p90	Hybritech
HLA-DR "framework"	OKIa 1		Ortho

ture and thereby reveal the cell lineage to which they are affiliated.

The results of differentiation induction by in vivo DC culture and in vitro suspension culture are given in Tables 2 and 3. No lineage-specific marker expression was found on the cells prior to culture.

The DC culture system, which has previously been shown to support proliferation and differentiation along the various myeloid (Hoelzer et al. 1977, 1981) and lymphoid (Lau et al. 1979) cell lineages, promoted lymphoid differentiation in two of five patients with null-AL (patients 1 and 2), leading to the expression of cALLA and of cytμ, respectively. Differentiation along the B cell lineage was probably already determined in the original blast cells of both patients, a supposition supported by the lack of expression of T cell markers during culture and recent findings by Korsmeyer et al. (1983) of rearranged μ heavy chain genes in the blast cells of most patients with cALLA-negative non-T, non-B ALL. In patient 1, the expression of markers in the in vitro suspension culture paralleled the results of DC culture, whereas myeloid (B 4.3) (Tetteroo et al. 1984) and stem cell markers (RFB-1) (Bodger et al. 1982) in addition to the lymphoid markers were induced in the cells of patient 2 only during suspension culture. In addition, the expression of 82H5, reported as a myeloid but also as a pluripotent stem cell marker (Janowska-Wieczorek et al. 1984), was further enhanced, indicating that a common lymphoid-myeloid progenitor might have been involved in the leukemic process in this particular case.

In addition to 82H5, during DC culture the cells of patient 3 sequentially expressed both lymphoid and myeloid markers, possibly due to sequential proliferation and maturation of two separate cell populations along two different lineages, whereas the cells of patient 4 mainly expressed 82H5 and lymphoid and myeloid markers were found only on a small number of cells. In patient 4 the growth pattern in DC culture was paralleled in suspension culture, where there was a marked increase in cells reactive with RFB-1 and 82H5 and appear-

Table 2. Differentiation induction in diffusion chamber (DC) culture[a]

Pt	Days in culture	Cells/DC ($\times 10^{-5}$)	% Positive cells OKIa	BA-1	BA-2	cALLA	cyt μ	82H5	B4.3	B13.9
1	0	8.3	98	89	–	–	–	–	–	–
	7	2.5	99	45	18	58	4	–	–	–
	14	2.0	79	–	29	53	–	–	–	–
2	0	7.5	61	44	–	–	–	60	–	–
	7	1.0	40	42	–	–	17	66	5	–
	14	0.8	41	10	NT	4	60	77	4	3
3	0	5.5	45	97	–	–	–	15	–	–
	7	2.6	25	47	49	4[b]	–	10	9	–
	14	8.2	24	–	–	–	–	82	78	42
4	0	8.0	90	–	73	–	–	9	–	–
	7	6.0	98	11	14	11	14	32	11	13
	14	5.8	98	3	–	8	5	68	10	2
5	0	5.1	–	–	–	–	–	–	–	–
	7	2.3	–	–	–	–	–	25	13	–
	14	2.6	–	–	–	–	–	36	38	–

[a] The percentage of blast cells on day 0 were 98% for patient 1; 95% for patient 2; 80% for patient 3; 97% for patient 4; and 99% for patient 5; cells were negative for RFB 1, OKT 6, OKT 3, MO 2, C 17.28, VIE G4

[b] 50% cALLA-positive on day 1

NT, not tested

Table 3. Differentiation induction of null-AL(L) cells in suspension culture

Pt	Days in culture	Agent	Cells/ml ($\times 10^{-5}$)	% Positive cells OKIa	BA-1	BA-2	cALLA	cyt μ	RFB 1	82H5	B4.3
1	0	–	10.0	98	89	–	–	–	–	–	–
	3	–	8.9	87	50	–	59[a]	28	–	–	–
	3	TPA	3.6	91	35	–	33[a]	–	3	–	–
2	0	–	10.0	61	44	–	–	–	–	60	–
	3	–	11.2	97	8	48	42[a]	–	44	100	26
	3	TPA	6.6	72	18	90	7[a]	NT	65	100	52
4	0	–	10.0	90	4	73	–	–	–	9	–
	3	–	11.0	74	–	–	8[a]	–	31	39	8
	3	TPA	3.0	93	–	–	18[a]	–	38	55	26

[a] Weak but positive reaction on mononuclear cells

NT, not tested

ance of small but significant percentages of cells reactive with anti-cALLA and B 4.3, consistent with a differentiation arrest at the level of the lymphoid-myeloid progenitor cell. Finally, in patient 5 only myeloid markers, of doubtful significance, were found after DC culture.

The exposure of the cells to TPA in patients 1, 2, and 4 increased the percentage although not the absolute number of cells carrying myeloid markers (B4.3); however, the expression of cALLA was not influenced. Only in patient 2 did TPA induce the de novo expression of RFBI. While

PDGF, X308-CM, and RA did not significantly alter cell growth or marker expression, BA had a profound cytotoxic effect.

Incubation of the cells in glutaraldehyde prior to cell surface analysis, as used here, has been shown to increase the sensitivity of cALLA detection substantially (Kranz et al. 1984), which could explain the demonstration of cALLA in our studies as opposed to earlier ones. In vitro experiments have not previously succeeded in inducing expression of cALLA or cytoplasmic immunoglobulins in null-AL cells (Cossmann et al. 1982; LeBien et al. 1982; Nadler et al. 1982). The reason for successful induction of cALLA and cytoplasmic immunoglobulins reported here might be related to the conditions of the in vivo DC culture system used and to the differences in the in vitro suspension cultures, e.g., the different culture media, as well as to differences in the nature of the cells under investigation.

The induction experiments reported here reveal the heterogeneity within this group of unclassified leukemias, with some cases expressing only lymphoid or myeloid markers and other cases which, upon culture, simultaneously develop markers of lymphoid-myeloid progenitor cells as well as of both lymphoid and myeloid cells. Since we do not have selective markers for pluripotent stem cells and their malignant counterparts, and therefore have to rely on the behavior of the cells in culture (Greaves et al. 1983), expression of both lymphoid and myeloid markers could well imply that in these cases common lymphoid-myeloid progenitor cells were involved in the malignant transformation event with subsequent block of differentiation.

References

Bodger MP, Francis GE, Delia D, Granger SM, Janossy G (1981) A monoclonal antibody specific for immature human hemopoietic cells and T lineage cells. J Immunol 127: 2269–2274

Cossman J, Neckers LM, Arnold A, Korsmeyer SL (1982) Induction of differentiation in a case of common acute lymphoblastic leukemia. N Engl J Med 307:1251–1254

Greaves MF, Bell R, Amess J, Lister TA (1983) ALL masquerading as AUL. Leuk Res 7:735 –746

Heit W, Vetter KU, Sato N, Carbonell F, Burrichter H, Stein H, Heimpel H (1983) Colony-stimulating factor (GM-CSF) and somatomedin (SM) production by cell lines derived from Hodgkin's disease (HD) and Burkitt's cell leukemia (BL). Exp Hematol 11 [Suppl 14]:229

Hoelzer D, Kurrle E, Schmücker H, Harriss EB (1977) Evidence for differentiation of human leukemic blood cells in diffusion chamber culture. Blood 49:729–744

Hoelzer D, Harriss EB, Carbonell F (1981) Maturation of blast cells in acute transformation of chronic myeloproliferative syndrome. In: Neth R, Gallo RC, Graf T, Mannweiler K, Winkler K (eds) Modern trends in human leukemia, vol 4. Springer, Berlin Heidelberg New York, pp 261–264

Janowska-Wieczorek A, Mannoni P, Turner AR, McGann LE, Shaw ARE, Turc JM (1984) Monoclonal antibody specific for granulocytic lineage cells and reactive with human pluripotent and committed haematopoietic progenitor cells. Br J Haematol 58:159–168

Korsmeyer SJ, Arnold A, Bakhshi A, Ravetch JV, Siebenlist U, Hieter PA, Sharrow SO, LeBien TW, Kersey JH, Poplack DG, Leder P, Waldmann TA (1983) Immunoglobulin gene rearrangement and cell surface antigen expression in acute lymphocyte leukemias of T cell and B cell precursor origin. J Clin Invest 71:301–313

Kranz BR, Thierfelder S (1984) More normal and leukemic cells express common lymphoblastic leukemia antigen using double sandwich immunocytochemistry and glutaraldehyde fixation. Exp Hematol 12:394

Lau B, Jäger G, Thiel E, Rodt H, Huhn D, Pachmann K, Netzel B, Böning L, Thierfelder S, Dörmer P (1979) Growth of the REH cell line in diffusion chambers: evidence for differentiation along the T- and B-cell pathway. Scand J Haematol 23:285–290

LeBien TW, Boue DR, Kersey JH (1982) Studies of human leukemic lymphoid progenitor cell differentiation with the phorbol ester TPA. In: Baum SJ, Ledney GD, Thierfelder S (eds) Experimental hematology today 1982. Karger, Basle New York, pp 171–178

Liszka K, Majdic O, Bettelheim P, Knapp W (1983) Glycophorin A expression in malignant hematopoiesis. Am J Hematol 15:219 –226

Morich FJ, Momburg F, Moldenhauer G, Hartmann KU, Bross KJ (1983) Immunoperoxidase slide assay (IPSA) – a new screening method for hybridoma supernatants directed against cell surface antigens compared to other binding assays. Immunobiology 164: 192–202

Nadler LM, Ritz J, Bates MP, Park EK, Anderson KC, Sallan SE, Schlossman SF (1982) Induction of human B cell antigens in non-T cell acute lymphoblastic leukemia. J Clin Invest 70:433–442

Tetteroo PAT, Lansdorp PM, Leeksma OC, von dem Borne AEGK (1983) Monoclonal antibodies against human platelet glycoprotein IIIa. Br J Haematol 55:509–522

Tetteroo PAT, Lansdorp PM, Geurts van Kessel AHM, Hagemeijer A, von dem Borne AEGK (1984) Serological and biochemical characterization of human myeloid-associated antigens and their expression on human-mouse cell hybrids. In: Bernard A, Boumsell L, Dausset J, Milstein C, Schlossman SF (eds) Leucocyte typing. Human leucocyte differentiation antigens detected by monoclonal antibodies. Springer, Berlin Heidelberg New York, Tokyo, pp 419–423

Haematology and Blood Transfusion Vol. 29
Modern Trends in Human Leukemia VI
Edited by Neth, Gallo, Greaves, Janka

Evidence of Sternberg-Reed Cells Being Derived from Activated Lymphocytes

H. Stein[1], J. Gerdes[1], H. Lemke[2], and D. Y. Mason[3]

A. Introduction

The nature and origin of Sternberg-Reed (SR) cells remains obscure despite numerous studies of this topic. In recent experiments we raised monoclonal antibodies against the Hodgkin's disease-derived cell line L428, with the aim of producing reagents specific for SR cells. Three monoclonal antibodies (designated Ki-1, Ki-24, and Ki-27; Stein et al. 1982, 1983) were obtained in the course of this study, and their reactivities are detailed in Table 1.

Monoclonal antibody Ki-1 differed from the other two reagents in that it detected a subpopulation of large cells, preferentially distributed around the margin of B cell follicles (Stein et al. 1982). This population of cells does not correspond to any cell type previously recognized using other monoclonal antibodies. Since the earliest site of lymph node involvement in Hodgkin's disease is the perifollicular region (as has been recognized previously from conventional histology and can also be shown by immunolabelling with Ki-1 antibody), we proposed that this population of Ki-positive cells in normal lymphoid tissue may represent the physiological counterpart of SR cells. However, it is not clear whether the subpopulation represents a novel cell lineage or simply a differentiation stage within one or more cell lineages. To study this question further, the expression of Ki-1 antigen, and also of the antigens detected by antibodies Ki-24 and Ki-27, was investigated in a wide range of lymphoid tissue samples, including fetal material and peripheral blood lymphocytes stimulated by a variety of mitogenic agents.

B. Material and Methods

I. Cases

Fresh unfixed biopsies of lymphoma and other tissues were obtained from the Hospital of the University of Kiel Medical School and the John Radcliffe Hospital, Oxford, England.

II. Phytohemagglutinin (PHA)-Stimulated and Virus-Transformed Human Peripheral Blood Cells

Cells (1×10^6 per ml) were cultured in the presence of 0.25 μg PHA/ml. Cells were harvested after 72 h and centrifuged onto glass slides. HTLV II transformed peripheral blood cells were a gift from Dr. I.Y. Chen. These cells had been transformed by co-cultivation with irradiated Mo-T cells, as described elsewhere (Chen et al. 1983). EBV transformed blood cells were prepared by in vitro infection as recently described (Moss et al. 1978).

1 Institute of Pathology, Klinikum Steglitz, Free University of Berlin, FRG
2 Institute of Biochemistry, University of Kiel, FRG
3 Nuffield Department of Pathology, John Radcliffe Hospital, Oxford, UK

Table 1. Reactivity of three monoclonal antibodies (Ki-1, Ki-24 and Ki-27) raised against the Hodgkin's disease-derived cell line L 428

Antibody	Normal lymphoid tissue	L 428 cell line	Sternberg-Reed cells
Ki-1	Scattered large perifollicular cells	+	+
Ki-24	None, or a very few scattered cells	+	+
Ki-27	Vessels, sinus lining cells, and no or only occasional lymphoid cells	+	+

III. Immunolabelling of Sections and Cytocentrifuged Cells

Immunolabelling was performed using either the alkaline phosphatase: antialkaline phosphatase (APAAP) method (Cordell et al. 1984) or the three-stage immunoperoxidase method (Stein et al. 1982).

C. Results and Discussion

The results obtained are summarized in Tables 2–5. The non-reactivity of Ki-1 antibody with fetal liver, fetal and adult bone marrow and fetal and postnatal thymus makes it unlikely that Ki-1-positive cells found in normal tissue represent precursors of T, B or monocyte/macrophage origin. This conclusion is supported by the fact that the other two SR-cell-associated antigens (Ki-24 and Ki-27) were also absent from these tissues.

Each of the three SR-cell-associated antigens (Ki-1, Ki-24 and Ki-27) could be induced on peripheral blood lymphocytes by exposure to PHA or by infection with HTLV or EBV (Table 3), although the proportion of positive cells differed for each antigen. Expression of each antigen was consistently accompanied by the appearance of the activation-associated antigens, i.e. the IL2 receptor (detected by anti-Tac, TÜ69 and ACT1).

These findings suggest the possibility that SR cells may represent activated T lymphocytes. To explore this possibility we analysed SR cells in situ by staining tissue sections for T cell and B cell antigens and activation-associated antigens using a newly developed highly sensitive immunalkaline phosphatase method (the APAAP technique). This analysis revealed that at least some of the SR cells in the majority of non-lymphocyte-predominant types of Hodgkin's disease express a variety of T cell antigens (T1, T3, T4 and T11). It was also possible to demonstrate strong staining for IL2 receptor in the majority of cases. However, a surprising finding was that a varying proportion of SR cells in many of these cases expressed B cell antigens, usually associated with T cell antigens but occasionally alone (Table 4).

These observations provide evidence that SR cells may indeed be activated T lymphocytes. However the expression of B cell antigens by SR cells in some cases requires explanation. One possible hypothesis is that the anti-B cell antibodies are only specific for this cell lineage when resting lymphoid cells are analysed, and this specificity may be lost when lymphocytes undergo transformation. Hence activated T cells may aberrantly express apparently B cell-specific markers.

The expression of B cell-associated antigens in some SR cells (and also the absence of T cell-associated antigens from cases of lymphocyte-predominant Hodgkin's disease) prompted us to investigate the possible B cell nature of SR cells in Hodgkin's disease further. For this purpose we analysed the expression of J chain, since this molecule has been shown to be a reliable marker for cells of the B lineage and numerous studies in the past have failed to demonstrate its expression in T lymphoid cells. As shown in Table 5 and Fig. 1, SR cells in all cases of

Table 2. Antibody Ki-1 reactivity in tissue containing myeloid and/or lymphoid precursor cells

Tissue	Ki-1 positive
Fetal tissue	
Liver (2)[a]	None
Bone marrow (2)	None
Thymus cortex (2)	None
Postnatal tissue	
Liver (6)	None
Bone marrow (6)	None
Thymus cortex	None

[a] Number of samples are given in parenthesis

Hodgkin's disease of nodular sclerosing, mixed cellularity and lymphocyte-depleted types were negative for J chain. However, SR cells in the majority of cases of lymphocyte-predominant disease of nodular subtype were J chain positive. This is in keeping with a previous report in the literature (Poppema 1980), in which J chain expression by SR cells was described in a single case of lymphocyte-predominant Hodgkin's disease.

Our working hypothesis (Table 6) based upon these results is that Hodgkin's disease represents the neoplastic proliferation of

Table 3. Antigen profile of peripheral blood lymphocytes following stimulation or transformation with PHA without or with IL2, HTLV or EBV

Stimulating transforming agent	Ki-27	Ki-24	Ki-1	T3	SIg	To15 B 4	Tac	TU69
None	0	0	0	82	12	15	0	0
PHA	3	6	15	93	10	14	97	98
PHA plus IL2	15	80	20	100	0	NA	100	100
HTLV	0	98	97	95	0	0	96	97
EBV	0	100	100	0	100	100	10	15

Table 4. Patterns of antibody reactivity of Sternberg-Reed cells of Hodgkin's disease established in 35 cases

Ki-1	HLA-DR	T3/T11	B4/To15	Tac	TU69
+	+	–	–	+/–	+/–
+	+	+	–	+/–	+/–
+	+	+	+	+/–	+/–
+	+	–	+	+/–	+/–

Table 5. Reactivity of Sternberg-Reed cells of Hodgkin's disease for J chain and granulocyte antigen detected by 3C4 or C3D-1

Histological type	No. of cases	J chain	Granulocyte antigen
Nodular sclerosis	9	0	9
Mixed cellularity	8	0	6
Lymphocyte depletion	6	0	4
Lymphocyte predominance (nodular subtype)	29	↗ 22	0
		↘ 0	5

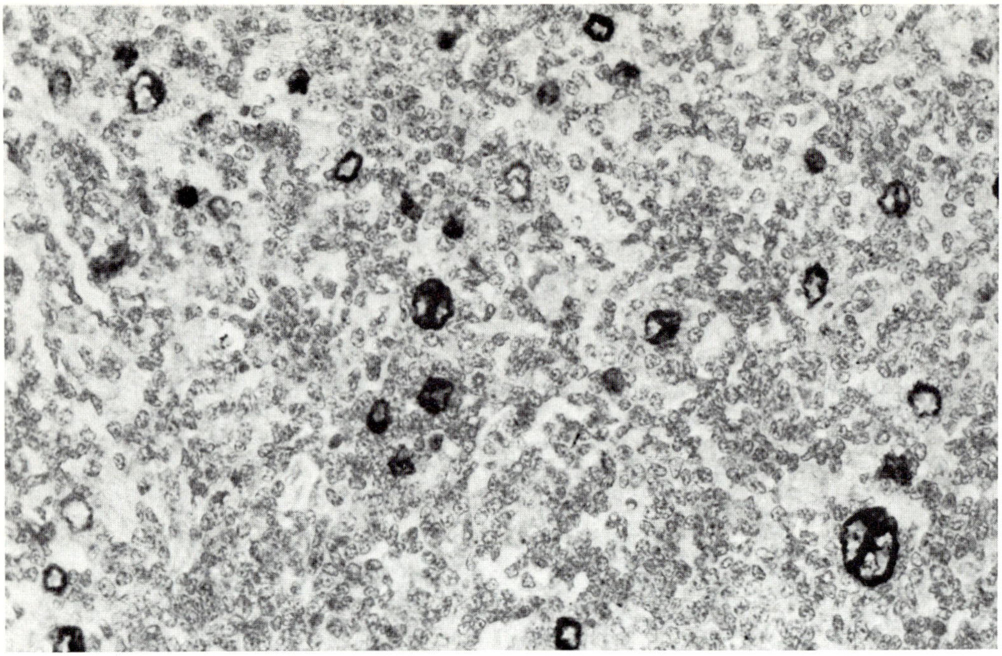

Fig. 1. Hodgkin's disease, lymphocyte predominance, nodular subtype immunostained with an anti-J-chain antiserum. The Sternberg-Reed cells are strongly positive (APAAP)

activated lymphoid cells, but that the histological type of the disease may be related to whether these cells are of T cell or B cell origin. Neoplasms of activated T cells show the histological appearances of nodular sclerosing, mixed cellularity and lymphocyte-depleted Hodgkin's disease. In contrast, the more rarely encountered neoplasms of activated B cell give rise to lymphocyte-predominant disease.

Table 6. Putative origin of Sternberg-Reed cells in Hodgkin's Disease

Origin	Histological appearance
Activated T cell	Nodular Mixed cellularity Lymphocyte depletion
Activated B cell	Lymphocyte predominance, nodular subtype (J chain positive)

References

Chen ISY, Quan SG, Golde DW (1983) Human T-cell leukemia virus type II transforms normal human lymphocytes. Proc Natl Acad Sci USA 80:7006–7009

Cordell JL, Falini B, Erber WN, Ghosh AK, Abdulaziz Z, MacDonald ST, Pulford KAF, Stein H, Mason DY (1984) Immunoenzymatic labeling of monoclonal antibodies using immune complexes of alkaline phosphatase and monoclonal anti-alkaline phosphatase (APAAP complexes). J Histochem Cytochem 32:219–229

Moss DJ, Rickinson AB, Pope JH (1978) Long-term T cell-mediated immunity to Epstein-Barr virus in man. I: Complete regression of virus transformation in culture of seropositive donor leukocytes. Int J Cancer 22:662–668

Poppema S (1980) The diversity of immunohistological staining pattern of Sternberg-Rees cells. J Histochem Cytochem 28:788–791

Stein H, Gerdes J, Schwab U, Lemke H, Mason DY, Ziegler A, Schienle W, Diel V (1982) Identification of Hodgkin and Sternberg-Reed cells as a unique cell type derived from a newly detected small cell population. Int J Cancer 30:445–459

Stein H, Gerdes J, Schwab U, Lemke H, Diel V, Mason DY, Bartels H, Ziegler A (1983) Evidence for the detection of the normal counterpart of Hodgkin and Sternberg-Reed cells. Hematological Oncology 1:21–29

Haematology and Blood Transfusion Vol. 29
Modern Trends in Human Leukemia VI
Edited by Neth, Gallo, Greaves, Janka

Production and Characterization of Monoclonal Antibodies Against the Human Leukemic Cell Line K562 *

B. Micheel, V. Böttger, and S. Hering

A. Introduction

The cell line K562 was originally established from a patient with chronic myeloid leukemia (CML) in terminal blast crisis [1]. The cells have the potential of self-renewal and pluripotency to differentiate into progenitors of different blood cells [2]. The aim of the present paper was to produce monoclonal antibodies which might be useful as indicators for the earliest differentiation stages of hematopoiesis and for leukemias transformed at this stage.

B. Reactivity of Monoclonal Anti-K562 Antibodies with Different Cell Lines and Normal Blood Cells

Monoclonal antibodies were produced according to the method of Köhler and Milstein [3] by immunization of BALB/c mice with K562 cells and fusing the spleen cells with X63-Ag.8.653 myeloma line. The first screening by radioimmunobinding assay resulted in 24/90 hybridomas positive for K562 cells. Three antibodies were selected which showed a restricted reactivity pattern when tested against different cell lines and normal blood cells (Table 1).

Antibody Y which was specific for K562 cells reacted with 30%–50%, antibody H with 40%–45%, and antibody C with 60% –64% of the K562 cells. Cloning experiments with K562 cells showed that stable cell clones can be established which express low or high concentrations of the antigen detected by antibody Y.

C. Reactivity of Monoclonal Anti-K562 Antibodies with Human Leukemic Cells of Different Origin

The antibodies Y, H, and C were also tested for reactivity with different human leukemic cells (Table 2). According to the tests summarized in Table 2, antibody Y showed a selective reactivity to myeloid leukemias. This reactivity was especially pronounced in myeloid blast crisis of CML, but not in the chronic phase or lymphoid blast crisis.

D. Future Directions

Further experiments are necessary to clarify whether the antigen detected by antibody Y is a leukemia-associated antigen or a differentiation antigen present on a low percentage of bone marrow stem cells. A comparison with anti-K562 monoclonal antibodies produced by other groups [4, 5] must also be performed to show which antibodies detect identical molecular entities. The practical relevance of the antibodies needs to be proven.

E. Summary

Of the anti-K562 monoclonal antibodies produced in our group:

* Department of Experimental and Clinical Immunology, Central Institute of Cancer Research, Academy of Sciences of the GDR, 1115 Berlin-Buch, Lindenberger Weg 80, GDR

Table 1. Reactivity of three monoclonal anti-K562 antibodies against several cell lines and normal cells of human origin by radioimmunoassay or fixed-cell immunofluorescence

Cells	ZIK-C1-A/D9 (Y)	ZIK-Cl-A/H5 (H)	ZIK-C1-A/C5 (C)
K562	+	+	+ + +
HMy2, NC 37	–	–	+ +, + + +
Reh, SKW-3	–	+, (+)	+ +, + + +
HL-60, Molt-4	–	–, (+)	–, (+)
Mononuclear blood and bone marrow cells	–	+	+ +
Granulocytes	–	+ +	(+)
Erythrocytes	–	–	–

Table 2. Reactivity of three monoclonal anti-K562 antibodies against human leukemic cells

Diagnosis	ZIK-C1-A/D9 (Y)	ZIK-C1-A/H5 (H)	ZIK-C1-A/C5 (C)
T-ALL, T-CLL	0/12[a]	(4)/7	10/11
AUL	(1)/18	(10)/15	(7)/15
0-ALL	0/3	0/1	0/1
B-ALL, B-CLL	0/5	(4)/5	(2)/5
ANLL (mainly AML)	8+(4)/15	7+ (3)/11	7+(1)/9
CML	6+(5)/20	6+(11)/19	3+(4)/15

[a] Number of positive cases divided by total cases tested, weakly positive cases in parentheses

ZIK-C1-A/D9 (Y) reacted exclusively with K562 cells and most AML and CML cells in myeloid blast crisis.
ZIK-C1-B/H5 (H) reacted with K562, AML, and CML cells, and with normal granulocytes and some mononuclear cells.
ZIK-C1-A/F5 (C) reacted with K562 cells and cells of the lymphatic lineage.

References

1. Lozzio CB, Lozzio BB (1975) Blood 45:321
2. Lozzio BB, Lozzio CB, Ichiki AT, Kalmaz GD, Bamberger EG. In: Killmann S-A, Cronkite EP, Müller-Berat CN (eds) Haemopoietic stem cells. Munksgaard, Copenhagen, p 323
3. Köhler G, Milstein C (1975) Nature 256:495
4. Schienle HW, Müller-Ruchholtz W (1981) J Cancer Res Clin Oncol 101:109
5. Young NS, Hwang-Chen SP (1981) Proc Natl Acad Sci USA 78:7073

Immunological Aspects in Malignancy

Haematology and Blood Transfusion Vol. 29
Modern Trends in Human Leukemia VI
Edited by Neth, Gallo, Greaves, Janka

Lymphocyte and Lymphoma Receptors Utilized in Differentiation, in Homing, and in Lymphomagenesis *

I. L. Weissman, M. S. McGrath, R. A. Reichert, W. M. Gallatin, S. Ezine, P. Fink, E. C. Butcher, J. Marian, and H. C. O'Neill

A. Normal Thymic Maturation

The thymus is believed to be the major, if not the sole site of differentiation of T lymphocytes [1, 2]. During fetal development the thymus receives a bolus of precursors of T cells from the hematopoietic organs, probably the fetal liver and/or the yolk sac [3, 4]; these populations subsequently undergo self-renewal as well as maturation [5]. In adult life the thymus receives cells from the bone marrow at a very low level, but in times of stress, or after irradiation, there is a massive renewal of cells in the thymus from bone marrow precursors [2].

The thymus is divisible into a cortex and a medulla. The cortex contains about 85% of the total lymphocyte population, whereas the medulla harbors the remaining 15%. The outer cortical region has a layer of self-renewing blast cells that also gives rise to the majority if not all of the cells in the cortex, as well as to a population that resides in the medulla [1, 6]. The thymus turns over its lymphoid population (at least in the cortex and partially in the medulla) every 3–5 days [1, 2]. Yet the thymus exports only about 1% of the cells in the thymus per day at 4 weeks of life, and 0.1% of the total thymic content at 6 months of age [5].

The "conventional wisdom" about thymus maturation is that the cortex contains functionally immature lymphocytes and that medullary cells are the functionally mature population [7]. Treatment of an animal with cortisone results in disappearance of the lymphoid cortex, while the medulla appears to remain intact. The cell types that are present in the medulla after cortisone share surface phenotypic markers (PNA^{lo}, $H\text{-}2K^{hi}$, TL^{-}) with medullary cells in the intact thymus, and it has been assumed that cortisone-resistant thymocytes = medullary thymocytes = immunocompetent T cells. Here we demonstrate that this notion is wrong, and that what really happens is more complex.

Peripheral, recirculating, immunocompetent T and B lymphocytes bear cell-surface *homing receptors* which specify their adherence to specialized cells lining high-walled endothelial venules (HEV) in peripheral lymphoid organs [8]. At least two *independent* homing receptors have been characterized, one for Peyer's patch HEV and one for lymph node HEV [8]; the latter contains an epitope detected by the monoclonal antibody MEL-14 [9]. In contrast to most peripheral lymphocytes, only 2%–5% of thymocytes are capable of homing to the periphery or binding to the HEV of these peripheral lymphoid organs. The fluorescence-activated cell sorter profile of MEL-14-stained thymocytes showed that about 3% of the cells in the thymus stained brightly and at levels equivalent to most peripheral T cells, while about 85% of the cells stained at 10% of that amount per cell and the remaining 5%–15% had no detectable stain. Where are these homing-competent thymocytes located? According to conventional wisdom, they should be in the medulla.

---

* Dept. of Pathology, Stanford, California 94305, USA

Immunohistochemical analysis of thymic frozen sections reveal, contrary to conventional wisdom, that the MEL-14^{hi} cells in the thymus are in the cortex rather than in the medulla. Do these cells give rise to the thymus cell migrants? Direct intrathymic infusion with fluorescein isothiocyanate labels thymic cells randomly, and allows detection of thymic emigrants. The cells that had homed into the lymph nodes or to the spleen were at least 80%–85% MEL-14^{hi}, and they came from a population of cells (that is, the thymus) in which only 1%–3% of the cells stained at such levels. Since it occurred within 3 h after intrathymic infusion, we concluded that the cells in the thymus which give rise to the major population of emigrants are the MEL-14^{hi} *cortical* cells. The MEL-14^{hi} cells within the thymus are mainly PNA^{lo} and $H\text{-}2K^{hi}$, similar to peripheral T cells (and medullary cells) [10]. Thus, MEL-14^{hi} thymocytes are cortical in location yet express the mature T cell phenotype. To test the *functional* capability of these MEL-14^{hi} thymic cells we did limiting dilution analysis of thymocytes to test their ability to recognize an MHC class I alloantigen by giving rise to clones of cytolytic T cells. The overall frequency of thymic cells which can give rise to allospecific cytolytic clones is about 1 : 10 000 cells. In the MEL-14-highest 2% of cells in the thymus it is 1 : 600, in the MEL-14-lowest 50% of cells, less than 1 : 100 000 [11]. Thus, most of the thymic allospecific cytolytic T cell precursors are MEL-14^{hi} cortical cells.

It appears that the cells in the thymus which are capable of responding to antigen and are capable of giving rise to thymus cell migrants are in the cortex rather than in the medulla. How can we resolve the paradox that 2–5 days after cortisone treatment the thymus contains only a population of cells restricted to the medulla which are immunologically competent, which when put into the bloodstream will home perfectly well, and which includes precursors of killer cells and of helper cells? Following cortisone treatment the *percentage* of cells that are MEL-14^{hi} increases dramatically, but the absolute number of MEL-14^{hi} cells only changes slightly [10]. We proposed that the MEL-14^{hi} cells in the cortex are cortisone-resistant and that most of the other cells in the thymic cortex are cortisone-sensitive. In fact, the thymus of hydrocortisone-treated mice undergoes massive pyknosis for 1–2 days, but among the cells in the thymus which survive are the MEL-14^{hi} subset. By 2 days the surviving MEL-14 cells reside in the medulla [10]. While it seems likely that MEL-14^{hi} cells in the cortex account for a significant proportion of the cortisone-resistant cells which end up in the medulla, we cannot rule out the possibility that there are some cortisone-resistant cells in the medulla which respond to hydrocortisone by becoming MEL-14^{hi} and immunologically competent.

The major set of problems that we have to solve next about thymus cell maturation has to do with *determination* of cells. At what point in their life history do thymic lymphocytes (or their precursors) become *determined* to express a particular surface phenotype (e.g., T4 or T8 in man, or L3T4 or Lyt-2 in the mouse)? At what stage(s) do they rearrange and express the T cell antigen receptor α- and β-chain genes? If these events occur before T cell precursors enter the thymus, the thymus will be mainly a selective microenvironment, whereas if they occur after arriving in the thymus the thymus could also be involved in generating receptor diversity amongst a population of noncommitted cells. At what point do they gain MHC restriction? Self/non-self discrimination? When do they commit to function (help, kill, suppress)? For all these questions we need a way of isolating clones of pre-T cells to follow their progeny in terms of each of these various commitments. We think we have found a way to clone them in vivo. To do this we combine small numbers of bone marrow cells from mice that are genetically Thy-1.2 with a large number of bone marrow cells from mice that are genetically Thy-1.1, and inject them into lethally irradiated mice. The Thy-1.2 cells are present in limiting numbers to allow rare thymus-entering cells to give rise to clonal outgrowths within these thymuses. We identify such clonal outgrowths by immunohistochemical localization of Thy-1.2 foci in host thymuses 3 weeks to 6 months after injection. In

80%–90% of focal (presumably clonal) repopulations, the focus spans both cortex and medulla. In 6/85 cases we found a medulla-only repopulation, and only in one thymus lobe. The medulla in these cases contains cells expressing medullary levels of Thy-1; cortical thymocytes always have about two to three times the amount of Thy-1 that medullary thymocytes have [12]. We have one case of cortex-only repopulation. The incidence of single foci does not change significantly for up to 2 months, and so it appears that a focus, once established, is self-renewing and unlikely to be displaced by another. These experiments show that it is technically feasible to look at clonogenic populations of cells that enter the thymus and reconstitute one region vs another [13]. Thus, it is now feasible to test in vivo at what stage and in which thymic microenvironment T cells gain their various commitments.

B. Receptor-Mediated Lymphogenesis

How is it possible that a retrovirus injected into a susceptible mouse strain will give rise to tumors that arise only in the thymus in a thymus-dependent fashion and after a latent period that can last up to 9 months after injection of the virus? One model that Baird, McGrath, and Weissman developed and tested was based on the receptor-mediated leukemogenesis hypothesis [14, 15]. In that model, these noncytopathic retroviruses selectively infect and transform the subset of those cells within the thymus that have antigen-specific (and/or growth factor) receptors directed against the virus. All clonal progeny of that particular infection and transformation would be cells having high levels of antigen-specific receptors directed against the envelope glycoproteins of the virus that induced them. Proliferation of normal T cells is usually dependent on two events. The first event is engagement of the T cell antigen-specific receptor with antigen, followed by transition of the cells from G_0 to G_1. At least one subset of T cells which engage antigen make a T cell growth factor, TCGF, now called interleukin 2 (IL-2). As a function of antigen recognition at least one other subset of T cells express the IL-2 growth factor receptor, and then proliferate. So proliferation of T lymphocytes depends on antigen recognition for all cell types, and IL-2 recognition by at least a subset of these cells. We proposed that retroviruses cause leukemias by using the normal mitogenic pathway, so that the virus which binds to that antigen-specific receptor can both infect the cell and cause it to undergo blastogenesis. Thus, the daughter cells would continually produce the same virus for which they have antigen-specific receptors, and triggering of these antigen-specific receptors would be an essential part of the mitogenic pathway. By cell-to-cell interaction or virus–cell interaction these daughter cells would be in a positive feedback loop of proliferation. This was (I think) the first autocrine hypothesis. Of course, it is entirely possible that the infected cell is an antigen-presenting cell, and in that context in vivo there would be a *microenvironment-dependent* malignant proliferation of lymphoid cells. We have performed several experiments to try to test (or rule out) the hypothesis, which cannot be explained by any of the cellular oncogene activation models alone (promoter-insertion-mediated oncogene activation, pX-mediated oncogene activation, or enhancer-mediated oncogene activation). More information on these experiments follows:

Is it possible that every T cell lymphoma in fact is a clone of cells having on their surface receptors with a high degree of specificity for the virus that induces the tumor? To test that prediction of the hypothesis we fluoresceinated (or rhodaminated) a number of leukemogenic retroviruses and used the FACS to assay the tumors for virus-binding receptors. Of over 40 T lymphomas examined, all bind their inducing retrovirus, and always with a high degree of specificity [15–17]. Although the high degree of specificity described here matches the diversity of antigen receptors, demonstration of specificity alone does not prove that the binding sites are the T cell receptors.

In a second set of experiments we wanted to determine the relevance of these kinds of receptors to lymphomagnesis in vivo. To study this, we assayed the thymuses of AKR mice (which regularly get tumors somewhere between 6 and 12 months of age) for binding with these various retroviruses. Very few receptors could be found in either the neonatal or the preleukemic period. Receptor-positive thymuses could always transfer donor-derived leukemias to congenic AKR/Thy-1.2 mice, whereas receptor-negative thymuses could not. In some cases, during preleukemic thymic involution the residual cells in the thymus were 50%–85% virus-binding population. FACS sorting of virus-binding cells in these cases gave rise to donor-derived leukemias upon transfer; virus-nonbinding cells from the same thymuses failed to give rise to donor-derived leukemia [17]. Whatever these receptors are, they are a clear diagnostic sign for leukemia cells.

Is virus binding required for lymphoma cell proliferation? We raised a number of monoclonal antibodies directed against AKR lymphoma cell surface determinants to check for those that would block virus binding. Four antibodies were found that blocked virus binding. Three of the four were directed against the Thy-1 determinant. The four antibodies that block virus binding were also antiproliferative; up to 1:10 000 dilution of them blocked 90% of thymidine incorporation into AKR lymphoma cells, while antibodies to other cell surface determinants could not [18]. Presaturation of the surface of these cells with high concentrations of purified cognate retrovirus allowed the cells to proliferate in the presence of the blocking antibodies. Other viruses that bind less well to the cell surface do not protect against the antiproliferative effect. Antibody inhibition of proliferation has been shown with KKT-2 cells [18] and S49 cells [19]. It is difficult to explain this finding by any other retrovirus leukemogenesis hypothesis.

C. Are the Virus Receptors on Lymphoma Cells Antigen Receptors?

Allison was the first to produce a monoclonal antibody that identifies the antigen-specific T cell receptor heterodimer, using a particular T cell tumor called C6VL [20]. C6VL is a RadLV-induced tumor. The anti-T cell receptor antibody, Mab124-40, was a clonotypic antibody; it recognized a variable region determinant on the C6VL T cell receptor. Mab124-40 – C6VL T cell receptor immune complexes were used to raise a rabbit antibody, 8177, which recognizes T cell receptors on many different T cells [21]. To test C6VL-RadLV/C6VL interactions we developed a plate-binding assay in which a microtiter plate is precoated with dilutions of retrovirus and then cells are added for binding; the washed plates are poststained for cells with Rose Bengal. C6VL cells bind to RadLV/C6VL at high virus dilutions, to RadLV/VL3 slightly less well, and to KKT-2 SL (an AKR leukemia virus) only poorly. The clonotypic antibody Mab124-40 significantly blocks binding of the cells to the plate over a 30-fold dilution range, as does 8177. Antibodies to H-$2D^b$ determinants on these cells do not block binding. These experiments indicate that virus receptors do exist on C6VL cells, and that the virus receptor is *at* or *near* the T cell antigen-specific receptors for this lymphoma.

We have strong evidence in two other systems that retrovirus binding is to an antigen-specific receptor. One of these systems is the B cell lymphoma, called BCL_1, described by Slavin and Strober [22]. BCL_1 is a B cell tumor which expresses high levels of IgM and low levels of IgD, and grows in animals as a spleen-dependent tumor [23, 24]. The in vivo BCL_1 tumor dies rapidly in vitro as a lymphoid cell suspension, but in vitro it persists in clusters with $I\text{-}A^+$ surface-adherent cells. The BCL_1 lymphocytes produce no retrovirus, but the adherent cells produce high levels of particles with the classical retrovirus polypeptide profile. BCL_1 X NS1 hybridomas produce and secrete the BCL_1 immunoglobulin. Plate-bound BCL_1 hybridoma immunoglobulin binds the retrovirus produced by those adherent cells, while other myeloma immunoglobulins of the same class do not. Anti-μ, anti-BCL_1 anti-idiotype, and even anti-gp70 antibodies block virus binding to this purified immunoglobulin. The anti-idiotype antibodies also block binding of the virus to the cell. Thus BCL_1 is one case in which the virus binding entity is an immunoglobulin on the cell surface.

The best example of what appears to be insertion activation of cellular *myc* genes is the avian leukosis system. We expected that these avian leukosis virus-induced bursal lymphomas would not have immunoglobulins that bound ALV, but that is probably wrong. We obtained from J.M. Bishop a bursal tumor called SC2L, induced by RAV ALV. Labeled RAV virus binds well to SC2L cells, and added cold RAV blocks in the binding as expected. Isolated SC2L chicken immunoglobulin stuck to a plate binds labeled RAV, and that binding is blocked with cold RAV or with Max Cooper's monoclonal anti-chicken light chain antibodies. The same antibodies block RAV binding to SC2L cells, whereas anti-Ia antibodies do not (Ia is abundant on SC2L cells). The anti-light chain antibodies also block RAV binding to bursal lymphomas as they arise in vivo, using samples provided by G. Gasic and W. Hayward. The large bursal cells which are abundant in the preleukemic period do not bind RAV. If one believes that the virus binding shown has relevance to the leukemogenic process, these experiments show that virus binding does not drive preleukemic bursal cell proliferation. Thus, as in the AKR model, the appearance of cells bearing high levels of leukemogenic retrovirus receptors heralds the leukemic state.

Finally, in preliminary experiments we have done binding studies with HTLV. ATL cells bind it well, and this binding can be blocked with cold HTLV. Although we have evidence that monoclonal antibodies to a number of T cell determinants do not inhibit HTLV binding to ATL cells, we have not completed that analysis and do not yet have antibodies to the human T cell receptor heterodimer.

References

1. Weissman I (1967) Thymus cell migration. J Exp Med 126:291
2. Cantor H, Weissman IL (1976) Development and function of subpopulations of thymocytes and T lymphocytes. Prog Allergy 20:1
3. Jotereau FV, LeDouarin NM (1982) Demonstration of a cyclic renewal of lymphocyte precursor cells in the quail thymus during embryonic and perinatal life. J Immunol 129:1869
4. Weissman I, Papaioannou V, Gardner R (1978) Fetal hematopoietic origins of the adult hematolymphoid system. In: Clarkson B, Marks PA, Till JE (eds) Cold Spring Harbor Meeting on Differentiation of Normal and Neoplastic Hematopoietic Cells. pp 33–47
5. Scollay R, Butcher E, Weissman IL (1980) Thymus cell migration. Quantitative aspects of cellular traffic from the thymus to the periphery in mice. Eur J Immunol 10:210
6. Weissman I (1973) Thymus cell maturation: studies on the origin of cortisone-resistant thymic lymphocytes. J Exp Med 137:504
7. Scollay R, Shortman K (1983) Thymus 5:245
8. Butcher EC, Weissman IL (1984) Lymphoid tissues and organs. In: Paul WE (ed) Fundamental immunology. Raven, New York, pp 109–127
9. Gallatin WM, Weissman IL, Butcher EC (1983) A cell surface molecule involved in organ-specific homing of lymphocytes. Nature 304:30
10. Reichert RA, Gallatin WM, Butcher EC, Weissman IL (1984) A homing receptor-bearing cortical thymocyte subset: implications for thymus cell migration and the nature of cortisone-resistant thymocytes. Cell 38:89
11. Fink PJ, Gallatin WM, Reichert RA, Butcher EC, Weissman IL (1985) Homing receptor-bearing thymocytes: an immunocompetent cortical subpopulation. Nature 3/3:233
12. Fathman CG, Small M, Herzenberg LA, Weissman IL (1975) Thymus cell maturation. II: Differentiation of three "mature" subclasses in vivo. Cell Immunol 15:109
13. Ezine SV, Weissman IL, Rouse RV (1984) Bone marrow cells give rise to distinct cell clones within the thymus. Nature 309:629
14. Weissman IL, Baird S (1977) Oncornavirus leukemogenesis as a model for selective neoplastic transformation. In: Koprowski H (ed) Neoplastic transformation: mechanisms and consequences. (Life sciences research report no. 7)
15. McGrath MS, Weissman IL (1978) A receptor mediated model of viral leukemogenesis: hypothesis and experiments. In: Clarkson B, Marks PA, Till JE (eds) Cold Spring Harbor Meeting on Differentiation of Normal and Neoplastic Hematopoietic Cells. pp 577–589
16. McGrath MS, Pillemer E, Kooistra D, Weissman IL (1980) The role of MuLV receptors

on T lymphoma cells in lymphoma cell proliferation. Contemp Top Immunobiol 11: 257–284
17. McGrath MS, Weissman IL (1979) AKR leukemogenesis: identification and biological significance of thymic lymphoma receptors for AKR retroviruses. Cell 17:65
18. McGrath MS, Pillemer E, Weissman IL (1980) Murine leukemogenesis: monoclonal antibodies to cell determinants which arrest T lymphoma cell proliferation. Nature 285:259
19. McGrath MS, Jerabek L, Pillemer E, Steinberg RA, Weissman IL (1981) Receptor-mediated murine leukemogenesis: monoclonal antibody-induced lymphoma cell growth arrest. In: Neth R (ed) Modern trends in human leukemia, vol 4. Springer, Berlin Heidelberg New York (Haematology and blood transfusion, vol 26)
20. Allison JP, McIntyre BW, Bloch D (1982) J Immunol 129:2293
21. McIntyre BW, Allison JP (1983) Cell 34:739
22. Slavin S, Strober S (1977) Spontaneous murine B cell leukemia. Nature 272:624
23. Knapp MR, Jones PO, Black SJ, Vitetta ES, Slavin S, Strober S (1979) Characterization of the spontaneous murine B cell leukemia (BCL_1). I: Cell surface expression of IgM, IgD, Ia, and FCR. J Immunol 123:1000
24. Kotzin B, Strober S (1980) Role of the spleen in the growth of a B cell leukemia. Science 208:259

Haematology and Blood Transfusion Vol. 29
Modern Trends in Human Leukemia VI
Edited by Neth, Gallo, Greaves, Janka

Quantitative Expression and Function of Differentiation Antigens on Normal and Malignant Lymphoid Cells

E. A. Clark [1], L. M. Rose [1], G. Shu [1], P. A. Dindorf [2], I. D. Bernstein [2], and J. A. Ledbetter [1]

A. Introduction

As lymphocytes differentiate, the expression of certain cell surface polypeptides can change both quantitatively and qualitatively. A classic example of quantitative variation is murine Thy-1 which decreases over five- to tenfold in density as thymocytes differentiate into mature T cells. What functions these quantitative variations may play for the most part is not known. However, variations in Ia antigen densities can profoundly affect immune responsiveness, and this has been postulated to play a central role in immunoregulation [12]. During lymphoid cell activation, the amount of certain antigens such as CD3 (T3) may decrease dramatically [21], while densities of other antigens may increase [15]. It has been suggested that IL-2 receptors increase in density after T cell activation as a means of promoting autocrine-induced proliferation [11].

A standard method for analyzing normal and malignant lymphoid cell phenotypes is to detect the presence or absence of various cell surface antigens with monoclonal antibodies (MoAb) and immunofluorescent or immunoperoxidase methods. A model put forward by Greaves at the last Wilsede meeting [7] and by others is that lymphoid malignancies suffer "maturational arrest" and that the heterogeneity observed for lymphoid leukemias and lymphomas reflects different stages of normal differentiation. The importance of considering quantitative as well as qualitative differences in leukemia or lymphoma phenotypes has been noted [6, 8], but not uniformly applied. Recently, quantitative flow cytometry and two-color immunofluorescence have been used to phenotype normal lymphocyte populations into more discrete subsets [14, 16, 17]. Here we present a summary of our structural and functional studies of lymphocyte surface structures on normal and malignant B and T cell populations using quantiative two-color flow cytometry.

B. Materials and Methods

I. Antibodies

The MoAb to B cell-associated antigens used in this study have been described [2, 4, 13]. They include 2H7 and 1F5 specific for the pan-B cell antigen Bp32; 2C3 anti-μ chain; δ-TA4-1 anti-δ chain; HB10a anti-HLA-DR; H616 anti-p76 B cell antigen; 3AC5 anti-p220 pan-leukocyte antigen; and 24.1 anti-p100, CD10 (cALLA) antigen. T cell-specific MoAb described according to the international nomenclature [1, 9] were G19-4 anti-Tp19-29, CD3; G3-7 anti-Tp41, CD7; 9.6 anti-Tp50, CD5 (E receptor); 10.2 anti-Tp67, CD2; G19-2 anti-Tp55, CD4 ($T_{h/i}$); G10-1 anti-Tp32, CD8 ($T_{s/c}$); and 9.3 anti-Tp44. The antibodies were purified and conjugated with fluorescein (green) or phycoerythrin (PE) (red) as described [15, 17].

1 Genetic Systems Corporation
2 Pediatric Oncology Program, Fred Hutchinson Cancer Research Center, Seattle, Washington 98121,USA USA

II. Cell, Preparation, Staining, and Flow Cytometry

Lymphoid cells were purified on Ficoll density gradients and stained with directly conjugated MoAb as described [5, 17]. Because only directly conjugated antibodies of high affinity were used, for cell populations of relatively uniform size, fluorescence intensity is a good indicator of antigen density. For two-color flow cytometry, a FACS IV with a single laser to excite fluorescein or PE was used [15].

C. Results and Discussion

I. Normal B Lymphocyte Populations

The quantitative expression of certain B cell surface polypeptides differs in different lymphoid tissues. For example, both HLA-DR and B4 antigens are expressed at higher densities on splenic and tonsillar B cells than on circulating blood B cells [19, 15]. The pan-B antigen Bp32 is expressed over a range of densities on tonsillar B cells [15]. Using two-color methods, we have found that B cells in tonsils can be classified into three phenotypes: $Bp32^{bright}$ ($Bp32^{bri}$) $IgM^{dull/neg}$ cells, $Bp32^{dull}IgM^{bri}IgD^{-}$ cells, and $Bp32^{dull}IgM^{bri}IgD^{+}$ cells. B cells found in the germinal center of secondary follicles are $Bp32^{bri}IgM^{dull/neg}$ while B cells in the mantle zones are $Bp32^{dull}IgM^{bri}IgD^{+}$ [16]. B cells expressing Tp67 (T1 or Ly1) are of great interest since chronic lymphocytic leukemias (CLL) are $Tp67^{+}$ [18] and $Ly1^{+}$ B cells are elevated in mice with lupus-like autoimmune disease [10]. Using the sensitive two color systems, we have not been able definitively to identify Tp67 B cells in B cell-enriched fractions of cord blood, adult blood, spleen, tonsils, lymph nodes, or bone marrow. If $Tp67^{+}$ B cells are present in normal lymphoid tissues, they are in quite small numbers, are localized in certain areas, or are expressed only at certain times in development.

II. Malignant B Cell Phenotypes

The intensity of antigen expression on chronic lymphocytic leukemias (CLL) and a variety of non-Hodgkin's lymphomas was evaluated [15]. As summarized in Table 1, for CLL antigen, densities for Bp32, sIgM, and HLA-DR vary over roughly a 10- to 25-fold range. The same markers generally are expressed at higher density and vary over a 100- to 500-fold range for the more heterogeneous non-Hodgkin's lymphomas. The Tp67 antigen in contrast is expressed at higher density on CLL than lymphomas. Five of the $Bp32^{+}sIgM^{+}$ samples (16%) expressed significant but low levels ($\geqq 2.0$) of the Tp50 Er marker. In our screen of normal adult lymphoid tissues, we did detect either Er^{+} or $Tp67^{+}$ B cells. Using two-color analyses with Tp67, Bp32, or HLA-DR as markers, at least three distinct phenotypes for CLL were detectable [15].

A small number of non-T, non-B ALL were screened using two-color IF (Figs. 1 and 2). The most informative combination for phemotyping $cALLA^{-}$ ALL was measuring p220 levels versus HLA-DR expression (Fig. 1); three phenotypes were evident: $p220^{bri}DR^{dull/bri}$ (ALL 1); $p220^{bri}DR^{bri}$ (ALL 2); and $p220^{-}DR^{bri}$ (ALL 3). The $cALLA^{+}$ ALL generally had higher levels of HLA-DR and lower levels of p220 than the $cALLA^{-}$ ALL (Table 1). Using green-anti-cALLA versus red-anti-Bp32 or HLA-DR, several phenotypes were detected (Fig. 2). Patient 4's leukemic cells were $cALLA^{dull}Bp32^{dull/neg}$ and HLA-DR^{bri}; patients 5 and 6 both had $cALLA^{bri}Bp32^{dull/neg}$ leukemic cells. However, ALL 5 cells were uniformly DR^{bri} while ALL 6 cells displayed a range of DR densities.

These results show that monoclonal leukemias can be quite heterogeneous in the patterns of surface antigen intensities they display. Apparently, phenotypes indicative of more than one stage of differentiation can be expressed. Two major tasks remain: (a) to relate malignant phenotype to normal lymphoid cell phenotypes – thus far we have not been able to identify the normal cell counterparts of many of our malignant cell phenotypes; and (b) to classify a battery of leukemias and lymphomas based on two-color phenotypes and assess the prognostic value of the classification.

Fig. 1. Quantitative two-color phenotypes of cALLA$^-$ non-T, non-B acute lymphocytic leukemias. Data of 25 000 cells plotted cell number (*vertical axis*) and log green fluorescence (anti-p220) versus log red fluorescence (anti-DR) (*upper left*). About every 4–5 *dots* represents a doubling of fluorescence. ALL 1, a leukemia with p220^{bri}DR$^{dull/bri}$ cells; ALL 2, a second leukemia with p220^{bri}DR^{bri} cells; ALL 3, a third leukemia with p220$^-$DR^{bri} cells

III. Normal T Cells

Two-color cytofluorographic methods have also been used to phenotype new T cell populations. We have conjugated a large panel of MoAb with FITC or PE and tested a variety of two-color combinations. The expression of so-called pan-T cell antigens on CD4$^+$ (T4) T helper/inducer ($T_{h/i}$) cells,

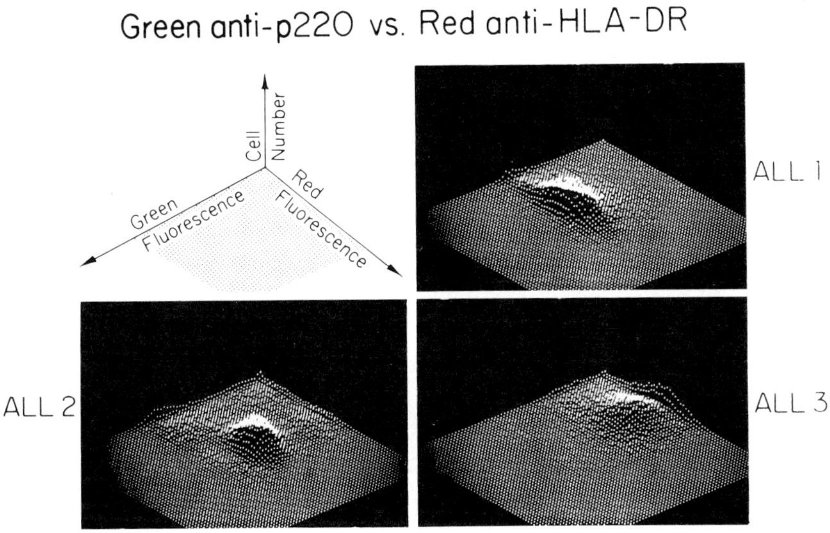

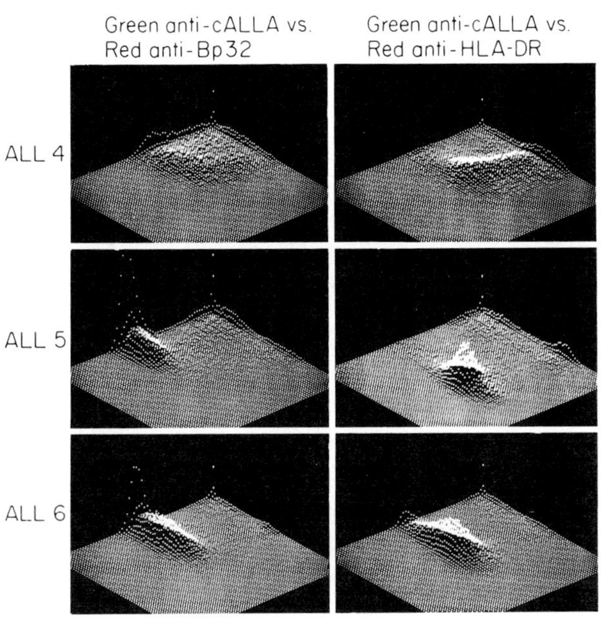

Fig. 2. Quantitative two-color phenotypes of cALLA$^+$ non-T, non-B acute lymphocytic leukemias. *Left column,* green cALLA versus red-Bp32; *right column,* green cALLA versus red-HLA-DR. Each *row* is a different leukemia. ALL 4, cALLA^{dull}Bp32$^{dull/neg}$DR$^{dull/bri}$ cells; ALL 5, cALLA^{bri}Bp32$^{dull/neg}$ DR^{bri} cells; ALL 6, cALLA^{bri} Bp32$^{dull/neg}$DR$^{neg/bri}$ cells

Table 1. Relative antigen expression on B and T cell malignancies

Condition	No.	Mean relative fluorescence intensity[a] (range) using Ab to:										
		Bp32	SIgM	DR	cALLA (CD10)	p220	Tp67 (CD5)	Tp50 (CD2)	Tp19 (CD3)	Tp41 (CD7)	Tp55 (CD4)	Tp32 (CD8)
CLL	15	19.1 (3–49)	1.8 (1–6)	81.3 (8–209)			18.5 (2–42)	2.8 (1–26)				
Non-Hodgkin's lymphomas	16	80.6 (11–189)	65.0 (1–451)	243.3 (19–1154)			5.9 (1–23)	1.5 (1–4)				
ALL												
Non-T, B cALLA$^-$	4	1.0	1.0	19.5 (8–37)	1.4 (1–2)	32.6 (2–63)						
Non-T, B cALLA$^+$	5	2.6 (1–5)	1.6 (1–2)	103.3 (36–215)	54.4 (3–112)	11.5 (3–22)						
T	10	1.1		1.3 (1–2)[b]			8.4 (1–17)	24.1 (1–184)	4.6 (1–22)	98.7 (2–239)	7.3 (1–31)	10.2 (1–56)
Normal PBL-B	3	275.3 (246–314)	15.1 (5–20)	74.5 (54–100)			1.3 (1–2)	1.0				
T		1.4	1.0	1.2			67	47	93	49	51	179

[a] Fluorescence intensity is a ratio of brightness of peak of malignant cells/brightness of peak of negative control Ab-stained cells (autofluorescence). For all experiments, direct IF was used and measured on a FACS IV cell sorter

[b] One Er^+ sample, DR = 177

$CD8^+$ (T8) T cytotoxic/suppressor ($T_{s/c}$) cells, and Fc receptor$^+$ (T_γ) T cells on normal periphery was examined [17]. The pan-T cell antigens split into four groups: (a) markers expressed on all $CD4^+$ cells and on $CD8^{bri}$ cells, but not on $CD8^{dull}$ or T_γ cells – CD3 (T3), CD5 (Tp67), and 9.3 (Tp441); (b) markers expressed on all $CD4^+$ and $CD8^+$ cells, but not all T_γ cells – CD2 (Er); (c) markers expressed on all $CD8^+$ and T_γ^+ cells, but not all $CD4^+$ cells – CD7; and (e) markers expressed on all T cell subsets – Tp90. The $T_{h/i}$, $T_{c/s}$, and T_γ cell subsets could be further divided into distinct subpopulations with appropriate two-color combinations (Rose et al., in preparation).

IV. T Cell Malignancies

A panel of ten T cell ALL displayed a range of antigen intensities (Table 1). As reflected by our studies with normal T cells, the most common or widely distributed marker in this panel was the CD7 antigen; CD7 also was consistently expressed at high densities, while many of the other antigens were expressed at lower levels than detected on normal T cells.

V. Functions of Bp32 and Tp32 Polypeptides

The functions of most B and T cell surface antigens are not known; insights into the functions of these molecules may assist in helping us understand leukemogenesis better and may help us design new approaches for diagnosis and therapy. Recently, we have focused on the functions of the B cell-specific polypeptide Bp32 and the $T_{s/c}$-specific polypeptide Tp32, and not solely because we like the number 32 [16]. Monoclonal antibodies to the Bp32 antigen, either alone or in conjunction with T cell factors, stimulate B cells to proliferate. The MoAb act directly on B cells and do not appear to require accessory cells. Anti-μ blocks this effect, suggesting that Bp32 may have to interact with the Ig receptor to activate B cells. Thus, like the CD3 (T3) molecule for T cells, the Bp32 structure plays a role in B cell activation.

The Tp32 molecule is thought to play some role in class I recognition by $T_{c/s}$ cells [20]. Recently, we have demonstrated for the first time that Tp32 molecules physically associate with the class I T cell differentiation antigen Thy,p45 (CD1) on thymocytes [16]. Tp32 appears to be an alternative structure for β_2-microglobulin (β_2M) and class I molecules since β_2M is not associated with the Tp32–Thy,p45 complex. We believe that Tp32 associates with different class I molecules during the course of differentiation and selection/education of cortical thymocytes into mature T cells. At each stage, it is possible that Tp32 plays an important role in allowing or promoting class I recognition.

Acknowledgments. This work was supported by Genetic Systems Corporation and National Institutes of Health Grants CA34199, AI20432, and CA09351.

References

1. Bernard A, Boumsell L, Dausset J, Milstein C, Schlossman SF (eds) (1984) Leukocyte typing. Springer, Berlin, 814 pp
2. Braun MP, Martin PJ, Ledbetter JA, Hansen JA (1983) Blood 61:718–725
3. Clark EA, Yokochi T (1984) In: Bernard A, Boumsell L, Dausset J, Milstein C, Schlossman SF (eds) Leucoyte typing. Springer, Berlin, pp 339–346
4. Clark EA, Shu G, Ledbetter EA (1985) Proc Nat Acad Sci USA 82:1766–1770
5. Clark EA, Ledbetter JA, Holly RD, Shu G, Dindorf P, Sturge JC (1985) Hum Immunol (in press)
6. Godal T, Lindmo T, Ruud E, Heikkila R, Henriksen A, Steen HB, Marton PF (1981) Haematol Blood Transfus 26:314–319
7. Greaves MF (1983) Haematol Blood Transfus 28:3–10
8. Greaves MF, Robinson JB, Delia D, Ritz J, Schlossman S, Sieff C, Goldstein G, Kung P, Bollum FJ, Edwards PAW (1981) Haematol Blood Transfus 26:285–304
9. Hansen JA, Martin PJ, Beatty PG, Clark EA, Ledbetter JA (1984) In: Bernard A, Boumsell L, Dausset J, Milstein C, Schlossman SF (eds) Leukocyte typing. Springer, Berlin, pp 195–212
10. Hayakawa K, Hardy RR, Parks DR, Herzenberg LA (1983) J Exp Med 157:202–218
11. Hemler ME, Brenner MB, McLean JM, Strominger JL (1984) Proc Nat Acad Sci USA 81:2172–2175

12. Janeway CA Jr, Bottomly K, Babich J, Conrad P, Conzen S, Jones B, Kaye J, Katz M, McVay L, Murphy DB, Tite J (1984) Immunol Today 5:99–105
13. Kuritani T, Cooper MD (1982) J Exp Med 155:839–848
14. Lanier LL, Loken MR (1984) J Immunol 132:151–156
15. Ledbetter JA, Clark EA (1985) Human Immunol (in press)
16. Ledbetter JA, Tsu T, Clark EA (1985) J Immunol (in press)
17. Ledbetter JA, Tsu T, Draves K, Clark EA (1985) Perspectives in Immunogenetics and Histocompatibility 6 (in press)
18. Martin PJ, Hansen JA, Nowinski RC, Brown MA (1980) Immunogenetics 11:429–439
19. Nadler LM, Anderson KC, Marti G, Bates M, Park E, Daley JF, Schlossman SF (1983) J Immunol 131:244–250
20. Reinherz EL, Meuer SC, Schlossman SF (1983) Immunol Today 4:5–8
21. Zanders ED, Lamb JR, Feldmann M, Green N, Beverley PC (1983) Nature 303:625–628

Haematology and Blood Transfusion Vol. 29
Modern Trends in Human Leukemia VI
Edited by Neth, Gallo, Greaves, Janka

Development of B Cell Subpopulations in Humans and its Relevance to Malignancy

G. Janossy [1], F. Caligaris-Cappio [2], M. Bofill [1], D. Campana [1, 2], and M. Janossa [3]

A. Introduction

B cell lineages are influenced by antigen-independent development and by immune activation when antigens stimulate the development of both memory B and plasma cell clones. It is difficult to investigate the origin of B cell malignancies without knowing the details of these physiological events. In 1974, Salmon and Seligmann [1] suggested that the various types of B lymphoid malignancies may derive from normal cells representing different levels of maturation. In addition, the degree of differentiation which takes place within the malignant clone also seems to be variable: some malignant cells, e.g. chronic lymphocytic leukaemia (CLL), are apparently "fixed" and unable to differentiate further, while in another disease, e.g. myeloma, the lymphoid or lymphoplasmacytoid "target cells" of malignancy differentiate into plasma cells. In our study we have, therefore, decided to approach the origin of B lymphoid disorders with a simple approach by asking the following questions:

1. What are the phenotypic features of B lymphocytes as they emerge in the normal bone marrow (BM) during childhood? The main aim here has been to find an answer to the question whether B cell populations in the BM versus peripheral lymphoid organs have mutually distinctive features.

2. How do B cells develop in the normal fetus? Do B cells at different sites show distinct phenotypic features? In this part of the study samples of fetal BM, para-aortic lymph nodes and spleen have been studied.

3. Can B cell types (and the corresponding B cell malignancies) change their features when stimulated in vitro?

There have been many previous clues about the early stages of B cell differentiation both in humans and animals (reviewed in [2, 3]). Small to medium-sized lymphoid cells with terminal transferase (TdT) enzyme activity are the likely precursors of larger pre-B cells which synthesize small amounts of cytoplasmic (Cy) μ heavy chain first, but no light chain [4, 5]. These pre-B cells, in turn, give rise to B cells with membrane IgM, but no IgD expression, and probably also to a proportion of IgM^+, IgD^+ B cells during the next stage of development [2, 6]. But these latter cells constitute a mixture: some of them (particularly during secondary responses) appear to return to the BM from the peripheral lymphoid organs [7]. Our aim has been to establish the reactivity of these cell types using a wide range of monoclonal antibodies (MoAb) against various non-Ig membrane antigens in combination with the analysis of Ig isotype expression. Thus, the purpose of the study is to endow the hypothetical differentiation scheme with further discriminating reagents. Clearly, Ig isotype expression alone is not sufficient for clear discrimination; e.g. mature B cells lose IgD [6]; IgM^+, IgD^- cells, without

1 Department of Immunology, Royal Free Hospital School of Medicine, London, NW3 2QG
2 Clinica Medica I, University of Turin, Italy
3 1st Department of Medicine, Semmelweiss University, Budapest, Hungary

further markers, cannot be affiliated to a given (early or late) maturation stage.

B. Methods

"Double-marker" methods were used with green fluorescein (FITC)- and red rhodamine (TRITC)-labelled antibodies in various combinations [4, 8]. For example, the reactivity of MoAb was studied on TdT$^+$ cells (labelled with rabbit anti-TdT) and μ^+ as well as δ^+ B cells (labelled with an anti-IgM and anti-IgD antisera, heavy chain specific, respectively). The overall proportion of μ^+, δ^- and μ^+, δ^+ cells was also determined in each sample. In histology the same double-immunofluorescence technique [8] and immunoperoxidase was used together with haematoxylin counterstaining on sections of frozen biopsies.

The induction of differentiation changes using 12-*O*-tetradecanoylphorbol-13-acetate (phorbol ester: TPA) was an empirical method to assess links between cells expressing different phenotypes. The concentration of TPA in experiments with cell lines was 10^{-7} *M* and with leukaemic cells was 1.6×10^{-8} *M* [9, 10].

The samples used were from normal child BM or regenerating samples taken from cessation of chemotherapy for AML or ALL. The fetal tissues were from medically approved abortions. All suspensions, including samples from patients with chronic lymphocytic (CLL), hairy cell leukaemia (HCL) and blood samples from normal donors, were separated on Ficoll–Hypaque gradients.

C. Results

I. Phenotypic Differences Between B Cells in the BM and Peripheral Lymphoid Organs

The MoAb used are shown in Table 1. The important common feature of B1, To15, RFB-4, RFB-6 and Y29/55 is that, when tested in double-marker combination with IgM in suspensions of blood and tonsil, these reagents react with >92% of IgM$^+$ B cells. These are, therefore, pan-B reagents by these criteria. Still, when these antibodies were tested on BM B cells, a heterogeneity emerged which was related to the cells' Ig isotype. While the IgM$^+$, IgD$^+$ cells showed the characteristic pan-B staining (>92% IgD$^+$ cells positive) with all these antibodies, the IgM$^+$, IgD$^-$ population was, in contrast, essentially negative with To15, RFB-4 and RFB-6 and had only about 50% reactivity with Y29/55. In addition, pre-B cells and the TdT$^+$ BM precursors were also negative with this set of B reagents (Table 2). These results can be interpreted to indicate that membrane antigens appear during B cell development in an orderly fashion. B1 is an "early marker" positive on the whole lineage starting from TdT$^+$ cells [11]. Other markers such as Y29/55 appear halfway through the generation of IgM$^+$ cells, and additional markers To15, RFB-4 and RFB-6 are expressed when IgM$^+$ cells also acquire IgD$^+$ and become functionally mature B cells. (This confirms previous results with RFA-2 and RFA-3; [12].)

There are two additional facts to support this scheme. First, another antibody, AL-1, showed a complementary pattern: strongly positive on TdT$^+$ and pre-B cells, weaker on IgM$^+$, IgD$^-$ cells, but negative on the mature IgD$^+$ B cells of peripheral lymphoid tissue (Table 2). Second, the antigens To15 and RFB-4, albeit absent from the cell membrane of pre-B and IgM$^+$, IgD$^-$ cells, can be found in the cytoplasm of the same cells. As Campana et al. [9] have recently shown, blast cells in fresh cases of common acute lymphoblastic leukaemia and permanent cell lines of non-T, non-B and pre-B type (KM3, REH and NALM-6) also show a cytoplasmic, but no membrane, expression of To15 and RFB-4. The interesting additional result is that these lines start expressing membrane To15 and RFB-4 when incubated with TPA for 48–72 h. It seems therefore that not only cytoplasmic μ can change to membrane IgM during B cell development, but some other molecules also demonstrate a similar sequence of events [9].

II. Investigations of Fetal BM

Around the 17th gestational week the BM contains large numbers (40%) of lymphoid-

Table 1. Antibodies and heterologous antisera used in this study

Name	Source	Reactivity	Species and class	Molecular weight
Monoclonal Ab-s				
AL-1	A. M. Lebacq	Pre-B, B	Rat IgG_2	120 k
BA-1	T. LeBien and Hybritech (Cat. No. 0452)	Pre-B, B, polymorph	Mouse IgM	30 k
B1	Coulter (Cat. No. 6602140)	Few pre-B, B	Mouse IgG_2	32 k
To15	D.Y. Mason and Dakopatt (Cat. No. M708)	B	Mouse IgG	140 k
RFB4	Royal Free Hospital	B	Mouse IgG_1	140 k
RFB6	Royal Free Hospital	B	Mouse IgG_1	180 k
Y29/55	H.K. Forster	B	Mouse IgG_2	
Anti-Tac	Drs. Uchiyama & Waldmann	IL-2 receptor	Mouse IgG	
SHCL-3	Dr. G. Schwarting	Hairy cell leukaemia, monocytes	Mouse IgG	
Heterologous antisera				
Anti-Hu IgM – $F(ab')_2$	Kallestad (Cat. No. 140)		Goat	900 k
Anti-Hu IgD – $F(ab')_2$	Kallestad (Cat. No. 138–148)		Goat	190 k
Anti-Ia	Royal Free Hospital		Chicken	28 + 33 k
Anti-TdT	F. J. Bollum and Supertech (Cat. No. 004)		Rabbit	67 k

Table 2. The reactivity of pre-B and B cells in the infant (4 samples) and regenerating bone marrow (4 samples) with B cell-specific Ab[a]

Ab	TdT^+	Pre-B	$sIgm^+$ B cells Total	$sIgD^{+b}$
Heterologous antisera				
sIgD	<1	<1	33±7	100
Monoclonal antibodies				
AL-1	70±5	80±9	83 ±5	53±2
BA-1	80±6	98±1	98 ±1	92±3
B1	10±2	98±1	97 ±3	98±1
To15	<1	<1	24 ±10[c]	98±1
RFB-4	<1	<1	25 ±4[c]	94±3
RFB-6	<1	<1	23 ±6[c]	92±4
Y29/55	<1	<1	71.3±3[c]	98±0.5

[a] Results are expressed as percentage of cells membrane-labelled with MoAb within the given population. The ranges of these populations in the samples are: TdT^+ cells 0.5%–12%; pre-B cells ($cy\mu^+$) 0.1%–1.5%; $sIgM^+$ B cells 5%–10% of Ficoll-Triosil-separated cells

[b] These cells also express IgM ($sIgM^+$, IgD^+) and represent a subset (33%±7%) of all $sIgM^+$ cells

[c] Within the $To15^+$, $RFB\text{-}4^+$, $RFB\text{-}6^+$ and $Y29/55^+$ populations the following percentages are $sIgD^+$: 91%, 85%, 92% and 57%

[d] The $sIgM^+$ B cells in the fetal bone marrow at 17–20th gestational week are largely (>90%) $sIgD^-$, $AL1^+$, $BA1^+$, $B1^+$, and $To15^-$, $RFB4^-$, $RFB6^-$ (see [13])

Table 3. B cell subpopulations in the developing human fetus[a]

Phenotype of relevant cells	Gestational week			
	Bone marrow 16–22	Spleen 16–22	Lymph node 16	Lymph node 17–22
Precursor TdT$^+$, IgM$^-$	5–20 (scattered)	<5	NT	NT
TdT$^-$, IgM$^+$, IgD$^-$, T1$^-$	70–80	10–20	95 (both rows)	<10
B IgM$^+$, IgD$^+$, T1$^-$	2– 5	80–90		In diffuse areas >90
IgM$^+$, IgD$^+$, T1$^+$	0.1–0.9	1–2	<5	In clusters >90 (Fig. 1)[b]
T cells IgM$^-$, T1$^+$ (T3$^+$, T11$^+$)	1%–2.5% of mononuclear cells	In separate T areas	In diffuse lymphoid zone (Fig. 1)	

[a] The results shown refer to the percentage of cells within the B lineage (unless otherwise indicated), determined by the following labelling combinations: TdT/IgM; IgM/IgD; IgM/RFT1 (T1 antigen; 67 k); IgM/UCHT1 (T3 antigen; 19 k); IgM/RFT11 (T11 antigen; 50 k). In the 16-week-old LN samples only IgM/RFT1 and IgM/UCHT1 combinations were tested

[b] The clusters are formed around follicular dendritic reticulum cells

looking cells. Of these 15%–25% were TdT$^+$ and a further 5%–10% were cytoplasmic IgM$^+$ pre-B cells; the majority of B lineage cells were membrane sIgM$^+$, sIgD$^-$ B lymphocytes. It was confirmed in tissue section that these populations were indeed predominantly negative for To15, RFB-4 and RFB-6 antigens [13]. Thus, the BM B cells in the fetus represent "early" types of B cells, as expected on the basis of findings in the infant BM (Table 2).

Further studies were performed to identify the T-lineage cells in the fetal BM. Two antibodies, OKT3-like (UCH-T1) and OKT1-like (RFT1) were used, the latter in double combination with anti-IgM. T cells (T3$^+$, T1$^+$) were rare (0.5%–1%) in 17-week-old fetal BM, and these were IgM$^-$ (Table 3). The proportion of RFT1$^+$, IgM$^+$ double-labelled cells was very low: 0.1%–0.9% amongst the IgM$^+$ population (0.02%–0.15%) of all BM cells. This contrasts with the findings observed in fetal lymph nodes (see Sect. C.IV).

III. Analysis of Fetal Spleen

In the samples of fetal spleen taken at the 18th gestational week 4–5 times more B cells were found than T cells. Of all cells, 4%–6% were IgM$^+$ and another 1%–2% T3$^+$. The T cell population was clustered around small blood vessels, and the B cells formed a loose band of cells at the edge of the splenic red pulp. No follicular dendritic reticulum cells were seen.

There were two important findings about the splenic B cells. First, these splenic B cells have clearly shown a "peripheral B cell" phenotype: 80%–90% were IgM$^+$, IgD$^+$ and virtually all (>95%) B cells clearly reacted with MoAb RFB-4, To15 and RFB-6. On the other hand, we could not observe significant numbers of IgM$^+$, IgD$^-$ B cells. This is interesting because in the adult human (and rat) spleen a clearly visible population of IgM$^+$, IgD$^-$ cells is present in the marginal zone [14], but these are probably mature cells in a relatively late stage of development. Second, immunohistological techniques were used to identify B cells expressing T cell-associated markers such as T1 and only a few (1%–2% of IgM$^+$ cells) appeared to express the T1 antigen (Table 3) up to the 23rd week when more T1$^+$, IgM$^+$ cells appeared [13].

IV. Analysis of Fetal Lymph Nodes

In the earliest lymph nodes found (at 16th gestational week) T and B cell areas were

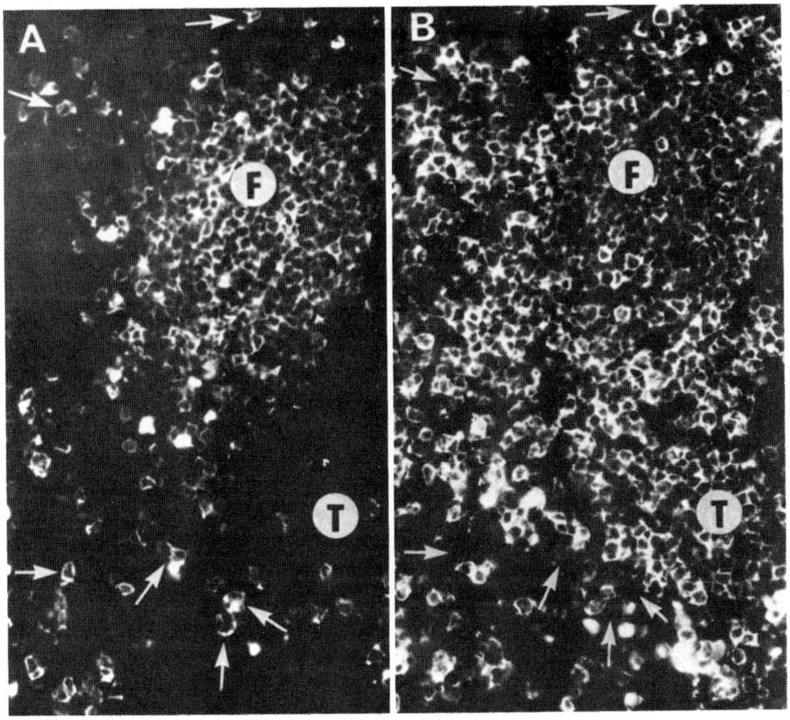

Fig. 1 A, B. B lymphocytes within the primary lymphoid nodules of fetal lymph nodes (20th gestational week) show double staining for IgM (**A**) and the T cell-associated antigen T1 (**B**). These B cells are accumulating around dendritic reticulum cells [13]. The rare B cells diffusely distributed in the paracortical T area are strongly IgM^+ and $T1^-$ (*arrows*). This B cell population is dominant in the fetal spleen (Table 2; [13])

not yet separated. T lymphocytes ($T1^+$, $T3^+$) as well as the IgM^+ B cells (30% of lymphocytes) were diffusely mixed. No $T1^+$, IgM^+ double-labelled cells were seen. In the lymph node samples taken at 18th week tight clusters of lymphocytes appeared accumulating 100–200 cells around follicular dendritic cells (FDR cells; identified by RFD-3 antibody) and uniformly showed a peculiar phenotype. All these cells were IgM^+, IgD^+ (moderately strongly), expressed BA-1 positivity and reacted with RFB-4, To15 as well as RFB-6 (B cells of peripheral type). In addition, the B cells in the clusters were invariably $T1^+$ (moderately strongly; Fig. 1) but HLA-DR positive and T3 negative. The T lymphocytes ($T3^+$, $T1^+$,$HLA\text{-}DR^-$, IgM^-) were found in the diffuse lymphoid area and showed a much stronger $T1^+$ staining. Finally, it is important to point out that within the small B lymphoid follicles no large germinal centre blasts were seen, and the $BA\text{-}1^-$, weak IgM^+, IgD^- central population seen in the germinal centres of adult lymph nodes were absent.

V. Malignant B Cells

TdT^+ cells are present in large proportions amongst the lymphoid cells of fetal liver [11, 15] and fetal BM [13, 15]. These cells lack a number of other B cell markers such as Y29/55 [16], RFB-6, or show only cytoplasmic, but no membrane expression of RFB-4 or To15. The phenotypic features of these TdT^+ cells are similar to the blast cells seen in common acute lymphoblastic (cALL) and pre-B ALL [9, 11, 15–17].

As we recently emphasized [13], the $T1^+$, IgM^+, IgD^+ cells with peripheral B cell features ($Y29/55^+$, $RFB\text{-}6^+$, $RFB\text{-}4^+$,

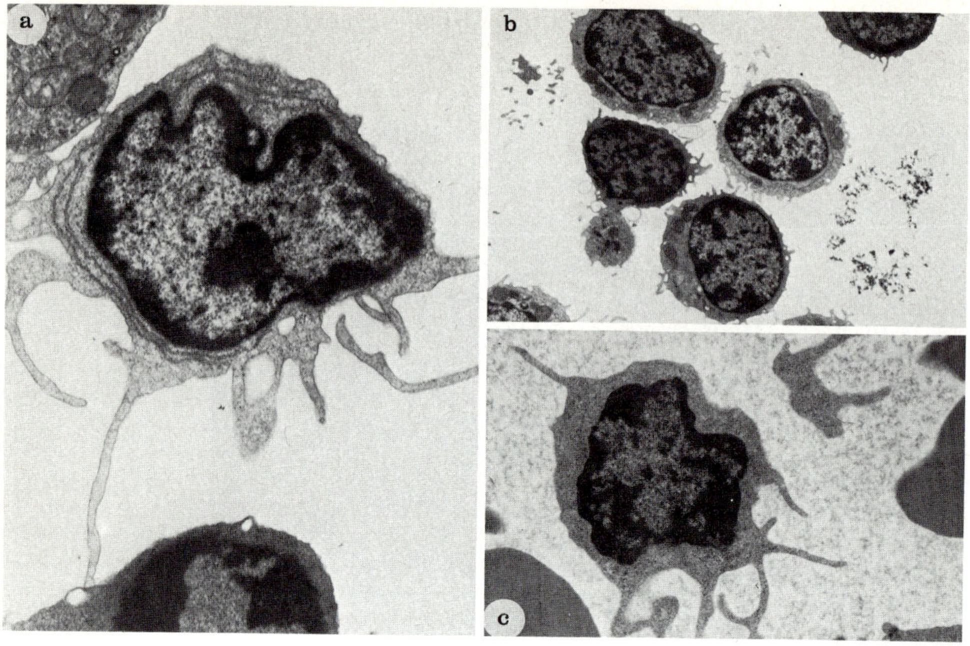

Fig. 2a–c. B-CLL cells after 72 h TPA stimulation develop "hairs" (**a** ×10 000). Cells in the control unstimulated B-CLL culture have smoother surface (**b** ×6000) and normal B cells in the presence of TPA also remain smooth (not shown; but see [23]). For comparison hairy cell leukaemia is shown (**c** ×8000). From [10] with permission

To15⁺) which cluster around follicular dendritic reticulum cells in fetal lymph nodes (see Sect. C.IV) are very similar, by phenotypic criteria, to two B cell malignancies: centrocytic lymphoma [18] and B-type chronic lymphocytic leukaemia (B-CLL; [19]). The further distinctive phenotypic features of these malignancies are the reactivity of Tü-33 Mo-Ab with centrocytic lymphoma and that of Tü-1 Ab with B-CLL [18]. Indeed, the normal equivalent $T1^+$, IgM^+ cells in the primary nodules of normal fetal LN samples are also heterogeneous in respect of Tü-33 and Tü-1 expression [13]. Thus, centrocytic lymphoma and B-CLL might originate from the Tü-33^+ and Tü-1^+ B cells of primary nodules, respectively.

The exact origin of hairy cell leukaemia (HCL) is nevertheless still unknown. This disease, in its typical form, is a B cell malignancy with the following features: (a) SmIg expression and Ig gene rearrangements [20]; (b) characteristic membrane protrusions and veils; (c) strong cytoplasmic tartrate-resistant acid phosphatase activity (TRAP; [21]); (d) reactivity with MoAb to interleukin-2 receptor (anti-Tac; [20]); and (e) reactivity with MoAb to SHCL3 antigen, a membrane moiety not expressed by B-CLL [22]. As the "normal equivalent" cell of HCL has so far been elusive, we have investigated whether any known malignant B cells can be transformed into HCL. The details will be published elsewhere [23] and the salient observations are as follows.

First, it has been observed that the expression of TRAP enzyme activity can be readily induced by TPA in *normal* tonsil B cells and their mouse rosetting subset [23] during a 72-h culture period (60% and 18% positivity, respectively). A few SHCL3-positive B cells were also generated in the same cultures (25% and 7%, respectively). Only very few Tac^+ B cells were seen, however, and these were best generated in 6- or 7-day cultures stimulated by PWM (Ig^+ blasts; 5% Tac^+). Thus, with the possible

Table 4. TPA-induced changes in B-chronic lymphocytic leukaemia (B-CLL) and hairy cell leukaemia (HCL)[c]

Phenotype	B-CLL (16 cases), incubated for		HCL (4 cases), incubated for	
	0 h	72 h with TPA[b]	0 h	72 h with TPA
A. Morphology	Small ly	Hairy cells[c]	Hairy cells	More adherent
B. HCL-associated features				
SHCL3^{+d}	3.3±2.1[e]	(3) 5 ±3[f] (13) 74 ±11	87±7	44±4
Anti-Tac$^+$	(15) 4.0±2 (1) 80	(7) 5.1±2.1 (9) 64 ±21	84±4	47±8
Tartrate-resistant acid phosphatase (TRAP)	< 5	65–85	60±5	50–70
C. B-CLL-associated features				
M-rbc$^+$ (rosettes)	61±8	< 5	33±4	
Tl (p67) antigen	87±6	79±11	1.5, 1, 3, 65	1, 2, 3, 60
sIg$^+$	80±3 (weak)	< 10 (very weak)	22± ¨	< 5
Cytoplasmic Ig$^+$	< 10	(12) > 50 (4) < 10	15±5	> 40

[a] 16 cases of B-CLL and 4 cases of HCL were studied. There has been no change in the features of B-CLL and HCL cultures for 72 h without TPA (except a slight decrease in M-rbc rosetting). For further details see [23]
[b] TPA (12-*O*-tetradecanoylphorbol-13-acetate) was used for 72 h at 1.6×10^{-8} *M* concentration
[c] See Fig. 2
[d] A MoAb from Dr. Schwarting [22]
[e] Percentage (± standard error) of cells reacting with each marker
[f] Numbers in parentheses refer to numbers of cases

exception of membrane irregularities, the features of HCL are not fully leukaemia specific. Next, various *leukaemias* were "induced" by TPA. These included 16 cases of B-CLL (Tl$^+$, sIgM$^+$, weak), 4 cases of prolymphocytic leukaemia and "mantle zone" lymphoma (strongly Ig$^+$ positive; Tl mostly negative) and 2 cases of common ALL (TdT$^+$, sIg$^-$).

We have reported previously that TPA-induced B-CLL cells developed membrane perturbations characteristic of hairy protrusions (Fig. 2; [10]). Clearly, other "HCL-associated" features could also be observed in the majority of cases. Of 16 cases, 13 had > 50% SHCL3$^+$ cells, and 9 showed strong Tac positivity in 64%±21% of activated B-CLL cells; 60%–85% of cells were TRAP$^+$ (Table 4). These "HCL-like" features on activated B-CLL cells were much stronger than on any of the TPA-activated normal B cell populations, including the mouse rosetting subpopulation. Similar HCL-like features (e.g. membrane irregularities and SHCL3 positivity) have not been recorded in the other leukaemias, although cases of PLL and mantle zone lymphoma did develop Tac positivity (45%–80%; results not shown, but see [23]). Finally, cases of HCL (four patients) when activated with TPA, did not show major phenotypic changes, and have not developed CLL-like features [23].

D. Discussion

The two main findings about emerging B cells during fetal development are that: (a) the "early" B cells (pre-B and IgM$^+$, IgD$^-$ B)

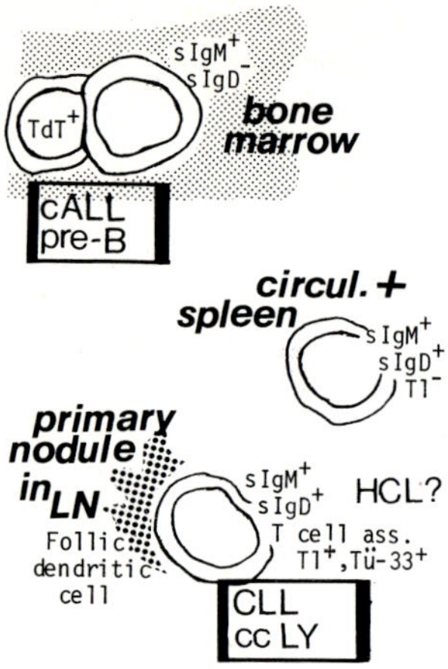

Fig. 3. The three main B cell types observed in the fetus. In the bone marrow pre-B and B cells are IgM^+, IgD^-, $AL\text{-}1^+$ and do not express membrane RFB-4, To15, RFB-6. On the periphery strongly Ig^+ (IgM^+, IgD^+) cells circulate in blood and are seen in the spleen while B cells in the primary nodules in the lymph node show weaker IgM^+ and IgD^+ and express T cell-associated antigen such as T1 and Tü-33. For further details see also [9, 13]

in fetal bone marrow are different, by a number of criteria, from peripheral B cells [9]; and (b) there is a dichotomy amongst the peripheral B cell populations [13]. This leads to emphasizing the existence of three major B cell types in the fetus: one in the BM, and two in the periphery (Fig. 3). To this heterogeneity further forms (e.g. germinal centre blasts, and plasma cells) are added when the individual is exposed to extrinsic antigens during later life. This scheme is similar to those presented by Galton and MacLennan [14] and also indicated by Stein et al. [18] on the basis of lymphoma heterogeneity. Indeed, the new findings here support the existence of normal B cells (most probably virgin peripheral B lymphocytes of primary lymphoid nodules) which express some T cell-associated markers such as T1 and Tü-33. These B cells are also present in adults [19], but only in smaller numbers, perhaps because they are "diluted out" by other newly emerging cell types.

The finding of IgM^+, $T1^+$ normal B cells in the primary nodules may explain two unrelated puzzling phenomena. First, certain B cell malignancies express T cell-associated features with some regularity. The T1 antigen on B-CLL, T1 plus Tü-33 on centrocytic lymphoma (Kiel classification; [18]) are the obvious examples (see Sect. C.), but T3 as well as T11 molecules were also seen in a few cases of B-CLL and B lymphomas, in spite of the fact that these showed monoclonal ($\varkappa$ or λ) light chain, IgM as well as HLA-DR [24–27]. Similarly, Cawley et al. [28] have emphasized that HCL were capable of expressing T cell features (sheep erythrocyte rosetting) during certain stages of disease progression. The derepression of T cell genes may be more frequent in the recently identified $T1^+$, IgM^+ cells or their malignant counterparts than in the other B cell subsets.

At least a subgroup of HCL might also be related to the B-CLL group. This is indicated by the observations of "inducing" HCL-like features in B-CLL cells with TPA (Table 4). Taken at face value, these results and those described by Caligaris-Cappio [10, 23] show that TPA-induced B-CLL and HCL both have abnormal membrane characteristics in terms of "hair" formation, which is not demonstrated in the equivalent normal cells. In other respects, HCL appears to be an activated variant of B-CLL or that of a closely related cell type. An alternative explanation is that the HCL-associated markers (Tac expression, TRAP and SHCL3 positivity) are nonspecific features which appear on unrelated B cell types. Clearly, more work is needed in this area, but it is already clear that other B cell malignancies such as prolymphocytic leukaemia, mantle zone lymphoma and pre-B ALL (and the corresponding cell lines) do not develop HCL-like features when induced by TPA [23]. Thus, the CLL–HCL link has so far appeared to be a rather special one. The possibility of the CLL–HCL link is also supported by the existence of leukaemias showing circulating HCL together with B-CLL-like histological pattern [29, 30].

Second, it has been demonstrated in the mouse that $Ly\text{-}1^+$, IgM^+ B cells are also present and, in the NZB strain, contribute to autoantibody synthesis [31]. The observation of frequent autoantibody formation in B-CLL [32] raises the possibility that in these patients the whole T1$^+$, IgM$^+$ lineage is hyperactive and the monoclonal malignancy might be just one of the later, although dramatic, consequences of this dysregulation. This is an interesting possibility from the point of view of preventing a malignant disease. Similarly, further studies are necessary to investigate this B cell population in autoimmune disorders. It will be interesting to see whether the increased numbers of circulating mouse rosetting B cells in rheumatoid arthritis [33] also show the T1$^+$, IgM$^+$ phenotype.

Acknowledgements. This work was supported by the Leukaemia Research Fund of Great Britain (G.J. and D.C.) by PFCCN-CNR of Italy (F.C.C. Grant No. 830075296) and by an Armour Pharmaceutical Scholarship (M.B.). We ware grateful to Dr. M. Chilosi, Verona, for TRAP staining and to Dr. G. Schwarting, Berlin, for SHCL3 antibody.

References

1. Salmon SE, Seligmann M (1974) B cell neoplasia in man. Lancet 2:1230–1233
2. Vogler LB (1982) Bone marrow B development. Clin Haematol 11:509–529
3. McKenzie IFC, Zola H (1983) Monoclonal antibodies to B cells. Immunol Today 4:10–14
4. Janossy G, Bollum FJ, Bradstock KF, McMichael A, Rapson N, Greaves MF (1979) Terminal transferase positive human bone marrow cells exhibit the antigenic phenotype of common acute lymphoblastic leukemia. J Immunol 123:1525–1529
5. Gathings WE, Lawton AR, Cooper MD (1977) Immunofluorescent studies of the development of pre-B cells, B lymphocytes and immunoglobulin isotype diversity in humans. Eur J Immunol 7:804–810
6. Moller G (ed) (1977) Immunoglobulin D: structure, synthesis, membrane representation and function. Immunol Rev 37
7. Benner R, Hijmans W, Haaijman JJ (1981) The bone marrow: the major source of serum immunoglobulins, but still a neglected site of antibody formation. Clin Exp Immunol 46:1–8
8. Janossy G, Thomas JA, Bollum FJ, Granger S, Pizzolo G, Bradstock KF, Wong L, Ganeshaguru K, Hoffbrand AV (1980) The human thymic microenvironment: an immunohistological study. J Immunol 125:202–212
9. Campana D, Janossy G, Bofill M, Trejdosiewicz LK, Ma D, Hoffbrand AV, Mason DY, Lebacq A-M, Forster H (1985) Human B cell development. I. Phenotypic differences of B lymphocytes in the bone marrow and peripheral lymphoid tissue. J Immunol 134:1524–1529
10. Caligaris-Cappio F, Janossy G, Campana D Chilosi M, Bergui L, Foa R, Delia D, Giubellino MC, Preda P, Gobbi M (1984) Lineage relationship of chronic lymphocytic leukaemia and hairy cell leukaemia: studies with TPA, Leuk Res 8:567–578
11. Hokland P, Rosenthal P, Griffin J, Nadler L, Daley J, Hokland M, Schlossman SF, Ritz J (1983) Purification and characterization of fetal hematopoietic cell that express the common acute lymphoblastic leukaemia antigen (CALLA). J Exp Med 157:114–129
12. Gobbi M, Caligaris-Cappio F, Janossy G (1983) Normal equivalent cells of B cell malignancies: analysis with monoclonal antibodies. Br J Haematol 54:393–403
13. Bofill M, Janossy G, Janossa M, Burford GD, Seymour GJ, Wernet P, Kelemen E (1985) Human B cell development. II. Subpopulations in the human fetus. J Immunol 134:1530–1537
14. Galton DAG, MacLennan ICH (1982) Clinical patterns in B lymphoid malignancy. Clin Haematol 11:561–587
15. Bodger MP, Janossy G, Bollum FJ, Burford GD, Hoffbrand AB (1983) The ontogeny of terminal deoxynucleotidyl transferase. Blood 61:1125–1131
16. Hirt A, Baumgartner C, Forster HK, Imbach P, Wagner HP (1983) Reactivity of acute lymphoblastic leukemia and normal bone marrow cells with the monoclonal anti-B-lymphocyte antibody, anti-Y29/55. Cancer Res 43:4483
17. Nadler LM, Anderson KC, Marti G, Bates M, Park E, Daley JF, Schlossman SF (1983) Human B lymphocyte-associated antigen expressed on normal mitogen-activated and malignant B lymphocytes. J Immunol 131: 244–258
18. Stein H, Gerdes J, Mason DY (1982) The normal and malignant germinal centre. Clin Haematol 11:531–559
19. Caligaris-Cappio F, Gobbi M, Bofill M, Janossy G (1982) Infrequent normal B lymphocytes express features of B-chronic lymphocytic leukaemia. J Exp Med 155:623–628
20. Korsmeyer SJ, Hieter PA, Ravetch JV, Poplack DG, Waldmann TA, Leder P (1981) Developmental hierarchy of immunoglobin gene rearrangements in human leukaemic pre-B cells. Proc Natl Acad Sci USA 78:7096–7100

21. Ly CY, Yam LT, Lam KW (1970) Acid phosphatase isoenzyme in human leucocytes in normal and pathologic conditions. J Histochem Cytochem 18:473
22. Schwarting G, Stein H (1985) Reactivity of SHCL3 antibody (in press)
23. Caligaris-Cappio F, Pizzolo G, Chilosi M, Bergui L, Campana D, Morittu L, Gobbi G, Janossy G (1985) Phorbol ester induces abnormal CLL cells to express features of hairy cell leukaemia. Blood (in press)
24. Aisenberg AC, Bloch KC, Wilkes BM (1981) Malignant lymphoma with dual B and T cell markers. Analysis of neoplastic cells with monoclonal antibodies directed against T cell subsets. J Exp Med 154:1709–1714
25. Habeshaw JA, Bailey D, Stansfeld AG, Greaves MF (1983) The cellular content of non-Hodgkin lymphomas: a comprehensive analysis using monoclonal antibodies and other surface marker techniques. Br J Cancer 7:327–351
26. Schroff RW, Foon KA (1982) Heterogeneity in a lymphoid tumour: co-expression of T and B markers. Blood 60:373–380
27. Sitia R, Sciariada L, Zicca A, Leprini A, Ghio R, Ferrarini M (1983) Expression of a receptor for sheep erythrocytes by B lymphocytes from a CLL patient. Clin Immunol Immunopathol 27:210–222
28. Cawley JC, Burns GF, Nash TA et al. (1978) Hairy cell leukaemia with T cell features. Blood 51:61–69
29. Palatke M, Tabaczka P, Mirchandani I, Goldfarb S (1981) Lymphocytic lymphoma simulating hairy cell leukaemia. Cancer 48:2047
30. Neiman RS, Sullivan AL, Jaffe R (1979) Malignant lymphoma simulating leukemic reticuloendotheliosis. Cancer 43:329
31. Hayakawa K, Hardy RP, Parks DR, Herzenberg LA (1982) The "Ly-1 B" cell subpopulation in normal, immunodefective and autoimmune mice. J Exp Med 157:202–220
32. Seligmann M (1984) Human lymphocyte subsets in health and disease. Prog Immunol 5:1047–1051
33. Room GRW, Plater-Zyberk C, Maini RN (1983) Mouse rosetting cells in rheumatoid arthritis. Rheumatol Int 23:141

Haematology and Blood Transfusion Vol. 29
Modern Trends in Human Leukemia VI
Edited by Neth, Gallo, Greaves, Janka

Genetic Determination of the Cytolytic T Lymphocyte Receptor Repertoire

L. A. Sherman[1]

A. Introduction

The immune system has evolved a number of sophisticated molecular mechanisms that assure the maintenance of a highly diverse repertoire of lymphocyte receptors. In view of the vast potential for V region diversity, the immune system must judiciously choose specificities that are of greatest value for expression in the lymphocyte receptor repertoire. Indeed, the challenge to immunologists no longer lies in explaining the generation of diversity, but rather in understanding the basis for variable region selection at the genomic level and receptor selection at the environmental level. This is, of course, also the ongoing challenge to the immune system.

Our interest in understanding the basis for repertoire selection led us to develop an experimental system that could be used to assess the influence of a variety of genetic, environmental, and developmental factors on expression of the receptor repertoire of cytolytic T lymphocytes (CTL). This entails antigenic stimulation of a large number of CTL clones under limiting dilution culture conditions, followed by identification of the receptor specificity of each clone by fine specificity analysis [1–4]. The murine H-2K^b antigen is uniquely suited to such an approach owing to the availability of a large number of H-2K^b mutants that provide a panel of heterologous targets required for fine specificity analysis.

The results of such an analysis of the B10.BR response to H-2K^b is given in Table 1. It is clear that the response against a single alloantigen is highly diverse. In this examination of 78 independently derived primary CTL clones, we observed 34 different receptor specificities, each defined by a different reactivity pattern (RP) on the panel of K^b mutants. The existence of such a large repertoire, coupled with the limited size of sampling that is feasible, precludes comparison of repertoires on the basis of the presence or absence of particular specificities. Fortunately, superimposed on such diversity is the existence of a small number of highly recurrent specificities. We believe these to be analogous to public idiotypes in antibody responses insofar as they recur frequently among individuals within an inbred strain and, as such, are phenotypic markers for the purpose of repertoire comparisons. Within the B10.BR response there are three specificities which are recurrent, RP23, RP39, and RP87 [2].

B. The Role of the MHC in Repertoire Determination

Having established a basis for repertoire comparison, it is possible to assess the contribution of a particular genetic region to repertoire expression by performing a comparable analysis of the genetically distinct murine strain in question. Of particular interest is the role of MHC in altering repertoire expression. There is a vast literature presenting evidence of the profound effect of MHC on T cell responsiveness; reviewed in [5]. The strategy used by the immune

1 Department of Immunology, Scripps Clinic and Research Foundation, La Jolla, California 92037

Table 1. The B10.BR anti-K^b CTL repertoire[a]

				bm9	+	+	+	+	−	−	−	−
				bm10	+	+	−	−	+	+	−	−
				bm11	+	−	−	+	+	−	−	+
bm8	bm1	bm3	bm4									
+	+	+	+		11	·	·	·	1	·	·	·
+	+	−	+		1	3	·	·	·	·	·	·
+	−	−	+		·	·	·	·	·	1	1	·
+	−	+	+		1	1	·	1	·	·	·	·
−	+	+	+		·	·	·	1	·	·	·	1
−	+	−	+		1	·	1	·	·	3	·	·
−	−	−	+		·	5	7	·	·	12	1	·
−	−	+	+		1	·	1	·	·	·	·	·
+	+	+	−		·	·	·	1	·	·		
+	+	−	−		·	·	·	·	·	·	·	·
+	−	−	−		·	·	·	·	·	·	3	1
+	−	+	−		·	·	·	1	·	1	·	2
−	+	+	−		1	·	·	·	·	·	·	·
−	+	−	−		·	·	1	·	·	·	·	·
−	−	−	−		·	1	2	·	·	·	3	·
−	−	+	−		·	·	1	4	·	·	·	1

[a] Each number represents the total number of clones observed which gave the indicated reactivity pattern (RP) [2]

system to focus on cellular presented antigens is the requirement for MHC-restricted recognition. The particular alleles recognized are determined by the MHC antigens expressed by the thymus [5, 6]. Is this predilection for "self" reflected within the receptor repertoire? Other types of MHC-directed effects on T cell responsiveness include tolerance and immune response gene (IR) phenomenon. Unlike restriction phenotype, which is a form of positive selection, both IR and tolerance are manifested as the loss of responsiveness associated with a particular MHC haplotype and therefore would be reflected as a negative effect on repertoire.

Figure 1 lists all such recurrent specificities that appear in the H-$2K^b$-specific response of B10.BR and B10.D2. It may be seen that each of these MHC-disparate, yet otherwise genetically identical strains expresses different recurrent specificities. In order to determine if these differences are reflective of negative or positive MHC-directed influences we next examined the repertoire of (B10.BR×B10.D2) F_1 hybrids. These results (Fig. 1) indicate that some specificities, such as RP47, are maintained within an F_1 environment, whereas others, such as RP87 and RP39, are represented at a much reduced level. Therefore, both positive and negative MHC influences are apparent.

This discussion has made an important assumption which is not necessarily warranted. Specifically, we assumed that all MHC effects are extracellular in origin and not determined by the MHC genotype of the T cell, but rather by the MHC phenotype of the environment. If this assumption is correct, we would anticipate that, having matured in the identical environment, cells of either H-2^d or H-2^k origin should be capable of expressing the identical repertoire. To test this prediction, we constructed double chimeras by repopulating lethally irradiated (B10.D2×B10.BR) F_1 mice with a mixture of fetal liver stem cells of B10.BR and B10.D2 origin. At 8 weeks after reconstruction, individual mice were killed and their spleen cells divided in half and treated with either anti-H-2^k or anti-H-2^d antibodies in the presence of complement. This procedure provides lymphocytes of different MHC genotype that have matured in an identical environment. Each repertoire was independently assessed (Fig. 2). Unlike the results already described, de-

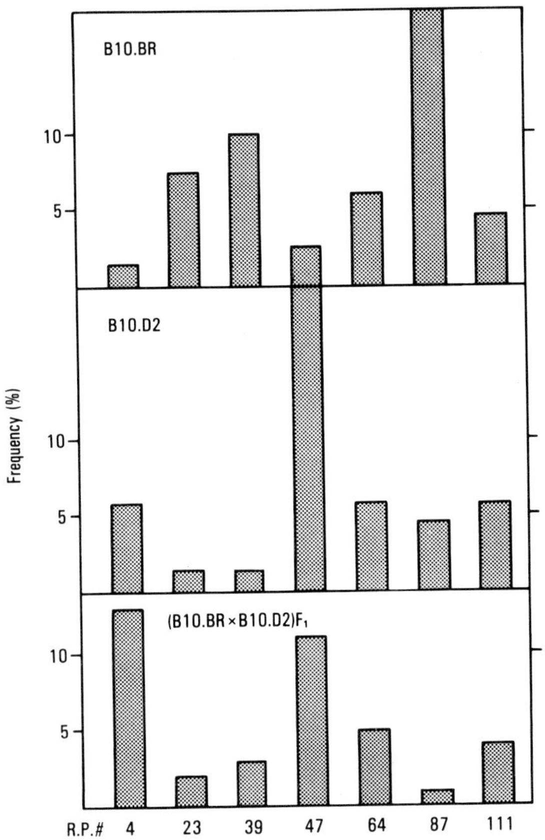

Fig. 1. Comparison of recurrent specificities exhibited by MHC congeneic strains and their F_1 hybrids. Data represent analysis of over 20 individually analyzed mice [2]

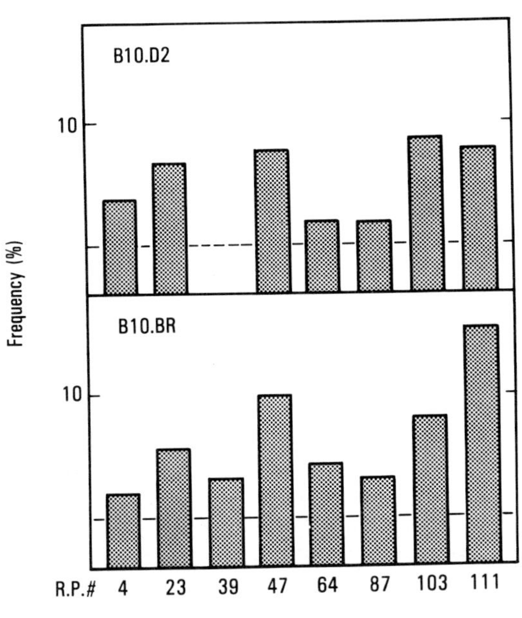

Fig. 2. Analysis of the repertoire of B10.D2 and B10.BR cells obtained from double-radiation chimeras

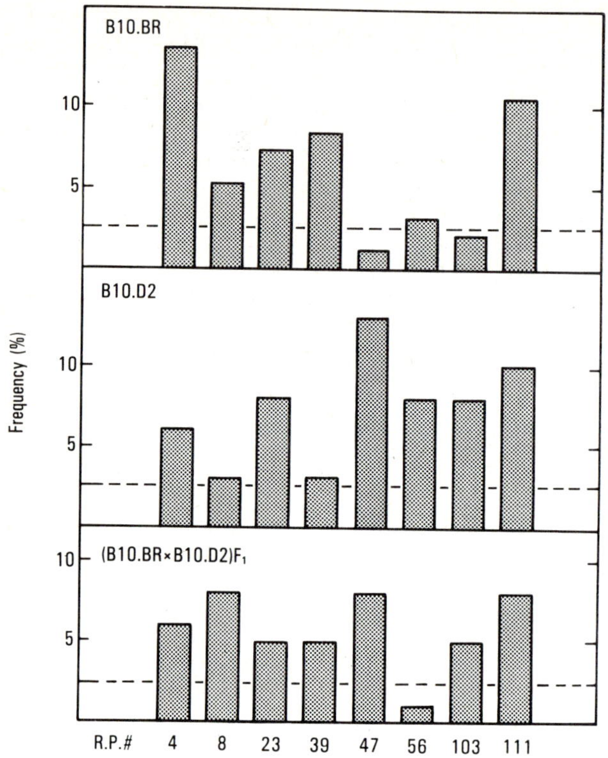

Fig. 3. Comparison of recurrent specificities exhibited by 10- to 14-day-old neonates [3]

spite their MHC differences, the repertoires of both cell types were very similar. Seven of eight recurrent specificities were comparably expressed by both cell types. Therefore, the effect of MHC observed in this system is essentially environmental in origin.

Another type of environmental influence which could be present in the splenic repertoire would be the effect of continual exposure to antigen in the context of self-MHC. This could yield a repertoire skewed toward self-recognition and would therefore be perceived as an MHC-linked environmental influence. To assess the contribution of post-thymic effects on repertoire we investigated the neonatal CTL response [3]. The rationale for this study is that neonates have experienced far less exposure to antigen. Indeed, as shown in Fig. 3, B10.D2 and B10.BR neonates demonstrate a significant number of repertoire similarities. In addition, it is clear that some recurrent specificities are unique to each strain and, most significantly, RP39 is unique to B10.BR in both the neonate and adult, whereas RP47 is unique to B10.D2. These RP, therefore, represent potential examples of positive selection in the thymus. Finally, it should be apparent that, unlike the adult F_1 hybrid, in most cases, neonates express the admixture of both parental (neonatal) repertoires. This indicates that coexpression of most parental specificities is permitted in an F_1 environment and, therefore, few effects of tolerance are evident inthe neonatal F_1 repertoire as judged by the H-2K^b specificity repertoire. This again suggests that many of the repertoire features characteristic of the adult may be the result of post-thymic effects.

C. The Role of IgH-Linked Genes in Repertoire Determination

Having observed a profound influence of MHC on the expressed T cell repertoire, we

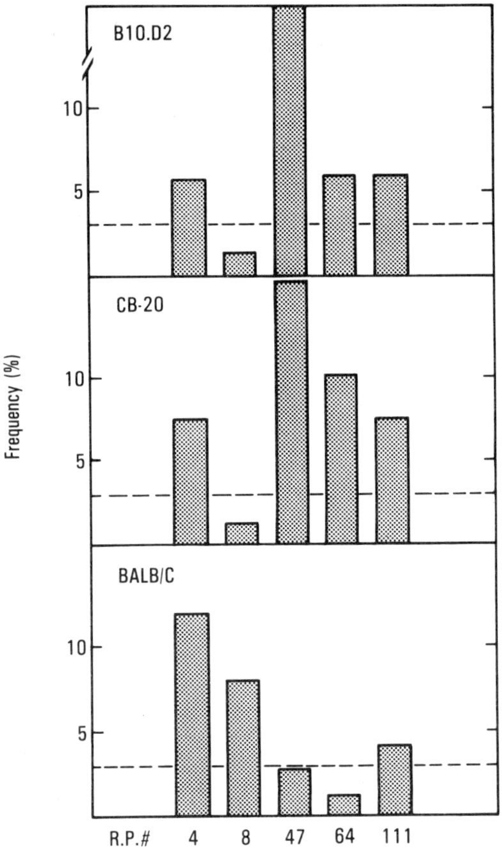

Fig. 4. Recurrent specificities representative of MHC-identical mice with different IgH allotypes. B10.D2 and CB-20 both express Igh^{b}. BALB/c expresses Igh^{a}

next wished to determine if other polymorphic genetic loci affect receptor expression. Inasmuch as numerous laboratories have reported the presence of Igh-linked idiotypic determinants on T cell products, this polymorphic region is an obvious candidate.

But what about other polymorphic loci? In order simultaneously to screen the effect of numerous polymorphic genes on T repertoire expression, we compared the H-2K^{b}-specific responses of two strains which share both MHC and Igh yet are otherwise of independent origin, CB-20 and B10.D2 [4]. Both strains are H-2^{d}, Igh^{b} yet CB-20 is of BALB/c origin and therefore broadly differs from B10.D2. The results of this analysis are presented in Fig. 4. It may be seen that the same recurrent specificities are observed in both repertoires. This implies the polymorphic differences between these two genetic backgrounds other than MHC and IgH are, in general, of little consequence to the expression of the H-2K^{b} specificity repertoire. In contrast, the allotype-congeneic strains CB-20 (Igh^{b}) and BALB/c (Igh^{a}) reveal a large number of significant repertoire differences. Most prominent is the decreased expression of RP47 and RP64 and the increased expression of RP8 in BALB/c. Therefore, allotype-linked genes profoundly influence the expressed T cell repertoire.

A variety of mechanisms could account for Igh-linked repertoire differences. To help narrow down the possibilities, it was necessary to determine if variable or constant region-linked genes were involved. To address this question, we took advantage of two strains in which recombination within the Igh locus has occurred. BAB-14 has the same variable region genes as BALB/c (Igh-V^{a}) yet the constant region is Igh-C^{b}. CBB 7904 is the reciprocal recombinant, Igh-V^{b}-C^{a}. The frequency of RP8, RP47, and RP64 in these strains is given in Fig. 5. These results suggest the levels of expression of these particular specificities are determined primarily by Igh-V-linked genes.

Although our data are consistent with the possibility that T cell receptor V regions are linked to Igh-V, in view of the susceptibility of repertoire to environmental regulatory events it is also possible to explain these data as a result of immunoregulatory selection by immunoglobulin variable regions [8, 9]. We are currently distinguishing between these two possibilities by examining the repertoire of allotype-different cells originating from double chimeras in which cells of Igh-V^{a} and Igh-V^{b} type are permitted to mature together.

In conclusion, we have identified two genetic regions that influence expression of the T cell receptor repertoire, MHC- and Igh-V-linked genes. It is important to note that our methods assess only the contributions of polymorphic genetic loci. Accordingly, we would predict that any other genetic region that participates in receptor expression is either nonpolymorphic be-

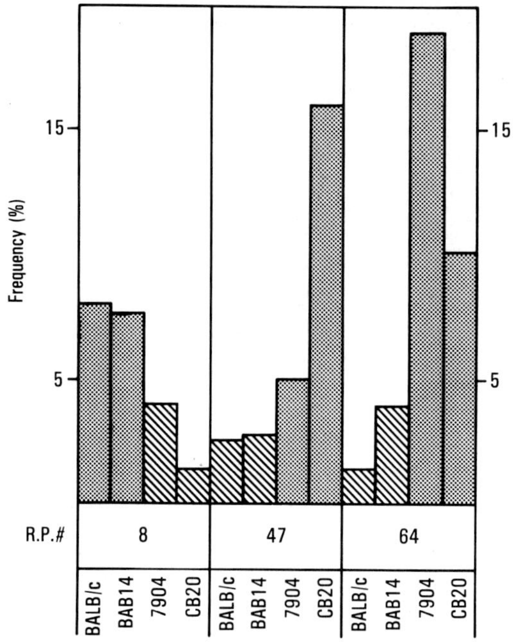

Fig. 5. The effect of recombination within Igh on expression of recurrent specificities

tween the BALB/c and B10 backgrounds, or its polymorphism is of limited consequence to repertoire expression.

Acknowledgments. This work was supported by National Institutes of Health Grant AI-20026 and grant IMM-324 from the American Cancer Society.

References

1. Sherman LA (1980) Dissecting the B10.D2 anti-H-2K^b receptor repertoire. J Exp Med 151:1386
2. Sherman LA (1982) The influence of the major histocompatibility complex on the repertoire of allospecific cytolytic T lymphocytes. J Exp Med 155:380
3. Sherman LA (1982) Genetic and regulatory contributions of the major histocompatibility complex to the developing cytolytic T lymphocyte repertoire. J Immunol 128:1849
4. Sherman LA (1982) Genetic linkage of the cytolytic T lymphocyte repertoire and immunoglobulin heavy chain genes. J Exp Med 156:294
5. Zinkernagel RM, Doherty PC (1979) MHC restricted cytotoxic T cells. Adv 27:51
6. Fink PJ, Bevan MJ (1978) H-2 antigens of the thymus determine lymphocyte specificity. J Exp Med 148:766
7. Schwartz R-H (1978) A clonal deletion mode for IR gene control of the immune response. Scand J Immunol 7:3
8. Rajewsky K, Takemori T (1983) Genetics, expression and function of idiotypes. Ann Rev Immunol 1:569
9. Miller JFAP, Morahan G, Walker ID (1983) T cell antigen receptors: fact and artifact. Immunol Today 4:141

Haematology and Blood Transfusion Vol. 29
Modern Trends in Human Leukemia VI
Edited by Neth, Gallo, Greaves, Janka

Internal Activity of the Immune System and its Physiologic Significance

A. Coutinho[1], D. Holmberg[1], C. Martinez-A.[2], A. de Freitas[1], E.-L. Larsson[1], P. Pereira[1,2], and A. Bandeira[1]

A. Introduction

After the introduction of Jerne's network theory 10 years ago, modern views of the immune system have been strongly influenced by the ideas of *autonomy* previously developed by those working on complex systems such as the brain. This "new immunology" attempts to describe the normal immune system as it is, the fundamental characteristics of its organization and, in the words of Francisco Varela, "the landscape of its eigen behaviours." Within this perspective, the study of the internal activity of the immune system, of the generation and decay of its cellular and molecular components, is likely to provide more relevant information as to the physiology of immune activity than the study of immune responses to the injection of large doses of antigen, as in classical approaches. Obviously, we aim to describe and understand the basis for this inner life of the immune system, embedded as it is in a multitude of molecular components that constitute the "self" of the individual, and exposed to the surrounding "noise" of the environment. We do not use artificial priming with antigen, neither antibodies nor antiidiotypes as surrogates of antigens in the induction of immune responses. On the other hand, the interpretation of such internal activity, as well as any hypothesis on the internal mechanisms inducing effector cells and their specificity, must necessarily rely on detailed knowledge of lymphocyte physiology: the mechanisms by which lymphocytes are turned on and turned off, and how their proliferation and maturation to effector functions are regulated as well as the nature of the functionally relevant molecules expressed at the surface of these cells.

In a meeting on human leukemia, what we have to say risks being completely out of place. We neither work with human cells, nor are we concerned with leukemia. Moreover, our perspectives and approaches may well lead us nowhere. The profound motivation to follow them is our dissatisfaction with current approaches to biologic systems, particularly within immunology, and their failure to solve problems (such as that of cancer and autoimmune pathology) within classical frameworks of thought and experimentation. We have provided detailed references in a previous publication [1].

B. Organizational Closure in the Normal Immune System

I. Internal Activity

It has now become clear that the normal immune system does not need environmental stimulation to be directed into relatively high levels of activity. This activity can be measured not only at the level of production and decay of lymphocytes, but also in the generation of effector cells.

1 Laboratory of Immunobiology, Department of Immunology, Pasteur Institute, Paris, France
2 Department of Immunology, Clinica Puerta de Hierro, Madrid, Spain

Thus, germ-free mice maintained on low molecular weight, chemically defined diets, possess in their spleens numbers of immunoglobulin-secreting cells that are quite similar, if not superior, to those found in the spleens of conventionally bred and infected mice. Interestingly, such mice have no plasma cells in the lymph nodes, an observation which actually provides a control for the "antigen-free" state of these mice. The ontogenic development of "natural plasma cells" in the spleen of these mice is perfectly comparable to that of mice born from normal mothers and bred in an infected environment with a normal diet [2]. It would appear, therefore, that at least within the spleen compartment, the immune system shows an activity of its own, which leads to the generation of large numbers of high rate immunoglobulin-secreting cells. Such an environment-independent activity is also observed in the other lymphocyte compartments. As we have recently shown, normal mice contain in their spleens activated effector cells of both the helper and the suppressor type, in roughly the same numbers as background effector cells of the B lymphocyte lineage. It is yet to be determined whether or not such "natural" generation of effector T cells is truly internal, by studying "antigen-free" mice, but we think it very likely that this is indeed the case. It is obvious, however, that even those carefully maintained animals are not antigen free, as the immune system is in contact with its own antigens and with those constituting the soma.

II. A Formal Network of Idiotypes

We have therefore turned experimentally to the study of the mutual interactions among the molecular and cellular components of the immune system, as well as between the immune system and other molecules found in the internal environment. To this end, we have isolated large collections of hybridomas, both of B and T lymphocytes, from newborn untreated animals, aiming at obtaining representative samples of the lymphocytes that have been activated in the internal environment. The analysis of these collections has already provided the first experimental evidence for the existence of a formal idiotypic network in the developing immune system. Thus, natural antibodies isolated from a single newborn mouse show an astonishingly high frequency of mutual reactions, demonstrating a degree of *connectivity* and *redundancy* in the developing immune system which might be expected on theoretical grounds as an attribute of stable networks. We are thus far unable to decide on the functional relevance of such idiotypic interactions. Experiments are at present being carried out, trying to analyze these aspects.

III. Mutual Influence of the T and B Cell Repertoires

The detailed study of these collections of naturally activated cells in normal mice has led us to an interesting conclusion: the specificity repertoire of background-activated cells is unique to each individual, even if newborn mice from the same litter of an inbred cross are compared. On the other hand, we can of course expect that the diversity repertoire of individual mice is submitted to genetic constraints, that is, limited to the possibilities allowed by gene families such as immunoglobulins, MHC, and T cell receptors. Within these potentialities, however, the individuality of immune systems defined by available repertoires appears to be established somatically by the connectivity between its cellular elements. Bearing in mind such organizational closure and internal activity, we have paid particular attention to the influences that antibody repertoires might have on T cell repertoires and the reverse, that is, the influences that T cell repertoires of both the helper and cytolytic type (as well as MHC genes) might have on natural antibody repertoires. Three clear-cut examples already exist, supporting the existence of these mutual influences which determine the specificity of the internal activity of the immune system.

One such example is already a few years old. It described the H-2 *and* immunoglobulin allotype control of a function of the normal immune system which consists in reproducing increased circulating levels of a given idiotype upon injection of nanogram amounts of same idiotype. Since idiotypes that had this property of "autoreproduction" are consistently found as natural antibodies in the serum of normal mice, we have concluded that natural antibody repertoires may well be under the influence of H-2 and, consequently, are at least in part selected on the basis of T cell specificities and activities. We have further suggested that among natural antibodies (i.e., products of cells that were internally activated), a relatively high frequency of idiotypic profiles resembling MHC products could be expected on the basis of the predominant anti-H-2 specificities in the T cell compartment. This hypothesis has been recently confirmed by isolating natural idiotypes which are internal images of self-MHC antigens.

As a mirror image of this type of influence, we have also found that helper cell repertoires, particularly the expression of idiotypes on clonally distributed receptors, is controlled not only by MHC-linked genes, but also by immunoglobulin heavy-chain genes. We have further shown that the influence of immunoglobulin genes on such repertoires is indirect and results from internal complementarities established between the two repertoires, because helper cell idiotypic repertoires are profoundly altered in mice deprived from birth of the antibody/B cell system.

We conclude from all these observations that a normal immune system is characterized by a high degree of internal activity which results from mutual specific complementarities between T and B cell repertoires. Effector cells are induced in the internal environment and themselves regulate the levels of activity in the normal system and determine, within the "noise" that surrounds the immune system, what makes sense to it and can therefore perturb its equilibrium and modify its activity.

C. The Normality of Autoreactivity

A large body of evidence has accumulated over the last few years indicating the existence of immune reactivities directed to other components of the immune system itself. Thus, antibodies, helper cells, and cytolytic T cells have been shown to recognize idiotypic determinants on other antibodies or on T lymphocytes. Furthermore, normal autoreactivity of T lymphocytes that appears to be stimulated by self-I-A under some conditions, has led to a large number of descriptions of what is called autologous MLR. It appears, therefore, that autoreactivity is a normal component within the immune system itself, as one would expect from a complex autonomous system that is self-organized. For a number of years, quite independently from these observations, a considerable number of reports have dealt with the existence in normal individuals of lymphocyte precursors in the B cell lineage with specificities for determinants expressed on other proteins of the "self" internal environment. The prevalent concept, however, is that in the absence of effective helper activity which is thought to be eliminated (T cell tolerance to self-determinants is a widely accepted concept), such B cell precursors will not be induced to antibody formation in the normal immune system. Autoimmunity has invariably been considered as pathologic and the approaches to its pathogenesis have been the search for either the abnormal expression (qualitative or quantitative) of a self-antigen, or the abnormal occurrence of one or more lymphocyte clones that should have been "forbidden."

More recently, however, considerable evidence has accumulated for the existence of autoreactive antibodies in the pool of natural circulating immunoglobulin. In the analysis of natural antibodies in newborn mice, we have observed that a very large fraction of these internally induced antibodies show extensive reactions with self-antigens. Other observations in adult individuals, both mice and humans, have led Avrameas and his collaborators to infer the invariable presence of autoreactive antibodies in the normal serum of these species. It follows that the presence of autoantibodies is not correlated with autoimmune pathology, a conclusion that had already been suggested by some workers in the field of autoimmunity. It becomes important, therefore, to separate the *physiology* from the *pathology* of autoreactivity, and to evaluate its physiologic relevance. It also appears to us that the study of the internal activity of the normal immune system, which is formally more similar to pathologic situations due to autoreactivity, may be more likely to lead us to the solution of these problems than the study of immune responses, developed within systemic strategies and clonal patterns of lymphocyte behavior which are definitely very different from those that can be observed in the normal physiology of the immune system.

Reference

1. Coutinho et al. (1984) Immunol Rev 79:151–168
2. Benner R, personal communication

Haematology and Blood Transfusion Vol. 29
Modern Trends in Human Leukemia VI
Edited by Neth, Gallo, Greaves, Janka

Antigen Presentation by Liposomes

P. Walden, Z. A. Nagy, and J. Klein[1]

A. Introduction

T cells respond to foreign antigen only when the latter is presented on the surface of an antigen-presenting cell (APC) together with a molecule encoded in the major histocompatibility complex (MHC). The nature of this antigen presentation is poorly understood. The difficulty of demonstrating soluble antigen serologically on the surface of APC, the finding that in some cases peptides of a certain protein are more antigenic than the whole molecule [1], the observation that T cells respond to native and denatured antigen equally well irrespective of which form was used for priming [2], and the fact that cells can rapidly degrade the antigen have led to the concept of antigen processing. According to this hypothesis the antigen is internalized and structurally altered (possibly enzymatically degraded) by the APC, and is then redisplayed on the surface of this cell in association with MHC molecules. Only antigens thus converted are recognizable by T cells [3].

To determine whether antigen processing is necessary for T-cell activation, we constructed liposomes carrying a foreign protein antigen and MHC class II molecules, and tested whether these liposomes could activate antigen-specific class II-restricted T cells in the absence of APC. The results presented here demonstrate that T cells can recognize unprocessed, native antigen.

1 Max-Planck-Institut für Biologie, Abteilung Immungenetik, Corrensstr. 42, 7400 Tübingen, FRG

The protocol used to produce the liposomes is described in detail elsewhere [4]. A summary is given in Fig. 1. The liposomes produced by this procedure contain MHC molecules inserted into the lipid bilayer by their transmembrane portion and a protein antigen covalently bound to DPPE (dipalmitoylphosphatidylethanolamin) lipids via a disulfide bond.

B. Results and Discussion

Table 1 summarizes a series of experiments that were performed with a lactate dehydrogenase B (LDH_B)-specific A^b-restricted mouse T-cell clone. Under the conditions when the T cells did not proliferate to LDH_B without adding APC they could be stimulated by liposomes containing the antigen and the restriction molecule (A^b) but could not be stimulated by either liposomes containing only one of these two components or liposomes with LDH_B together with another class II molecule. A mixture of liposomes carrying the antigen and liposomes carrying the MHC molecule or a mixture of A^b-containing liposomes with soluble LDH_B were also ineffective. These results show that the antigen and the restriction molecule combined in the same membrane provide a sufficient signal for the activation of T cells. Thus an APC-dependent processing step is not required for antigen recognition by T cells. Apparently the antigenic site seen by the T cell is only determined by the molecular properties of the antigen and is not influenced by the APC.

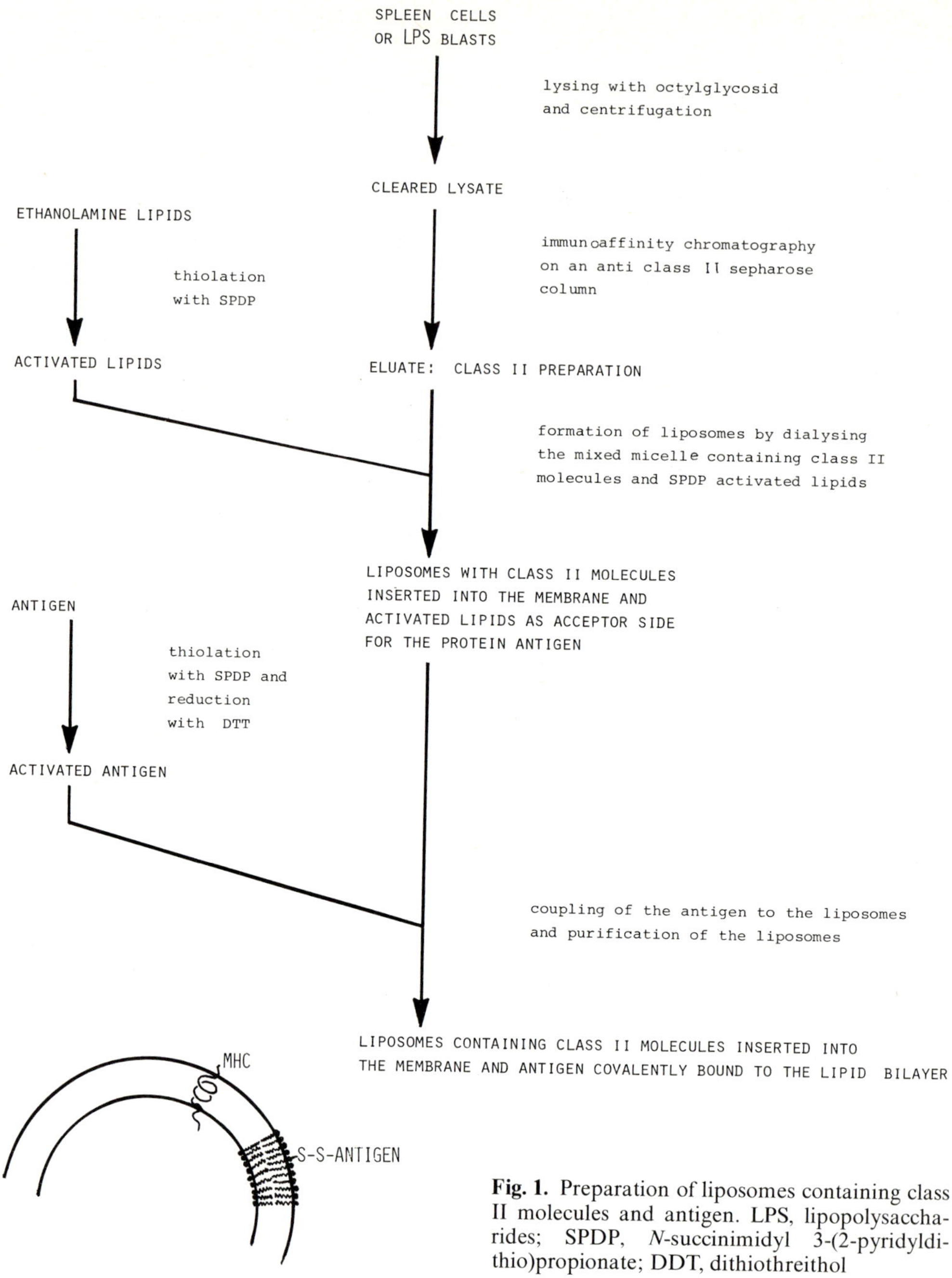

Fig. 1. Preparation of liposomes containing class II molecules and antigen. LPS, lipopolysaccharides; SPDP, *N*-succinimidyl 3-(2-pyridyldithio)propionate; DDT, dithiothreithol

Two further important observations could be made in these experiments. First, the physical properties of the liposome membrane influence the response dramatically. Liposomes composed of lipids that form a liquid crystalline bilayer at the incubation temperature (experiments 1, 2) have a much lower stimulatory capacity than rigid liposomes composed of lipids that result in a bilayer with a high phase-transition temperature (experiments 3, 4). Thus, the mobility of the two essential com-

Table 1. Proliferative response of the B6 anti LDH_B T-cell clone L_B-E8/G11 to liposomes containing MHC class II molecules and antigen (cpm)

Lipids in the liposomes	DPPC : DOPC : OPPC : SPDP-DPPE 5 : 1 : 3 : 1		DPPE : SPDP-DPPE 9 : 1	
Experiment No.	1	2	3	4
Response to				
SC + antigen LDH_B	31 296 ± 3 090	16 077 ± 1 141	6 496 ± 200	16 786 ± 1 822
SC + Con A	286 983 ± 74 058	ND	56 809 ± 3 413	64 505 ± 3 882
SC + CM	257 ± 125	576 ± 118	572 ± 116	672 ± 247
Antigen LDH_B	424 ± 170	396 ± 269	1 266 ± 40	514 ± 247
CM	315 ± 137	582 ± 127	637 ± 177	ND
Liposomes containing				
A^b and LDH_B	4 812 ± 1 252	3 900 ± 59	153 298 ± 5 600	103 971 ± 5 034
LDH_B	949 ± 63	893 ± 397	ND	5 025 ± 837
A^b	841 ± 152	1 252 ± 236	ND	3 625 ± 649
A^D and LDH_B	1 050 ± 649	1 315 ± 110	ND	ND
Mixture of A^b and LDH_B	ND	750 ± 242	ND	3 874 ± 812
A^b and free LDH_B	ND	1 266 ± 182	ND	ND
No protein	814 ± 387	ND	ND	8 437 ± 978

DPPC, dipalmitoylphosphotidylcholine; DOPC, dioleylphosphatidylcholine; OPPC, oleylpalmitoylphosphatidylcholine; SC, spleen cells; con A, concanavalin A; cm, culture medium; ND, not done

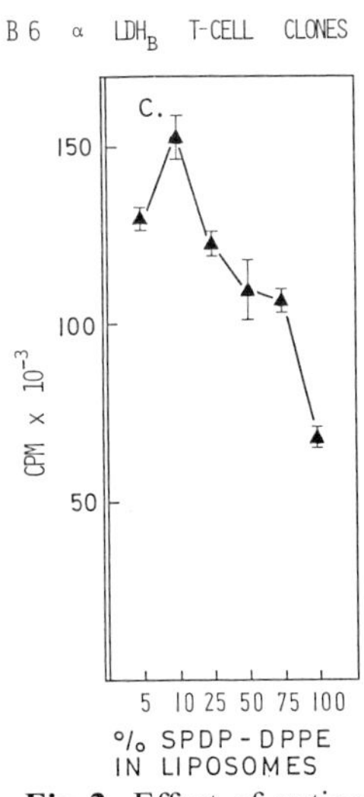

Fig. 2. Effect of antigen density on proliferative T-cell response. The liposomes were produced with DPPE containing different amounts (5%–100%) of SPDP-modified DPPE and A^B molecules. They were allowed to react with a large excess of SPDP-coupled LDH and were purified by sucrose-gradient centrifugation. Control values (cpm) for the response of the clone E8/G11 to: medium, 637 ± 177; LDH_B 1266 ± 40; syngeneic spleen cells 572 ± 116; spleen cells + LDH_B, 6496 ± 200. SPDP-DPPE, SPDP-modified DPPE

ponents appears to correlate negatively with the ability of the vesicles to trigger T cells. This result suggests that cross-linking of T-cell receptors may be a signal for T-cell activation. Second, the antigen density in the membrane with a constant amount of MHC molecule exhibits a sharp optimum (Fig. 2). The finding that high antigen densities, although increasing the probability of MHC-antigen interaction, result in decreased T-cell response, argues against the hypothesis that the formation of MHC-antigen complexes is a prerequisite for T-cell stimulation. Thus T cells may recognize antigen and MHC as separate entities.

That the MHC-antigen ratio in liposomes was critical for T-cell activation was observed also in other experiments: Fig. 3 shows a titration experiment with a pigeon cytochrome C specific B10.A(5R) T-cell hybridoma as an indicator system. In this case, liposomes that contain the antigen at a too high density to activate the T cells in the presence of the appropriate restriction element (here E^k) could trigger T cells in the absence of MHC molecules or in the presence of an irrelevant MHC molecule. This finding can be explained by the cross-linking model, namely, by assuming that

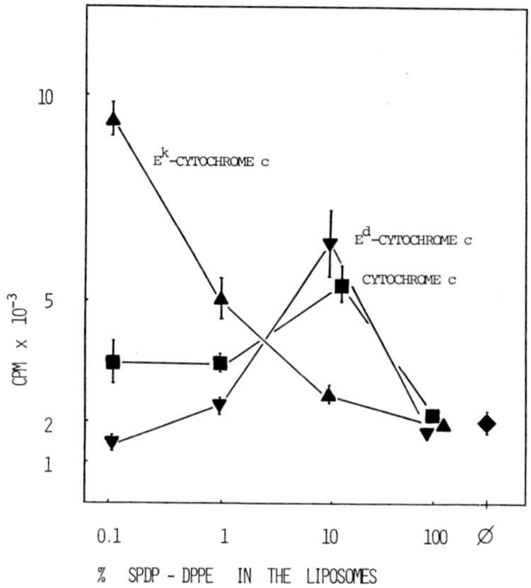

Fig. 3. Effect of antigen density on the induction of IL-2 by the B10.A (5R) anticytochrome c T-cell hybridoma line. The liposomes were produced with DPPE containing varying amounts (0.1%–100%) of SPDP-modified DPPE (efficiency of the modification, 1.7%) and E^k molecules. They were produced as described and tested for their capacity to induce IL-2 production by the T-cell hybridoma 4117 (B10.A[5R]); Heber-Katz et al.). Liposomes containing E^k and cytochrome c (▲), E^d and cytochrome c (▼), and cytochrome c (■) were used. Control values (cpm) for IL-2 production: feeder cells (B10.A), 542±88; antigen (cytochrome c), 2145±348; feeder cells and antigen, 74 680±7384. SPDP-DPPE, SPDP-modified DPPE

Table 2. Secondary response of T cells to liposomes containing MHC class II molecules and antigen (cpm)

Cell line	B10.D2 α KLH	B 6 α OVA	B 6 α Insulin	B10.A α HEL
Responses to				
SC + antigen	179 166 ± 16 012	81 237 ± 9 279	184 657 ± 12 134	29 479 ± 2 936
SC + Con A	299 335 ± 18 599	74 790 ± 4 487	161 640 ± 2 032	158 149 ± 6 271
SC + CM	6 829 ± 557	1 533 ± 632	1 756 ± 377	4 196 ± 513
Antigen	22 721 ± 1 136	881 287	1 536 ± 607	1 198 ± 402
Liposomes containing				
A^d and KLH	172 006 ± 2 916			
A^b and KLH	263 412 ± 21 747	1 413 ± 280		
KLH	247 183 ± 12 841			
A^b and OVA		27 724 ± 4 325	3 163 ± 358	
OVA		6 472 ± 518		
A^b and insulin			81 844 ± 8 074	
Insulin			173 661 ± 10 420	
A^k and HEL				121 273 ± 9 799
A^b and HEL				1 855 ± 312
HEL				4 768 ± 827
A^k and cytochrome c				1 911 ± 392
A^k				4 419 ± 688
A^b		1 178 ± 39	4 063 ± 72	
A^d	5 378 ± 41			
Mixture of liposomes containing				
A^b + Insulin			23 811 ± 1 059	
A^d + KLH	160 828 ± 12 074			
A^b + OVA		6 776 ± 978		
A^k + HEL				3 343 ± 697
A^b + free insulin			3 324 ± 582	
A^d + free KLH	28 715 ± 3 074			
A^b + free OVA		1 095 ± 289		
A^k + free HEL				7 236 ± 973
eeee	8 398 ± 1 696	1 546 ± 344	5 010 ± 512	2 090 ± 711

KLH, keyhole limpet hemocyanin; HEL, hen egg lysozyme; SC, spleen cells; cm, culture medium weak interactions can sum up to reach the threshold affinity for the initiation of the response.

The observations reported here can be generalized as shown by the experiments in Table 2. Short-term T-cell lines from different mouse strains that were specific for different antigens were used to test the liposomes. The findings are basically the same as those discussed above. With these polyclonal T-cell populations, we observed in several instances that liposomes containing only the antigen induced a T-cell response.

In conclusion, our data suggest that the most important function of APC is to provide a cell surface with the appropriate density of foreign antigen and MHC molecules for triggering of T cells. Thus the presence of antigen and MHC on the same membrane appears to be the only requirement to activate primed T cells. The results rule out the possibility that extensive processing is necessary to render foreign proteins antigenic for T cells. The question of possible additional functions of APC, such as the secretion of nonspecific mediators required for T-cell differentiation, is not addressed by this study.

References

1. Shimonkevitz R et al. (1983) J Exp Med 158:303–316
2. Chesnut RW et al. (1980) Clin Immunol Immunopathol 15:397–408
3. Unanue ER (1984) J Immunol 132:1–5
4. Walden P, Nagy ZA, Klein J (1985) Nature (in press)

Haematology and Blood Transfusion Vol. 29
Modern Trends in Human Leukemia VI
Edited by Neth, Gallo, Greaves, Janka

Thymic Dendritic Cells Present Blood-Borne Antigens to Medullary Thymocytes In Vivo: A Possible Role in the Generation of the T-Cell Repertoire

B. A. Kyewski [1]

A. Introduction

The thymus represents a crucial phase in the differentiation of T cells, from their earliest precursor committed to the T-cell lineage in the bone marrow, to the full array of peripheral T-effector cells. Specification of T-cell subsets, generation of receptor diversity, selection of self-MHC-restricted T-cell precursors, and induction of self-tolerance are thought to be largely or exclusively intrathymic events [24]. How such complex functional events relate to the relatively simple structure of the thymus is poorly understood. It has become apparent that the pattern of T-cell reactivity is selected by the environment [6, 26] in which T cells develop rather than being strictly genetically fixed; thus interest has focused on the definition of such selection sites. To this end direct cell–cell interactions between cells of the T-cell lineage and nonlymphoid stromal cells in the murine thymus have been characterized [25, 13, 14]. These interactions preexist in vivo, can be isolated as intact multicellular lymphostromal complexes by differential digestion of the thymus, and are thus amenable to analysis in vitro. At least three lymphostromal–cell interactions can be discerned: (1) between T cells and macrophages (M*Φ*), (2) between T cells and dendritic cells (DC) (both 1 and 2 referred to as thymocyte rosettes, *T-ROS*), and (3) between T cells and epithelial cells (thymic nurse cells, *TNC*). T-ROS and TNC are obtained as sequential fractions during digestion, thereby making possible a separate isolation of distinct complex types. A comparison between these interaction structures revealed the following salient points [25, 13–16, 7]. All three interactions seem to be obligatory steps for T-cell differentiation; their frequency correlates with ontogeny of T-cell maturation and is unaffected by the immune status of the animals. T-cell-stromal-cell recognition in vivo does not require syngeneity but occurs between fully allogeneic partner cells [16]. The T-cell subsets engaged in stromal-cell interactions (2%–3% of all thymocytes) are immature in surface antigen phenotype and enriched in cycling cells over unselected thymocytes. When the entry of donor bone marrow (BM)-derived Thy 1.1 pre-T cells was followed in the thymus of congenic Thy 1.2 hosts, they were found to interact first with macrophages, second with epithelial cells, and third with dendritic cells, indicating a temporal hierarchy of lymphostromal recognition during T-cell development. These kinetics do not necessarily imply a colinear maturation sequence since precursor product relationships are not known. By direct comparison of the appearance of donor T cells in lymphostromal-cell complexes after isolation in vitro, with the concomitant localization of donor T cells in situ, M*Φ*-ROS and TNC were located to the cortex and DC-ROS to the medulla (Kyewski, unpublished data).

Though the recognition structures governing these interactions are not known,

1 Institute for Immunology and Genetics, German Cancer Research Centre, Im Neuenheimer Feld 280, 6900 Heidelberg, FRG
Henry Kaplan Award for the best poster Immunological Session

Table 1.

Stromal cell type	Location	Expression of MHC antigens class		Tissue derivation	Antigen accessibility	Antigen presentation capacity	Kinetic order of T-cell interaction	Presumptive funcion
		I	II					
Macrophage	Inner cortex	Yes	No	Bone marrow	Secluded	Deficient	First	Growth and differentiation of early thymocytes
Epithelial cell	Outer cortex	Yes	Yes	Third pharyngeal pouch	Secluded	Deficient	Second	Selection according to self-MHC antigens
Dendritic cell	Medulla	Yes	Yes	Bone marrow	Accessible	Highly efficient	Third	Tolerance induction via corecognition of MHC and non-MHC self antigens

it is surmised from indirect evidence in radiation chimeras that self-MHC determinants at least in part specify these interactions [6, 26]. Given the observation that both cortical epithelial cells and medullary dendritic cells express high amounts of class II MHC-antigens constitutively in vivo (whereas cortical macrophages were found to be I-A/E negative), we tested whether non-MHC-antigens may have access to the thymus and be presented to maturing thymocytes during their maturation in vivo. This question bears particular relevance to the problem of where developing T cells expressing antigen-specific receptors are first confronted with non-MHC-self-antigens and where self-tolerance takes place. Recent evidence indicating that tolerance induction is MHC restricted would favor T-cell-accessory-cell interactions at such sites [8, 18, 19].

B. Results and Discussion

Intrathymic antigen presentation was assayed by coculture of antigen-specific I-A-restricted cloned T-helper cells with purified irradiated thymic lymphostromal-cell complexes [11, 15]. As antigens we used myoglobin, L-glutamic acid^{60}-L-alanine^{30}-L-tyrosine^{10} (GAT), and keyhole limpet hemocyanin (KLH). Proliferation of T cells was measured 72 h after culture in vitro by [^{3}H]thymidine uptake. Antigen was either injected intravascularly (i.v.) before isolation of the stimulator population or added to the culture in vitro. After injection of 0.5 mg myoglobin/g body weight i.v. into C57BL/Ka mice, T-ROS copurified with specific stimulation of I-A^b-restricted myoglobin-specific T-helper cells. This antigen-specific stimulation was a property of Thy-1.2-negative stromal cells (anti-Thy 1.2 antibody plus complement treatment did not alter the presentation capacity of *T-ROS*) and could be inhibited by more than 90% after pretreatment of the stimulator population with anti I-A^b monoclonal antibody and complement. Antigen traffic to the thymus in vivo was dose dependent within the range of 1.0–0.25 mg myoglobin/g body weight. Threshold doses for thymic and splenic antigen-presenting cells (APC) required to present antigen were similar, indicating no significant seclusion in vivo of APC enclosed in the T-ROS fraction. Similar results were obtained after injection of KLH (molecular weight 3×10^6) and GAT (molecular weight, 1×10^5) [15]. When kinetics of antigen persistence in the thymus were measured, antigen-specific stimulation of T cells was demonstrable up to 48 h after injection i.v. (Fig. 1A). The prolonged presence of antigen within the thymus argues

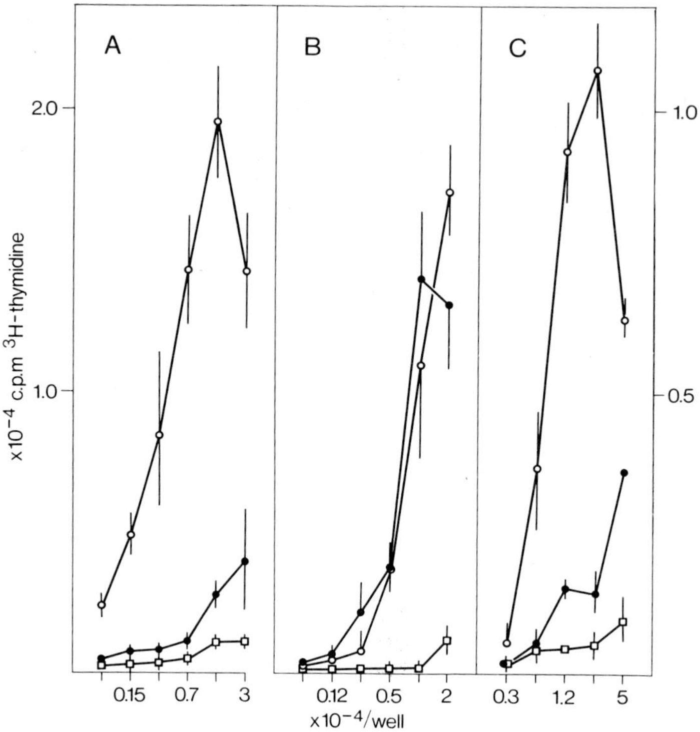

Fig. 1A–C. A Kinetics of antigen persistence in the thymus. C57BL/Ka mice were injected with 0.5 mg myoglobin/g body weight i.v. and 15 min (○) or 48 h (●) later nonadherent T-ROS were purified, irradiated, and cocultured with myoglobin-specific cloned T-helper cells (2×10^4/well). T-cell proliferation was measured after 72 h of coculture by [^{3}H]thymidine uptake. □ uninjected control; **B** Cellular characterization of thymic antigen-presenting cells. C57BL/Ka mice were injected with myoglobin (see **A**) and 2 h later T-ROS were isolated, fractionated, and cocultured with specific T-helper cells. ● unseparated T-ROS; ○ nonadherent T-ROS; □ adherent T-ROS; **C** Physiological turnover of thymic antigen-presenting cells. Nonadherent T-ROS were isolated from (C57BL/Ka×C3H/J)F_1 mice (○), (C57BL/Ka×C3H/J)F_1 BM→C3H/J newborn (●), and (Balb/c×C3H/ J) BM→C3H/J newborn (□) chimeras. Newborn mice were injected with 20×10^6 BM cells/day on days 0–4 and tested 2 weeks later. T-ROS were cocultured with cloned allo-anti I-A^b T-helper cells. *Values on abscissa* refer to numbers of stromal cells/well

against a trivial explanation of these results, namely the uptake of antigen by stromal cells (which were secluded in the intact organ), after disruption of the tissue context during the isolation procedure. Although myoglobin (molecular weight 17 000) is rapidly cleared from the circulation, the APC activity of T-ROS was unchanged when tested 15 min or 12 h after injection of antigen.

In further defining the cell type(s) responsible for uptake of antigen in vivo and presentation in vitro we separated T-ROS stromal cells into adherent and nonadherent fractions. More than 90% of adherent stromal cells are composed of I-A/E-negative, F 4/80-positive, phagocytic MΦ-like cells, whereas the nonadherent stromal cells contain 50%–80% nonphagocytic F 4/80-negative, I-A/E-positive DC-like cells [1, 14]. When separately tested for APC activity after injection of myoglobin i.v., the nonadherent fraction contained all functional APC, whereas the adherent-cell fraction even when pulsed with additional antigen in vitro remained nonstimulatory (Fig. 1B). Though this separation method needs further confirmation by enrichment protocols using strictly lineage-specific surface markers, it was reproducibly found that depletion of strongly adherent MΦ did not affect the ability of the T-ROS fraction to present antigen. The lack of class II MHC-antigen expression on cortical macrophages forming T-ROS is compatible with this result. In order to test DCs and TNCs separately for their accessibility and capacity to present antigen, we turned our attention to their different embryonic origins. DCs are strictly bone marrow derived whereas epithelial cells are derived from the third pharyngeal pouch. Thus, $P_1 \rightarrow (P_1 \times P_2)$ F_1 radiation chimeras were analyzed in which DCs were completely replaced by P_1-type cells and epithelial cells remained of the F_1 type. When antigen presentation by cells isolated from such animals was tested 10 weeks after reconstitution with T-helper cells restricted to P_2-type I-A antigens, no T-cell proliferation was measured using either purified T-ROS (that is bone-marrow-derived stromal cells) or epithelial cells as stimulators. The latter, however, expressed class II-MHC-determinants of P_2-type abundantly, as determined by fluorescence microscopy. This lack of antigen presentation by thymic epithelial cells after injection of myoglobin i.v. could not be overcome by providing optimal doses of antigen in vitro [15]. This result indicates an intrinsic deficiency of epithelial cells in stimulation of T-helper cells, rather than a seclusion from antigen in vivo. It is not clear to date whether the epithelial cells lack the ability to process antigen and/or fail to produce obligatory costimulation factors (e.g., interleukin-l). Interestingly, thymic epithelial cells have been successfully grafted across allogeneic barriers without being rejected [21]. Given the assumption that DCs are responsible for antigen presentation in the thymus, we further assessed the physiological turnover of thymic DCs (equivalent here to nonadherent T-ROS). To this end we used nonradiation chimeras. Newborn P_1 mice were given multiple injections with F_1 bone marrow cells at daily intervals. Such animals establish a stable bone marrow chimerism which is proportional to the dose of donor cells injected (Kyewski, unpublished data). In such "normal" hosts, without prior ablation of bone marrow-derived hemopoietic lineages, F_1-BM-derived cells establish stem-cell chimerism and replace host cells during physiological turnover. When nonadherent T-ROS from such $F_1 \rightarrow P_1$ newborn chimeras were cocultured with cloned T-helper cells restricted to P_2-type I-A antigens, specific proliferation was detected (Fig. 1C). This proliferative response amounted to about 10%–20% of the magnitude induced by normal F_1 mice-derived T-ROS, indicating a significant replacement in the thymus of host-type DCs by cells of donor origin. The result indicates that medullary DCs, in contrast to cortical epithelial cells, undergo a constant physiological turnover and replacement by extrathymic DCs. Thus, in addition to the direct entry of blood-borne antigens into the thymus, circulating antigen-laden-DCs may contribute to the spectrum of intrathymically presented antigens.

The described results, in concert with earlier studies on these cell interactions [25, 13–16, 7], indicate a strict compartmentalization of thymic stromal cells with regard to their accessibility to circulating antigens and their intrinsic capacity to present these antigens to T cells. Macrophages and epithelial cells (here isolated by virtue of their interactions with thymocytes in vivo) seem to be highly inefficient in presentation of soluble protein antigens and are presumably secluded from blood-borne antigens by a vascular blood-cortex barrier. In contrast, presenting DCs are strictly confined to the medulla, which in turn displays a vascular architecture permissive to the passage of macromolecules [20]. Thus, an important aspect of cortex/medulla dichotomy with regard to T-cell recognition resides in either the prevention or facilitation of T-cell encounters with non-MHC antigens in conjunction with self MHC-antigens.

In the following we speculate on the possible roles of the three recognition steps in the context of the development of the T-cell repertoire. Pre-T cells probably enter the thymus at the cortical side of the cortical-medullary junction and first interact with

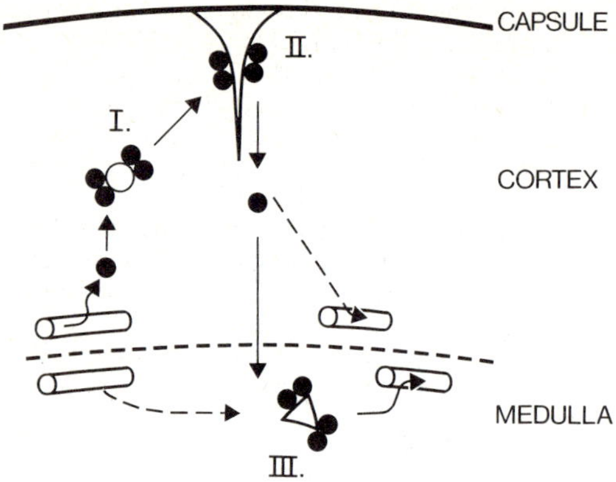

Fig. 2. *Solid arrows* indicate conjectural routes of intrathymic T-cell migration intercalated by lymphostromal recognition and selection steps between thymocytes and macrophages (*I*), epithelial cells (*II*), and dendritic cells (*III*). *Dashed arrows* indicate equally possible traffic routes

and proliferate around macrophages in the inner cortex (Fig. 2). The role of these macrophages may resemble those in hemopoietic islands in the bone marrow, in which they support the growth and differentiation of erythropoietic and granulopoietic cell lineages by direct cell–cell contact [2, 5]. This early stage of thymocyte–accessory-cell interaction may not yet involve the T-cell receptor for antigen recognition but may induce its expression. After this initial M*Φ*-induced growth and differentiation phase a second interaction with epithelial cells follows in the outer cortex. As proposed previously, this interaction may represent the recognition of self-MHC determinants expressed on epithelial cells by a minor selective set of clonally expressed T-cell receptors, thus determining the self-MHC restriction of cytotoxic and helper T cells [6, 26]. If correct, one would predict that all T cells associated with epithelial cells should have productively rearranged T-cell-receptor genes and express membrane-bound T-cell-receptors [12]. In the absence of non-MHC antigens this recognition step has to be different from the obligatory corecognition of MHC antigens and nominal antigens exhibited by mature T cells [23, 3]. A third type of intercellular recognition, now in the medulla between thymocytes and dendritic cells, displays the characteristic MHC-restricted recognition of non-MHC antigens, which enter this compartment and are presented here to maturing T cells. By conjecture this site may constitute a possible microenvironment where self-tolerance is induced. This proposition receives indirect support from the recent observation that thymic epithelial cells when grafted across allogeneic barriers do not induce T-cell tolerance to their own class II MHC antigens [21]. DC-thymocyte interactions would conform to the prediction that tolerance induction is MHC restricted [8, 18, 19]. In addition, the ontogeny of thymocyte-DC interactions parallels the induction of self-tolerance [17] (Kyewski, unpublished data). These considerations, however, leave the cellular and molecular mechanisms of how self-tolerance is induced and maintained completely unexplained. According to this model, recognition structures on stromal cells select for complementary receptors on T cells expressed at the respective stage of their interaction. With the advent of monoclonal antibodies and molecular probes specific for the T-cell-receptor certain predictions of this model may be tested [9, 10]. In the absence of direct evidence for a precursor–product relationship between the various interactions, and the unknown fate of the selected thymocytes, the developmental pathways of T cells still remain conjectural [22] (Fig. 2).

The outlined results and speculations depict the complexity of intrathymic T-cell maturation with regard to cell-to-cell communication, compartmentalization, and directed lymphocyte traffic. The possibly critical involvement of stromal cells in growth control of hematopoietic cell lineages has recently been reemphasized [4]. In view of the notion that some forms of acute T-cell leukemias may represent an arrest in differentiation rather than an irreversible transformation step, the analysis of the inductive signals responsible for T-cell growth and differentiation may aid our understanding of the mechanism of T-cell leukemogenesis. T-cell transformation, at least in the murine model, has been shown to be strictly dependent on an intact thymic microenvironment.

Acknowledgment. This work has been conducted under the stimulating guidance of the late Henry S. Kaplan, Cancer Biology Research Laboratory, Dept. of Radiology in collaboration with Dr. C. G. Fathman, Div. of Immunology, Dept. of Medicine, Stanford University Medical School. The author was supported by a postdoctoral fellowship of the DFG.

References

1. Austyn JM, Gordon S (1981) F4/80, a monoclonal antibody directed specifically against the mouse macrophage. Eur J Immunol 10: 805–811
2. Ben-Ishay Z, Yoffey JM (1972) Ultrastructural studies of erythroblastic islands of rat bone marrow. II Resumption of erythropoiesis in erythropoietically depressed rebound marrow. Lab Invest 26:637–647
3. Bevan MJ (1981) Thymic education. Immunol Today 2:216–219
4. Boettiger D, Anderson S, Dexter TM (1984) Effect of *src* infection on long-term marrow culture: increased self renewal of hemopoietic progenitor cells without leukemia. Cell 36:763–773
5. Cline MJ, Golde DW (1979) Cellular interactions in hematopoiesis. Nature 277: 177–181
6. Fink PJ, Bevan MJ (1978) H-2 antigen of the thymus determines lymphocyte specificity. J Exp Med 148:766–775
7. Fink PJ, Weissman IL, Kaplan HS, Kyewski BA (1984) The immunocompetence of murine stromal cell-associated thymocytes. J Immunol 132:2266–2272
8. Groves ES, Singer A (1983) Role of H-2 complex in the induction of T cell tolerance to minor histocompatibility antigens. J Exp Med 158:1483–1497
9. Haskins K et al. (1983) The major-histocompatibility-restricted antigen receptor on T cells. I. Isolation with a monoclonal antibody. J Exp Med 157:1149–1169
10. Hedrick S et al. (1984) Isolation of cDNA clones encoding T-cell-specific membrane-associated proteins. Nature 308:149–153
11. Infante AJ, Atassi MZ, Fathman CG (1981) T cell clones reactive with sperm whale myoglobin. Isolation of clones with specificity for individual determinants on myoglobin. J Exp Med 154:1342–1356
12. Kavaler J, Davis MM, Chien Y-H (1984) Localization of a T-cell receptor diversity-region element. Nature 310:421–423
13. Kyewski BA, Kaplan HS (1982) Lymphoepithelial interactions in the murine thymus: phenotypic and kinetic studies on thymic nurse cells. J Immunol 128:2287–2294
14. Kyewski BA, Rouse RV, Kaplan HS (1982) Thymocyte rosettes: multicellular complexes of lymphocytes and bone-marrow-derived stromal cells in the murine thymus. Proc Natl Acad Sci USA 79:5646–5650
15. Kyewski BA, Fathman CG, Kaplan HS (1984a) Intrathymic presentation of circulating non-major histocompatibility complex antigens. Nature 308:196–199
16. Kyewski BA, Travis M, Kaplan HS (1984b) Intrathymic lymphopoiesis: stromal cell-associated proliferation of T cells is independent of lymphocyte genotype. J Immunol 133:1111–1116
17. Lu C-Y, Beller DI, Unanaue E (1981) During ontogeny, Ia-bearing accessor cells are found early in the thymus but late in the spleen. Proc Natl Acad Sci USA 77:1597–1601
18. Matzinger P, Zamoyska R, Waldmann H (1984) Self tolerance is H-2 restricted. Nature 308:738–741
19. Rammensee, H-G, Bevan MJ (1984) Evidence from *in vitro* studies that tolerance for self-antigens is MHC-restricted. Nature 308: 741–744
20. Raviola E, Karnovsky MJ (1972) Evidence for a blood-thymus barrier using electron opaque tracers. J Exp Med 136:466–498
21. Ready AR, Jenkinson EJ, Kingston R, Owen JJT (1984) Successful transplantation across major histocompatibility barrier of deoxyguanosine-treated embryonic thymus expressing class II antigens. Nature 310: 231–233
22. Scollay R (1983) Intrathymic events in the differentiation of T lymphocytes: a continuing enigma. Immunol Today 4:282–286
23. Von Böhmer H, Haas W, Jerne NK (1978) Major histocompatibility complex-linked immune-responsiveness is acquired by lymphocytes of low-responder mice differentiating in thymus of high-responder mice. Proc Natl Acad Sci USA 75:2439–2442
24. Wagner H, Röllinghoff M, Pfitzenmaier K (1982) The influence of the thymus on the generation of T cell repertoire. Behring Inst Mitt 70
25. Wekerle H, Ketelsen U-P, Ernst M (1980) Thymic nurse cells. Lymphoepithelial cell complexes in murine thymus: morphological and serological characterization. J Exp Med 151:925–944
26. Zinkernagel RM et al. (1978) On the thymus in the differentiation of "H-2 self recognition" by T cells: evidence for dual recognition. J Exp Med 147:882–896

Haematology and Blood Transfusion Vol. 29
Modern Trends in Human Leukemia VI
Edited by Neth, Gallo, Greaves, Janka

Natural Defense and Chemical Carcinogenesis

I. P. Witz[1], M. Efrati[1], R. Ehrlich[1], B. Gonen[1], L. Kachlon[1], O. Sagi[1], E. Sahar[2], L. Shochat[1], N. I. Smorodinsky[1], S. Yaakov[1], M. Yaakubowicz[1], and I. Yron

A. Introduction

It is becoming increasingly clear that chemical, physical, and biologic carcinogens are immunosuppressive. Most of the available information on the immunosuppressive activity of oncogenic agents concerns adaptive immunity [17]. Recent studies have indicated that exposure of laboratory animals to various carcinogenic insults affected also certain expressions of innate, natural immunity such as natural killer (NK) activity (for review see [2]).

In previous studies, we demonstrated that the chemical carcinogen dimethylbenzanthracene (DMBA) exerted a severe suppressive effect on NK activity of mouse splenocytes [3, 4]. In the present study, we addressed the following questions:

1. Is the decrease in NK activity of DMBA-treated mice restricted to the spleen, or is this decrease also evident in other lymphocyte-containing compartments? To answer this question, we compared the NK activity of peripheral blood leukocytes (PBL) from untreated and DMBA-treated mice. We also performed adoptive transfer experiments in which we tested the NK activity of splenocytes from lethally irradiated recipients reconstituted with syngeneic bone marrow from either untreated or from DMBA-treated donors.

2. Is the decrease in NK activity of DMBA-treated animals due to a functional defect or is it due to a reduction in the size of the NK cell population? This was answered in the present study by performing a flow cytometry analysis of cells expressing asialo-GM-1- (a ganglioside expressed on the membrane of certain lymphocyte subpopulations, especially NK cells [7]), in the spleen of DMBA-treated animals.

3. Are other cells of the immune system also affected by DMBA? We have begun to answer this by performing mixed lymphocyte reactions (MLR) in which lymphocytes of DMBA-treated animals served as responders.

4. Is the activity of natural antitumor antibodies (NATA) affected by carcinogen treatment? We have compared NATA activity of untreated mice with that of urethane- or DMBA-treated ones.

B. Results

I. The NK Activity of PBL from DMBA-Treated BALB/c Mice

Table 1 shows that the NK activity of PBL from DMBA-treated BALB/c mice is considerably lower than that of untreated age- and sex-matched syngeneic controls. These results indicate that the effect of DMBA on

1 Departments of Microbiology
2 Biotechnology, The George S. Wise Faculty of Life Sciences, Tel Aviv University, Tel Aviv, Israel

Table 1. The NK activity of PBL from DMBA-treated BALB/c mice

Effector : target	Cytotoxicity index ± standard deviation [a]	
	Untreated controls [b]	DMBA-treated [c]
100 : 1	10.0±4.6	6.1±3.9
50 : 1	7.4±5.1	4.3±2.7
25 : 1	4.9±4.0	2.9±2.0
12.5 : 1	3.4±2.8	2.0±1.3

[a] $\text{Cytotoxicity index} = 100 \times \frac{\text{cpm released in experimental well} - \text{spontaneous release}}{\text{total cpm incorporated} - \text{spontaneous release cpm}}$

Mean cytotoxicity index ± standard deviation given by PBL obtained from the tail vein from 30–50 mice tested individually in 3 experiments. YAC-1 cells were used as targets

[b] 8 to 10-week-old females

[c] Age and sex-matched mice were treated intragastrically with 1 mg/week DMBA (Sigma) dissolved in corn oil; 4 weekly treatments were given; NK activity was tested 21 days after the last DMBA treatment

NK activity was systemic and not restricted to the spleen.

II. The NK Activity of Splenocytes from Lethally Irradiated BALB/c Mice Reconstituted with Bone Marrow Cells from DMBA-Treated Donors

In this series of experiments, we assayed the ability of adoptively transferred bone marrow cells from DMBA-treated mice or from untreated controls to reconstitute splenic NK activity of syngeneic BALB/c mice irradiated with 950 rad. The results shown in Table 2 indicate that DMBA treatment, under the experimental conditions utilized in this study, impaired the ability of bone marrow precursors to reconstitute NK activity in lethally irradiated recipients.

In order to find out whether or not DMBA was selectively toxic toward lymphatic cells such as NK cells, we compared spleen colonies of irradiated mice which received an adoptive transfer of bone marrow cells either from DMBA-treated mice or from untreated controls. We detected no qualitative or quantitative differences between the two groups. DMBA also failed to affect the ability of bone marrow cells to produce colonies in soft agar. These results suggest that DMBA acts selectively on lymphocyte precursors in the bone marrow.

III. Flow Cytometry Analysis of Splenocytes from DMBA-Treated BALB/c Mice

The percentage of Thy-1, Lyt-1, Lyt-2, and asialo-GM-1-positive cells in the spleen of untreated or DMBA-treated animals was determined by flow cytometry using commercially available fluorescently tagged antibodies. The results presented in Table 3 indicate that the percentage of the total T cell population and the two major T cell subpopulations were not affected by DMBA. The percentage of asialo-GM-1-positive NK cells was however drastically reduced. It should be remembered that the size of the spleen in DMBA-treated mice was reduced by about 50% [4]. The absolute number of T cells in the spleen was therefore reduced by the same factor whereas that of asialo-GM-1-positive cells was reduced by a much larger factor. These results suggest that DMBA was selectively toxic toward asialo-GM-1-positive cells with NK activity. However, sorting of asialo GM-1 positive cells originating in spleens or PBL of control or DMBA-treated animals (results not shown) indicated that the decreased NK activity observed in the

Table 2. The NK activity of splenocytes from lethally irradiated BALB/c mice reconstituted with bone marrow cells from untreated or DMBA-treated donors

	Cytotoxicity index ± standard deviation (% of nonirradiated controls)[a]	
	Source of bone marrow cells[b]	
Effector : target	Untreated donors	DMBA-treated
100 : 1	78	45
50 : 1	81	51
25 : 1	84	58
12.5 : 1	85	52

[a] See footnote [a] Table 1. The NK activity of splenocytes from nonirradiated, untreated controls was taken as the 100% baseline. The values represent the percentage activity (given by the indicated group) of such controls. The cytotoxicity index given by the NK cells of the control group ranged from 14 at an effector : target ratio of 12.5 : 1 to 32 at an effector : target ratio of 100 : 1. Average values of 12 experiments

[b] 8 to 10-week old female BALB/c mice were irradiated with 950 rad and reconstituted intravenously the same day with 5×10^6 bone marrow cells either from donors treated with 6 mg DMBA (1 mg/week see footnote [c] Table 1) or from age and sex-matched untreated donors. NK activity was assayed 1 month after irradiation and cell transfer. YAC-1 cells served as targets

Table 3. Flow cytometry of splenocytes from DMBA-treated BALB/c mice

	Splenocytes from DMBA-treated mice[a] (% of untreated controls)[b]	
Marker	3 mg DMBA	6 mg DMBA
Thy-1[d]	106 ± 13 (5)[c]	97 ± 8 (5)[c]
Lyt-1[d]	88 ± 4 (3)	94 ± 13 (3)
Lyt-2[d]	92 ± 10 (3)	90 ± 9 (3)
Asialo-GM-1[e]	48 ± 18 (3)	41 ± 30 (3)

[a] Splenocyte suspensions were freed of erythrocytes by osmotic shock and then passed through nylon wool columns. The nonadherent fraction was used

[b] The percentage of marker-positive cells in spleens of untreated controls was taken as the 100% baseline. Nonadherent splenocytes of such untreated controls contained 62% Thy-1-positive cells, 72% Lyt-1-positive cells, 21% Lyt-2-positive cells, and 4.4% asialo-GM-1-positive cells

[c] Numbers in parentheses indicate the number of experiments performed. A pool of spleens from 3–4 mice was tested in each experiment. The mice were tested 2–4 weeks after the last DMBA treatment (see footnote [c] to Table 1)

[d] Cells were directly stained with FITC-conjugated monoclonal antibody directed against the appropriate marker

[e] Cells were first treated with rabbit IgG directed against asialo-GM-1 and then stained with FITC-conjugated affinity-purified goat antibody against rabbit IgG

Table 4. The ability of splenocytes from DMBA-treated BALB/c mice to respond to alloantigens[a] in one-way mixed lymphocyte reactions

Treatment	Average[b] stimulation index	(% of untreated controls)
None	24.5 ± 13.3	100
3 mg DMBA	11.1 ± 7.4	45
6 mg DMBA	9.6 ± 6.3	39
None	9.6 ± 5.1	100
Irradiation + adoptive transfer[c] of bone marrow cells from untreated donors	3.6 ± 1.3	37
Irradiation + adoptive transfer of bone marrow cells from DMBA-treated donors	2.1 ± 0.4	22

[a] C3H/eB cells (H-2^k) served as stimulators. Stimulator cells were treated with mitomycine C

[b] $\text{Stimulation index} = \frac{\text{cpm in allogeneic MLR}}{\text{cpm in syngeneic MLR}}$

An average of 8–12 experiments is presented

[c] For details see footnote [b] Table 2

latter mice was due to a reduction in the size of the NK cell population rather than to a functional defect of these cells.

IV. The Ability of T Cells from DMBA-Treated BALB/c Mice to Respond in the Mixed Lymphocyte Reaction

As we have seen, the marker analysis of splenic T cells of DMBA-treated mice showed no difference between the treated mice and untreated controls. We carried out experiments to find out whether DMBA, while not affecting the number of T cell populations, had some effects on their responder function in MLR. The results of assays in which splenocytes from DMBA-treated or from untreated BALB/c (H-2^d) mice were allowed to react against C3H/eB(H-2^k) antigens, are given in Table 4. It was shown that DMBA administration reduced the ability of BALB/c mice to respond to the assayed alloantigens by an average of 50%.

Adoptive transfer experiments in which bone marrow from untreated or from DMBA-treated animals was transferred to lethally irradiated recipients were performed. The results of these experiments indicated (Table 4) that bone marrow precursors were also affected by DMBA in their capacity to reconstitute MLR responder activity.

V. Lymphoma-Reactive Natural Antibodies in Untreated and in Carcinogen-Treated BALB/c Mice

In a previous study [19] we found that sera from young normal BALB/c mice contain IgM antibodies able to mediate complement-dependent lysis of certain syngeneic or allogeneic tumor target cells. The titer of such naturally occurring antitumor antibodies (NATA) was found to increase with aging.

A longitudinal serologic study comparing the cytotoxicity potential of NATA from normal and from urethane-treated BALB/c mice was performed. It was found that urethane-treated mice that did not develop primary lung adenomas within the duration of the experiment had significantly lower NATA titers against the L5178-Y lymphoma than urethane-treated animals that developed lung adenomas. This difference was evident in two independent experiments. The results suggested that the

Table 5. The binding pattern of naturally occurring lymphoma-reactive antibodies

		Binding index of indicated monoclonal[a]				
		1.67	1.80	3.88	2.2	1.91
Lymphomas	L5178-Y	+ + +	+ + +	+ +	+ +	+ +
	Eb	–	–	+ + +	–	+ + +
	Esb	–	–	+ + +	–	+ + +
	YAC-1	–	+ + +	+ + +	+	+ +
	RL♂1	+ +	+ + +	+ + +	–	+
Lymphatic cells	Bone marrow	+	+	+	+	+
	Thymocytes	+ +	–	+	+	+
	Splenocytes	+	–	–	–	–
	Peritoneal macrophages	–	–	+	–	+
Nonlymphatic normal	Embryonic fibroblasts	+ + +	–	+ + +	–	–
	Erythrocytes (MRBC)	+	–	–	+	+
	Bromelain-treated MRBC	+ +	–	+ +	+ + +	+ +

[a] The binding pattern was established by calculating the binding index (BI). This is the ratio between the binding (cpm) to the indicated cell of the tested monoclonal and the nonspecific binding of the radioactive reagent. + + + BI = > 10; + + BI = 5–10; + BI = 1.5–5; – BI = < 1.5

lower antibody activity of the urethane-treated mice that did not develop tumors existed even before exposure to the carcinogenic insult. The results of preliminary experiments suggest that a similar situation also exists with DMBA carcinogenesis. These findings raise the possibility that certain populations could be segregated according to their natural antibody profile into those individuals which will develop primary tumors within a certain period if exposed to a subthreshold amount of carcinogen, and those which will not. Furthermore, the results indicated that these naturally occurring lymphoma-reactive antibodies may play a biologic role in the development of certain primary tumors.

In order to study these antibodies and the antigens they react with, we prepared hybridomas from lymphocytes of LPS-stimulated, but otherwise untreated BALB/c mice. These hybridomas were screened for secretion of antibodies which bind to L5178-Y lymphoma cells. Some binding characteristics of five of the L5178-Y lymphoma-reactive natural monoclonals are given in Table 5. It can be seen that two of the five natural hybridomas secrete antibodies which bind primarily to lymphoid tissues.

C. Discussion

Natural defense mechanisms are considered by several investigators to be the first line of defense against developing neoplasia [10]. If this is indeed the case, then suppression of such defense mechanisms, for example by cancer-inducing agents, might enhance the proliferation and progression of transformed cells toward a fully fledged malignancy. There are numerous investigations showing that exposure to cancer-inducing agents such as chemicals [4], irradiation [8, 15], or hormones [12] causes a depression in one or more of the expressions of natural immunity.

The major part of the present study is an extension of previous findings, showing that the chemical carcinogen DMBA causes a severe suppression of NK activity shortly after administration and long before the appearance of palpable tumors [4]. In this study, we demonstrated that the effect is systemic and that bone marrow precursors are affected. The results also proved that the decreased NK activity was due to a selective toxic effect toward NK precursors and perhaps also to mature NK (asialo-GM-1-positive cells), but not due to a functional defect of such cells. We do not know, as yet, if the NK deficiency of DMBA-treated mice contributes toward tumor development.

The mode of induction of naturally occurring-antibodies, their physiologic role, and the mechanisms regulating their levels and functions are largely unknown.

It seems that the repertoire of naturally occurring antibodies is rather large, equaling perhaps that of adaptively induced antibodies. Among the epitopes recognized by naturally occurring antibodies are many expressed on normal cells [6, 21], on malignant cells [13, 14], or on various oncoviruses [9, 16]. None of these epitopes is restricted to these cells or viruses. However, even in this situation, naturally reacting antibodies directed against epitopes expressed on malignant cells could function as regulators of the progression of malignancy. This could occur at several levels by various mechanisms such as binding to and neutralization of oncogenic viruses [1, 11], opsonizing transformed or nascent malignant cells, lysing them by complement activation, or arming of naturally occurring Fc receptor-positive killer immunocytes [18, 20]. It is also possible that natural antibodies may enhance tumor growth and development by direct or indirect mechanisms [5]. Our previous studies suggested that certain lymphoma-reactive natural antibodies may play a role in chemical carcinogenesis.

The characterization of these antibodies is an essential prerequisite in order to establish the physiologic function of such antibodies and the role they play in controlling primary tumor development. Establishing hybridomas secreting tumor-reactive antibodies is the first step toward this goal.

Acknowledgments. This work was supported by a grant awarded by Concern Foundation in conjunction with the Cohen–Appelbaum–Feldman Families Cancer Research Fund, Los Angeles, California. Isaac P. Witz is the incumbent of the David Furman chair of Immunobiology of Cancer

References

1. Bentvelzen P, Creemers PC (1977) Natural immunity to murine mammary tumor viruses. Contemp Top Immunobiol 6:229
2. Ehrlich R, Witz IP (1982) Natural killer cells and naturally occuring antibodies as representatives of natural tumor immunity. Pathobiol Ann 12:85
3. Ehrlich R, Efrati M, Bar-Eyal A, Wollberg M, Schiby G, Ran M, Witz IP (1980) Natural cellular reactivities mediated by splenocytes from mice bearing three types of primary tumors. Int J Cancer 26:315
4. Ehrlich R, Efrati M, Malatzky E, Shochat L, Bar-Eyal A, Witz IP (1983). Natural host-defence during oncogenesis. NK activity and dimethylbenzanthracene carcinogenesis. Int J Cancer 31:67
5. Feldman JD (1972) Immunological enhancement: A study of blocking antibodies. Adv Immunol 15:167
6. Guilbert B, Dighiero G, Avrameas S (1982) Naturally occurring antibodies against nine common antigens in normal humans. 1. Detection, isolation and characterization. J Immunol 128:2779
7. Habu S, Okumura K (1982) Cell lineage of NK cells: Evidence for T cell lineage. In: Herberman RB (ed) NK cells and other natural effector cells. Academic, New York, p 209
8. Haller O, Wigzell H (1977) Suppression of natural killer activity with radioactive strontium: effector cells are marrow dependent. J Immunol 118:1503
9. Hanna MG Jr, Ihle JN, Batzing BL, Tennant TW, Schenley CK (1975): Assessment of reactivities of natural antibodies to endogenous RNA tumor virus envelope antigens and virus-induced cell surface antigens. Cancer Res 35:164
10. Herberman RB, Holden HT (1978) Natural cell mediated immunity. Adv Cancer Res 27:305
11. Ihle JN, Aurthur LO, Fine DL (1976) Autogenous immunity to mouse mammary tumor virus in mouse strains of high and low mammary tumor incidence. Cancer Res 36: 2840
12. Kalland T (1980) Reduced natural killer activity in female mice of neonatal exposure to diethylstilbestrol. J Immunol 124:1297
13. Martin SE, Martin WJ (1975) Anti-tumor antibodies in normal mouse sera. Int J Cancer 15:658
14. Menard S, Colnaghi MI, Della Porta G (1977) Natural antitumor serum reactivity in BALB/c mice. I. Characterisation and interference with tumor growth. Int J Cancer 19:267
15. Parkinson DR, Brightman RP, Waksal SD (1981) Altered natural killer cell biology in C57BL/6 mice after leukomogenic split-dose irradiation. J Immunol 126:1460

16. Snyder HW Jr, Fleissner E (1980) Specificity of human antibodies to oncovirus glycoproteins: Recognition of antigen by natural antibodies directed against carbohydrate structures. Proc Natl Acad Sci USA 77:1622
17. Stutman O (1975) Immunodepression and cancer. Adv Cancer Res 22:261
18. Wakefield JD, Batchelor JR (1966) The effect of natural antibody in guinea pig serum on mouse lymphoma cells in vitro and in vivo. Immunology 11:441
19. Witz IP, Yaakubowicz M, Gelernter I, Hochberg Y, Anavi R, Ran M (1984) Studies on the level of natural antibodies reactive with various tumor cells during Urethane carcinogenesis in BALB/c mice. Immunobiology 166:131
20. Wolosin LB, Greenberg AH (1979) Murine natural anti-tumor antibodies. I. Rapid in vivo binding of natural antibody by tumor cells in syngeneic mice. Int J Cancer 23:519
21. Wolosin LB, Greenberg AH (1981) Genetics of natural antitumor antibody production: Antibodies to MHC-linked determinants detected in the serum of unstimulated mice. J Immunol 126:1456

Haematology and Blood Transfusion Vol. 29
Modern Trends in Human Leukemia VI
Edited by Neth, Gallo, Greaves, Janka

Genes and Antigens Controlling Tumor Metastases *

L. Eisenbach and M. Feldman

A. Introduction

The generation of metastases by neoplastic cells constitutes the main problem in tumor malignancy. Metastasis is a multistep process, in which each of the sequential steps is controlled by different properties of the disseminating tumor cells. The host's capacity to recognize metastatic, as against nonmetastatic, cells of the tumor cell population could exert a controlling effect on each of the stages culminating in the progressive growth of metastases. Recognition of cell-surface antigenic epitopes on metastatic cells via T lymphocytes would be restricted by cell-surface class 1 glycoproteins coded by the major histocompatibility complex (MHC). In mice, such glycoproteins are coded by the *H-2D* and *H-2K* genes of the MHC, and differences in their expression on metastatic, as distinct from nonmetastatic, cells of a given tumor could therefore elicit different T cell effector responses, which would then determine the fate of the disseminating tumor cells. The feasibility of an MHC control of the metastatic process attracted us during investigations of the unique properties of a metastatic carcinoma originated in a C57BL ($H\text{-}2^b$) mouse, the 3LL Lewis lung carcinoma. Following transplantation in syngeneic animals, the 3LL carcinoma generates spontaneous lung metastases while growing locally at any site of transplantation. However, this tumor differs from all normal tissues and from many other tumors in its capacity to grow in allogeneic recipients. Yet, metastases were generated only when the tumor grew in syngeneic animals [1]. The allograft response elicited by the local tumor could not arrest the local growth, but was sufficiently powerful to prevent the growth of metastatic lung nodules. Subsequent experiments indicated that the spontaneous lung metastases behaved as "secondary" grafts, being rejected by the alloreactive T cells that had been elicited by the local graft [2]. When the 3LL cells were injected intravenously to similar allogeneic mice, lung tumors developed as "primary" grafts and these did grow progressively [2]. It thus appeared that in an allogeneic recipient the local tumor can resist an immune response, which prevents the growth of its spontaneous lung metastases. This raised the question as to whether an immune response elicited by the growing local tumor in *syngeneic* recipients could similarly prevent the progression of spontaneous metastases in syngeneic animals and whether the probability of forming metastases by individual tumor cells grown in syngeneic mice is a function of their immunogenic properties, which in turn might be a function of the expression of the restricting class 1 MHC antigens on the neoplastic cells.

* Department of Cell Biology, The Weizmann Institute of Science, Rehovot 76100, Israel

B. The Relative Expression of H-2K^b/H-2D^b on Clones of the 3LL Tumor is Correlated with Their Metastatic Competence

Our approach to the question as to whether differences in the expression of H-2D^b ver-

Table 1. Metastases and H-2 expression of 3LL subclones

Clone	Percent positive cells[a]				Ratio K^b/D^b		Lung weight (mg)[b]	
	Gain 4		Gain 8		Gain 4	Gain 8	Mean	Range
	K^b	D^b	K^b	D^b				
A9A5	1±0	1± 0	5± 0	5± 0	1.0	1.0	243± 58	126– 361
A9FH5	2±2	2± 3	6± 4	8± 3	1.0	0.75	217± 35	163– 271
A9FJ1	3±1	4± 1	13± 2	15± 2	0.75	0.87	230± 62	187– 378
A9C3	11±3	25± 6	33± 6	60±15	0.44	0.55	233± 25	195– 273
A9E2	13±6	28± 8	43± 9	55±18	0.46	0.78	220± 41	172– 278
A9G3	10±6	31±10	35±10	54±16	0.32	0.65	229± 27	180– 263
A9H3	14±4	26±11	30± 4	42± 9	0.54	0.71	224± 21	178– 237
A9H6	16±5	53±15	40±13	67±14	0.30	0.60	236± 91	174– 478
A9J2	16±6	37± 9	53±10	73±14	0.43	0.73	218± 28	185– 264
A9FA1	22±6	37±10	45± 2	55±12	0.59	0.82	192± 28	145– 227
A9FA6	16±4	37± 0	43± 8	70± 4	0.43	0.61	208± 14	182– 224
A9FI1	9±3	21± 8	35± 9	47±12	0.43	0.74	201± 18	180– 239
A9FJ2	14±0	65± 0	47± 0	87± 0	0.22	0.54	236± 30	193– 273
A9FJ3	18±7	50±10	44±16	75±18	0.36	0.59	214± 31	183– 278
3LLFI6	23±5	30± 3	61±11	61± 6	0.70	1.0	219± 39	173– 290
A9E6	11±6	47± 2	34± 9	84± 8	0.24	0.40	259± 73	215– 458
A9L2	14±0	69± 0	42± 0	89± 0	0.20	0.47	284± 23	252– 320
A9FE2	5±2	23±16	14± 6	45±16	0.22	0.31	367±300	233–1159
3LLFA5	9±9	51±20	25± 9	63±13	0.18	0.40	310±188	204– 767
3LLFL1	14±8	35±10	30±41	57±13	0.40	0.53	294±159	185– 588
A9FG6	7±3	43±17	15± 7	71±23	0.16	0.21	429±395	205–1311
A9FJ4	7±3	29± 9	14± 7	56±19	0.24	0.25	451±361	168–1355
3LLFA3	2±0	41±10	11± 6	56±18	0.05	0.20	437±347	175–1226
3LLFB4	8±7	45±10	15± 7	61±10	0.18	0.25	947±243	662–1409
3LLFC1	6±0	87± 0	22± 0	96± 0	0.07	0.23	641±220	486–1073
3LLFC6	7±2	32±15	11± 8	47±17	0.13	0.23	492±224	336–1226
3LLFL5	2±3	42±13	9± 6	62±12	0.05	0.15	567±387	193–1290
3LLFL6	4±4	26± 6	6± 5	52±13	0.15	0.12	662±367	233–1158
3LLFM2	4±3	28± 7	19± 8	72± 8	0.14	0.26	518–191	236– 735

[a] Tumor cells $2\text{–}4 \times 10^6$ were incubated at 4 °C for 30 min in purified anti-K^b (28-13-3) monoclonal antibody or anti-D^b (28-14-8) antibody, washed twice in phosphate-buffered saline with 1% bovine serum albumin and 0.2% sodium azide, and reincubated in fluorescein isothiocyanate-labeled rabbit anti-mouse Ig. Fluorescence-activated cell sorter II analysis was performed with photomultiplier tube set at 550 V

[b] In 10 C57BL/6J male mice, 10^5 cells were inoculated i.f.p. When the primary tumors reached 8 mm in diameter tumor-bearing legs were amputated. Metastatic load was determined 30 days after amputation

sus H-$2K^b$ glycoproteins (the class 1 antigens of the mouse MHC) control the metastatic potency of 3LL cells was triggered by earlier experiments in our laboratory. In these we aimed at determining the minimum genetic identities between the tumor strain of origin and the host's phenotype that are required for the generation of metastases. We found that identities at the *H-2D^b* gene and the non-MHC background are sufficient for metastasis formation, whereas the H-2K phenotype of the recipient was completely irrelevant [1]. It then turned out that identity at the H-$2K^b$ was unnecessary, because the 3LL tumor hardly expressed the H-$2K^b$ on its cell surface [3].

Table 2. The effect of interferon and retinoic acid on MHC cell surface expression and metastasis

Treatment	Antibody binding (cpm/10^4 cells)[a]				Spontaneous metastases: Lung wt (mg±SD)
	Anti-K^b 28-13-3	Anti-K^b 20-8-4	Anti-D^b 28-14-8	K^b-D^b (28-13-3/ 28-14-8)	
A9 clone					
–	13 028±1 022	25 529± 402	17 224±1 441	0.76	249± 66
Interferon	23 854±1 214	55 141±4 342	77 424±2 218	0.31	410±205
Retinoic acid	12 518± 853	22 276±1 524	48 537± 983	0.26	519±270
D122 clone					
–	2 610± 123	3 300± 211	13 200± 459	0.20	536±176
Interferon	5 329± 327	6 500± 259	44 000±1 320	0.12	794±236
Retinoic acid	1 958± 73	2 800± 322	12 800± 924	0.15	620±178

Treatment was performed with 10^5 tissue culture-propagated cells transferred to 100-mm petri dishes in 10 ml Dulbecco's modified Eagle's medium supplemented with 10% fetal calf serum (FCS), 1% glutamine, 1% sodium pyruvate, 1% nonessential amino acids, and 1% antibiotics in the presence of 100 units/ml interferon (α and β, 10^7 units/mg) or 10^{-6} mol/liter retinoic acid. The cells were grown to confluency (1 week), with twice-weekly changes of growth medium

[a] Direct radioimmunoassay: 10^6 living cells were incubated with 50 µl ^{125}I-labeled antibody, 0.1–1.5 µg protein A-Sepharose-purified (28-14-8 and 20-8-4), or 0.5–7.5 µg semipurified antibody (28-13-3). Binding was done for 1 h at 4 °C in a 300-µl final volume of phosphate-buffered saline (PBS), 5% FCS, after which plates (24 wells) were washed four times in PBS-FCS and cells were collected into tubes and monitored in a gamma counter. The saturation values of a dose-dependence curve are given

The question which thus arose was whether the absence of H-2K^b expression concomitant with the presence of *H-2D^b* determined the metastatic potency of the tumor cell population. To answer this question we cloned 3LL cells in soft agar and tested the metastatic potency of individual clones. We found that the clones differ in their capacity to generate spontaneous lung metastases when grown intrafootpad (i.f.p.) in syngeneic animals. As previously demonstrated for other tumors [4], this tumor cell population varied in the metastatic potency of its individual cells. To test whether there is a correlation between the metastatic properties of individual clones and the expression of MHC genes, we used monoclonal antibodies 28-13-3 and 20-8-4, which identify H-2K^b molecules, and antibody 28-14-8, which identifies H-2D^b molecules [5]. We analyzed 30 clones by direct radioimmunoassay and with the fluorescence-activated cell sorter. We found (Table 1) that *the lower the H-2K^b/H-2D^b ratio, the higher was the metastatic potential of the cloned cells* [6].

C. Induced Alterations of H-2K/H-2D Ratio Alters the Metastatic Phenotype

To examine whether the relative expression of class 1 antigens of the MHC was *causally* related to its metastatic phenotype, we attempted to alter the H-2K^b/H-2D^b ratio, and then to test whether such alteration will change the metastatic potency of the cells. For this purpose we treated in vitro-cloned tumor cells with either interferon $\alpha+\beta$ (a stimulator of H-2 synthesis) or with retinoic acid. Cells of two clones were used in these experiments: The low metastatic A9 clone that expresses both the H-2K and the H-2D glycoproteins, and the high-metastatic D122 clone that expresses the H-2D^b molecules but lacks H-2K^b expression. It was found that interferon caused an increase in both K and D expression of both A9 and D122 cells, yet the net increase in H-2D^b expression was significantly higher than that of H-2K^b expression, thus lowering the H-2K/H-2D ratio (Table 2). These changes were associated

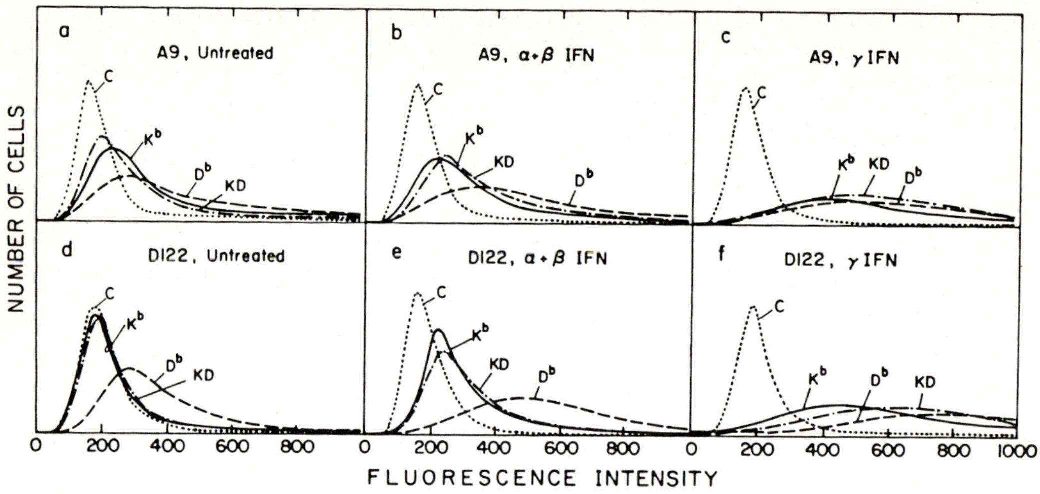

Fig. 1a–f. Effect of interferons on cell surface expression of H-$2K^b$ and H-$2D^b$ alloantigens of clones A9 and D122. Quantities of 2×10^5 tissue culture-propagated cells were transferred to 100-mm petri dishes in 10 ml Dulbecco's modified Eagle's medium supplemented with 10% fetal calf serum, 1% glutamine, 1% sodium pyruvate, 1% nonessential amino acids, and 1% antibiotics. The cells were grown for 5 days in the presence of no interferon (**a**, **d**); interferon $\alpha+\beta$ 500 units/ml, 10^7 units/mg (**b**, **e**); or γ-interferon 100 units/ml, 12×10^7 units/mg (**c**, **f**). Cells were treated with monoclonal antibody 28-13-3 (anti-K^b), 20-8-4 (anti-K^bD^b, reacts mainly with K^b molecules), or 28-14-8 (anti-D^b) and analyzed by the FACS II

with a significant increase in the metastatic load produced by both the A9 clone and the D122 clone. Treatment with retinoic acid did not affect H-2K expression, but increased significantly H-$2D^b$ production, lowering the H-2K/H-2D ratio even further. This again increased the metastatic load produced by D122 cells, and converted the low metastatic A9 clone to a high metastatic phenotype (Table 2).

Thus far we have not found a chemical signal which would cause an increase in the H-2K/H-2D ratio and thereby effect a decrease in the metastatic potency of the cells. Very recent experiments with γ-interferon have indicated that this interferon is more effective than interferon $\alpha+\beta$ in induction of the cell surface expression of H-$2D^b$ and, especially, of H-$2K^b$ molecules on A9 and D122 tumor cells (Fig. 1). While testing for spontaneous lung metastases we observed no changes in the low metastatic phenotype of A9 clone and a reduction in the number of metastatic nodules formed by the high metastatic D122 clone.

D. The Relative Expression of H-2K/H-2D Molecules is Correlated with the Immunogenic Properties of the Cloned Cell Populations

We then considered whether the low H-2K/H-2D ratio determines a metastatic phenotype because it confers a low immunogenic potency on the neoplastic cells.

I. Growth and Metastasis in Allogeneic Recipients

As stated above, the parental 3LL cell population, manifesting a low H-2K/H-2D ratio, can grow across H-2 barriers although metastases are not formed in allogeneic mice. We also tested whether the nonmetastatic A9 clone (K^+D^+) and the D122 clone (K^-D^+) differed in their capacity to grow in allogeneic recipients. Whereas the D122 grew locally without generating metastases in BALB/c (H-2^d) and C3H (H-2^k)

mice, the nonmetastatic A9 clone was rejected by allogeneic recipients [7]. The metastatic potential in syngeneic mice was thus correlated with the immunogenic effect determining growth in allogeneic mice.

II. Growth and Metastasis in Congenic Recipients

Clone A9 behaves as a regular incompatible immunogenic allograft in allogeneic mice. To test whether the class I antigens alone on the A9 clone could elicit rejection of the grafted tumor, 10^5 A9 or D122 cells were inoculated to groups of H-2-recombinant mice on a C57BL/10 background [7]. We used B10.HTG (K^dD^b), B10.D2 (K^dD^d), and B10.A(4R) (K^kD^b) mice. Clone A9 (K^bD^b) grew in 9/10 B10.HTG mice at a slower rate than in C57BL/6J mice. Only partial and slow growth was observed in B10.D2 mice (5/11), and the A9 clone grew in only one of nine mice of the B10.A(4R) strain. In contrast, D122 grew in C57BL/6J and in the three recombinant strains at a similar rate. Testing for metastases, we found that D122 metastasized in C57BL/6J (K^bD^b), B10.HTG (K^dD^b), and B10.A(4R) (K^kD^b), but not in B10.D2 (K^dD^d) mice. The K^b-positive A9 cells grew partially in recombinant mice, while D122 grew progressively and metastases were rejected only in B10.D2 (D^d) mice. Thus, the higher immunogenic effect of clone A9, compared with the D122 clone, is a function of an immune response elicited by the H-2K determinant.

III. Clone A9, Unlike Clone D122, is Immunogenic in Syngeneic Mice

In view of the differences in growth pattern of A9 and D122 clones in allogeneic and H-2-recombinant mice [7], we asked whether the higher immunogenicity of the A9 clone was also effective in the syngeneic host, and whether this could account for the inability of the A9 clone to metastasize. C57BL/6J mice were immunized by three intraperitoneal injections of 10^7 irradiated A9, D122, or 3LL cells at 1-week intervals. Ten days after the last injection, immunized mice and controls were challenged by A9 or D122 cells. We found that immunization by A9 cells significantly slowed the growth rate of a second A9 tumor but did not affect the growth rate of the metastatic D122 tumor. Immunization by clone D122 or by 3LL did not retard the growth of a second A9 or D122 tumor. Similar results were obtained when mice were intradermally immunized with living A9 or D122 cells.

IV. Cytotoxic Activity of Lymphocytes Sensitized In Vivo to A9 and D122 Tumor Cells

Following the in vivo observations, we tested the cytotoxic T lymphocyte (CTL) responses evoked by cells of A9 and D122 clones in syngeneic hosts. C57BL/6J mice received 5×10^4 or 10^5 A9 or D122 tumor cells by intradermal injection. At 12 days after the immunization, spleen cells were removed and stimulated in vitro for 5 days on monolayers of irradiated and mitomycin C-treated A9 or D122 cells. The cytotoxic activity of these spleen cells was assayed against A9 and D122 target cells in a 16-h indium-111 release assay. Figure 2 demonstrates that A9 induced high levels of cytotoxic activity, which was manifested against A9 cells and to a lesser extent against D122 target cells. D122 cells induced a lymphocyte population that manifested low cytotoxic activity against D122 or A9 target cells. Thus, the in vitro interaction of immune lymphocytes with nonmetastatic A9 cells led to the destruction of the tumor cells, whereas lymphocytes interacting with D122 cells were significantly less efficient in destroying the tumor cells.

E. Molecular Nature of MHC Gene Products in 3LL Clones

Low metastatic clones such as A9 were shown to bind anti-H-$2K^b$ and anti-H-$2D^b$ antibodies, while high metastatic clones such as D122 bound only H-$2D^b$ antibodies (Table 2). We tested the molecular similarity of the MHC glycoproteins to H-2^b

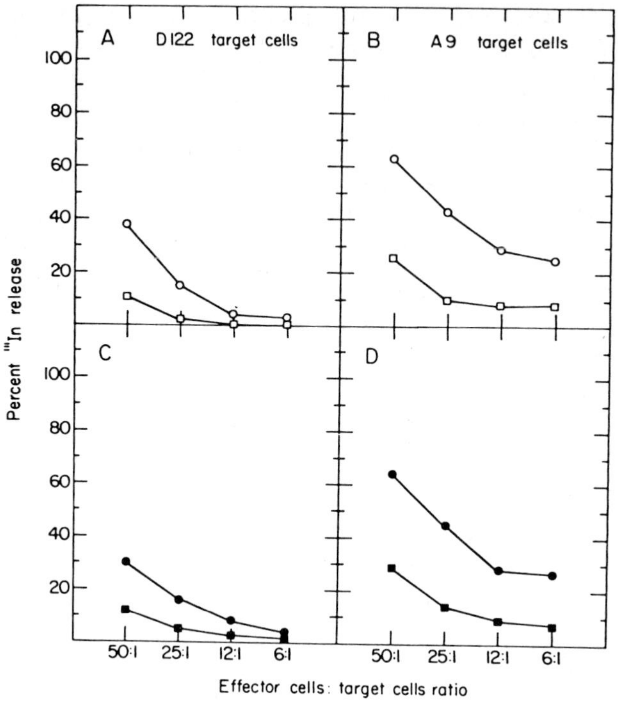

Fig. 2A–D. Correlation of *H-2K* gene expression on 3LL clones with ability to stimulate cytotoxicity and susceptibility to cell-mediated cytolysis. C57BL/6J mice were immunized intradermally with 5×10^4 A9 cells (●——●), 1×10^5 A9 cells (○——○), 5×10^4 D122 cells (■——■), or 1×10^5 D122 cells (□——□). On day 12, spleens were removed and lymphocytes were restimulated in vitro on irradiated and mitomycin-treated A9 or D122 cells. Indium-111-labeled A9 (**B**, **D**) or D122 (**A**, **C**) cells reacted with these lymphocytes in a 16-h assay

molecules of C57BL/6J spleens. Immunoprecipitation of ^{125}I cell surface-labeled and ^{35}S-methionine-labeled extracts of A9 and D122 clones showed a strict correlation between synthesis and cell surface expression. In D122 and in the parental 3LL cells, but not in A9, synthesis of K^b molecules was suppressed [6]. The 45K proteins precipitated by anti-H-2^b serum or monoclonal anti-H-$2K^b$ (from clone A9) were similar in migration to molecules precipitated from C57BL/6J splenocytes, and a 12K β2-microglobulin molecule was coprecipitated. Separation on lentil-lectin Sepharose showed that most of the H-2^b-encoded proteins were in their glycosylated form [6]. To obtain a better understanding of the transcriptional level of the *K* gene suppression in metastatic clones, we used Northern blot hybridization to analyze the mRNA from clones A9, D122, and 3LL as compared to liver mRNA and RNA extracted from metastatic and nonmetastatic clones of another metastatic tumor, the T10 sarcoma (T10 sarcoma is an F_1 (H-$2^b\times$H-2^k) tumor that expresses only D end products of the MHC). We used four probes: (a) a genomic K^b, 5′ region probe, H8Pst8 [8]; (b) a cDNA, H-2^d, 3′ region probe, pH2IIa [9]; (c) a cDNA, H-2^d, 5′ region probe, pH2III [9]; and (d) a human HLA-B9 cDNA probe. All these probes hybridize to both K and D end transcripts. Figure 3 shows that the normal H-2 transcript of 2 kb that is expressed in the liver is also expressed at a high level in clone A9 and in the 3LL line. A lower level of transcription of the 2-kb mRNA is observed in clone D122 and in the T10 sarcoma clones, as both D122 and all T10 clones lack expression of K end products. Besides the normal 2-kb transcripts, an abnormal RNA of 5.5–6 kb was observed in all tumor clones [10]. This transcript hybridized to the three 5′ region probes but not to the 3′ region probe. The origin of this large RNA is not yet known, but it may result from the insertion of a foreign DNA into the *H-2K* gene of the tumors. In this event the large RNA could represent a transcript contain-

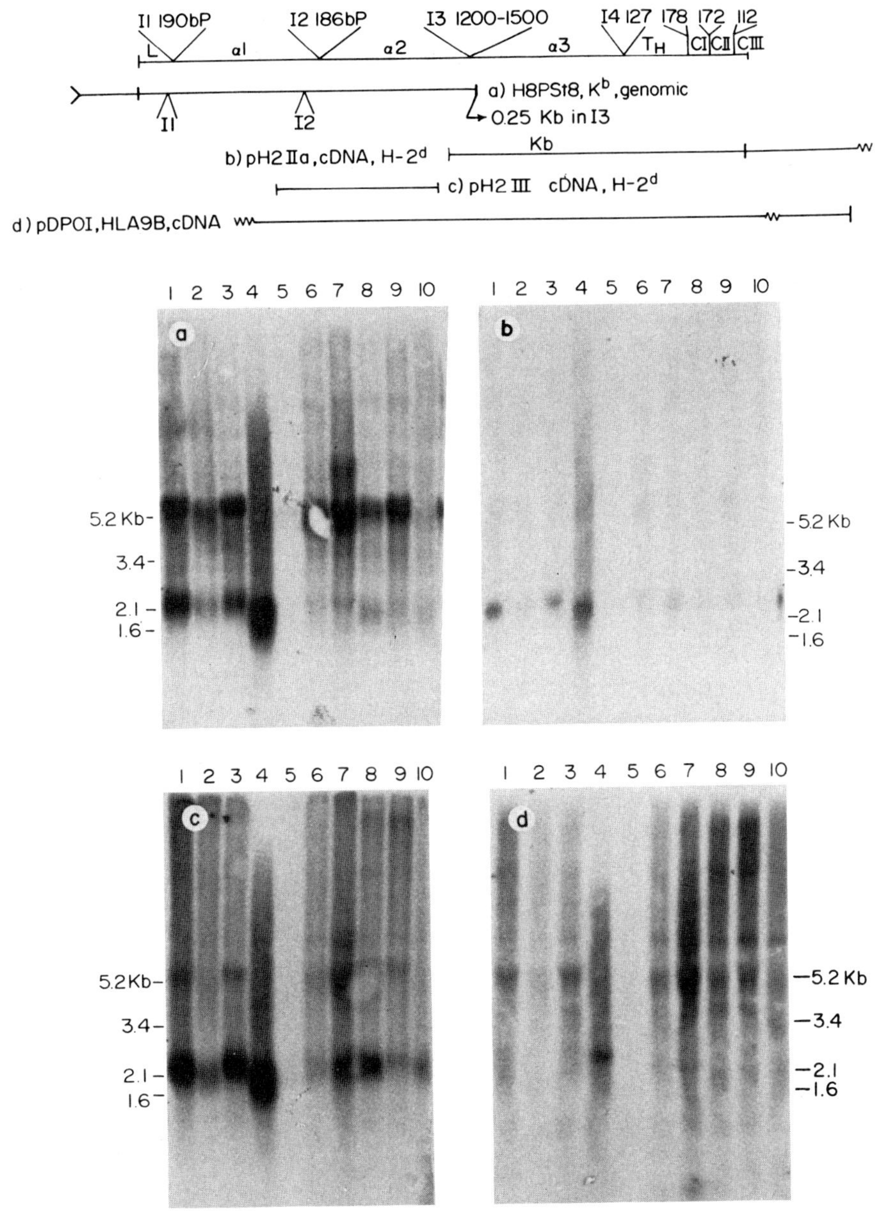

ing H-2 sequences plus other sequences, and this could explain the inactivation of the *H-2K* gene.

Southern blot analysis, although very complex, revealed new fragments hybridizing to the H-2 probes when the genomic DNA from tumor clones was digested with EcoRI, BamHI, XbaI, or SStI and compared with liver DNA of the same mouse

Fig. 3a–d. Transcription of MHC class I genes in tumor clones. Northern hybridization performed with poly(A)$^+$ RNAs from 3LL carcinoma and T10 sarcoma. *1*, A9, low metastatic, 3LL; *2*, D122, high metastatic, 3LL; *3*, 3LL, parental; *4*, liver; *5*, IC9, nonmetastatic, T10; *6*, D6 moderately metastatic, T10; *7*, IB9, high metastatic, T10; *8*, IE7, high metastatic, T10; *9* and *10*, T8, T40, parental T10. Probes used: **a** H8PSt8, **b** H-2IIa, **c** H-2III, and **d** PDPOI

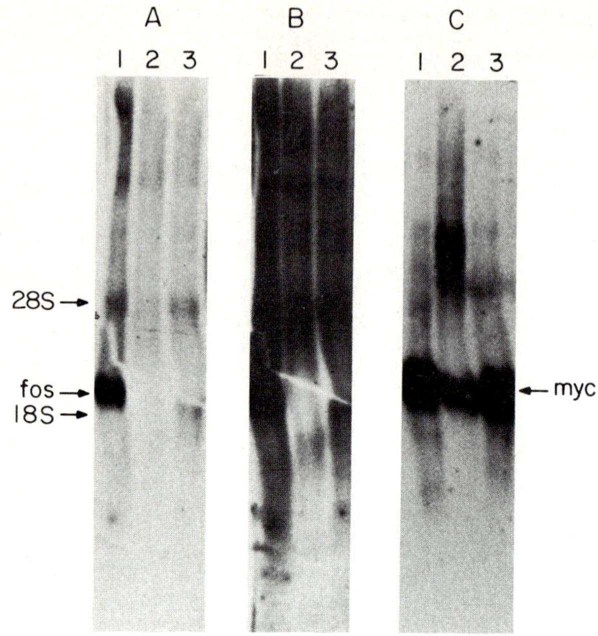

Fig. 4A–C. Expression of c-*myc* and c-*fos onc* genes in 3LL clones. Polyadenylated mRNA was selected on oligo-dT cellulose and electrophoresed on formaldehyde-agarose gels. RNA was then transferred onto nitrocellulose filters which were subsequently hybridized with a ^{32}P-labeled nick-translated c-*myc* probe, washed, and exposed to x-ray film. The same blot was cleaned of the c-*myc* probe and rehybridized to a *fos* probe. *1*, mRNA from low metastatic A9 clone; *2*, mRNA from high metastatic D122 clone; *3*, mRNA from parental 3LL line. **a** Hybridization to *fos*, blots exposed for 1 day; **b** hybridization to *fos*, blots exposed for 3 days; **c** hybridization to *myc*, blots exposed for 1 day

strains (C57BL for 3LL clones and F_1 for T10 clones). Differences were also observed between clones A9 and D122. The possibility that a mutation or insertion in *H-2K* genes might result in the loss of expression of an H-2 molecule, giving rise to clones insensitive to the host immune system, is investigated.

F. The Metastatic Phenotype Might Represent a Lower Level of Molecular Differentiation: Expression of c-*fos* Gene

The co-expression of the two class I antigens, which characterizes the low or nonmetastatic clones of 3LL, also characterizes most nucleated normal somatic cells, whereas both early embryonal cells and nondifferentiated teratocarcinoma cells lack expression of H-2 molecules. Do other gene products of the metastatic versus the nonmetastatic phenotypes signify differences in state of differentiation? Of particular interest from this viewpoint is the *fos* gene. Expression of c-*fos*, the cellular counterpart of the FBJ osteosarcoma viral *onc* gene, was shown to correlate with the induction of differentiation in human myeloid leukemia line WEHI-3B [11]. Transfection of F9 teratocarcinoma cells by a cloned *fos* gene was shown by Muller and Wagner to induce differentiation of teratocarcinoma cells to endoderm-like cells [12]. In a recent study of the organization and expression of *onc* genes in metastatic and nonmetastatic clones we observed that the c-*fos* proto-*onc* gene is expressed in the low metastatic clone A9 at high levels, while the high metastatic clone D122 does not contain c-*fos*-related m-RNA (Fig. 4). A low level of c-*fos* transcription was also observed in parental 3LL cells. Expansion of these results showed that other low metastatic 3LL clones also expressed c-*fos*. In addition, we found that the c-*myc* oncogene was amplified 60-fold in all 3LL clones. Thus, the level of c-*myc* mRNA is very high in A9 and D122 clones, as well as in the parental 3LL line. Figure 4 demonstrates, using the same Northern blot, that while c-*myc* is expressed in all three cell types, c-*fos* is expressed mainly in the low metastatic A9 clone.

Is the expression of *fos* gene product and a full expression of H-2K and H-2D gene products an indication of a more differentiated state of the A9 low metastatic clone than of the metastatic D122 clone, and is such a differentiation step crucial in the control of metastatic spread by the host? We are currently investigating these questions.

Acknowledgments. This investigation was supported by PHS grant no. CA 28139 awarded by the National Cancer Institute, DHHS, USA.

References

1. Isakov N, Feldman M, Segal S (1981) Control of progression of local tumor and pulmonary metastases of the 3LL Lewis lung carcinoma by different histocompatibility requirements in mice. J N C I 66:919
2. Isakov N, Feldman M, Segal S (1982) An immune response against the alloantigens of the 3LL Lewis lung carcinoma prevents the growth of lung metastases but not of local allografts. Invasion and Metastasis 2:12
3. Isakov N, Katzav S, Feldman M, Segal S (1983) Lewis lung carcinoma cells possess immunogenic H-2D^b region gene products but lack H-2K^b region products. J N C I 71:139
4. Fidler IJ, Kripke ML (1977) Metastasis results from pre-existing variant cells within a malignant tumor. Science 197:893
5. Ozato K, Sachs DH (1981) Monoclonal antibodies to MHC antigens. Hybridoma antibodies reacting to antigens of H-2^b haplotype reveal genetic control of isotype expression. J Immunol 126:317
6. Eisenbach L, Segal S, Feldman M (1983) MHC imbalance and metastatic spread in Lewis lung carcinoma clones. Int J Cancer 32:113
7. Eisenbach L, Hollander N, Greenfeld L, Yakor H, Segal S, Feldman M (1984) The differential expression of H-2K versus H-2D antigens, distinguishing high-metastatic from low-metastatic clones, is correlated with the immunogenic properties of the tumor cells. Int J Cancer 34:567
8. Weiss E, Golden L, Zakut R et al. (1983) The DNA sequence of the H-2K^b gene: Evidence for gene conversion as a mechanism for the generation of polymorphism in histocompatibility antigens. EMBO J 2:453
9. Steinmetz M, Erelinger JG, Fisher D et al. (1981) Three cDNA clones encoding mouse transplantation antigens: Homology to immunoglobulin genes. Cell 24:125
10. Eisenbach L, Hollander N, Segal S, Feldman M (1985) The differential expression of class I major histocompatibility complex antigens controls the metastatic properties of tumor cells. Transplantation Proc 17:729
11. Gonda TJ, Metcalf D (1984) Expression of myb, myc and fos proto-oncogenes during the differentiation of a murine myeloid leukaemia. Nature 310:249
12. Muller R, Wagner GF (1984) Differentiation of F9 teratocarcinoma stem cells after transfer of c-fos proto-oncogenes. Nature 311:438

Haematology and Blood Transfusion Vol. 29
Modern Trends in Human Leukemia VI
Edited by Neth, Gallo, Greaves, Janka

Killer Cells in Leukemia *

H. W. L. Ziegler-Heitbrock, B. Emmerich, H. Theml, W. Siegert, and G. Riethmüller

A. Introduction

Killer cells can be analyzed in the context of human leukemia in three different ways:

1. The cytotoxic potential of nonleukemic cells found in a leukemic sample can be analyzed.
2. The leukemic cells can serve as targets for cytotoxic cells.
3. Leukemias can represent transformants of killer cells. In the following we will summarize in brief our results on these separate topics.

B. Materials and Methods

Leukemic cells from peripheral blood, classified by morphology, cytochemistry, and immunologic markers, were used either fresh or after storage in liquid nitrogen. Analysis with monoclonal antibodies (MoAb) was done in indirect immunofluorescence and cytotoxicity was studied by chromium release.

C. Results and Discussion

In chronic lymphocytic leukemia (CLL), the deficiency of the immune system appears to be of utmost importance for the outcome of the disease, since infections and secondary malignancies are major causes of death. When the nonleukemic cells were isolated from peripheral blood samples of CLL patients, the natural killer (NK) cell activity was found to be profoundly defective in a large portion of patients [1]. At the cellular level, this might be explained: (a) by the presence of functionally defective mature effector cells; or (b) by the absence of the effector cells. Using the MoAb HNK-1 [2] which detects mostly early inactive NK cells plus some active NK cells, and the MoAb VEP13 [3] which detects active NK effector cells only, we found that in patients with defective NK cell activity the VEP13$^+$ cells were absent while the HNK-1$^+$ cells were increased [4] (Fig. 1a). We suggest that there might be a block in differentiation of the NK cells in CLL, which results in accumulation of precursor cells.

In analyzing acute leukemia cells as target cells, we were able to demonstrate that the cell-mediated killing of these cells can be greatly enhanced by a short preincubation with actinomycin D [5]. The allogeneic effector cells responsible for this lysis could either be T cells, monocytes, or NK cells. Using the MoAb VEP13, we were able to demonstrate the NK cell nature of the effector cells [6] (Fig. 1b). The results point to a possible cooperation of cytostatic drug and the immune system and further studies will have to test this possibility in autologous combinations.

We have developed a system that allows for measurement exclusively of cytotoxic monocytes against tumor cells in a short-term (7 h) assay with whole peripheral blood mononuclear cells [7]. For the analysis of clonal killer monocytes, we used cells

* Institut für Immunologie, Goethestr. 31, 8000 München 2

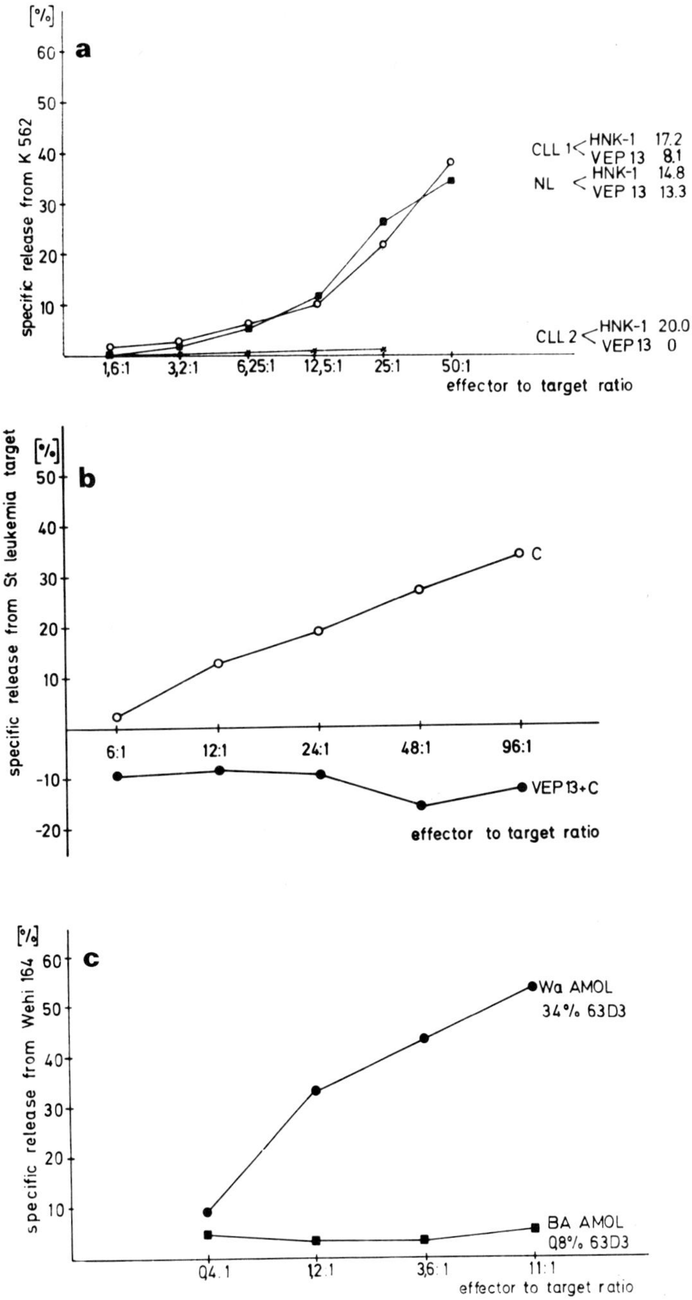

Fig. 1a–c. **a** NK cell activity of nonleukemic cells obtained after BA-1 plus complement treatment from two CLL patients and one control; **b** Phenotype of spontaneous killer cells active in enhanced killing of allogeneic leukemia cells. Interferon-treated effector cells lyse actinomycin D-treated leukemia cells. Killing is abrogated by treatment with VEP13 plus complement; **c** Cytotoxicity of monoblastic leukemia cells against a monocyte-specific fibrosarcoma cell

from acute monoblastic leukemia (AMoL) patients and we found that AMoL cells can exert high cytotoxicity which is linked to the expression of a MoAb-defined cell surface marker (63D3) [8, 9] (Fig. 1c). In conclusion, analysis of killer cells in leukemia can increase our understanding of the normal regulation of these important effector cells of the immune system and at the same time it can provide information useful for the management of the disease and for designing new therapeutic strategies.

References

1. Ziegler HWL, Kay NE, Zarling JM (1981) Deficiency of natural killer cell activity in patients with chronic lymphocytic leukemia. Int J Cancer 27:321
2. Abo T, Miller CA, Balch CM (1984) Characterization of human granular lymphocyte subpopulations expressing HNK-1 (Leu 7) and Leu 11 antigens in the blood and lymphoid tissues from fetuses, neonates and adults. Eur J Immunol 14:616
3. Rumpold H, Kraft D, Obexer G, Böck G, Gebhard W (1982) A monoclonal antibody against a surface antigen shared by human large granular lymphocytes and granulocytes. J Immunol 127:1024
4. Ziegler-Heitbrock HWL, Rumpold H, Kraft D, Wagenpfeil C, Munker R, Abo T, Balch CM, LeBien TW (1985) Patients with a deficiency of natural killer cell activity lack the VEP13 positive lymphocyte subpopulation. Blood 65:65
5. Ziegler-Heitbrock HWL, Erhardt J, Riethmüller G (1983) Treatment of fresh human leukaemia cells with actinomycin D enhances their lysability by natural killer cells. Br J Cancer 48:507
6. Ziegler-Heitbrock HWL, Fütterer A, Rumpold H, Kraft D, Munker R, Riethmüller G (1984) The use of VEP13 monoclonal antibody for definition of natural killer cells: spontaneous killer cells directed against fresh human leukemia cells carry the VEP13 antigen. Clin Exp Immunol 58:470
7. Ziegler-Heitbrock HWL, Riethmüller G (1984) A rapid assay for cytotoxicity of unstimulated human monocytes. J Natl Cancer Inst 72:23
8. Ugolini V, Nunez G, Smith RG, Stastny P, Capra JD (1980) Initial characterization of monoclonal antibodies against human monocytes. Proc Natl Acad Sci USA 77:6764
9. Ziegler-Heitbrock HWL, Munker R, Thiel E, Krebs I, Riethmüller G (1985) Killer cell activity of human monoblastic leukemia cells as detected with a monocyte specific target cell. Blood 65:8

Haematology and Blood Transfusion Vol. 29
Modern Trends in Human Leukemia VI
Edited by Neth, Gallo, Greaves, Janka

Influence of Colchicine and Cytochalasin B on Pinocytosis, Phagocytosis, and Antibody-Dependent Cell-Mediated Cytotoxicity

A. Piasek[1] and P. Obłąkowski[2]

A. Introduction

The cytoskeleton is an organelle of eukaryotic cells engaged in organization and external and internal cell movements, e.g., endocytosis. Our previous experiments proved that colchicine (an antitubular drug) and cytochalasin B (cyt B, an antimicrofilament agent) have significant influence on the development of the process [8, 9]. Reports on the inhibiting effect of the development of antibody-dependent cell-mediated cytotoxicity (ADCC) are inconsistent. The aim of the present work was to examine the influence of colchicine and cyt B on the development and mutual dependence of pinocytosis, phagocytosis, and cytotoxic effect.

Peritoneal resident cells (PRC) isolated from Swiss mice were used as effector cells in our experiments. Macrophages constituted 60%–80% of this cell population. PRC at a concentration of 4×10^6/ml were incubated 2 h in MEM in 37 °C, 5% CO_2 with addition of: (a) colchicine 10^{-6} *M*; (b) cyt B 4 μg/ml; and (c) pure medium (control).

B. Pinocytosis

After 2 h of incubation, 0.5 ml MEM containing horseradish peroxidase (HRP) at a concentration of 3 mg/ml was added to the culture. After 90 min incubation, the cells were centrifuged, washed five times and after sonication in the presence of 0.05% Triton X-100, HRP was determined according to Karnowsky's method [4].

C. Phagocytosis

After 2 h of incubation as described, opsonized sheep red blood cells (SRBC) were added to the effector cell culture. The cultures were incubated "under" standard conditions for 90 min. The cells were centrifuged and supernatants were collected for determination of released hemoglobin (Hb). Nonphagocytized erythrocytes were removed by means of double lysis with 0.5 *M* NH_4Cl solution. After additional washing with PBS, the cells were sonicated in the presence of 0.05% Triton X-100. The Hb content in homogenates was determined as a measure of the effectiveness of phagocytosis. Phagocytosis was also examined using ^{51}Cr-labeled SRBC and measuring the radioactivity of the effector cells at the end of the experiment. Phagocytosis was also confirmed by morphological observations.

D. ADCC

In supernatants collected from PRC cultures with opsonized SRBC, Hb was determined according to a modified Karnowsky's method. When ^{51}Cr-labeled SRBC were used as the target cells, the

1 Department of Histology and Embryology, Institute of Biostructure, Medical School, Chałubińskiego 5, 02-044 Warsaw, Poland
2 Department of Medicine, Institute of Haematology, Chocimska 5, 00-957 Warsaw, Poland

radioactivity of the ^{51}Cr released was determined in a gamma scintillation counter. Full details of this assay procedure are described elsewhere [11, 12].

E. Results and Discussion

We have observed that cyt B and colchicine decreased pinocytosis of HRP by PRC by more than 30% (Table 1). In the case of colchicine treatment, phagocytosis was inhibited similarly to pinocytosis, but the process was completely stopped by cyt B (Table 2).

The results of endocytized Hb determination were identical with the determination by the isotope method. Analogously, ADCC activity was found to be identical with both methods (Hb or ^{51}Cr). PRC colchicine treatment had no influence on the development of ADCC, but cyt B treatment almost completely stopped the reaction (Table 3). The literature shows that a cytotoxic effect may be caused by enzymes [1, 2, 5–7]. This role is ascribed to lysosomal hydrolases released to the environment or to the enzymes producing oxygen radicals (superoxide) and hydrogen peroxide. It is considered that endo- and exocytosis are in constant dynamic balance. In both processes, the same cellular organelles: actin microfilaments and microtubules, take part. It was suggested in this and other work that the strong inhibition of pinocytosis and phagocytosis after microtubule destruction with colchicine might be connected with the strong decrease of enzyme release.

Table 1. Influence of colchicine and cyt B on pinocytosis

Medium	Number of endocytized HRP (ng/mg protein)	Percentage of control ratio
MEM	3 300	100%
MEM + colchicine	2 125	64%
MEM + cyt B	2 046	62%

Table 2. Influence of colchicine and cyt B on phagocytosis

Medium	Number of phagocytized SRBC/ 10^6 PRC	Percentage of control ratio
MEM	2 112 000	100%
MEM + colchicine	1 221 000	58%
MEM + cyt B	Undetermined	–

Table 3. Influence of colchicine and cyt B on ADCC

Medium	Number of SRBC destroyed by 1×10^6 PRC	Percentage of control ratio
MEM	4 212 000	100%
MEM + colchicine	4 085 000	97%
MEM + cyt B	385 000	9%

The effect of this should be a decrease in ADCC activity. In our work, PRC colchicine treatment had no influence on the reaction. The second possibility concerning the role of oxygen radicals seems to be inadequate to explain the ADCC mechanism. There are reports on monocytes unable to produce hydrogen peroxide and oxygen radicals that show strong activity in ADCC [3]. Cyt B in the concentrations examined causes disorganization of movement in the cell membrane. The effect of this is capping inhibition on the lymphocyte surface [10]. The destruction of actin microfilaments caused almost complete inhibition of ADCC by PRC.

It is known that the cell movements and the movements of the cell membrane elements are connected with actin microfilaments. So it is possible that the specific configurations of these elements in the cell membranes of the PRC, together with hydrophobic domains that lyse the membranes of the target cells, are responsible for the PRC cytotoxic effect in ADCC. This mechanism would be similar to that of complement action during formation of the membrane attack complex.

References

1. Adams DO, Kao KJ, Farb R, Pizzo SU (1980) Effector mechanisms of cytolytically activated macrophages. II. Secretion of a cytolytic factor by activated macrophages and it's relationship to secreted neutral proteases. J Immunol 124:239–300
2. Currie GAW (1978) Activated macrophages kill tumor cells by releasing arginase. Nature 273:758–759
3. Fleer A, Van Schaik MLJ, Von Dem Borne AEGK, Engelfriet CP (1978) Destruction of sensitized erythrocytes by human monocytes in vitro: effects of cytochalasin B, hydrocortisone and colchicine. Scand J Immunol 8:515–524
4. Graham RC, Karnowsky MJ (1966) The early stages of absorption of injected horseradish peroxidase in the proximal tubules of mouse kidney: ultrastructural cytochemistry by a new technique. J Histochem Cytochem 14:669–684
5. Hibbs JB Jr (1974) Heterocytolysis by macrophages activated by Bacillus Calmette-Guerin: lysosomal exocytosis into the tumor cells. Science 184:468–471
6. Johnston RBJ, Godzik CA, Cohn ZA (1978) Increased superoxide anion production by immunologically activated and chemically elicited macrophages. J Exp Med 148:115–127
7. Nathan C, Cohn Z (1980) Role of oxygen-dependent mechanisms in antibody-induced lysis of tumor cells by activated macrophages. J Exp Med 152:198–208
8. Piasek A, Thyberg J (1979) Effects of colchicine on endocytosis and cellular inactivation of horseradish peroxidase in cultured chondrocytes. J Cell Biol 81:426–437
9. Piasek A, Thyberg J (1980) Effects of colchicine on endocytosis of horseradish peroxidase by rat peritoneal macrophages. J Cell Sci 45:59–71
10. Southwick FS, Stossel TP (1983) Contractile proteins in leukocyte function. Sem Hematol 20:305–320
11. Walker WS, Demus A (1975) Antibody-dependent cytolysis of chicken erythrocytes by an in vitro established line of mouse peritoneal macrophages. J Immunol 114:765–769
12. Walker WS (1977) Mediation of macrophage cytolytic and phagocytic activities by antibodies of different classes and class-specific Fc receptors. J Immunol 119:367–373

Haematology and Blood Transfusion Vol. 29
Modern Trends in Human Leukemia VI
Edited by Neth, Gallo, Greaves, Janka

In Vivo Studies with Covalent Conjugates of Cobra Venom Factor and Monoclonal Antibodies to Human Tumors

C.-W. Vogel[1], S. D. Wilkie[1], and A. C. Morgan[2]

A. Introduction

Cobra venom factor (CVF) is a nontoxic glycoprotein with $M_r \sim 140\,000$, obtained from cobra venom. CVF is a functional analog of C3b, the activated form of the third component of complement. Like C3b, CVF forms in serum with factor B of the alternative complement pathway an enzyme, the C3/C5 convertase [1]. The CVF-dependent enzyme is very stable and resistant to inactivation by control proteins. Therefore, once the enzyme is formed, it continuously activates C3 and C5.

We have previously shown that covalent conjugates of CVF with monoclonal antibodies to human tumor antigens are nontoxic by themselves, but elicit specific killing of antigen-positive tumor cells in the presence of serum complement in vitro [2]. We now wish to report our results of initial in vivo studies. We investigated the stability, the pharmacokinetics, and the tumor-suppressive activity of conjugates of CVF with the 9.2.27 murine monoclonal antibody to a human 250 000 daltons glycoprotein melanoma antigen [3].

1 Departments of Biochemistry and Medicine, and Vincent T. Lombardi Cancer Center, Georgetown University, Washington, DC 20007, USA

2 Monoclonal Antibody/Hybridoma Section, Biological Response Modifiers Program, National Cancer Institute, Frederick Cancer Research Facility, Frederick, Maryland 21701, USA

B. Materials and Methods

CVF was purified from lyophilized *Naja naja siamensis* venom (Miami Serpentarium Laboratories) by sequential column chromatography [4]. Covalent conjugates of CVF with the 9.2.27 monoclonal antibody were prepared as described [2] with three different heterobifunctional cross-linking reagents: *N*-succinimidyl-3-(2-pyridyldithio)propionate (SPDP) (Pharmacia), *m*-maleimidobenzoyl-*N*-hydroxysuccinimide ester (MBS) (Pierce), and iodoacetyl-*N*-hydroxysuccinimide ester (IAHS) (Fig. 1). IAHS was synthesized according to [5] with some modifications as described [6]. Prior to the coupling, CVF was radiolabeled with ^{125}I using immobilized chloramine-T (Pierce). For the pharmacokinetic studies, three female BALB/c mice each were injected i.v. with approximately 300 μg radiolabeled conjugates. At time intervals as indicated, the animals were bled and plasma samples were counted for radioactivity. Aliquots of the plasma samples were also subjected to 3%–9% gradient polyacrylamide gel electrophoresis in the presence of SDS with subsequent autoradiography.

C. Results

I. Pharmacokinetics and In Vivo Stability of Monoclonal Antibody–CVF Conjugates

Figure 2 shows a semilogarithmic plot of the elimination of the conjugates from mouse plasma. After an initial distribution

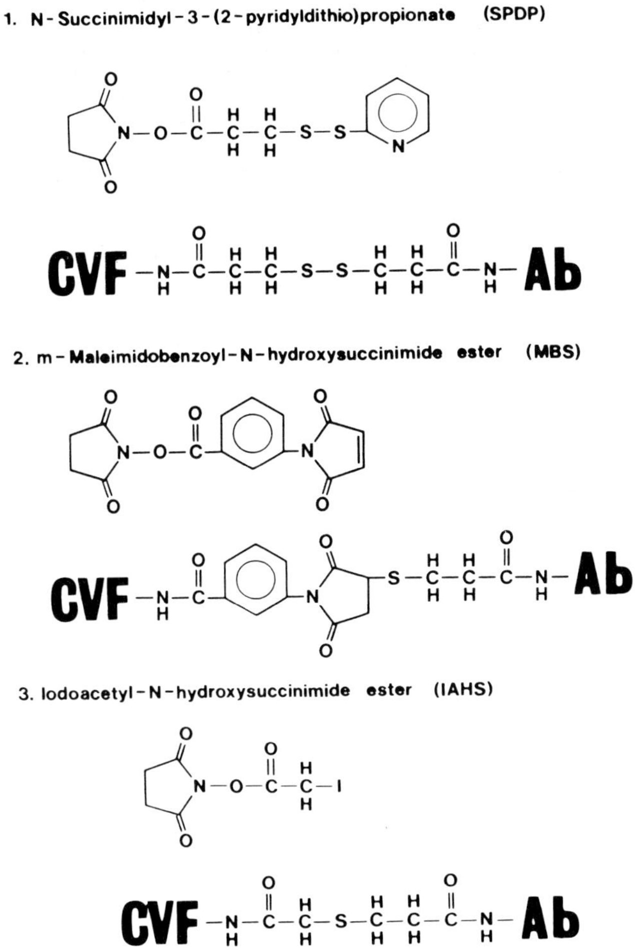

Fig. 1. Structures of the heterobifunctional cross-linking reagents and the resulting intermolecular cross-links. SPDP-linked conjugates contain a disulfide bond in the intermolecular cross-link while MBS-linked and IAHS-linked conjugates contain a thioether

phase of approximately 3 h, the SPDP-linked conjugates and IAHS-linked conjugates showed first-order elimination kinetics with plasma half-times of 23.5 and 25 h, respectively. In contrast, approximately 75% of the MBS-linked conjugates had been removed from the circulation within the first hour and continued to be eliminated with a half-time of 3.5 h. The fast removal of the MBS-linked conjugates was confirmed by the analysis of plasma samples by gradient gel electrophoresis and autoradiography. As shown in Fig. 3, MBS-linked conjugates were hardly detectable 10 h after injection while SPDP-linked and IAHS-linked conjugates were still present after 4 days. In addition, the higher oligomeric forms of the MBS-linked conjugates seemed to be preferentially removed.

Figure 3 also reveals that SPDP-linked conjugates underwent some degradation, as evidenced by an increasing amount of unconjugated CVF. However, this degradation was slow and the majority of the conjugates remained intact. A rather unexpected behavior was observed for the IAHS-linked conjugates. As evident from Fig. 3, the IAHS-linked conjugates exhibited in plasma a higher apparent molecular weight, suggesting a covalent interaction with plasma proteins.

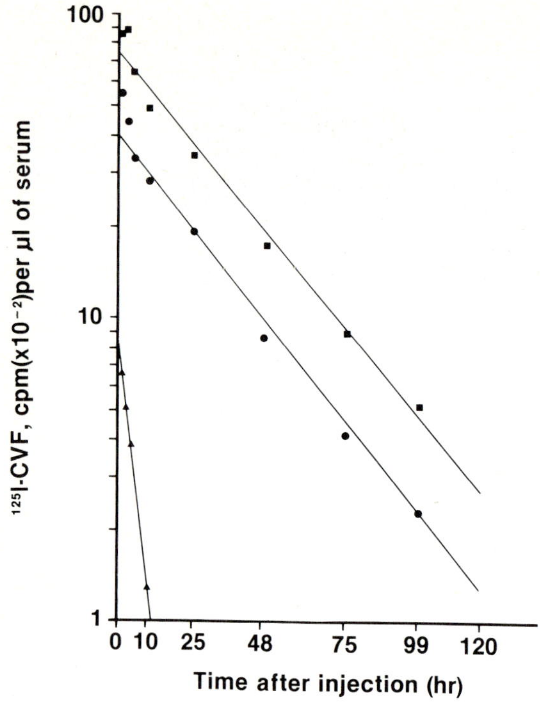

Fig. 2. Kinetics of elimination of 9.2.27 antibody-CVF conjugates from mouse plasma. Animals were bled at time intervals as indicated and plasma samples were counted for radioactivity (*squares* IAHS-linked conjugates; *circles* SPDP-linked conjugates; *triangles* MBS-linked conjugates)

II. Tumor-Suppressive Activity of Monoclonal Antibody–CVF Conjugates

Outbred nude mice with intraperitoneal transplants of human melanoma cells were used as a first model system to investigate the tumor-suppressive activity of monoclonal antibody-CVF conjugates. Mice were injected with 5×10^7 FEMX MET II cells. The animals received on the same day a single i.p. injection of 100 µg unconjugated 9.2.27 antibody or of SPDP-linked 9.2.27–CVF conjugates. Tumor growth, as evidenced by ascites formation, was delayed for approximately 2 weeks in animals treated with the 9.2.27–CVF conjugates compared with control animals treated with saline. The treatment with unconjugated 9.2.27 antibody was without effect.

D. Discussion

We synthesized covalent conjugates of the 9.2.27 monoclonal antibody with CVF, employing three different heterobifunctional cross-linking reagents. The stability and pharmacokinetics of these conjugates were investigated in mice. All three conjugates were, to a variable extent, stable in the circulation. Only the SPDP-linked conjugates, which contained a disulfide bond in the intermolecular cross-link, showed some degradation which is believed to occur by disulfide exchange or reductive cleavage (compare Fig. 1). However, the extent of this degradation does not preclude SPDP as a cross-linker for in vivo studies. MBS-linked conjugates were far more rapidly eliminated from the circulation than the two other conjugates. While the mechanism for this different kinetic behavior is not known, we believe that the hydrophobic nature of the MBS molecule may be responsible. IAHS-linked conjugates exhibited an interaction with plasma proteins, as demonstrated by their higher apparent molecular weight in plasma. This interaction with plasma proteins, which was also observed in vitro [7], must be covalent since it was resistant to boiling for 5 min in the presence of SDS. We are

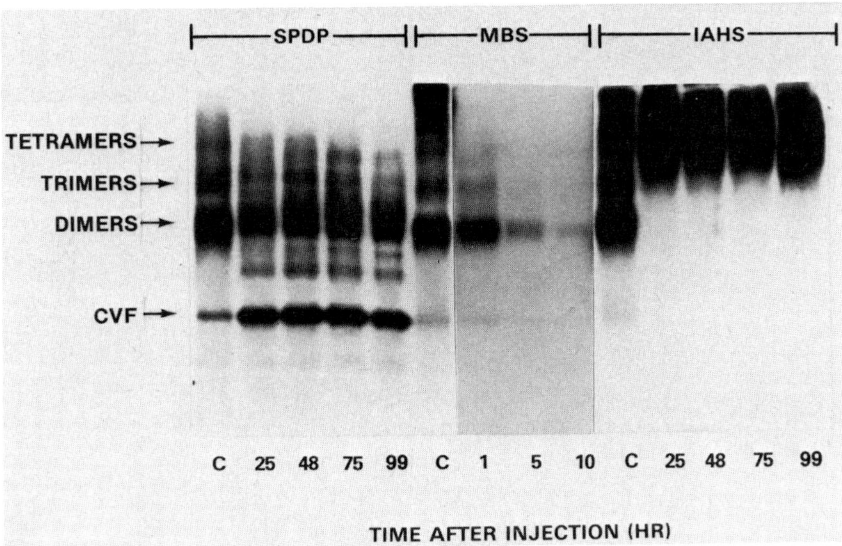

Fig. 3. Electrophoretic analysis of monoclonal antibody–CVF conjugates after injection into BALB/c mice. Shown is an autoradiogram of a 3%–9% gradient gel. *Control lanes* (marked *C*) show the injected material which contained dimeric, trimeric, and some higher oligomeric conjugates as well as small amounts of unconjugated CVF and antibody. Note that only CVF was radiolabeled

currently investigating whether unreacted IAHS groups remaining on the conjugates after the coupling reaction bind to plasma proteins containing free sulfhydryl groups or whether nascent C3b binds to the IAHS-linked conjugates through its reactive thioester.

Two important conclusions can be derived from our studies. First, stable conjugates of monoclonal antibodies with CVF exhibiting reasonable plasma half-times can be made. This finding now allows immunotherapeutic studies to be performed with such conjugates. Second, the nature of the heterobifunctional cross-linking reagent used for the synthesis of monoclonal antibody–CVF conjugates influences the pharmacokinetic behavior of the conjugates and, therefore, may have major impact on their distribution and immunotherapeutic effects.

We also performed an immunotherapeutic experiment in nude mice with intraperitoneally growing human melanomas. A single dose of 100 μg monoclonal antibody–CVF conjugates caused a significant delay of tumor growth after injection of a rather substantial inoculation of 5×10^7 melanoma cells. This promising result justifies further investigations of monoclonal antibody–CVF conjugates as potential agents for immunotherapy of cancer.

Acknowledgments. We thank Miss Alice H. Grier for injecting and bleeding the mice. This work was supported by NIH grant CA 35525 to C.-W. V.

References

1. Vogel C-W, Müller-Eberhard HJ (1982) J Biol Chem 257:8292–8299
2. Vogel C-W, Müller-Eberhard HJ (1981) Proc Natl Acad Sci USA 78:7707–7711
3. Morgan AC, Galloway DR, Reisfeld RA (1981) Hybridoma 1:27–36
4. Vogel C-W, Müller-Eberhard HJ (1984) J Immunol Methods 73:203–220
5. Rector E-S, Schwenk RJ, Tse KS, Sehon AH (1978) J Immunol Methods 24:321–336
6. Wilkie SD (1984) M. S. thesis, Georgetown University, Washington, D.C.
7. Wilkie SD, Vogel CV (1984) Fed Proc 43:1971

Subject Index